Clinical Anesthesiology II

Jonathan L. Benumof • Gerard R. Manecke
Editors

Clinical Anesthesiology II

Lessons from Morbidity and Mortality Conferences

Springer

Editors
Jonathan L. Benumof
Department of Anesthesiology
University of California
UCSD Medical Center
UCSD School of Medicine
San Diego, CA
USA

Gerard R. Manecke
Department of Anesthesiology
University of California
UCSD Medical Center
UCSD School of Medicine
San Diego, CA
USA

ISBN 978-3-030-12363-5 ISBN 978-3-030-12365-9 (eBook)
https://doi.org/10.1007/978-3-030-12365-9

This Springer imprint is published by the registered company Springer Nature Switzerland AG
The registered company address is: Gewerbestrasse 11, 6330 Cham, Switzerland

Preface

In 2014, we published a unique book, *Clinical Anesthesiology: Lessons Learned from Morbidity and Mortality Conferences*. We now present a logical companion to that book: Volume II, *Clinical Anesthesiology: Lessons Learned from Morbidity and Mortality Conferences*. An extension of its predecessor, this volume is a compilation of new selected cases presented at the weekly University of California San Diego (UC San Diego) Department of Anesthesiology Morbidity and Mortality (M + M)/Quality Improvement (QI) conferences. Case descriptions, relevant physiological and medical issues, and "lessons learned" have been written up in the form of chapters to create an easily accessible, clinically relevant compendium. Two main factors prompted us to create this new book. The first is that Volume I is very popular, with electronic access exceeding 111,000 "look-ups" since its publication. The publisher informs us that, for clinical medicine texts, this performance is excellent. Evidently, readers find the format of the book and teaching points valuable. Secondly, the "lessons" just keep coming! Our weekly conferences continue to be very high-quality case descriptions and discussions presented by a resident and moderated by a senior, learned faculty (often ourselves ☺). Each conference has teaching points brought forth by the moderator, other faculty during discussion, the presenting resident, and other attendees. Being a tertiary/quaternary care health system, UC San Diego has many critically ill patients, as well as numerous healthy patients undergoing "bread and butter" procedures. Thus, at UC San Diego, there is a virtually limitless supply of challenging anesthetics, complex surgeries, emergency calls, and unexpected events in the operating rooms, ICUs, and floor units – all with take-home lessons galore. Immediately upon the completion of Volume I, we recognized that we were rapidly accumulating important new clinical and teaching material for a Volume II.

These new case chapters are presented in the same format as in the first volume, with each consisting of a case description and "lessons learned," gleaned from either the case or the subsequent conference discussion. We believe this format is unique and informative, since it incorporates the case experience of the provider, the "clinical pearls" from the discussion of the group, the lessons provided by the moderator, and the important source information from the medical literature.

There are two significant differences between this volume and Volume I, however. The first is that in this text, we have asked the authors of each chapter to go into significant depth – there are very few superficial discussions in this book. The intent is for the reader to be able to obtain detailed, up-to-date information on a clinical problem, condition, or case scenario, without having to consult other sources. Source references are, of course, provided, should the reader desire to delve even deeper or understand the background and data supporting each chapter. The second difference involves the grouping and ordering of the chapters. In the first volume, the chapters were grouped according to general physiologic systems or areas of anesthetic practice (e.g., respiratory, circulatory, obstetric, pain, and regional). In this volume, the chapters seemed to be organized according to the impact or potential impact on the patient (e.g., death, major morbidity, minor morbidity, no morbidity but clinically challenging). We have thus grouped them by those categories.

Although all the cases in this volume are new, there is necessarily some overlap in the material provided in this volume and the previous one. Items such as hypoxemia, ventilation problems, hypotension, dysrhythmias, obstructive sleep apnea, coagulopathies, and potential for airway fire are recurring themes in our practice and discussions. Thus, they are found in both volumes, in one form or another. There are other chapters in Volume II that cover new and difficult subjects such as death during monitored anesthesia care, drug administration error, massive pulmonary hemorrhage, and abdominal compartment syndrome.

We have both learned a great deal in compiling this text and believe that the reader will likewise learn and benefit from it. We are even so bold as to suggest that the reader's patients will benefit as well. In the preface to Volume I, we pointed out the unique nature of the approach, saying "Try it, you'll like it." You *did* try it, and you *did* like it. With this volume, we say "Try it again, you'll like it again!"

San Diego, CA, USA

Jonathan L. Benumof, MD
Gerard R. Manecke, MD

Contents

Contributors

Thomas Archer, MD Department of Anesthesiology, University of California, San Diego, CA, USA

Richard Bellars, MD Department of Anesthesiology, University of California, San Diego, CA, USA

Jonathan L. Benumof, MD Department of Anesthesiology, University of California, UCSD Medical Center, UCSD School of Medicine, San Diego, CA, USA

Alyssa Brzenski, MD Department of Anesthesiology, University of California, San Diego, CA, USA

Leon Chang, MD Department of Anesthesiology, University of California, San Diego Medical Center, San Diego, CA, USA

John J. Finneran IV, MD Department of Anesthesiology, University of California, San Diego, CA, USA

Deborah L. Fretwell, MD Department of Anesthesiology, University of California San Diego Health System, San Diego, CA, USA

Mark Greenberg, MD Department of Anesthesiology, University of California, San Diego, CA, USA

Brittany Grovey, MD Department of Anesthesiology, University of California, San Diego, CA, USA

Seth Herway, MD Department of Anesthesiology, University of California, San Diego, CA, USA

Department of Anesthesia, Mountain West Anesthesian, St. George, UT, USA

Ryan W. Hill, MD Department of Anesthesiology, University of California, San Diego, CA, USA

Jessica G. Hollingsworth, MD Department of Anesthesiology, University of California, San Diego, CA, USA

Bjorn Benjamin Jensen, BS, MD Department of Anesthesiology, University of California, San Diego, CA, USA

Martin Krause, MD Department of Anesthesiology, University of Colorado, Denver, Aurora, CO, USA

Gerard R. Manecke, MD Department of Anesthesiology, University of California, UCSD Medical Center, UCSD School of Medicine, San Diego, CA, USA

Kevin D. Marcus, MD Department of Anesthesiology, Mission Hospital – Mission Viejo, Mission Viejo, CA, USA

Anush Minokadeh, MD Department of Anesthesiology, University of California, San Diego, CA, USA

Christopher Nguyen, MD Department of Anesthesiology, University of California, San Diego, Orange, CA, USA

James Phillips, BA, MD Department of Anesthesia, Community Anesthesia Providers, Clovis, CA, USA

Kimberly A. Pollock, MD Department of Anesthesiology, University of California, San Diego, CA, USA

Karim T. Rafaat, MD Department of Anesthesiology, University of California, San Diego, CA, USA

Asheen Rama, MD Department of Anesthesiology, University of California, San Diego, CA, USA

Luis M. Rivera, MD, MSEE Department of Anesthesiology, University of California, San Diego, CA, USA

Kimberly S. Robbins, MD Department of Anesthesiology and Critical Care Medicine, University of California, San Diego, CA, USA

Ramon Sanchez, MD Department of Anesthesiology, University of California, San Diego, CA, USA

Sonya M. Seshadri, MD Department of Anesthesiology, Southern California Permanente Medical Group, San Diego, CA, USA

Daniel J. Sisti, MD Department of Anesthesiology, University of California, San Diego, CA, USA

Claire Soria, MD Department of Anesthesiology, University of California, San Diego, CA, USA

Ryan Suda, MD Department of Anesthesiology, University of California, San Diego, CA, USA

Preetham J. Suresh, MD Department of Anesthesiology, University of California, San Diego, CA, USA

Lawrence Weinstein, BA, MD Department of Anesthesiology, University of California, San Diego, CA, USA

Part I
Cases Resulting in Perioperative Death

Chapter 1
Death During Monitored Anesthesia Care

Kevin D. Marcus and Jonathan L. Benumof

The patient was a 69-year-old, 155 cm, 68 kg female with a calculated BMI of 28.3 kg/m^2, who presented with significant right-upper-quadrant pain. Work-up on the patient revealed choledocholithiasis with evidence of cholecystitis. The patient was subsequently scheduled for endoscopic retrograde cholangiopancreatography (ERCP) **(L-1)** in the endoscopy suite.

Prior medical history was significant for obesity, now several years status-post laparoscopic gastric band surgery. There was otherwise no significant past medical, surgical, or medication history. A preoperative chest X-ray and EKG were unremarkable. Blood work showed mildly elevated liver enzymes and a hemoglobin and hematocrit of 10.8 gms/dl and 33%. Vital signs were as follows: BP = 135/73 mmHg, HR = 81 bpm, and S_pO_2 = 97% on room air. The patient was deemed to be ASA class II, with mild systemic disease, and taken to surgery with plans for a MAC anesthetic **(L-2)** with propofol sedation **(L-3)**.

The patient was positioned prone with O_2 via nasal cannula at 5 L/min. A noninvasive blood pressure cuff, EKG/HR, and S_pO_2 were used to monitor the patient. Continuous CO_2 monitoring was not employed, and an anesthesia machine was not in the endoscopy suite **(L-4, 5)**. However, an American Heart Association (AHA) ACLS "crash" cart was located 50 ft down a hallway.

Anesthesia was induced with an initial propofol bolus of 70 mg, and over the next 40 min, an additional 310 mg was given in intermittent, divided doses ranging

K. D. Marcus (✉)
Department of Anesthesiology, Mission Hospital – Mission Viejo, Mission Viejo, CA, USA

J. L. Benumof
Department of Anesthesiology, University of California, UCSD Medical Center, UCSD School of Medicine, San Diego, CA, USA

J. L. Benumof, G. R. Manecke (eds.), *Clinical Anesthesiology II*,
https://doi.org/10.1007/978-3-030-12365-9_1

from 30 to 70 mg. A total of 380 mg of propofol was given during the course of the 40-min ERCP **(L-6)**.

Minutes after the final dose of propofol was given, the anesthesia provider noticed an approximately 50% decrease in the patient's blood pressure, heart rate, and pulse oximeter values. A code was called. The patient was then turned supine and bag mask ventilation was instituted. The decision was made to intubate the patient, and direct laryngoscopy by the anesthesiologist revealed what was thought to be a grade I view of the larynx, and an endotracheal tube (ETT) was passed. One to 2 min after the tracheal intubation attempt, an emergency department (ED) physician arrived on the scene with a portable colorimetric CO_2 monitor (Easy Cap detector), but this monitor was not utilized at this time. There was no CO_2 confirmation of correct ETT placement **(L-7)**.

Several minutes after the ETT was placed, the patient's peripheral pulses were lost to continuous palpation by the ED physician, and there were no audible breath sounds on auscultation or color change on the colorimetric CO_2 detector. The ETT was removed, and a repeat laryngoscopy was performed with placement of a second ETT. This time, there was portable exhaled CO_2 colorimetric confirmation of correct ETT position within the trachea **(L-8)**. However, the patient was unable to be resuscitated despite administration of ACLS during the code blue.

Lessons Learned

L-1: What Is an ERCP?

ERCP stands for endoscopic retrograde cholangiopancreatography and is an invasive procedure performed primarily by gastroenterologists for both diagnostic and therapeutic purposes related to the biliary and pancreatic ductal systems. An endoscope is passed through the mouth and past the stomach into the duodenum where the opening to the biliary and pancreatic ducts, the ampulla of Vater, is located (Fig. 1.1a). A catheter is then advanced through this ampulla and into the biliary and pancreatic ducts, at which point the ductal anatomy can be explored, usually by way of injection of radiopaque dye, which is seen on fluoroscopy.

Therapeutic interventions are also possible, such as removal of stones. The sphincter of Oddi, a circular band of muscle that surrounds the ampulla of Vater, can sometimes present a barrier to access. This is solved with a sphincterotomy (Fig. 1.1b), which can be stimulating and painful to the patient. Removal of stones by deployment of a distal basket or balloon (Fig. 1.1c) can also prove to be painful as the stones are swept out of the ducts. Careful attention must be paid to these portions of the procedure as they may require adjustment in the level of sedation.

Common indications for ERCP include obstructive jaundice, choledocholithiasis, pancreatic tumors, dilation of strictures, and insertion of stents.

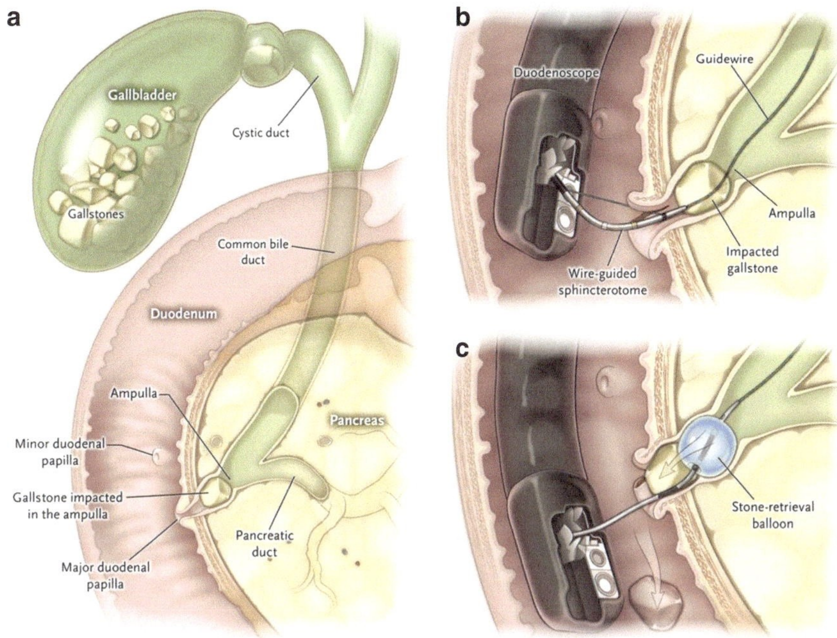

Fig. 1.1 Anatomy of the biliary and pancreatic ductal systems, during ERCP. (**a**) Biliary system anatomy depicting impacted common bile duct gallstone. (**b**) Sphincterotomy for passage of catheter into common bile duct. (**c**) Inflation of distal balloon for gallstone removal. (Reprinted from Fogel and Sherman [18]. With permission from Massachusetts Medical Society)

L-2: What Is a "MAC" Anesthetic? (Fig. 1.2)

Monitored anesthesia care, or MAC, is a "specific anesthesia service in which an anesthesia provider has been requested to participate in the care of a patient undergoing a diagnostic or therapeutic procedure" [1]. The MAC service includes all aspects of anesthesia care, including a pre-procedure visit, intra-procedure care, and post-procedure anesthesia management [2]. Relief of pain, treatment of complications, or diagnosis and treatment of coexisting medical problems are just a few examples of what the MAC service might entail.

According to the ASA position statement on MAC, "monitored anesthesia care may include varying levels of sedation, analgesia and anxiolysis as necessary" [2]. This means that the anesthetic during a MAC may range from local anesthesia without sedation to deep sedation and even general anesthesia. Even if a patient is thought to require only minimal sedation for a procedure, they may need a MAC service because there is the potential for adverse effects, either secondary to the sedation given or the procedure itself, which would require intervention from an anesthesia provider ranging from resuscitation to general anesthesia [3].

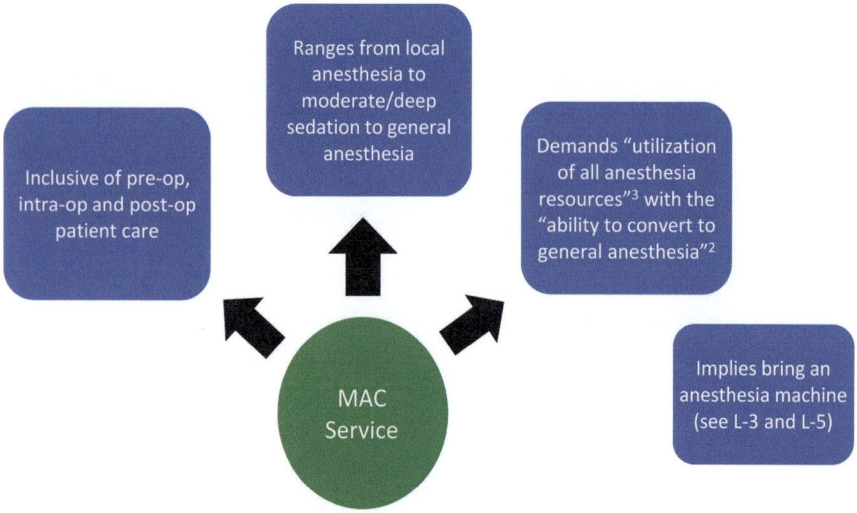

Fig. 1.2 Components of MAC anesthesia service

Therefore, MAC is an anesthesia service and does not imply a specific type of anesthesia being administered.

It should be apparent from the above that a central tenant from the ASA regarding MAC is that the anesthetic provider "must be prepared and qualified to convert to a general anesthetic when necessary" [2]. This fact is key to differentiating MAC from "moderate sedation," as non-anesthesia personnel can often provide moderate sedation (see L-3). MAC service allows for safe administration of a maximal depth of sedation in excess of what can be provided during moderate sedation, by personnel equipped to provide general anesthesia. There is also an ASA expectation that a provider of a MAC service must be able to "utilize all anesthesia resources to support life" [3]. This directive further differentiates "moderate sedation" from a MAC service.

The statements "utilize all anesthesia resources to support life" [3] and "be prepared and qualified to convert to general anesthesia" [2] strongly imply that an anesthesia machine, or the component parts of the anesthesia machine, be immediately available to anyone who provides a MAC service (Fig. 1.2).

L-3: What Are the Different Levels of Sedation?

The ASA defines four distinct levels of sedation or anesthesia, namely, minimal sedation, moderate sedation, deep sedation, and general anesthesia [1] (Table 1.1). The commonly used term "conscious sedation" is synonymous with a moderate sedation level.

Table 1.1 ASA definition of levels of sedation and general anesthesia in terms of various clinical parameters

Clinical parameter	Minimal sedation	Moderate sedation	Deep sedation[a]	General anesthesia
Responsiveness	Normal response to verbal stimuli	Purposeful response to verbal or tactile stimuli	Purposeful response following repeated painful stimuli	Unarousable even with painful stimulus
Airway patency	Unaffected	No intervention required	Intervention may be required	Intervention often required
Spontaneous ventilation	Unaffected	Adequate	May be inadequate	Frequently inadequate
Cardiovascular function	Unaffected	Usually maintained	Usually maintained	May be impaired

Based on data from Ref. [1]

[a]If a provider is planning deep sedation, they must be prepared to provide a general anesthetic according to the ASA position statement. This may include the probability of needing an anesthesia machine

As depicted in the above table, the various levels of sedation and anesthesia are largely defined by the patient's response to various stimuli during the course of their sedation.

Minimal sedation is defined as a "drug-induced state during which patients respond normally to verbal commands" [1]. Cognitive function and physical coordination may be slightly impaired.

Moderate sedation, or "conscious sedation," is defined as "drug-induced depression of consciousness during which patients respond purposefully to verbal commands, either alone or accompanied by light tactile stimulation" [1]. Purposeful responses do not include reflex withdrawal. Non-anesthesia providers can give moderate sedation to patients but must be trained to also recognize deep sedation, manage its consequences, and adjust the level of sedation to a moderate or lesser level.

Deep sedation is defined as a "drug-induced depression of consciousness during which patients cannot be easily aroused, but respond purposefully following repeated or painful stimulation" [1]. It is during deep sedation that spontaneous ventilation may become compromised, requiring an airway intervention by the provider. It is for this reason that in cases where deep sedation may be required, a MAC service is essential for the reasons discussed in the previous lesson (see L-2).

General anesthesia is defined as a "drug-induced loss of consciousness during which patients are not arousable, even by painful stimulation" [1]. It is at this point that spontaneous ventilation is often inadequate and airway intervention is frequently required, although general anesthesia does not mandate use of an advanced airway.

The ASA's position statement on the various levels of sedation comments that the level of sedation is fluid and can rapidly fluctuate from one level to another and that it is often not possible to predict an individual's response to sedative or hypnotic medications. For this reason, it is recommended that a provider of sedation be able to rescue and treat a patient who becomes one level deeper than expected [1]. For instance, if a provider is planning "deep sedation," they must be prepared to provide a general anesthetic and all that accompanies this service, which may include the probability of needing an anesthesia machine.

L-4: What Are the Standard ASA Monitors?

The ASA last published practice guidelines on the standards for basic anesthetic monitoring in 2010, with an effective date of July 1, 2011. These standards were meant to apply to all anesthesia care, including general anesthesia, regional anesthesia, and monitored anesthesia care. The overall standard is that "the patient's oxygenation, ventilation, circulation and temperature be continually evaluated" [4].

Oxygenation

To adequately ensure blood oxygenation, it is required that a quantitative method of assessing oxygenation, such as pulse oximetry, be used for all anesthetics. It is not enough just to use a pulse oximeter; a variable pitch pulse tone, which changes with specific O_2 saturation levels, and low threshold alarm must also be audible to the anesthesiologist. For general anesthetics utilizing an anesthesia machine, it is also required that an oxygen analyzer with a low O_2 concentration alarm be used to assess the oxygen concentration in the breathing circuit (Table 1.2).

Table 1.2 Monitoring requirements for each clinical parameter listed in the ASA practice guideline for basic anesthetic monitoring during moderate/deep sedation and general anesthesia

<table>
<tr><th>Clinical parameter to be monitored</th><th>Mandatory monitors</th><th>Additional/supplementary monitors</th></tr>
<tr><td rowspan="2">Oxygenation</td><td>Pulse oximeter with audible alarms</td><td rowspan="2">None, all monitoring mandatory</td></tr>
<tr><td>Oxygen analyzer with low [O_2] alarm</td></tr>
<tr><td rowspan="2">Ventilation (also see Table 1.3)</td><td>Continual exhaled CO_2 detection</td><td rowspan="2">Quantitative monitoring of volume of expired gas[b]</td></tr>
<tr><td>Audible alarm for detecting circuit leaks[a]</td></tr>
<tr><td rowspan="5">Circulation</td><td>Continuous ECG tracing</td><td>Palpation of pulse</td></tr>
<tr><td rowspan="4">BP and HR every 5 min</td><td>Auscultation of heart sounds</td></tr>
<tr><td>Arterial line pressure tracing</td></tr>
<tr><td>Ultrasound peripheral pulse monitoring</td></tr>
<tr><td>Pulse plethysmography[c]</td></tr>
<tr><td>Body temperature</td><td colspan="2">Must be monitored when clinically significant changes are intended, anticipated, or suspected</td></tr>
</table>

[a]Only when ventilation is controlled by mechanical ventilator
[b]Strongly encouraged by ASA during general anesthesia
[c]At least one of the listed additional circulation monitors must be used in addition to the mandatory monitors

Ventilation

The practice guidelines to ensure adequate ventilation depend on the type of anesthesia that is being provided. The anesthesia provider need only assess the qualitative clinical signs of adequate ventilation during regional or local anesthesia performed without sedation (Table 1.3). These qualitative clinical signs may include chest excursion, observation of the reservoir breathing bag, or auscultation of breath sounds [4]. However, during moderate, deep sedation and general anesthesia, the "adequacy of ventilation *SHALL* be evaluated by the presence of exhaled CO_2 unless precluded or invalidated by the nature of the patient, procedure or equipment" [4]. These preclusions might include cardiopulmonary bypass, operations on the nose and mouth, or machine malfunctions mid-operation, all of which may affect the ability to accurately interpret exhaled CO_2.

For general anesthesia with an endotracheal tube (ETT) or laryngeal mask airway (LMA), correct positioning must be verified by clinical assessment and exhaled CO_2. Additionally, continuous end-tidal CO_2 using capnometry, capnography, or mass spectroscopy must be in use from the time of placement of the airway device to the time of removal.

Table 1.3 ASA statement on the requirements for adequate monitoring of ventilation

Depth of anesthesia +/− airway	Regional or local anesthesia without sedation	Moderate or deep sedation	General anesthesia without airway	General anesthesia with ETT or LMA
Quote from the ASA on the type of monitoring required for ventilation based upon the depth of anesthesia	"The adequacy of ventilation shall be evaluated by continual observation of qualitative clinical signs[a]" [4]	"The adequacy of ventilation shall be evaluated by continual observation of qualitative clinical signs[a] and monitoring for the presence of exhaled carbon dioxide" [4]	"Every patient receiving general anesthesia shall have the adequacy of ventilation continually evaluated… continual monitoring for the presence of exhaled CO_2 shall be performed" [4]	"Continual end-tidal CO_2 analysis, in use from the time of ETT/LMA placement until extubation/removal… shall be performed using a quantitative method such as capnography, capnometry or mass spectroscopy" [4]
Qualitative clinical signs	YES	YES	YES	YES
Qualitative CO_2 monitoring[b]	NO	YES	YES	NO
Quantitative CO_2 monitoring	NO	NO	NO	YES

[a]Qualitative clinical signs may include chest excursion, assessment of the reservoir breathing bag movement, or auscultation of breath sounds
[b]For example, colorimetric CO_2 detection devices

Note that the essential difference between regional and/or local anesthesia without any sedation given and moderate or deep sedation is that with no sedation given, a provider need only monitor qualitative signs of adequate ventilation; however, if *any* sedation is given, one must also utilize, at a minimum, qualitative exhaled CO_2 monitoring.

Circulation

To ensure adequate circulation during all anesthetics, multiple monitoring components must be satisfied. First, every patient must have a continuously displayed electrocardiogram from the beginning to the end of the anesthetic. Secondly, arterial blood pressure and heart rate must be assessed at least every 5 min. Lastly, circulation must also be assessed by at least one of the following in addition to the mandates above: palpation of pulse, auscultation of heart sounds, intra-arterial pressure tracing, ultrasound peripheral pulse monitoring, or pulse plethysmography or oximetry [4].

Body Temperature

In order to enable the anesthesia provider to maintain appropriate patient body temperature during anesthesia, every patient must have their temperature monitored when clinically significant changes are intended, anticipated, or suspected [4].

The ASA has issued a separate statement on standards for appropriate respiratory monitoring that has specific implications to the case presented in this chapter. It states that "exhaled CO_2 *should* be conducted during endoscopic procedures in which propofol alone or in combination with opioids and/or benzodiazepines" are utilized for sedation [5]. The statement clearly emphasizes that special attention needs to be paid to ERCP procedures performed in the prone position.

In summary, the basic monitors required for all anesthetics are pulse oximetry, exhaled CO_2 (except when no sedation given), continuous electrocardiography, arterial blood pressure monitoring (usually via noninvasive cuff pressures), heart rate display (usually via ECG, pulse oximetry, or noninvasive blood pressure), and temperature. In this case, the provider failed to adequately assess ventilation by not having a means of monitoring exhaled CO_2. They also failed to appropriately confirm placement of their ETT with exhaled CO_2 (see L-7).

L-5: What Are the Advantages of Having an Anesthesia Machine at Out-of-the-OR Locations?

Many times, anesthesia providers are asked to administer sedation and/or general anesthesia in locations other than the operating rooms. These out-of-OR locations may include endoscopy suites, interventional radiology, interventional cardiology,

MRI or CT scanners, or even ICU beds. Providing anesthesia in these remote locations can be an unfamiliar and even dangerous experience, if not properly prepared.

In a review of the ASA Closed Claims database, it was determined that overall, patients receiving anesthesia in remote locations were older, had higher ASA classifications, and more often underwent emergent procedures than those patients in the OR [6]. The most common anesthetic technique at remote locations was MAC, whereas general anesthesia was the most common anesthetic technique in the OR. Although adverse respiratory events were the most common mechanism of injury at both locations, they occurred roughly twice as commonly in remote locations [6]. Furthermore, the proportion of deaths in outlying locations was nearly twice as what occurred in the OR [6] (Fig. 1.3). In-depth analysis of these closed claims cases revealed that injuries at these remote locations were more often judged to be preventable by better monitoring of patients.

Based upon the prior data, it would stand to reason that having all available supplies to administer general anesthesia, despite whatever the initial plan for anesthesia was, would be a prudent decision. Having a fully stocked anesthesia machine with attached monitors, drawers, and ventilators is of great value, especially when considering that an unanticipated anesthetic urgency or emergency might occur.

Some of the advantages of a fully stocked anesthesia machine include:

1. Continuous CO_2 waveform: usually in the form of a capnograph, continuous CO_2 is important for breath-to-breath confirmation of adequate ventilation. It is also useful for confirmation of appropriate ETT placement and adequacy of chest compressions and return of spontaneous circulation during cardiac arrest (see L-8).
2. Additional airway supplies: drawers in the anesthesia machine will typically have multiple additional laryngoscopes in various sizes and shapes. There is also

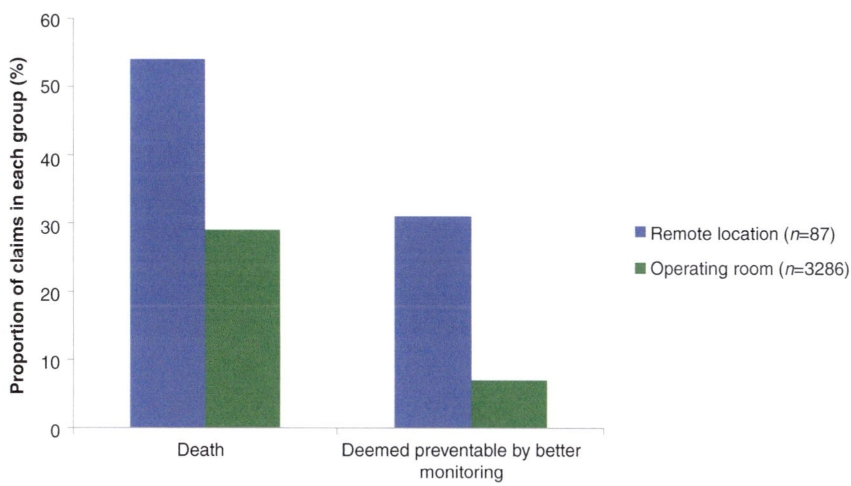

Fig. 1.3 Proportion of claims in remote locations vs. operating rooms including death and total proportion of claims that were thought to be preventable by better monitoring. (Based on data from Ref. [6])

typically a bougie, as well as LMAs, oral/nasal airways, and other devices necessary to complete the difficult airway algorithm.

3. Mechanical ventilator: various modes of ventilation can be helpful in situations where sedation is rapidly converted to general anesthesia with the need for mechanical ventilation. There is also the added benefit of known minute ventilation and the ability to set tidal volumes, respiratory rates, and respiratory modes.
4. Additional O_2 source: all anesthesia machines will have an extra E-cylinder of oxygen attached. This can prove invaluable in the event of loss of wall pressure or other malfunction. Having a backup O_2 source is one of the absolute requirements for providing out-of-OR anesthesia [8].
5. Touch-sensitive reservoir bag: provides tactile feedback when providing positive pressure ventilation and/or assisting spontaneous ventilation. The bag is also useful for determining changes in lung compliance/resistance and can even help in detecting early esophageal intubation in the hands of a skilled provider.
6. Volatile anesthetics: in the event of conversion to a general anesthetic, having the option of providing volatile anesthesia is an advantage.
7. N_2O tank: readily available on most anesthesia machines is an E-cylinder of nitrous oxide, which can be used to provide additional inspired analgesia with minimal decrement in respiratory drive and minute ventilation.
8. Suction: provides life-saving capability should the need arise for intubation in a patient with copious secretions, active vomiting, or a bloody airway. This is another mandatory item for providing anesthesia in out-of-the-OR locations according to the ASA [8].
9. O_2 flush valve: allows rapid filling of the anesthesia machine bellows and reservoir bag.

Although most of these supplies may also be found in anesthesia work rooms and collected prior to providing anesthesia in an out-of-OR location, having the complete anesthesia machine saves time and also prevents possible oversight that can happen when trying to assemble all of the necessary components listed above. Especially in an emergency situation, familiarity with your workstation and knowing you have all of the necessary equipment can mean the difference between a close call and a disaster.

L-6: What Are the Guidelines for the Use of Propofol During MAC Anesthesia?

Propofol is an alkylphenol compound that is formulated as an egg lecithin emulsion commonly used for intravenous induction and maintenance of anesthesia. Once injected, propofol produces rapid hypnosis, usually within 40 s, and has a blood-brain equilibration half-time of 1–3 min [7]. Because propofol is a rapid-acting sedative-hypnotic, it is a very popular medication to administer for both general anesthesia and sedation cases (Table 1.4).

Table 1.4 Propofol dosing recommendations for sedation cases based upon intermittent bolus dosing or continuous infusion

Method of administration	Induction of sedation	Maintenance of sedation
Intermittent bolus dosing	0.5 mg/kg over 3–5 min	10–20 mg individual doses titrated to clinical effect
Continuous infusion	100–150 μg/kg/min for period of 3–5 min	25–75 μg/kg/min and adjusted to clinical response

Current recommendations for the dosing of propofol for sedation cases can be found in the above table [7]. However, no patient or procedure is exactly the same. Therefore, as with any other anesthetic agent, propofol must be carefully titrated by the anesthesia provider to achieve the desired sedative effects while minimizing the undesired side effects, such as cardiorespiratory depression. During sedation with propofol, side effects such as hypotension, hypopnea, apnea, and oxyhemoglobin desaturation are more common with intermittent bolus dosing [7]. For this reason, it is recommended by the manufacturers that a variable rate infusion method be used for maintenance of sedation instead of intermittent boluses [7]. If intermittent bolusing of propofol is to take place, it is recommended that the anesthesia provider wait a period of 3–5 min to allow for the peak drug effect of the previous dose to be observed clinically before administering another dose so as to minimize the risk of overdosing [7].

Like nearly all anesthetic agents, propofol requires special consideration when being administered to the elderly (age >55 years) and debilitated patient populations. Due to decreased clearance rates and a decreased volume of distribution, the elderly population can be expected to have increased blood concentrations of propofol after equivalent doses in the younger population. This contributes to increased sedative and cardiorespiratory depressant effects in the elderly. Therefore, the manufacturers of propofol have stated that, in the elderly (age >55 years), "repeat bolus administration should not be used for MAC sedation" and that the dosage "should be reduced to approximately 80% of the usual adult dosage" [7].

In the case presented herein, it is clear that the anesthesiologist did not follow several of the package insert recommendations for the administration of propofol for MAC sedation in an elderly patient (Fig. 1.4).

L-7: Use of Exhaled CO_2 to Confirm Placement of Endotracheal Tubes

Confirmation of correct placement of an endotracheal tube (ETT) within the trachea by presence of exhaled CO_2 is mandated by several guidelines for the safe practice of anesthesia [4, 9, 10]. Visualization of the ETT passing through the vocal cords, although helpful, does not take the place of objective confirmation by exhaled CO_2. Multiple methods exist for accurate confirmation of the exhaled CO_2 after instrumentation of the airway.

- Intermittent bolus dosing was used in an elderly patient despite recommendation for continuous infusion
- The dose of propofol was not reduced to the recommended 80% of maximum for an elderly patient
- 30-70 mg bolus doses were used instead of the recommended 10-20 mg doses for maintenance of sedation
- 70 mg (~1 mg/kg) induction dose was administered instead of the recommended 0.5 mg/kg induction of sedation dose
- The 68 kg patient received a total of 380 mg over 40 min, which calculates out to 140 μg/kg/min continuous infusion rate. The package insert for propofol states that a range between 150 – 200 μg/kg/min should be used for 10–15 min after induction of general anesthesia, followed by a 30–50% reduction in dose. At a calculated total dose of 140 μg/kg/min given for 40 min, it is clear that the provider in this case administered a general anesthetic dose of propofol for a planned sedation case

Fig. 1.4 Deviations from propofol package insert recommendations found in the case presented in this chapter

One method for determination of exhaled CO_2 is a colorimetric device that changes color depending on the presence of CO_2. These devices are relatively inexpensive, portable, and qualitative in nature, allowing for fast and efficient confirmation of CO_2, even in remote locations where anesthesia is performed. The detector houses a pH-sensitive paper that changes color from purple to yellow with the presence of exhaled CO_2, allowing for easy visual confirmation. Studies have shown that these detectors are reliable indicators of properly positioned ETTs, with sensitivity approaching 100% [11, 12] (Fig. 1.5).

In contrast to the portable and qualitative nature of colorimetric CO_2 detection devices are the more standard and traditional means of exhaled CO_2 quantification via capnometry. This refers to the numerical representation of a CO_2 concentration that can be displayed continuously during both inspiration and exhalation, usually via a capnograph. This technique relies upon either infrared absorption spectrophotometry or mass spectrometry to quantify the concentration of exhaled CO_2. The main advantages of this method are the quantifiable nature of CO_2 concentration and the graphical representation of these numerical values. Analysis of this information allows the anesthesiologist to make judgments on physiologic changes that can arise in a patient under anesthesia, in addition to serving as a method of accurate confirmation of ETT placement within the trachea. Some of the causes of changes in end-tidal CO_2 ($EtCO_2$) can be found in Fig. 1.6 below.

L-8: What Is the Value of Exhaled CO_2 Monitoring During Cardiac Arrest?

As seen in the previous figure, one cause for the precipitous decrease and eventual loss of $EtCO_2$ is cardiac arrest. During arrest, cardiac output goes to zero, and there is no mechanism for the return of CO_2 to the pulmonary circulation to allow for

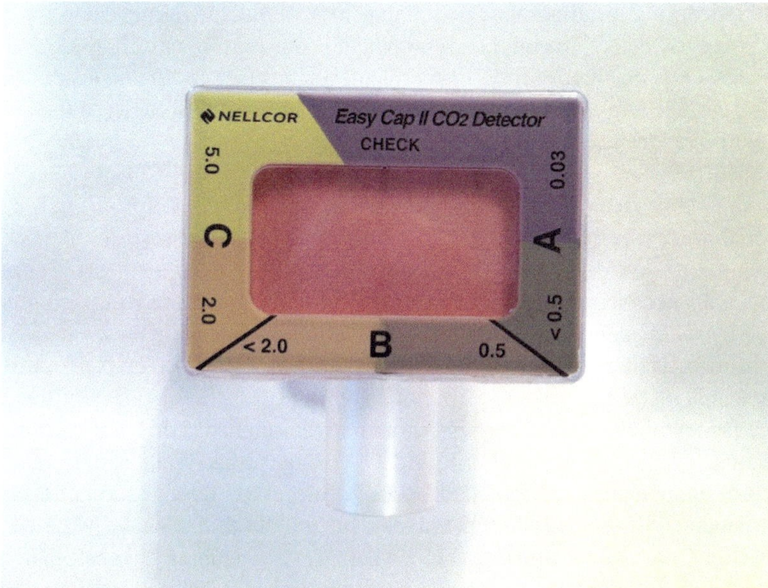

Fig. 1.5 Nellcor Easy Cap II qualitative, colorimetric CO_2 detection device. The purple pH-sensitive paper in the center will change to a yellow/gold color as indicated on the perimeter of the device as increasing levels of CO_2 are detected

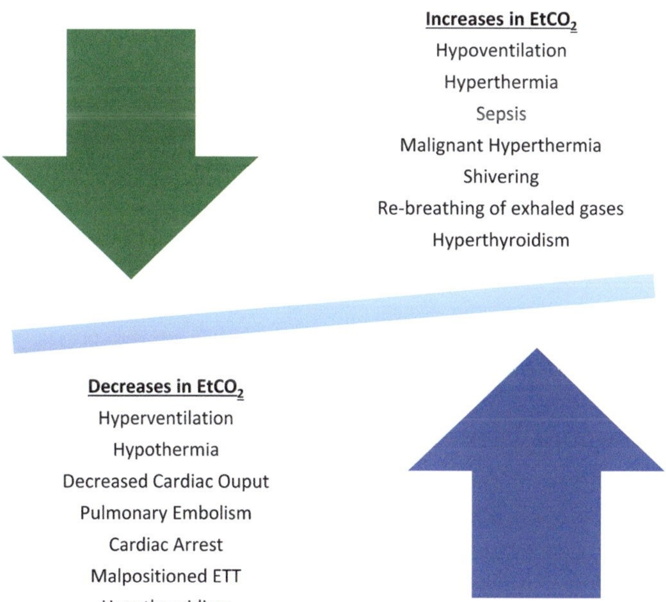

Fig. 1.6 Common causes of changes in quantitative end-tidal CO_2 ($EtCO_2$) concentration during anesthesia. (Based on data from Ref. [13])

exhalation during ventilation. The reliable loss of $EtCO_2$ during such an arrest allows for early detection and intervention and is one reason why continuous monitoring of CO_2 is mandatory for all general anesthetics (see L-4). The loss of $EtCO_2$ during a cardiac arrest does not, however, relieve the anesthesiologist of the responsibility to continue monitoring for exhaled CO_2.

In fact, there are several reasons why monitoring exhaled CO_2 during cardiac arrest and subsequent resuscitation attempts can prove very helpful. First, during cardiopulmonary resuscitation (CPR), chest compressions serve as a means of augmenting cardiac output/blood flow through the body when the heart is arrested. $EtCO_2$ varies in concordance with changes in cardiac output. As a result, continuous monitoring of changes in exhaled CO_2 concentrations has been shown to coincide with the effectiveness of chest compressions during CPR [16]. The AHA currently recommends that if the [$EtCO_2$] <10 mmHg during CPR, the adequacy of the depth and frequency of chest compressions should be reevaluated [10].

Second, another use of monitoring $EtCO_2$ during cardiac arrest is to evaluate for the return of spontaneous circulation (ROSC). Successful resuscitation of a cardiac arrest patient will yield an abrupt increase in the concentration of exhaled CO_2 approaching normal values (Fig. 1.7) [10]. Certain studies suggest that these increases in $EtCO_2$ are often the first clinical indicator of ROSC [14, 16]. A corollary to this fact is that persistently low $EtCO_2$ (<10 mmHg) during resuscitative efforts have been associated with worse outcomes and the inability to resuscitate patients [14–16]. Third, once there is ROSC, $EtCO_2$ once again becomes the primary determinant for setting the minute ventilation in a patient. Finally, administration of sodium bicarbonate during cardiac arrest and the subsequent conversion of HCO_3^- to CO_2 are easily detected by spikes in $EtCO_2$ and can help to guide therapy.

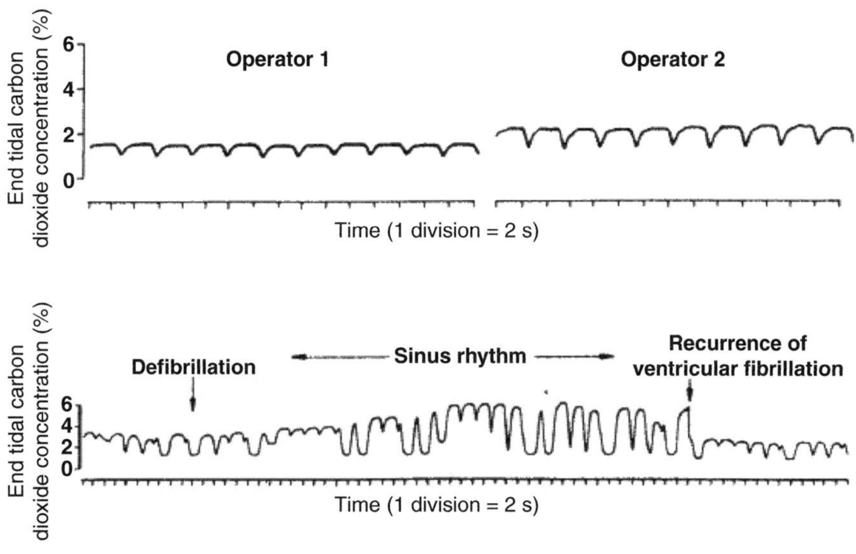

Fig. 1.7 The top panel shows an increase in CO_2 concentration when a second provider begins more adequate chest compressions. The bottom panel shows an increase in CO_2 concentration for a brief period after ROSC and sinus rhythm. (Reprinted from Benumof [17]. With permission from Elsevier)

References

1. American Society of Anesthesiologists. Continuum of depth of sedation: definition of general anesthesia and levels of sedation/analgesia. Last amended October 15, 2014.
2. American Society of Anesthesiologists. Position on monitored anesthesia care. Last amended October 16, 2013.
3. American Society of Anesthesiologists. Distinguishing monitored anesthesia care ("MAC") from moderate sedation/analgesia (conscious sedation). Last amended October 21, 2009 and reaffirmed on October 16, 2013.
4. American Society of Anesthesiologists. Standards for basic anesthetic monitoring. Last amended October 20, 2010, with an effective date of July 1, 2011.
5. American Society of Anesthesiologists. Statement on respiratory monitoring during endoscopic procedures. Last amended October 15, 2014.
6. Metzner J, Domino KB. Risks of anesthesia care in remote locations. Anesth Patient Saf Found Newsl. 2011. 26(1).
7. Diprivan ® [package insert]. Wilmington: Zeneca Pharmaceuticals; 1999.
8. American Society of Anesthesiologists. Statement on non-operating room anesthetizing locations. Last amended October 16, 2013.
9. American Society of Anesthesiology. Practice guidelines for management of the difficult airway: an updated report by the ASA task force on management of the difficult airway. Anesthesiology. 2013;18(2).
10. Field JM, et al. American Heart Association guidelines for cardiopulmonary resuscitation and emergency cardiovascular care. Circulation. 2010;122:640–56.
11. Hayden SR, et al. Colorimetric end-tidal CO2 detector for verification of endotracheal tube placement in out-of-hospital cardiac arrest. Acad Emerg Med. 1995;2(6):499–502.
12. MacLeod BA, et al. Verification of endotracheal tube placement with colorimetric end-tidal CO2 detection. Ann Emerg Med. 1991;20(3):267–70.
13. Barash PG, et al. Clinical anesthesia. 6th ed. Philadelphia: Lippincott Williams & Wilkins; 2009.
14. Garnett AR, et al. End-tidal carbon dioxide monitoring during cardiopulmonary resuscitation. JAMA. 1987;257(4):512–5.
15. Sanders AB, et al. End-tidal carbon dioxide monitoring during cardiopulmonary resuscitation: a prognostic Indicator for survival. JAMA. 1989;262(10):1347–51.
16. Falk JL, et al. End-tidal carbon dioxide concentration during cardiopulmonary resuscitation. N Engl J Med. 1988;318:607–11.
17. Benumof JL, editor. Anesthesia for thoracic surgery. 2nd ed: Elsevier Health Sciences; 1995.
18. Fogel EL, Sherman S. ERCP for gallstone pancreatitis. N Engl J Med. 2014;370:150–7.

Chapter 2
Anesthesia During Liver Transplant: Hepatic Function, TEG, Massive Transfusion, Stages of Liver Transplantation, and MELD Scoring

Kevin D. Marcus and Jonathan L. Benumof

The patient was a 52-year old, 175 cm, 80.9 kg Korean male with a calculated BMI of 26.3 kg/m^2 and a past medical history significant for hepatitis B (HBV) and alcoholic liver cirrhosis, who was scheduled for orthotopic, cadaveric liver transplantation **(L-1)**. In light of his history of prolonged HBV infection, the patient also developed hepatocellular carcinoma (HCC), which furthered the patient's candidacy for transplantation. Additional medical history revealed stable esophageal varices and prior pleural effusion **(L-2)**.

The patient had undergone extensive prior work-up and treatment for his liver failure and HCC, including two transarterial chemoembolization procedures, radiofrequency ablation of liver tumors, as well as a right hepatic lobectomy. The patient was being medically treated with the antiviral drug entecavir. He had no known drug allergies. All preoperative laboratory values (including creatinine, liver function enzymes, bilirubin, albumin, and coagulation parameters) were within normal limits except for a low platelet count of 136×10^9/L **(L-2)**. The calculated biologic MELD score was 7 **(L-3)**, with a MELD exception score for HCC of 31 **(L-4)**. Vital signs were as follows: BP = 133/85 mmHg, HR = 74 bpm, and S_pO_2 = 97% on room air.

The patient was brought to the operating room where, after application of standard ASA monitors, general anesthesia was induced. After induction, radial and femoral arterial lines were placed in addition to a right internal jugular (IJ) and left subclavian vein 9 French introducer sheaths. A pulmonary arterial catheter was placed through the right IJ introducer sheath, and finally, a transesophageal echocardiography (TEE) probe was inserted into the esophagus. A Belmont rapid infuser system was connected to the two 9 French sheaths, and a dedicated perfusionist was available to assist with transfusion of blood products and arterial blood gas

K. D. Marcus (✉)
Department of Anesthesiology, Mission Hospital – Mission Viejo, Mission Viejo, CA, USA

J. L. Benumof
Department of Anesthesiology, University of California, UCSD Medical Center, UCSD School of Medicine, San Diego, CA, USA

J. L. Benumof, G. R. Manecke (eds.), *Clinical Anesthesiology II*,
https://doi.org/10.1007/978-3-030-12365-9_2

measurements. Appropriate line placement was confirmed with intraoperative X-ray prior to surgical incision.

Anesthesia was maintained with isoflurane and intermittent fentanyl boluses while the surgeons proceeded to dissect down to the existing liver through the fairly dense adhesions that were present as the result of previous surgery. During this dissection period, prior to removal of the patient's liver, there was significant blood loss and development of a coagulopathy. The hematocrit decreased from 36% to 21% over the course of 29 min despite treatment with aggressive transfusion of packed red blood cells (PRBC). Three units were given by the anesthesia provider in addition to approximately 12 units by the perfusionist via the rapid infuser system during this time. Platelets and fresh frozen plasma (FFP) were also given in response to the coagulopathy that was observed clinically as well as on a thromboelastograph (TEG) tracing **(L-5)**. Hypocalcemia was treated with a background infusion of calcium chloride as well as intermittent boluses. In addition to infusion of blood products for volume, hemodynamic stability was maintained with titration of a phenylephrine infusion.

Eventually, the surgeons removed the liver, marking the beginning of the anhepatic stage of transplantation, and began the process of sewing in the donor liver. Once adequate portal venous and hepatic arterial anastomoses were complete, the liver was reperfused. Calcium chloride, sodium bicarbonate, and dilute epinephrine boluses were used to combat the hemodynamic instability and profound acidosis that accompanies liver reperfusion **(L-6)**.

After reperfusion, there was ongoing severe coagulopathy and blood loss requiring massive transfusion of blood products by the anesthesia providers and perfusionist via the rapid infusion system **(L-8, 9)**. Increasing doses of vasopressors were also required to maintain adequate mean arterial pressures. Evaluation of the newly reperfused liver revealed separation of the capsule from the liver surface with development of a subcapsular hematoma and increasing superficial hemorrhage. In light of the worsened appearance of the liver, continued hemorrhage, and severe coagulopathy, the surgeons made the determination that there was primary nonfunction of the donor liver **(L-7)**. A plan was made to perform a total hepatectomy with temporary portacaval shunt while re-listing the patient for repeat transplantation, in the hopes of securing a second donor organ.

While this plan was implemented, aggressive resuscitation of the patient continued with massive transfusion of various blood products **(L-8, 9)**. Throughout the course of the case, a total of 92 units of PRBC, 7 units of platelets, 45 units of FFP, 4 units of cryoprecipitate, and 2 doses of prothrombin complex concentrate were given. Despite maximal transfusion efforts, the hematocrit reached a nadir of 8%.

Once the nonfunctional donor liver was removed, the abdomen was packed, and the patient was transported to the ICU with ongoing transfusion of blood products via the rapid infuser system and three vasopressor infusions. Upon arrival to the ICU, plans were made to continue massive transfusion and to begin continuous renal replacement therapy (CRRT) to combat continued acidosis and fluid overload while waiting for a second donor liver. Unfortunately, prior to a new organ becoming available, the patient developed a malignant arrhythmia and passed away 4 h after admission to the ICU, despite attempted resuscitation.

Lessons Learned

L-1: What Are the Primary Functions of the Liver in a Healthy Patient?

The liver is the largest solid organ in the body and accounts for several physiologic functions that are integral for regulation of homeostasis. The dual blood flow to the liver is a major characteristic that accounts for its unique ability to affect so many physiologic mechanisms (Fig. 2.1). The hepatic artery branch off of the celiac artery supplies the liver with oxygenated blood and vital substrates for the organ's intrinsic function. Additional blood supply to the liver arises from the portal vein, which is a confluence of the venous drainage from the large majority of the splanchnic circulation. All told, the liver receives approximately 25% of the total cardiac output.

Primarily, the liver serves as a major metabolic resource for the body, participating in protein, carbohydrate, and lipid metabolism (Table 2.1). The breakdown of amino acids into component parts, including ammonia (see L-2), is one part of protein metabolism. Perhaps more important clinically are the multitude of proteins in the body that the liver is responsible for synthesizing. The principle among these are several parts of the coagulation cascade, including fibrinogen, prothrombin, protein C and S, as well as the vitamin K-dependent coagulation factors II, VII, IX, and

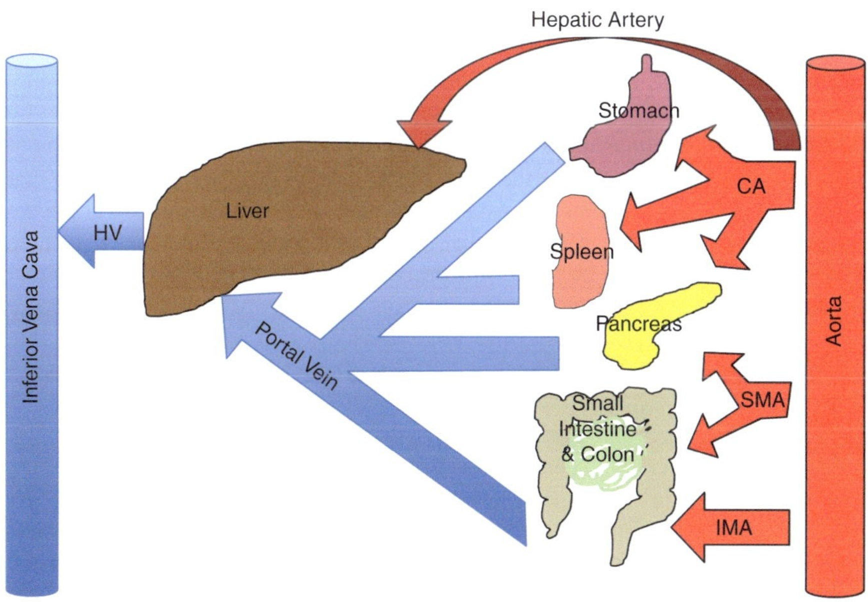

Fig. 2.1 Diagram depicting the blood flow to the liver including both systemic arterial and portal venous contributions. CA celiac artery, SMA superior mesenteric artery, IMA inferior mesenteric artery, HV hepatic vein. (Based on data from Ref. [1])

Table 2.1 Primary metabolic functions of the liver

Metabolic category	Liver functions
Protein metabolism	Amino acid breakdown
	Albumin synthesis
	Synthesis of many coagulation factors
Carbohydrate metabolism	Synthesis, storage, and breakdown of glycogen
	Gluconeogenesis
Lipid metabolism	Fatty acid oxidation
	Formation of lipoproteins (i.e., VLDL)
Bilirubin metabolism	Bilirubin conjugation and excretion
Drug metabolism	Inactivation of drugs via biotransformation
	Excretion into bile

X. The liver also produces albumin, a major circulating protein that contributes to the oncotic pressure in the blood. In terms of carbohydrate metabolism, the liver serves as the major store of the large polysaccharide glycogen, which can be broken down to circulating glucose during times of fasting. The liver can also participate in gluconeogenesis, the process of de novo glucose synthesis, when glycogen stores have been exhausted. Fatty acid oxidation and the formation of lipoproteins such as very-low-density lipoprotein (VLDL) are other metabolic functions of the liver. Additionally, the liver is the primary organ of bilirubin conjugation. Degraded red blood cells produce unconjugated bilirubin, which is difficult for the body to clear prior to conjugation in the liver and secretion into bile, which is yet another product of the liver.

Drug metabolism and biotransformation are other major functions of the healthy liver. Both orally and parenterally administered drug concentrations are affected by the liver due to its unique blood supply. Previously mentioned synthetic products of the liver, such as albumin, alter the bioavailability of drugs by acting as sinks that bind to the free form of the drug. Additionally, the liver also chemically alters the structure of drugs, usually rendering them inactive and making them water-soluble for excretion in either bile or urine. This process of inactivation, known as biotransformation, involves a series of reactions, classified as either phase I or phase II reactions. Phase I reactions involve the ubiquitous cytochrome P-450 system that participates in oxidation and reduction reactions. Phase II reactions further enhance the water solubility of drugs by way of conjugation with polar substances such as glutathione and glucuronic acid.

The liver also serves many additional complementary roles to the endocrine, immunologic, and hematologic systems. For instance, the liver is involved in biotransformation of various hormones such as insulin, thyroid hormones, aldosterone, and estrogens, which leads to alteration in endocrine function. Being a part of the reticuloendothelial system, the liver also plays a role in immunologic responses by acting as a "sieve" for antigens brought to it via the portal vein. Porphyrin metabolism in the liver also serves to facilitate heme synthesis, which supplements that which takes place in the bone marrow.

L-2: What Are the Common Complications of End-Stage Liver Disease?

It should be clear from the previous lesson that the liver plays important roles in several different organ systems throughout the body. It comes as no surprise then that when the liver fails, numerous physiologic consequences arise (Table 2.2).

From a cardiovascular standpoint, there is splanchnic and systemic vasodilation due to both excessive amounts of vasodilatory mediators such as nitric oxide and hyporesponsiveness to vasoconstriction [2]. Circulating blood volume is usually slightly elevated; however, due to unequal vasodilation between the splanchnic and systemic systems, there is a higher blood volume in the splanchnic circulation and a relative hypovolemia in the systemic circulation. These changes are accompanied by increased cardiac output, which is traditionally why liver failure is referred to as a "hyperdynamic" or "high-output" disease process. Mean arterial pressures, filling

Table 2.2 Consequences of liver failure according to organ system

Neurologic	Hepatic encephalopathy
Cardiovascular	Increased cardiac output
	Decreased systemic vascular resistance
	Increased arteriovenous shunting
	Decreased responsiveness to catecholamines
Pulmonary	Increased alveolar-arterial O_2 gradient
	Intrapulmonary shunting
	Hepatic hydrothorax/pleural effusions
	Portopulmonary hypertension
Gastrointestinal	Portal hypertension
	Esophageal and gastric varices
	Caput medusae
Hematologic	Decreased coagulation factor synthesis
	Hyperfibrinolysis
	Disseminated intravascular coagulation
	Quantitative and qualitative platelet
	Dysfunction
Endocrine	Abnormal glucose utilization
	Prone to hypoglycemia
	Gonadal dysfunction
	Increased growth hormone and glucagon levels
Renal	Ascites
	Prerenal failure
	Acute tubular necrosis
	Oliguria
	Hyponatremia

pressures in the heart, and heart rate are usually maintained in liver failure, but decompensation and development of cardiomyopathy are common in very-late-stage disease.

Hepatic encephalopathy (HE) is a generic term for the metabolic encephalopathy that can occur as a result of liver failure. Due to the major metabolic contributions of a healthy liver, products that are normally degraded and/or metabolized are allowed to reach higher concentrations during liver failure. Chief among these substances is ammonia, which is a by-product of protein catabolism. In fact, a high-protein diet has been shown to be a risk factor for development of HE in patients with liver failure, and protein restriction is recommended [3].

The pulmonary system also undergoes several alterations in liver failure. Hypoxemia is more common for a variety of reasons. First, there is increased arteriovenous shunting of blood due to dilation of the pulmonary vasculature. Second, impaired hypoxic pulmonary vasoconstriction and mechanical dysfunction related to ascites and pleural effusions lead to ventilation and perfusion mismatch. Third, there is decreased diffusion capacity due to increased fluid and development of portopulmonary hypertension [1].

Portal hypertension is a hallmark of liver disease and results from a pathologic increase in the portal venous pressures. This increased pressure is usually due to increased resistance to blood flow at the level of hepatic sinusoids and can lead to upstream consequences such as gastroesophageal varices (Fig. 2.1) and buildup of abdominal ascites. Variceal bleeding is a known complication of liver failure and usually requires individualized therapy as these patients also typically have concomitant coagulopathies.

The coagulopathies that are often seen in liver failure are the result of failure of the synthetic properties of the liver. Because the liver is the site of synthesis for all of the vitamin K-dependent coagulation factors and many other important coagulation proteins, bleeding diatheses are common. Additionally, during liver failure, there is a quantitative and qualitative thrombocytopenia, hyperfibrinolysis, and, oftentimes, disseminated intravascular coagulation (DIC).

The healthy liver also regulates many hormones and components of the endocrine system as previously discussed. With impaired liver function, patients are more prone to hypoglycemia due to interference with adequate gluconeogenesis and dysfunctional utilization of glycogen stores. Interestingly, glucose intolerance is also prevalent because of antagonism of insulin by increased levels of growth hormone and glucagon, as well as increased fatty acid concentrations [1]. Abnormal metabolism of sex hormones also causes feminization, gynecomastia, and impotence in men as well as oligomenorrhea or amenorrhea in women with liver failure.

Alterations in blood flow secondary to vasodilation discussed previously contribute to decreased renal blood flow, which is a major factor in the renal impairment that accompanies liver disease. Glomerular filtration rate (GFR) decreases due to this decreased perfusion. Secondary effects of the drop in renal perfusion pressure are increased circulating levels of renin and aldosterone, which leads to a reduction in the excretion of sodium and free water. However, a dilutional hyponatremia can occur quickly when fluid intake overwhelms the decreased ability of the kidneys to excrete free water. Furthermore, up to 10% of patients with liver failure will develop hepatorenal syndrome, which is a functional prerenal failure [1].

As one might expect, drug pharmacology is also significantly altered in liver failure. There are increased circulating amounts of bioavailable drug due to the decreased levels of albumin that would ordinarily bind to the drug. With portal hypertension, there is often collateral circulation via portosystemic shunts that allow oral medications to bypass the liver, which reduces first-pass metabolism of the drugs. Terminal half-lives of drugs are also increased in liver failure due to a reduction in total hepatic blood flow. Hypoalbuminemia and presence of ascites can also contribute to an increased volume of distribution in liver failure patients.

L-3: Diagnosis of Liver Failure and Classification for Transplantation

The diagnosis of liver failure is a clinical one, although many laboratory tests exist to assess the function of the liver and help guide this diagnosis. These tests are helpful in determining progression of disease but are sometimes nonspecific and need to be taken in the context of other comorbid conditions. The various blood tests used in the evaluation of the liver can also help to elucidate the differential causes of hepatic dysfunction. Table 2.3 below shows common blood tests that can be taken to evaluate the different functions of the liver or damage done to the liver.

Because of the variable nature of the previous laboratory values in the evaluation of liver failure, another method for classifying dysfunction was created for use in allocation of donor organs when considering transplantation. The Model for End-Stage Liver Disease (MELD) score was initially established as a way of predicting poor outcome after transjugular intrahepatic portosystemic shunt (TIPS) procedures [4]. The United Network for Organ Sharing (UNOS) has since adopted this scoring system as an acceptable means of stratifying patient's liver dysfunction prior to transplantation.

The MELD score calculation is based upon three laboratory parameters that become abnormal in patients with liver failure. The parameters are serum bilirubin, serum creatinine, and the international normalized ratio (INR). The actual MELD score involves mathematical manipulation of the mentioned laboratory values to arrive at an integer value. As liver disease progresses, there is typically a worsening of these laboratory values, such that the MELD score increases. Calculated MELD scores can be used to prognosticate about the 3-month mortality of patients with liver dysfunction [5] (Table 2.4). It is clear from this data that higher MELD scores portend much worse outcomes for patients with liver disease.

With regard to allocation of donor organs, UNOS utilizes a specific order in which organs will be offered to patients based upon several parameters including MELD score, the severity and acuteness of liver failure, age, location, and organ compatibility [9]. The MELD score is the major determinant of disease severity, and use of this primarily MELD-based allocation of donor organs has resulted in better 1-year survival rates posttransplantation [6].

Table 2.3 Laboratory indices of various hepatic functions

Hepatic function being assessed	Laboratory test	Change occurring in liver failure
Hepatocellular damage	Aspartate aminotransferase (AST)	Increased
	Alanine aminotransferase (ALT)	Increased
	Lactate dehydrogenase (LDH)	Increased
	Glutathione s-transferase (GST)	Increased
Bile flow obstruction	Bilirubin[a]	Increased
	Alkaline phosphatase	Increased
	γ-glutamyl transferase (GGT)	Increased
	5′-nucleotidase	Increased
Synthetic function	Albumin	Decreased
	Prothrombin time (PT)	Prolonged
	International normalized ratio[a] (INR)	Increased
Hepatic blood flow	Indocyanine green elimination	Decreased
Metabolic function	Monoethylglycinexylidide (MEGX) test of lidocaine metabolism	Decreased

[a]Used in conjunction with serum creatinine, a renal function test that also becomes abnormal in hepatic dysfunction, to calculate the MELD score

Table 2.4 Three-month mortality based upon MELD scores in patients with liver failure

Calculated MELD score	Three-month mortality
≤9	1.9%
10–19	6.0%
20–29	19.6%
30–39	52.6%
≥40	71.3%

Based on data from Ref. [5]

L-4: Why Does a Patient with HCC Have a Different MELD Score?

In the case presented at the beginning of the chapter, it is clear that the patient did not have an elevated biologic, or native, MELD score based upon the normal laboratory values of serum bilirubin, creatinine, and INR. The patient's calculated MELD score of 7 would have put him very far down on the list of recipients when an organ became available.

Due to the clinical nature of HCC, patients with early disease will often have preserved liver function and therefore normal, or near normal, laboratory values. However, patients with HCC often see morbidity associated with increased tumor burden, and not just intrinsic liver dysfunction [7]. Furthermore, the overall outcomes for patients with HCC are generally poor, with 5-year survival between 20%

and 40% [8]. It is clear that use of the biologic MELD score, which would be low in the setting of preserved liver function, for patients with HCC would severely limit their ability to receive a liver transplant that would be potentially curative of their disease process.

Due to this disparity between low MELD scores and need for transplantation, current guidelines for donor organ allocation utilize an exception MELD score for patients with HCC. The MELD exception score is based on, and directly proportional to, the total tumor burden. However, the MELD exception score will change over time. For instance, patients with T2 HCC who register for an exception receive a score equivalent to 15% probability of death within 3 months and additional MELD points equivalent to a 10% increase in mortality risk every 3 months they do not receive a donor organ [7]. This increases the likelihood of receiving a liver transplant for this subset of patients, who would otherwise endure significant and prolonged morbidity prior to qualifying.

In the case at the beginning of the chapter, the patient was assigned a MELD score of 22 upon registration for exception based upon the diagnosis of HCC. This score increased every 3 months until a donor organ was made available to him, at which time his MELD exception score for HCC was 31.

L-5: What Is a Thromboelastogram (TEG)?

Thromboelastography is a method for evaluation of the mechanical properties of a blood clot. The resultant thromboelastograph (TEG) provides information on all elements of the hemostatic process, including platelet aggregation, coagulation, and fibrinolysis, allowing the provider to make a decision on potential transfusion therapies. This is one advantage of the TEG over other tests of coagulation such as prothrombin time (PT) and partial thromboplastin time (PTT). These tests are commonly used to evaluate only one segment of the coagulation cascade, namely, the extrinsic and intrinsic pathways, respectively.

Completion of a TEG involves placing a small volume of whole blood into a sample cup and pin assembly while the cup continuously oscillates around the pin. The intrinsic viscoelastic properties of the blood change the interaction of the pin and cup as fibrin clot begins to form. A computer measures these changes and then develops a graphical representation of the mechanical properties of the clot (Fig. 2.2).

Several parameters are a part of the basic TEG, and each can be used to determine an individual aspect of coagulation and clot formation/degradation (Table 2.5). The initial parameter is the reaction time, or "R" time, which is the time until clot formation begins. This is dependent upon thrombin formation and is a reflection of the enzymatic reaction function of the coagulation cascade. Prolongation of the R time can be seen in coagulation factor deficiencies and presence of heparin, which inhibits thrombin. A shortened R time is present in hypercoagulable states, where feedback mechanisms may have been lost.

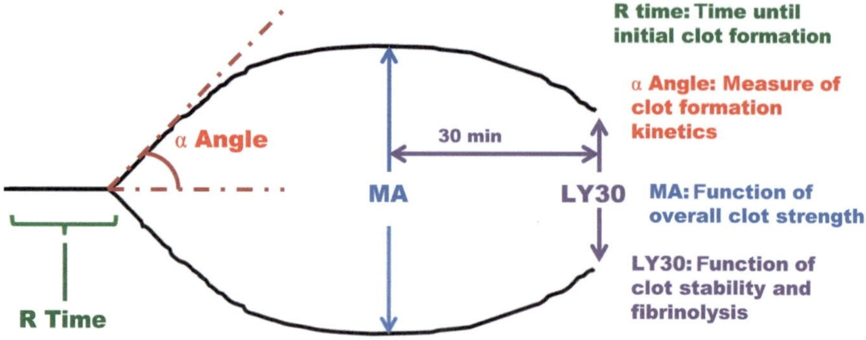

Fig. 2.2 Schematic of TEG tracing including the major parameters

Table 2.5 Major components of the thromboelastograph

Parameter	Definition	Coagulation parameter involved	Abnormalities	Possible treatments for abnormalities
R time	Time from start of TEG until initial clot formation	Coagulation cascade factors	Prolonged: factor deficiency, heparin	FFP, PCC, protamine
			Shortened: hypercoagulability	Various anticoagulants
K time	Time for TEG tracing to reach 20 mm	Fibrinogen	Prolonged: low fibrinogen level	FFP, cryoprecipitate
			Shortened: hypercoagulability	Variable
α-Angle	Measure of speed of clot formation	Fibrinogen	Increased: hypercoagulability	Variable
			Decreased: low fibrinogen level	FFP, cryoprecipitate
Maximum amplitude (MA)	Maximum clot strength dependent on platelets (80%)	Platelets[a]	Low: decreased or poor functioning platelets	Platelets
			High: excessive platelet activity	Antiplatelet therapy
"G" parameter (a function of MA)	Representation of clot strength and platelet function	Platelets	Similar to MA	Similar to MA
Coagulation index (CI)	Global index of hemostatic status	Coagulation index	CI >+3.0: hypercoagulable	Dependent on remainder of TEG
			CI <−3.0: hypocoagulable	
LY30/EPL	% decrease from MA and estimated rate of change	Clot stability	Excessive fibrinolysis: possible tPA or DIC	Antifibrinolytics (i.e., tranexamic acid, aminocaproic acid)

tPA tissue plasminogen activator, *DIC* disseminated intravascular coagulation
[a]Platelets are the major determinant of MA, although fibrinogen also contributes

The "K" time is the time it takes the TEG tracing to reach a width of 20 mm and is reflective of further clot formation and kinetics. It, too, is dependent on the rate thrombin generation in addition to the conversion of fibrinogen to fibrin as well as fibrin cross-linking with platelets. A prolonged K time is indicative of coagulation factor deficiencies or insufficient generation of fibrin from fibrinogen. Similar to the K time is the α-angle, which is also a measure of clot formation kinetics. Thrombin generation, conversion of fibrinogen to fibrin, and fibrin interaction with platelets are all reflected in the α-angle. A decreased α-angle is possible with low fibrinogen levels, platelet dysfunction, or insufficient thrombin generation. Increased α-angle can be seen in platelet hypercoagulability.

The maximum amplitude (MA) is the widest diameter that the TEG tracing achieves and is indicative of overall clot strength. Due to the composition of the clot, the MA is 80% dependent on platelets and 20% on fibrinogen. In most cases, derangements in the MA are simplified to reflect perturbations in platelet count or function. For instance, a low MA is usually due to thrombocytopenia or poor platelet function, whereas a high MA may indicate platelet hypercoagulability or excessive functionality. The "G" parameter is a mathematical conversion of the MA into units of dynes/cm^2 via the formula $G = (5000 \times MA)/(100 - MA)$. The G parameter describes an exponential relationship between clot strength and platelet function, compared to the linear relationship described by MA. This makes the G parameter more sensitive to changes in platelet function than the MA.

The coagulation index (CI) provides a linear combination of the kinetic parameters of clot development and clot strength. CI takes into account R time, K time, α-angle, and MA in order to give a global view on hemostatic status. Normal values for CI range from −3.0 to +3.0, with more positive values indicating hypercoagulability and more negative numbers indicating hypocoagulability.

Clot stability and fibrinolysis are also evaluated in a TEG with the LY30 and estimated percent lysis (EPL) values. LY30 is the percent decrease in amplitude 30 min after the MA is reached. EPL is the estimated rate of change in the amplitude after MA is reached. Elevated values for LY30 and EPL are indicative of increased fibrinolytic activity, which, if greater than clot formation, may contribute to increased bleeding.

Table 2.6 is derived from the basics of TEG presented in Table 2.5, showing common clinical coagulopathic scenarios and the corresponding abnormalities that would be found on TEG. The blood products that can be administered to counteract each coagulopathy are also shown, highlighting how specific TEG abnormalities can lead to more guided and specific transfusion therapy. Note that most TEG displays will have common laboratory ranges for all parameters listed to further guide interpretation of the TEG tracing (see Figs. 2.3, 2.4 and 2.5).

The appeal of the TEG is that a single laboratory test can provide a comprehensive analysis of hemostatic properties that have the ability to guide transfusion decisions. TEG-based algorithms have been used to successfully reduce transfusion requirements in cardiac surgery, liver transplantation, and massive trauma [10]. During the case presented earlier, several TEG studies were obtained (Figs. 2.3, 2.4 and 2.5).

Table 2.6 Common clinical coagulopathic states during massive transfusion and their findings on TEG

Coagulopathy	TEG abnormality	Blood product to give
Decreased coagulation factors	Prolonged R time	FFP, PCC
Thrombocytopenia	Decreased MA	Platelets
DIC with decreased fibrinogen	Low α-angle	Cryoprecipitate

FFP fresh frozen plasma, *PPC* prothrombin complex concentrate

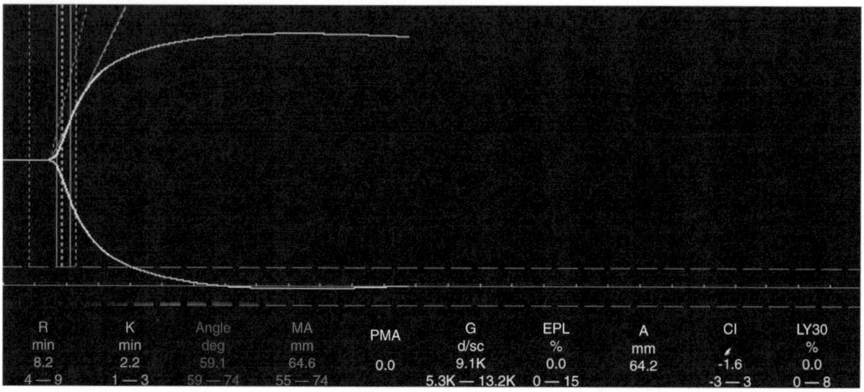

Fig. 2.3 Baseline TEG study obtained shortly after placement of hemodynamic monitors and prior to any significant bleeding or hemodynamic compromise

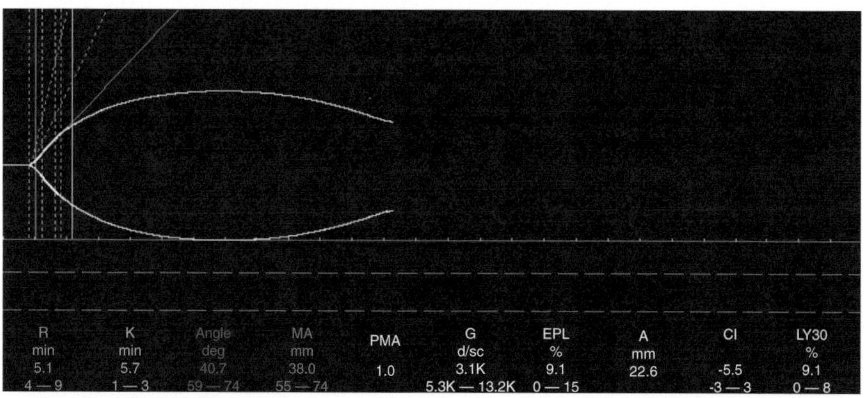

Fig. 2.4 Repeat TEG obtained prior to native liver excision but during a time of significant bleeding and clinical coagulopathy

Figure 2.3 shows the normal configuration of a TEG in the absence of coagulation abnormalities. This TEG was taken very early on in the case and is representative of the normal coagulation profile that this patient had, which correlates with the rest of his normal coagulation labs. All major TEG parameters are within the normal

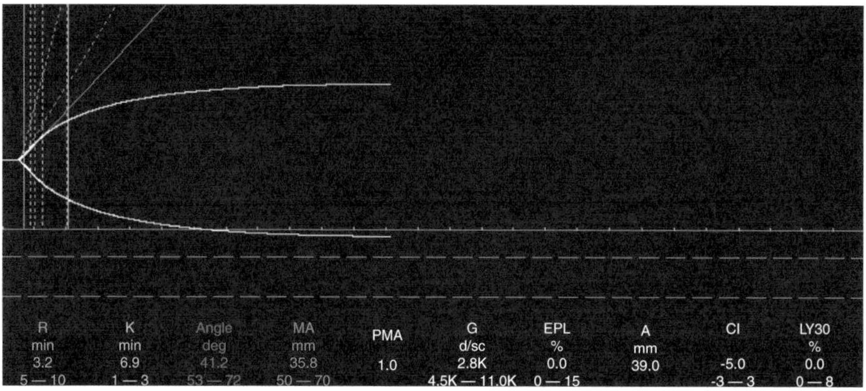

Fig. 2.5 TEG taken during continued massive hemorrhage and coagulopathy after donor liver reperfusion and just prior to decision to remove the newly transplanted organ for primary nonfunction of the graft

limits illustrated at the bottom of the figure. A repeat TEG is taken later in the case, during a time of significant bleeding, but prior to excision of the native liver (Fig. 2.4). It is clear when comparing Figs. 2.3 and 2.4 that there has been significant change. Figure 2.4 now shows a prolonged K time, decreased α-angle, decreased MA and G parameter, negative CI, and elevated LY30/EPL. This represents an overall state of hypocoagulability and lack of adequate fibrinogen and platelets and excessive fibrinolysis. In response to this TEG, platelets and FFP were given, followed shortly by cryoprecipitate.

Figure 2.5 shows another TEG that was taken just prior to the decision to remove the newly transplanted liver for primary graft nonfunction. At this time, massive hemorrhage was ongoing, and coagulopathy was obvious in the surgical field, an abnormality that is well represented in this TEG tracing. Again, there is a prolonged K time, decreased α-angle, decreased MA and G parameter, and a negative CI as in Fig. 2.4. Interestingly, the LY30/EPL have normalized, despite the decision not to administer an antifibrinolytic. Massive transfusion continued with platelets, FFP, cryoprecipitate, and prothrombin complex concentrate (PCC). The R time remained within normal limits, likely due to the transfusion of so many products containing coagulation factors (FFP, PCC).

L-6: What Are the Three Common Stages of a Typical Liver Transplant?

The liver transplant operation can be divided into three stages, the hepatectomy, or pre-anhepatic stage, the anhepatic stage, and, finally, the neohepatic stage. Each stage has unique considerations for both the surgical team and the anesthesia providers (Table 2.7).

Table 2.7 Surgical and anesthetic considerations for the three stages of liver transplantation

Stage of transplant	Definition	Surgical considerations	Anesthetic considerations	Anesthetic actions
Pre-anhepatic	Begins with skin incision and ends with removal of the native liver	Dissection to liver	Hyperglycemia	Administer insulin
		Adhesions from prior surgery	Hemorrhage	Transfuse PRBC to goal Hct
		Mobilization of liver	Coagulopathy	Use TEG to guide therapy
		Mobilization of vessels	↓ preload with IVC clamping	Administer IVF and/or blood products
Anhepatic	Begins with clamping of hepatic vessels, IVC, and removal of liver; ends with reperfusion of donor liver	IVC anastomosis	Hemorrhage	Transfuse PRBC to goal Hct
		Flushing donor organ	Coagulopathy	Use TEG to guide therapy
		Portal vein and hepatic artery anastomosis	Acidosis	AdministerNaHCO_3^-
			Hypocalcemia	Administer calcium
			Avoid volume overload	Follow CVP, PAC tracing, clinical appearance of surgical field
Neohepatic	Begins with unclamping of portal vein, hepatic artery, and IVC to reperfuse donor liver	Anastomotic inspection	Hypotension	Vasopressors, IVF, blood products
		Hemostasis	Bradycardia	Epinephrine, anticholinergics
		Cholecystectomy	↓ SVR	Administer α-agonist
		Bile duct reconstruction	Pulmonary HTN, RV failure	Check TEE, PAC; give inotropic agents
		Abdominal closure	Air and thromboembolism	Ensure adequate flushing of liver, monitor TEE for strain
			Hyperkalemia	Administer Ca^{++}, insulin, β-agonists
			Profound acidosis	AdministerNaHCO_3^-
			Hypokalemia	Administer calcium
			Hyperglycemia	Administer insulin
			Hypothermia	Warm IVF, forced air warming device

IVC inferior vena cava, *SVR* systemic vascular resistance, *HTN* hypertension, *RV* right ventricle, *Hct* hematocrit, *IVF* intravenous fluids, *Na*HCO_3^- sodium bicarbonate, *TEG* thromboeleastograph, *CVP* central venous pressure, *PAC* pulmonary artery catheter, *TEE* transesophageal echocardiography, Ca^{++} calcium

Beginning with surgical incision, the hepatectomy and pre-anhepatic portion of the case starts. This stage is characterized by surgical dissection down to the liver and mobilization of the various blood vessels and organ itself in preparation for excision. Depending upon the baseline physiology of the patient, this stage can be relatively well tolerated. However, things like severe portal hypertension, baseline coagulopathy, and prior abdominal surgeries complicate this stage with increased hemorrhage and difficulty of dissection. From an anesthesia standpoint, perturbations in venous return are common as the liver is manipulated and the IVC and portal veins are eventually clamped.

After clamping of the hepatic vessels and the IVC, the native liver is removed, and the anhepatic stage of the operation begins. Generally speaking, this stage involves sewing in the donor liver with all accompanying vascular anastomoses. Due to the absence of vascular flow out of the portal system, congestion of the abdominal organs is common, leading to decreased perfusion pressures. Special attention needs to be paid to the kidneys in order to minimize renal dysfunction. Increasing coagulopathy, hemorrhage, and acidosis are also considerations during this phase. Maintenance of adequate intravascular volume should be a goal; however, fluid overload can be detrimental during upcoming reperfusion and entry into the neohepatic phase.

Reperfusion of the donor liver at the beginning of the neohepatic stage is the time during a liver transplant that is the most complicated and requires excellent communication between all parties. This is due to the major hemodynamic changes and complications that can arise during this time period. In fact, post-reperfusion syndrome (PRS) is a recognized phenomenon involving significant decreases in mean arterial pressures occurring in the several minutes after un-clamping of the portal vein and IVC. Patients who experience PRS are more likely to develop postoperative renal failure and are also more likely to die in the 15 days posttransplant than those patients who did not have PRS [11]. Additional concerns during this vulnerable time include profound acidosis, hyperkalemia, hypothermia, pulmonary hypertension contributing to right ventricular failure, air embolism, bradycardia, and other arrhythmias. Proper correction of electrolytes and administration of sodium bicarbonate, vasopressors, and inotropic agents are all part of the anesthetic management of donor organ reperfusion. Once stabilized, the surgeon completes final anastomoses and hemostasis is achieved both surgically and via administration of continued blood products.

L-7: What Is Primary Nonfunction of the Liver?

Primary graft nonfunction (PGNF) is a life-threatening consequence after liver transplantation. UNOS defines PGNF as "irreversible graft function requiring emergency liver replacement during the first 10 days after liver transplantation" [12]. Other definitions relate PGNF to an aggravated form of reperfusion injury resulting in irreversible graft failure without detectable technical (e.g., surgical anastomoses failure) or immunological problems [14]. Clinical and laboratory markers for the diagnosis of PGNF vary depending on the source, ranging from liver transaminases, ammonia levels, bile production, prothrombin time (PT)/INR, lactate levels, need for clotting support, and even presence of encephalopathy [13].

The incidence of PGNF lies between 4% and 8% taken from the compiled data of various studies [13]. However, due to the significant impact on not only the patient but also medical resources, many have taken to attempting to define risk factors for PGNF in order to potentially reduce the incidence by means of better selection of donor and recipients. In one study, investigators determined that increasing age of donor (>40 years), split/partial grafts, donation after cardiac death, increased cold ischemia time, and the cause of brain death in donors all were associated with increased risk of liver graft failure [14].

L-8: What Is a Massive Transfusion Protocol?

Massive transfusion of blood products is a lifesaving practice that occurs in various situations in surgery and anesthesia: liver transplantation, obstetric emergencies, and trauma, to name a few. The definition of massive transfusion varies according to the source; some state >10 units PRBC in 24 h, others >20 units PRBC in 24 h [15, 16]. Others suggest a smaller time frame of >4 units PRBC in 1 h with ongoing need for transfusion [16]. Regardless of the exact definition, massive transfusion utilizes large amounts of medical resources and has the potential for significant morbidity and mortality. Therefore, many institutions have implemented some sort of a massive transfusion protocol to limit adverse events, such as dilutional coagulopathy (see L-9), and to also be able to respond quickly and efficiently to emergent situations.

At the University of California, San Diego (UCSD), the massive transfusion protocol is published by the blood bank. After the responsible physician makes the decision to utilize the massive transfusion protocol, the blood bank immediately makes available 45 units each of PRBC and FFP, in addition to 4–6 units of platelet apheresis (concentrated) units. The initial four units of PRBC may be type O negative and the FFP may be AB. After this first set, the blood bank releases a second set of six units PRBC, six units FFP, and one platelet unit. If the need continues, subsequent batches of products released from the blood bank will consist of ten units PRBC, ten units FFP, and one to two platelet units. While transfusion of the previously released batches of products is underway, the blood bank is continually reconfirming the patients' ABO/Rh blood type status, and the decision is made to switch to type-specific blood as soon as is feasible to do so.

After a review of several existing massive transfusion protocols, it was suggested by Malone et al. that massive transfusion protocols should have the following basic guidelines: initiate transfusion of plasma products early without compromising transfusion of PRBC, transfuse platelets to maintain a count $>50\times10^9$/L, and utilize a 10:10:1 ratio for PRBC/FFP/platelet (apheresis units) transfusion [15]. High ratios of FFP and platelets to PRBC administered early on in massive transfusion situations have been shown to not only decrease the amount of PRBC needed but also led to improved survival [17]. With regard to laboratory monitoring during massive transfusion, the ASA committee on blood management cautions that standard tests of coagulation (e.g., PT, PTT, INR, platelet count, and fibrinogen) may not provide an accurate assessment of current coagulation status and that utilization of TEG (see L-5) should be considered to guide hemostatic therapies during massive transfusion [16]. It has also been suggested that in the absence of ongoing, active bleeding, abnormal tests of coagulation should not be corrected with further transfusion of hemostatic agents (e.g., FFP, platelets, etc.) [15].

L-9: What Are the Complications Associated with Massive Transfusion?

Transfusion of blood products is by no means a benign process, and both the risks and proposed benefits should be carefully weighed prior to transfusion. Even the transfusion of a single unit of blood product carries with it the risk of infection, incompatibility reactions, anaphylaxis, and end-organ damage such as transfusion-related acute lung injury (TRALI). However, there are many other complications that can arise specifically from massive transfusion of blood products (Fig. 2.6), in addition to the risks associated with smaller transfusion volumes.

Dilutional coagulopathy (12 o'clock, Fig. 2.6) is one of the major consequences of massive transfusion of blood products. This is a process in which administration of large volumes of fluid that are devoid of platelets and clotting factors causes a relative dilution of these products that function in clot formation and stability. As a result, these processes are limited and a coagulopathy develops. Most commonly, the relative deficiency in clotting factors will develop prior to thrombocytopenia [1]. This is one reason why massive transfusion protocols are aimed at early administration of plasma-rich products such as FFP. Additionally, most massive transfusion protocols have also adopted a ratio for transfusion of PRBC to other products such as FFP and platelets (see L-8), so as to minimize the dilutional coagulopathy that can result from too much PRBC in the absence of other products. It is also recommended that the use of isotonic crystalloid solutions to aid in resuscitation from hypovolemia be limited as this can contribute further to dilutional coagulopathy [16].

During massive transfusion, the total volume of fluid administered can be quite large, up to many times the normal circulating blood volumes. Volume overload (2 o'clock, Fig. 2.6) can lead to major deleterious end-organ consequences. First, pulmonary and airway edema may occur, resulting in progressive hypoxia. Second, elevated venous pressures reduce end-organ perfusion pressures which can lead to ischemia.

Hyperkalemia (3 o'clock, Fig. 2.6) is another well-documented consequence of massive transfusion. Storage of PRBC causes the redistribution of potassium out of cells to maintain electric neutrality. The longer the blood is stored, cells begin to die

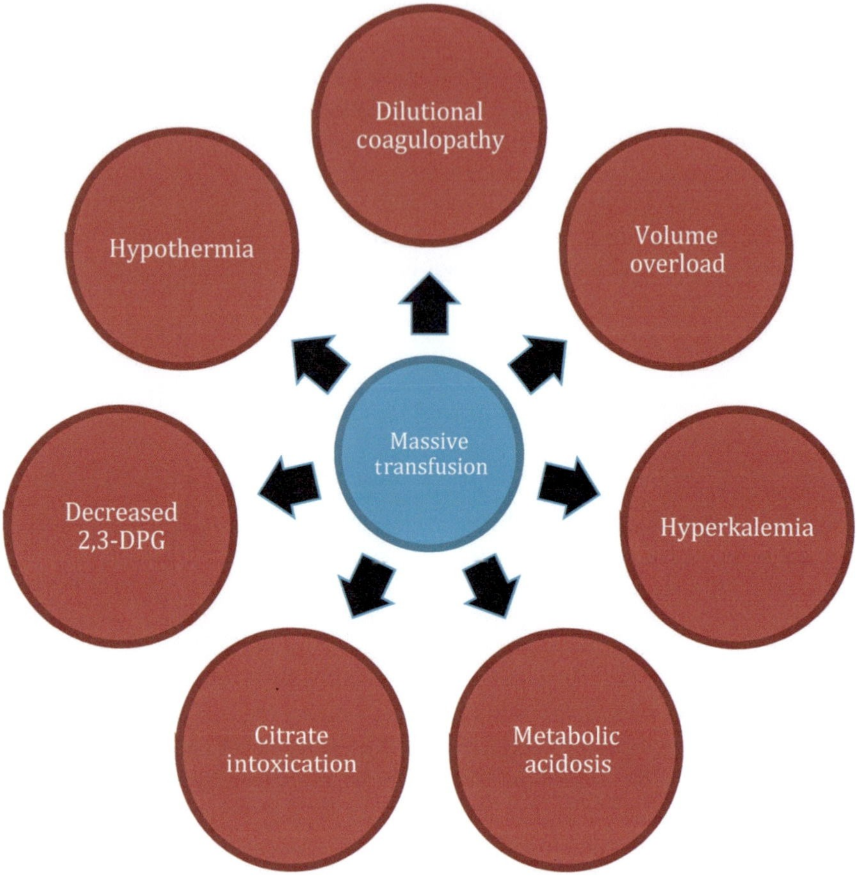

Fig. 2.6 Complications of massive transfusion of blood products. 2,3-DPG = 2,3-diphosphoglycerate

and release additional potassium, which can reach between 19 and 35 mEq/L in blood stored for 21 days [1]. Rapid administration of large quantities of stored blood can therefore lead to clinically significant hyperkalemia. This hyperkalemia is exacerbated by another consequence of massive transfusion, metabolic acidosis, which causes a transcellular shift of intracellular potassium to the extracellular space in exchange for extracellular hydrogen ions.

The metabolic acidosis (5 o'clock, Fig. 2.6) that accompanies massive transfusion is, again, largely related to the storage of blood. In order to lengthen the shelf life of blood, a citrate-phosphate-dextrose-adenine (CPDA) solution is added. This leads to an initial decrease in pH of the blood, which is exacerbated during storage by the anaerobic metabolism of glucose to lactate. At the end of 21 days in storage, the pH of the blood can be as low as 6.9 [1]. Transfusion of this acidic blood product may contribute to some acidosis during massive transfusion, although there is usually some degree of existing hypoperfusion and anaerobic metabolism causing a

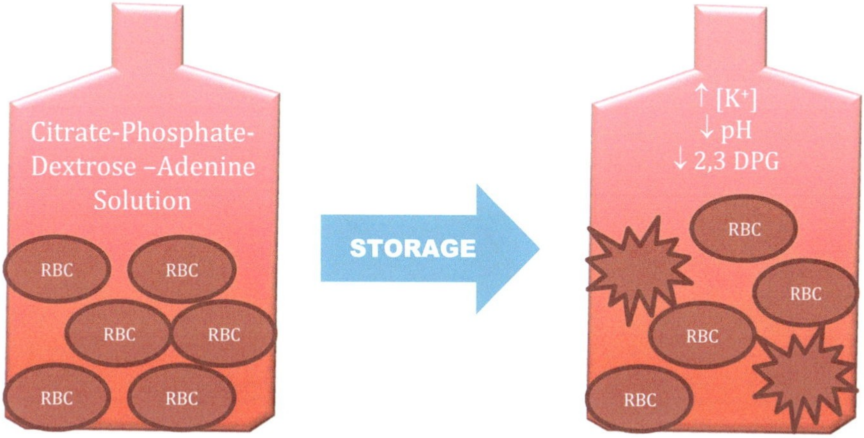

Fig. 2.7 Schematic representation of the changes that occur in packed red blood cells (PRBC) after storage in CPDA solution prior to transfusion

lactic acidosis in most patients that would require initiation of a massive transfusion to begin with (Fig. 2.7).

Another consequence of the storage of blood in CPDA solution is the concept of citrate intoxication (7 o'clock, Fig. 2.6). When rapidly administered during the course of massive transfusion, citrate has the ability to cause a temporary reduction in the amount of ionized calcium, leading to consequences associated with hypocalcemia. It is also worth mentioning that most citrate administered during transfusion comes from FFP, not PRBCs [1]. Normally, a healthy functioning liver is capable of metabolizing the citrate load unless it exceeds 1 ml/kg/min, or roughly one unit of blood every 5 min [1]. However, as in this case presentation, a compromised liver would lead to significantly increased risk of citrate intoxication and hypocalcemia.

2,3-Diphosphoglycerate (2,3-DPG) is a molecule present in red blood cells that has a high affinity for binding to deoxygenated hemoglobin, which facilitates the release of oxygen from hemoglobin to tissues. When blood is stored, the concentration of 2,3-DPG decreases (9 o'clock, Fig. 2.6) with time, such that the blood administered during massive transfusion is less efficient at off-loading oxygen to tissues, despite the increased hemoglobin concentration. This concept is represented by a left shift in the oxygen-hemoglobin dissociation curve (Fig. 2.8).

Hypothermia (10 o'clock, Fig. 2.6) commonly accompanies massive transfusion of blood products. The administration of one unit PRBC at 4 °C can reduce the core temperature of a 70 kg person by about 0.25 °C [1]. Hypothermia contributes to increased coagulopathy by slowing the enzymatic processes associated with hemostasis. There is also impaired tissue oxygenation as a result of a left shifting of the oxygen-hemoglobin dissociation curve and a decreased cardiac output with hypothermia. Warming of blood products is recommended and becomes especially important during massive transfusion.

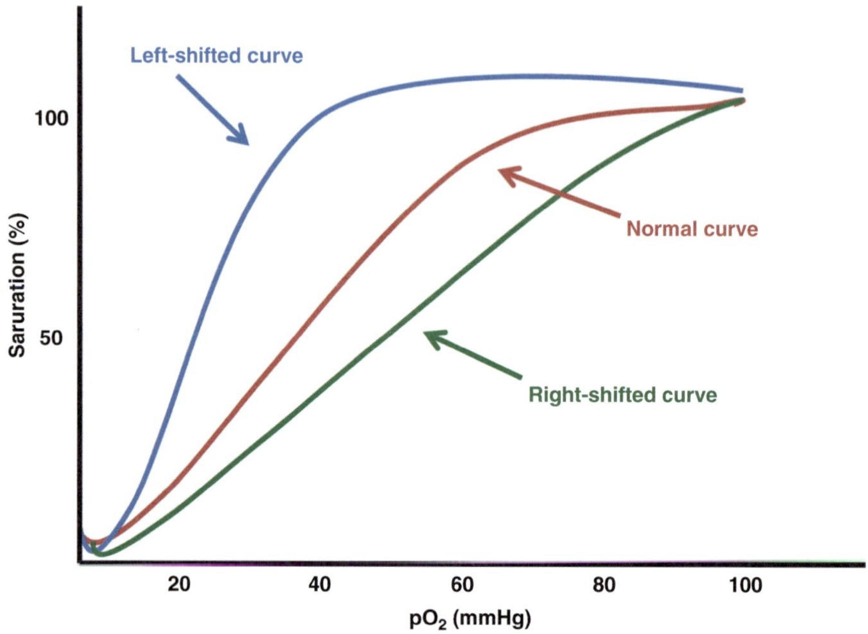

Fig. 2.8 Oxyhemoglobin dissociation curve showing the relationship between arterial saturation and partial pressure of oxygen under normal and abnormal conditions. Left-shifted curves represent increased affinity between oxygen and hemoglobin. Right-shifted curves represent decreased affinity between oxygen and hemoglobin

References

1. Barash PG, et al. Clinical anesthesia. 6th ed. Philadelphia: Lippincott Williams & Wilkins; 2009.
2. Colle I, et al. Hemodynamic changes in splanchnic blood vessels in portal hypertension. Anat Rec (Hoboken). 2008;291(6):699–713.
3. Iwasa M, Takei Y. Pathophysiology and management of hepatic encephalopathy 2014 update: ammonia toxicity and hyponatremia. Hepatol Res. 2015;45:1155–62.
4. Malinchoc M, et al. A model to predict poor survival in patients undergoing transjugular intrahepatic portosystemic shunts. Hepatology. 2000;31(4):864–71.
5. Wiesner R, et al. Model for end-stage liver disease (MELD) and allocation of donor livers. Gastroenterology. 2003;124(1):91–6.
6. Qiu J, et al. Liver transplantation in the United States. Clin Transpl. 2005:17–28.
7. Piscaglia F, et al. A new priority for patients with hepatocellular carcinoma awaiting liver transplantation within the model for end-stage liver disease system. Liver Transpl. 2007;13(6):857–66.
8. Duffy JP, et al. Liver transplantation criteria for hepatocellular carcinoma should be expanded. Ann Surg. 2007;246(3):502–11.
9. Questions and Answers for Transplant Candidates about Liver Allocation. www.unos.org/docs/Liver_patient.pdf, United Network for Organ Sharing.
10. Bollinger D, Seeberger MD, Tanaka KA. Principles and practice of thromboelastography in clinical coagulation management and transfusion practice. Transfus Med Rev. 2012;26(1):1–13.

11. Paugam-Burtz C, et al. Postreperfusion syndrome during liver transplantation for cirrhosis: outcome and predictors. Liver Transpl. 2009;15(5):522–9.
12. Chen H, et al. Initial poor graft dysfunction and primary graft non-function after orthotopic liver transplantation. Liver Biopsy Mod Med. 2011:183–206. ISBN: 978-953-307-883-0.
13. Lock JF, et al. Early diagnosis of primary nonfunction and indication for reoperation after liver transplantation. Liver Transpl. 2010;16:172–80.
14. Feng S, et al. Characteristics associated with liver graft failure: the concept of a donor risk index. Am J Transplant. 2006;6(4):783–90.
15. Malone DL, Hess JR, Fingerhut A. Massive transfusion practices around the globe and a suggestion for a common massive transfusion protocol. J Trauma. 2006;60(6):91–6.
16. Smith CE, et al. American Society of Anesthesiologists Committee on Blood Management. Massive Transfusion Protocol (MTP) for hemorrhagic shock. Transfus Med Rev. 2011;25(3):217–31.
17. Zink KA, et al. A high ratio of plasma and platelets to packed red blood cells in the first 6 hours of massive transfusion improves outcomes in a large multicenter study. Am J Surg. 2009;197(5):565–70.

Chapter 3
Obstructive Sleep Apnea: Falling Through Caregiver Cracks to Death

Christopher Nguyen and Jonathan L. Benumof

Case Narrative

A 53-year-old, 87 kg, 5′6″ tall, BMI 32.5, woman was seen by her primary care physician for excessive daytime sleepiness and loud snoring. The primary care physician ordered a sleep study, which revealed an apnea-hypopnea index (AHI) of 74.0/h ($A = 54.8$/h and $H = 19.1$/h), a low SpO2 of 74%, and a decrease in the AHI from 74.0 to 8/h with 15 cmH2O continuous positive airway pressure (CPAP); all three findings were entirely consistent with a diagnosis of severe obstructive sleep apnea (OSA) (L-1, L-2). The patient was placed on nightly CPAP at 15 cmH2O, and on this therapy the patient did very well for the next 5 years. The sleep specialist did all the OSA follow-up care, and the sleep study was filed away by the primary care physician, for whom the OSA essentially became a nonissue (Fig. 3.1a).

Over the next 5 years, the patient's OSA continued to be managed by the sleep specialist and remained well controlled with 15 cmH2O CPAP, despite the patient's weight increasing by 15 kg and BMI increasing from 32.5 to 37.6. At age 58, the patient presented to her primary care physician at her office early in the morning. She had signs and symptoms of an acute abdomen, which caused the primary care physician to admit her to the hospital. Unfortunately the admission history and physical by the primary care physician made no mention of OSA (Fig. 3.1b).

On admission, the consulting surgeon evaluated the patient and decided that an exploratory laparotomy was required. The surgeon saw no mention of OSA in the patient's history and physical, and he himself did not ask the patient about OSA. The patient herself, who was very ill at this point, did not volunteer information about

C. Nguyen (✉)
Department of Anesthesiology, University of California, San Diego, Orange, CA, USA

J. L. Benumof
Department of Anesthesiology, University of California, UCSD Medical Center, UCSD School of Medicine, San Diego, CA, USA

J. L. Benumof, G. R. Manecke (eds.), *Clinical Anesthesiology II*,
https://doi.org/10.1007/978-3-030-12365-9_3

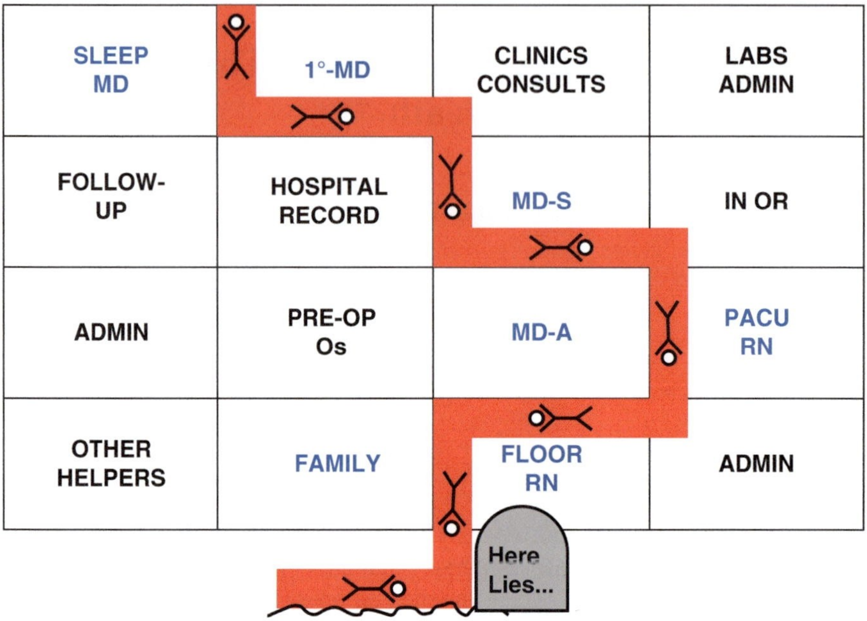

Fig. 3.1 Falling through caregiver cracks to death. This patient went through multiple transitions of care, and each point crucial information regarding her OSA failed to be relayed. (**a**) The primary care physician did not recognize OSA as a significant issue on admission. (**b**) The primary care physician did not relay OSA information to the surgeon. (**c**) The surgeon and the anesthesiologist did not discuss the possibility of OSA. (**d**) The anesthesiologist did not tell the PACU nurse about the patient's OSA. (**e**) The PACU nurse did not discuss OSA with the floor nurse. (**f**) The floor nurse and the family did not discuss the patient's OSA until it was too late

her OSA to the surgeon. The anesthesiologist evaluated the patient and did not ask about OSA before giving the patient midazolam and fentanyl and transporting her to the operating room (Fig. 3.1c). On the way to the OR, the patient told the anesthesiologist, "Oh, by the way, I used to have OSA but I now do very well with nightly CPAP." At this time, mid-transport to the operating room, the anesthesiologist made no attempt to determine the severity of OSA (L-3).

Once in the operating room, general anesthesia was induced, and the patient was intubated without any issues. Surgery proceeded with a large incision from the xiphoid process to the pubis, and an enormous (30 cm) ovarian cyst was removed. At the end of surgery, the patient was awakened and extubated. She was transported to the postanesthesia care unit (PACU), and care was transferred to the PACU nurse. There was no mention made from the anesthesiologist to the nurse about the patient's OSA (Fig. 3.1d). During the PACU stay, the nurse administered ordinary doses of analgesics and observed a few short episodes of apnea but did not think they were remarkable. The PACU nurse transferred the patient to the floor, making no mention of the apneic episodes or the possibility of OSA to the receiving floor nurse (Fig. 3.1e).

On the surgical ward, the patient was placed in a private room with no continuous monitors of any kind. Orders were written for intramuscular morphine 10 mg every

4 h as needed. The floor nurse did not know that the patient had OSA or used CPAP at home, so no CPAP or supplemental oxygen was started. Other than the family members in the room, the only observation the patient received was during vital sign checks every 4 h by nursing personnel (Fig. 3.1f). After a while the husband told the floor nurse that the patient had severe OSA and used CPAP at home; the nurse told him to go home and get the CPAP machine. Meanwhile, she intended to check on the patient but became busy, and so an hour passed before she instructed an LVN to gather vital signs on the patient. When the LVN entered the room 20 min later, the family was gathered at the foot of the bed playing cards (Fig. 3.1f). The LVN then found the patient blue, pulseless, and asystolic. Resuscitation was started per ACLS, but despite best efforts, the patient suffered severe hypoxic encephalopathy (L-4).

Lessons Learned

L-1: Patients with OSA Are a Multidimensional Problem for the Anesthesiologist

OSA is a multidimensional problem for anesthesiologists, causing important (A) intubation, (B) extubation, and (C) postoperative pain management problems. In the senior author's experience with over 50 OSA-related malpractice cases, the approximate distribution and incidence of problems were roughly equal among these three periods.

Intubation Problems

As stated in the ASA OSA guidelines [1], patients with OSA are best managed by following the ASA difficult airway guidelines [2]. A thorough assessment of the airway should be conducted according to the ASA difficult airway preoperative airway physical examination (Table 3.1). Airway management per se should be guided by the ASA difficult airway algorithm (Fig. 3.2). The first branch point in the algorithm is deciding whether to perform an awake intubation or intubation after induction of general anesthesia, based on the preoperative airway evaluation and the expected feasibility of ventilation and intubation. Should the practitioner decide to attempt intubation after induction of general anesthesia, it is critical to have identified and prepared multiple back-up plans prior to induction.

Extubation Problems

The primary goal that should guide management during emergence is maintaining control of the airway and not allowing the patient to determine when extubation occurs. This is particularly pertinent for the patient with OSA, given that they

Table 3.1 Preoperative airway physical examination

Airway examination component	Nonreassuring findings
1. Length of upper incisors	Relatively long
2. Relation of maxillary and mandibular incisors during normal jaw closure	Prominent "overbite" (maxillary incisors anterior to mandibular incisors)
3. Relation of maxillary and mandibular incisors during voluntary protrusion of cannot bring	Patient mandibular incisors anterior to (in mandible front of) maxillary incisors
4. Interincisor distance	Less than 3 cm
5. Visibility of uvula	Not visible when tongue is protruded with patient in sitting position (e.g., Mallampati class greater than II)
6. Shape of palate	Highly arched or very narrow
7. Compliance of mandibular space	Stiff, indurated, occupied by mass, or nonresilient
8. Thyromental distance	Less than three ordinary finger breadths
9. Length of neck	Short
10. Thickness of neck	Thick
11. Range of motion of head and neck	Patient cannot touch tip of chin to chest or cannot extend neck

Adapted from Apfelbaum et al. [1]. With permission from Wolters Kluwer Health, Inc.
This table displays some findings of the airway physical examination that may suggest the presence of a difficult intubation. The decision to examine some or all of the airway components shown in this table depends on the clinical context and judgment of the practitioner. The table is not extended as a mandatory or exhaustive list of the components of an airway examination. The order of presentation in this table follows the "line of sight" that occurs during conventional oral laryngoscopy

are more likely to be obese, are more prone to post-extubation pharyngeal obstruction, and are more likely to be difficult with regard to reestablishing the airway. In general, plan to extubate the patient fully awake and following commands. The key to a smooth emergence is having a simple, routine approach. Warn the patient preoperatively that they will be emerging in the operating room and will still have the endotracheal tube in place; although difficult to prove, in the senior author's experience, this preoperative warning seems to reduce the agitation seen during emergence. Other measures that help the patient tolerate the endotracheal tube include liberally applying lidocaine ointment to the distal end of the tube and cuff and using a laryngotracheal spray kit prior to intubation. Adequate analgesia at the end of the case is also important; typically opioids can be titrated to a respiratory rate of approximately 10–12 breaths per minutes. It is possible that the above measures may fail to prevent emergence agitation. Therefore, for all emerging OSA patients in whom it is desired to do an awake extubation, it is crucial that they be adequately restrained to prevent self-extubation. It is important to remember that these patients can be very strong, and if they are able to flex even a finger, they will be able to generate enough leverage to eventually free the arm and be out of the provider's control. Therefore, they should be restrained in full extension.

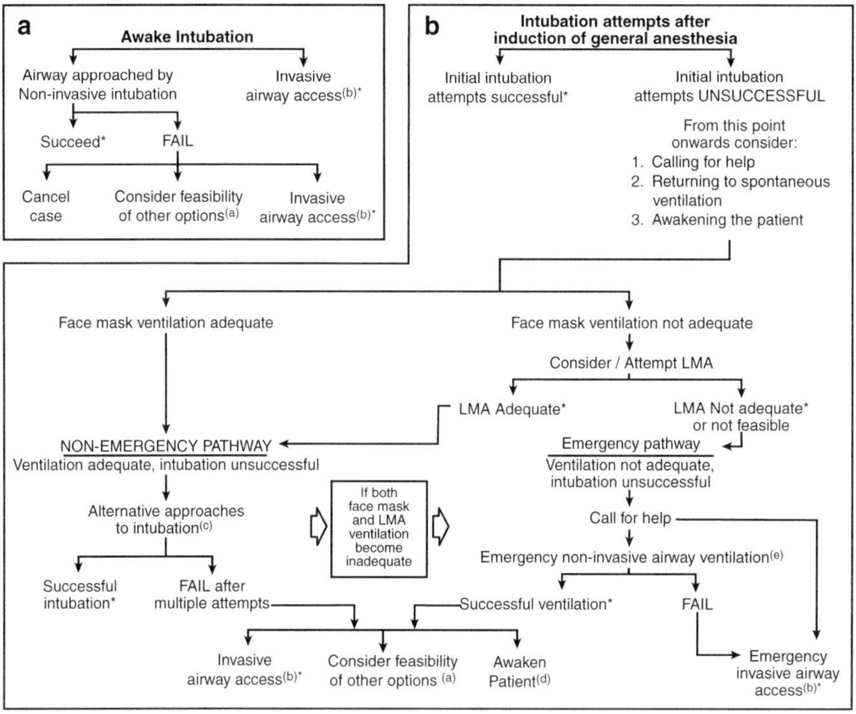

*** Confirm ventilation, tracheal intubation, or LMA placement with exhaled CO_2**

a. Other options include (but are not limited to): surgery utilizing face mask or LMA anesthesia, local anesthesia infiltration or regional nerve blockade. Pursuit of these options usually implies that mask ventilation will not be problematic. Therefore, these options may be of limited value if this step in the algorithm has been reached via the Emergency Pathway.

b. Invasive airway access includes surgical or percutaneous tracheostomy or cricothyrotomy.

c. Alternative non-invasive approaches to difficult intubation include (but are not limited to): use of different laryngoscope blades, LMA as an intubation conduit (with or without fiberoptic guidance), fiberoptic intubation, intubating stylet or tube changer, light wand, retrograde intubation, and blind oral or nasal intubation.

d. Consider re-preparation of the patient for awake intubation or canceling surgery.

e. Options for emergency non-invasive airway ventilation include (but are not limited to): rigid bronchoscope, esophageal-tracheal combitube ventilation, or transtracheal jet ventilation.

Fig. 3.2 ASA difficult airway algorithm. (Adapted from American Society of Anesthesiologists [2]. With permission from Wolters Kluwer Health, Inc.)

Postoperative Problems

The primary postoperative problem seen in OSA-related malpractice cases is that of finding the patient either near arrest, in arrest, or just stone-cold dead in bed by either a family member or caregiver. Many of these cases are due to the patient falling through caregiver cracks (Fig. 3.1). This means that some caregivers either did not transmit some important information, did not know or understand the significance of the information, or assumed the next caregiver would discover all the relevant information. The relevant information included such items as the patient was morbidly obese, had severe OSA, had an abdominal incision, was receiving narcotics, and was off CPAP and oxygen supplementation. This case chapter is about a patient who had all of these characteristics and passed between many caregivers, without a single caregiver putting together the big picture, leading to her death.

L-2: What Are the Implications of the Sleep Study in This Patient?

During this patient's sleep study, she had an average of 54.8 apneic episodes and 19.1 hypopneic episodes per hour, for a total apnea-hypopnea index (AHI) of 74.0/h. An apnea is defined as complete cessation of breathing, and a hypopnea is defined as a decrease of greater than 50% of the average awake tidal volume for longer than 10 s during which the SpO2 decreases more than 4%. According to the most recent guidelines from the American Academy of Sleep Medicine, mild OSA is diagnosed with an AHI of 5–15/h, moderate OSA with an AHI of 15–30/h, and severe OSA with an AHI greater than 30/h [3]. Of note, the ASA OSA guideline has different cutoffs for mild, moderate, and severe OSA, using the ranges of 6–20/h, 21–40/h, and >40/h, respectively [1]. Severe OSA is also defined as a lowest saturation below 80%; this patient's lowest recorded oxygen saturation was 74%. However, there were additional findings on this patient's sleep study that indicated the OSA situation was even more critical than was obvious. To understand this, first we will discuss some basic OSA pathophysiology.

The human pharynx consists of three anatomic divisions: the nasopharynx, oropharynx, and laryngopharynx (Fig. 3.3). The nasopharynx begins at the beginning of the soft palate and ends at the end of the soft palate (the tip of the uvula), and

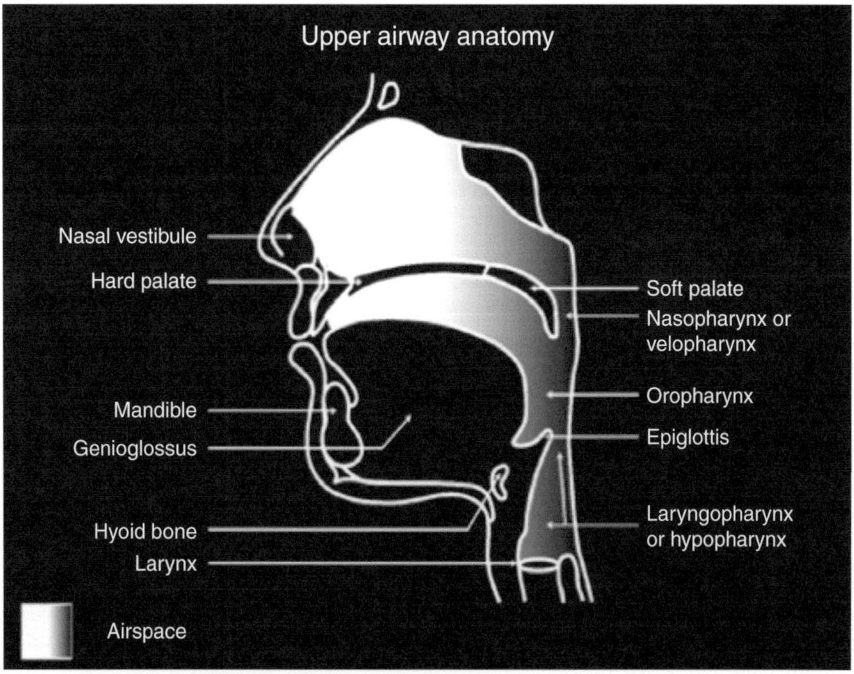

Fig. 3.3 Anatomic structures of the upper airway. The nasopharynx is retropalatal, the oropharynx is retroglossal, and the laryngopharynx is retroepiglottic

therefore the nasopharynx is a retropalatal pharynx (also called the velopharynx). The oropharynx begins at the tip of the uvula and ends at the tip of the epiglottis, and therefore the oropharynx is a retroglossal pharynx. The laryngopharynx begins at the tip of the epiglottis and ends at the vocal cords, and therefore the laryngopharynx is a retroepiglottic pharynx (also called the hypopharynx). The nasopharynx, oropharynx, and laryngopharynx make the upper airway a long soft-walled tube. The long soft-walled tube fulfills two functions that are uniquely human. First, this structure creates a chamber for the development of resonance and harmonics that allows humans to speak and sing. Second, the long soft-walled tube is soft and collapsible. The only way this space can stay patent is by the action of pharyngeal muscles (Fig. 3.4). The tensor palatine pulls the soft palate forward keeping the retropalatal nasopharynx open. The genioglossus pulls the tongue forward keeping the retroglossal oropharynx open. Small paired hyoid muscles pull the epiglottis forward keeping the retroepiglottic laryngopharynx open.

There are two stages of sleep, and they are called non-rapid eye movement (NREM) (which has substages 1, 2, 3, and 4) and rapid eye movement (REM) sleep. Deep and restorative sleep is considered to occur during REM sleep and NREM stages 3 and 4 (Fig. 3.5). Twenty percent of sleep should be in REM, and 20% should be in NREM 3 and 4. During sleep there is relaxation of all the muscles of the body, including the pharyngeal muscles. The pharyngeal muscle relaxation causes pharyngeal collapse. The deeper the sleep, the greater the degree of pharyngeal muscle relaxation and pharyngeal collapse. In an OSA patient, an increased degree of pharyngeal muscle collapse is caused by certain anatomic traits, including

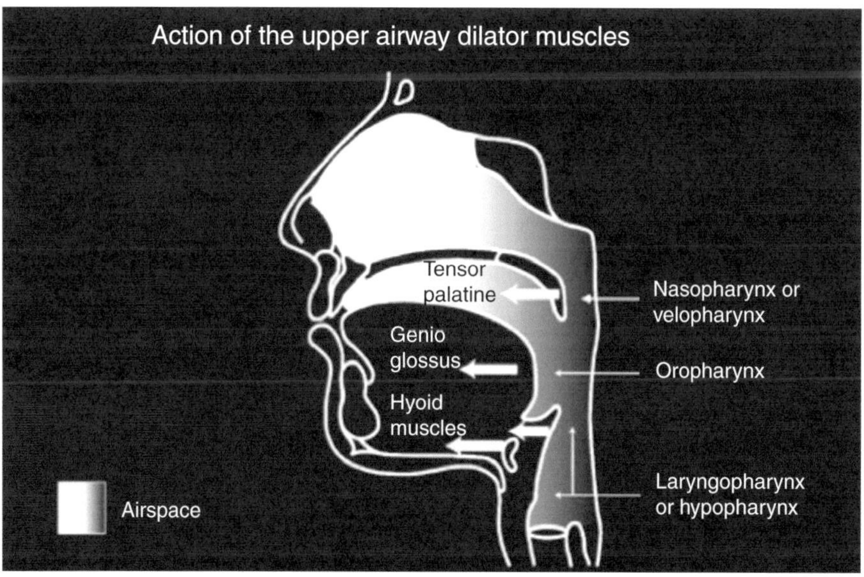

Fig. 3.4 The tensor palatine pulls the soft palate forward, the genioglossus pulls the tongue forward, and the hyoid muscles pull the epiglottis forward. These combined actions keep the entire pharynx open

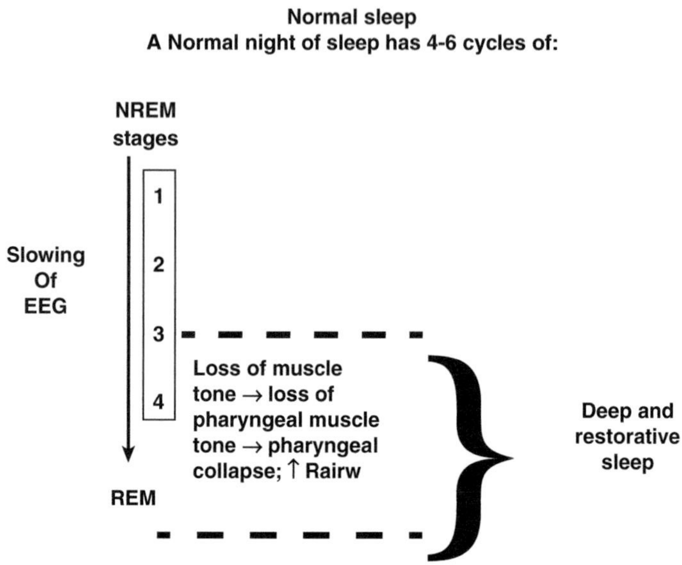

Fig. 3.5 A normal sleep cycle consists of REM sleep and 4 stages of NREM sleep. During deep and restorative sleep, which includes REM and NREM stages 2 and 3, there is loss of muscle tone leading to pharyngeal collapse and increased resistance to air movement through the airway

obesity-related changes (large tongue, pharyngeal fat [small pharynx], thick neck [extra weight on upper airway]) and other contributions such as large tonsils, uvula thickening, nasal obstruction, and retrognathia (Fig. 3.6).

If the degree of pharyngeal muscle relaxation and pharyngeal collapse is great enough to cause the inspired air to flutter around the uvula, tongue, and epiglottis, then there will be snoring and hypopnea. If the degree of pharyngeal muscle relaxation and pharyngeal collapse is enough to cause complete obstruction, then there be will no flow, silence, and apnea. In OSA, in order to overcome each and every one of the innumerable and repetitive obstructions during sleep, there has to be some sort of arousal. In the vast majority of situations, the arousal is a mini-arousal consisting of a burst of activity on the electroencephalogram (EEG) and externally manifesting as twitching, turning, extremity movement, and vocalization. The mini-arousal activates the pharyngeal muscles, opening the airway and allowing the patient to breathe again. Thus OSA consists of repetitive cycles of sleep, arousal, sleep, and arousal. Because the sleep is fragmented and the patient is robbed of deep and restorative sleep, the patient develops a sleep deficit that manifests as daytime sleepiness.

With this context, some details of our patient's sleep study take on a new light. Despite the high AHI index, very little of her sleep was spent in the deep and restoratives stages of sleep: 0% of the time was in NREM 3 and 4, and 0.2% was in REM. This indicates that her pharyngeal muscles were so prone to collapse and obstruction that she was symptomatic even during light sleep. We can expect that her

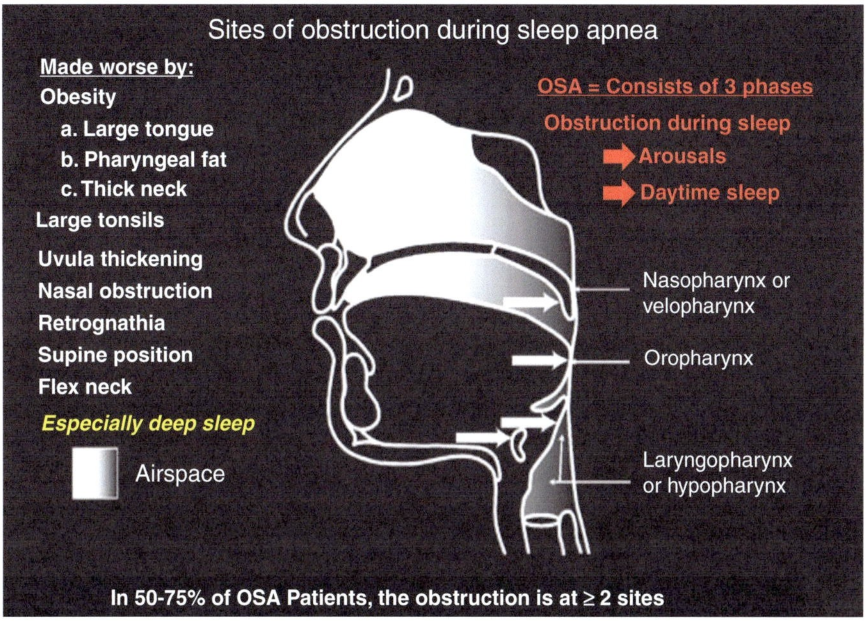

Fig. 3.6 Sites of obstruction during sleep apnea. The presence of any of the causes listed on the left side of the figure may cause obstruction during sleep (indicated by rightward arrows on the right side of the figure) and should raise the anesthesiologist's suspicion for OSA

OSA severity will only worsen with deeper sleep, whether from rebound sleep or artificially induced by medications, with increases in weight, or when the patient is off of CPAP. As we will see, all of these factors played a role in this patient's eventual demise.

L-3: What Does the ASA OSA Guideline Say About OSA Assessment and Management?

Understanding the ASA OSA guideline requires that we recognize how the logic of the guidelines dictates the specifics of the guideline (Fig. 3.7).

Causes of OSA

An anesthesiologist should know the causes of OSA (Fig. 3.6). The causes of OSA consist of obesity, large tongue, large tonsils, large uvula, obstructed nasal passages, retrognathia, supine position, and head flexion. Obesity causes OSA because fat is deposited in the tongue making the tongue bigger (and the airway smaller), fat is

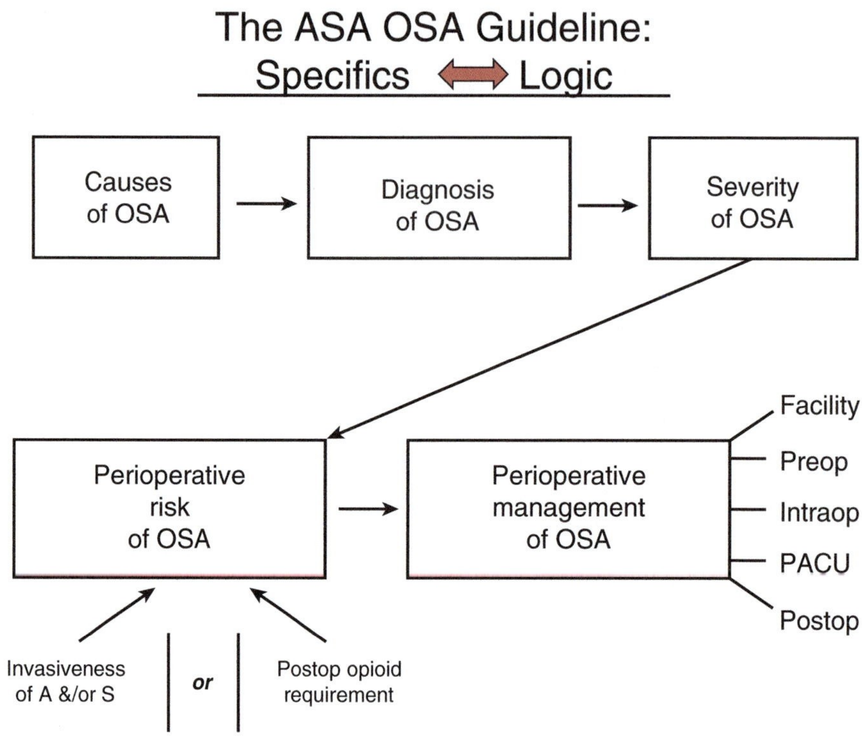

Fig. 3.7 Pathway for understanding the ASA OSA guideline. Following the logic of this pathway dictates what specifics are important to consider at each step

deposited in the pharynx making the oropharyngeal and laryngopharyngeal air spaces smaller, and fat is deposited in the neck causing compression of the long, soft-walled upper airway. Any disease process that makes the tongue bigger, like a glycogen storage disease or a lingual mass, will also cause OSA.

Diagnosing OSA

If a cause (or causes) of OSA is present, then the anesthesiologist should ask the patient whether they have OSA, and if the patient does not know, then the anesthesiologist should attempt to rule in or rule out a presumptive clinical diagnosis of OSA (Fig. 3.8). A presumptive clinical diagnosis of OSA can be made by asking the patient about obstruction during sleep (snoring, apnea, turning blue), arousals (turning, twitching, extremity movement, vocalization, and snorting), and daytime somnolence (easily falling asleep during quiet times). Having an automatically used questionnaire is encouraged and can serve as a partial surrogate for detecting the presence of OSA but does not replace a thorough clinical evaluation by a physician.

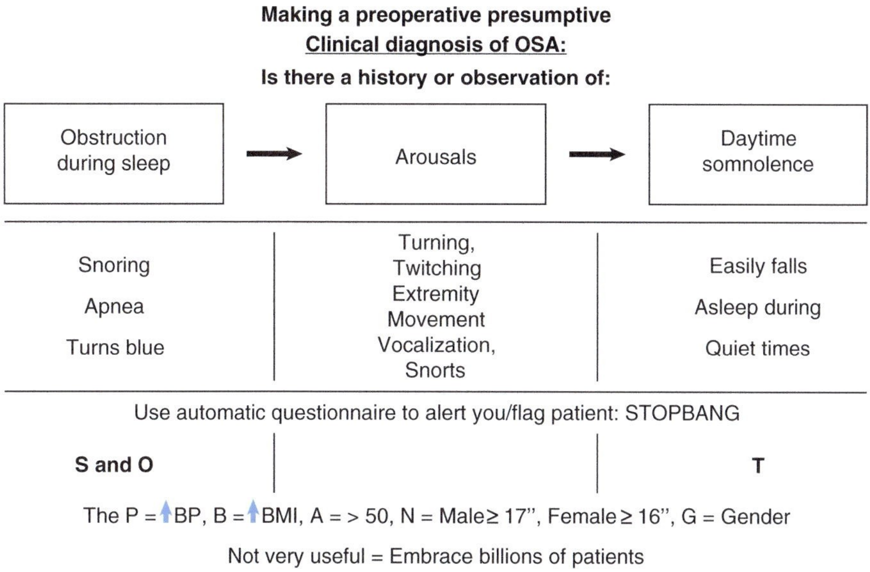

Fig. 3.8 Making a presumptive clinical diagnosis of OSA. The commonly used STOP-BANG questionnaire asks about snoring (S), tiredness (T), and observed apnea (O), but a complete assessment should ask about all the symptoms listed above. P blood pressure, B BMI, A age, N neck size, G gender

Assessing Severity

Once the diagnosis of OSA has been made, the next step is to determine the severity of the condition, either using clinical criteria or with a sleep study as previously described (see L-2). In order to understand how to diagnose mild, moderate, and severe OSA, it is useful to first polarize the issues in the diagnoses for mild versus moderate OSA (Table 3.2). Mild OSA can be recognized by the following features: these patients are usually obese, snore most of the time, do not have obvious episodes of arousal but do occasionally appear restless during sleep, occasionally fall asleep during quiet times of the day, and usually do not have significant cardiovascular disease. In contrast, severe OSA is characterized by patients who are morbidly obese, snore all of the time, have frequent apneic episodes, have frequent arousal during sleep, occasionally turn blue during apnea, fall asleep frequently during quiet times, and may have significant cardiovascular disease. Making a clinical diagnosis of moderate OSA requires judgment, and the physician can never take judgment out of the equation. If the OSA is not mild or severe, then call it moderate and move on; this determination is not a test of the physician. It is far more important to try to ballpark the severity so that the practitioner may formulate a rational plan of management.

Table 3.2 Characteristics of mild versus severe OSA. If a patient does not fit clearly in either category, they should be classified as having moderate OSA

	Occurrence	
Characteristics of OSA	Mild	Severe
Obesity	Obese	Morbidly obese
Snore	Supine – most of the time	All positions – all of the time
Stop breathing	No?	Yes
Turn blue	No	Yes
Arouse	Some	A lot
Daytime somnolence	Occasionally	A lot
Cardiovascular disease	None to?	Probably

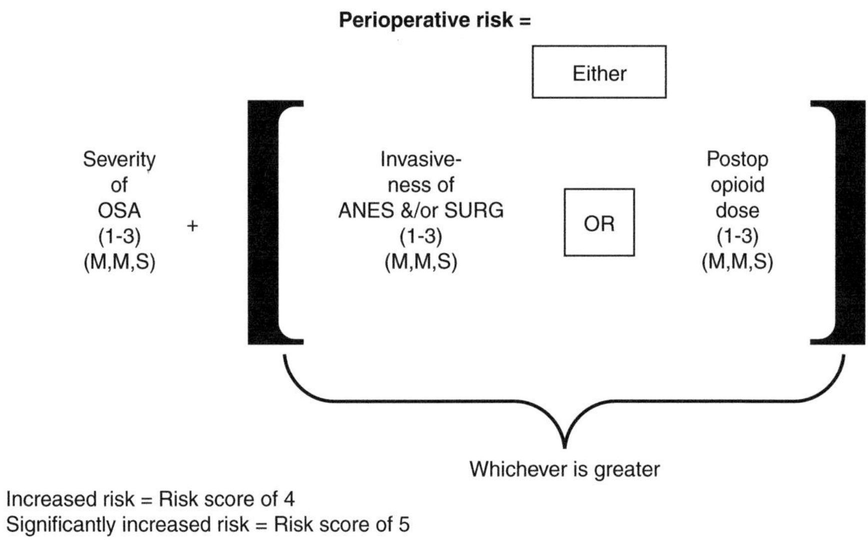

Fig. 3.9 Calculating the perioperative risk score. Severity of OSA earns from 1 to 3 points. For the second component, use whichever earns a higher score: invasiveness of the procedure and anesthetic versus post-op opioid dose. Per the ASA OSA guidelines, patients with a score of 5 or 6 should be done as inpatients. M, M, S mild, moderate, severe

Perioperative Risk Score

Once severity has been determined, using either clinical or sleep study criteria, a perioperative risk score can be calculated (Fig. 3.9). OSA severity is assigned a point value of 1, 2, or 3, corresponding to mild, moderate, or severe OSA. The other component considers the invasiveness of the surgical procedure and anesthetic or the postoperative opioid dose, whichever earns a higher point value. In terms of surgical invasiveness, a mild procedure (1 point) would be a superficial or peripheral procedure, with at most moderate sedation, whereas a major procedure (3 points) would be anything requiring a thoracotomy or large abdominal incision. A moderate procedure (2 points) would be anything else in between those extremes. In terms of post-op opioid dose, mild (1 point) would include low-dose oral opioids, and severe (3 points) would include high-dose oral opioids or parenteral opioids. Using this calculation, a risk score of 4 would indicate increased perioperative risk, while a risk score of 5 or greater would indicate significantly increased risk. The patient in the case being discussed, with severe OSA (3 points) and having a large abdominal incision (3 points), would have the highest possible risk with a score of 6.

Perioperative Management

Perioperative OSA risk should determine the specifics of perioperative management. The ASA OSA guidelines say patients with OSA risk scores of 5 and 6 should have their surgery as inpatients. All anesthesiologists would agree, as an absolute truth, that a morbidly obese patient with severe OSA receiving an abdominal surgery must be done as an inpatient case. However, there are no official guidelines regarding the appropriate facility for patients who approach these extreme outpatient surgery exclusion criteria. It will be up to the practitioner and their practice group to decide how far to back off the extreme outpatient criteria in terms of who can be done as an outpatient.

Preoperatively, the patient should be counseled to lose weight and to continue using CPAP nightly. Intraoperative considerations regarding intubation and extubation were previously described (see L-1). Postoperatively, both in the PACU and after PACU discharge, the patient should be closely watched. There are no replacements for human eyes, and it is critical that there be caregivers able to physically observe the patient for episodes of apnea or hypopnea. This, of course, must be supplemented with continuous electronic monitors such as pulse oximetry and capnography.

L-4: What Led to This Patient's Death?

The failure of the primary care physician to mention OSA in the history is the first of several events that can be traced to the patient's outcome. The primary care physician later explained that she did not mention OSA because the patient's OSA was very well controlled, the patient presented in the morning and sleep was not an active issue, the acute abdomen was the overriding primary concern, she had expected the other physicians to do their own complete history, and she had expected the patient to be a good historian with the other physicians. Each of these assumptions can be independently understandable, especially in the urgent clinical context of a patient with an acute abdomen, and it is entirely possible that some practitioners have made similar assumptions from time to time. Yet it is these assumptions that began the process of this patient eventually falling through the cracks to her death, underscoring the importance of recognizing and respecting the danger of OSA at every step in a patient's progress through the medical system.

Similarly, the consulting surgeon did not obtain a history from the patient regarding her OSA; it is expected that the surgeon would be preoccupied with assessing the surgical situation. As a result, the presence of severe OSA was not communicated to the anesthesiologist. The anesthesiologist was eventually made aware of the OSA by the patient but made no effort at the time of wheeling the patient into the operating room to assess the severity of the OSA. It is important to recognize that severity matters a great deal; the perioperative risks from OSA are directly proportional to severity. This failure to bring notice to the patient's severe OSA continued down the line, such that none of the subsequent caregivers (PACU nurse and floor nurse) were aware of the risk to the patient, thus directly leading to her death.

In summary, it is the responsibility of the anesthesiologist to recognize the perioperative risk from severe OSA and to make the decision of where the patient goes after discharge from the PACU. The presence of obesity or any of the other causes of OSA should trigger the anesthesiologist to rule in or rule out a presumptive clinical diagnosis of OSA. If a presumptive clinical diagnosis is made, or if it is known from other sources that the patient has OSA, then the severity should be assessed, either clinically or with a sleep study if available. A sleep study can offer useful information beyond the AHI; pay attention also to the patient's weight at the time of the study and depth of sleep. Only by having all this information can the anesthesiologist make a rational decision of where to send the patient after PACU. Ignoring this responsibility would otherwise mean you are asking the patient to blindly jump off a clinical cliff, possibly to their death.

References

1. Apfelbaum JL, Hagberg CA, Caplan RA, Blitt CD, Connis RT, Nickinovich DG, Hagberg CA, Caplan RA, Benumof JL, Berry FA, Blitt CD, Bode RH, Cheney FW, Connis RT, Guidry OF, Nickinovich DG, Ovassapian A, American Society of Anesthesiologists Task Force on Management of the Difficult Airway. Practice guidelines for management of the difficult airway: an updated report by the American Society of Anesthesiologists Task Force on Management of the Difficult Airway. Anesthesiology. 2013;118:251–70.
2. American Society of Anesthesiologists. Practice guidelines for the perioperative management of patients with obstructive sleep apnea: an updated report by the American Society of Anesthesiologists Task Force on Perioperative Management of Patients with Obstructive Sleep Apnea. Anesthesiology. 2014;120(2):268–86.
3. American Academy of Sleep Medicine Task Force. Sleep-related breathing disorders in adults: recommendations for syndrome definition and measurement techniques in clinical research. The report of an American Academy of Sleep Medicine Task Force. Sleep. 1999;22:667–89.

Chapter 4
Abdominal Compartment Syndrome and Pulmonary Aspiration

Deborah L. Fretwell and Luis M. Rivera

Case Description

We present the case of a 70-year-old man with a past medical history significant for HIV/AIDS (CD4 count 91 cells/mm^3), cirrhosis, asthma, and paroxysmal atrial fibrillation who was found obtunded in his skilled nursing facility (SNF).

The patient was brought to the emergency department (ED) from his SNF after being found unresponsive with a tense abdomen. The night before, he was seen by his spouse and at that time was at his baseline mental status. He reported early satiety but was not complaining of abdominal pain. He arrived to the hospital being mask-ventilated by emergency medical personnel. He was emergently intubated in the ED via rapid sequence intravenous induction with 20 mg of etomidate and 70 mg of rocuronium. A 7.5 mm endotracheal tube (ETT) was placed at a depth of 25 cm at the teeth (Wt 68 kg, Ht 6′1″). During the intubation, the ED physician noted emesis in the patient's airway and suctioned the emesis prior to placing the ETT. On auscultation, he was noted to have good bilateral breath sounds and exhaled CO_2 color change using a colorimetric CO_2 detector. A 16 French orogastric tube was then placed. His initial blood pressure was 57/32 mmHg, and heart rate and rhythm were sinus tachycardia at about 100–110 beats per minute (BPM). Lab results were significant for chronic hyponatremia (Na = 128 mEq/L) and coagulopathy related to his chronic liver failure (INR 1.6, PLT 112 × 10^9/L). A venous blood gas was consistent with severe acute hypercarbic respiratory failure with a metabolic alkalosis (pH 7.07, pCO_2 116 torr, pO_2 49 torr, HCO_3 33 mEq/L).

D. L. Fretwell
Department of Anesthesiology, University of California San Diego Health System, San Diego, CA, USA

L. M. Rivera (✉)
Department of Anesthesiology, University of California, San Diego, CA, USA
e-mail: LMRivera@ucsd.edu

J. L. Benumof, G. R. Manecke (eds.), *Clinical Anesthesiology II*,
https://doi.org/10.1007/978-3-030-12365-9_4

A central line was placed, and intravenous infusions of vasopressin, norepinephrine, and phenylephrine were started to support his blood pressure. An abdominal X-ray showed significant free air in the abdomen concerning for perforated bowel. The X-ray findings in conjunction with the patient's severely distended abdomen seen on physical exam and his hemodynamic instability led to the preliminary diagnosis of abdominal compartment syndrome **(L-1)**. He was taken to the operating room (OR) emergently for exploratory/decompressive laparotomy.

Upon arrival to the OR, the patient was disconnected from the transport ventilator and connected to the anesthesia circuit. Difficult ventilation **(L-2)** and several other ventilation issues arose simultaneously:

1. No end-tidal CO_2 ($ETCO_2$) was detected **(L-3).**
2. Hypoxemia (SpO_2 70–80%).
3. Elevated peak airway pressures (35–45 mm H_2O).
4. Low tidal volumes (125–150 mL).

The anesthesiology team proceeded with the assumption that several issues were impacting their ability to ventilate and oxygenate: aspiration pneumonitis **(L-4)**, ETT placed too deep, and his distended abdomen pushing on the diaphragm and preventing lung expansion.

While hand ventilating to assess compliance, the anesthesiologist asked the surgeons to open the abdomen expeditiously in order to relieve pressure against the diaphragm **(L-5)**. While waiting for the surgeons, the patient was positioned in a slight reverse Trendelenburg position, anticipating that this would worsen the patient's hypotension but aiming to further relieve pressure against the diaphragm and facilitate ventilation. One hundred milligrams of rocuronium was administered empirically to eliminate any muscle tone, which might also have been contributing to the high abdominal pressure.

Auscultation of the lungs revealed very diminished bilateral breath sounds. The ETT was suctioned, with no gastric contents, mucus plugs, or secretions found. Due to concern that the endotracheal tube was potentially too deep because of probable cephalad displacement of the diaphragm from the patient's distended abdomen, the ETT was empirically pulled back from 25 to 23 cm at the teeth. Later in the case, after the surgeons suctioned 2 L of ascites from the abdominal cavity, and with the ETT repositioned as stated above, a fiber-optic bronchoscopic examination confirmed placement of the ETT 3 cm above the carina.

During the case, the patient displayed shock physiology, with tachycardia at a heart rate of 110–120 BPM, and hypotension with a blood pressure in the 60s/40s mmHg range, despite high doses of three vasopressors (vasopressin 0.04 units/min, norepinephrine 30 mcg/min, and phenylephrine 125 mcg/min) and several boluses of the above vasopressors. An arterial line was placed, and the patient was managed with escalating doses of these vasopressors while using a minimal concentration of volatile agent. In order to improve hemodynamics, small boluses of epinephrine were administered (20 mcg). A continuous epinephrine infusion was prepared, and a 250 mL bolus of albumin was rapidly infused.

The surgeons found all the bowel to be viable, and the abdomen was left open with a wound vacuum in place. The patient remained critically ill in the surgical intensive care unit for the next several days. He continued to require vasopressin, norepinephrine, epinephrine, and phenylephrine while in multi-organ failure (acute renal failure requiring continuous renal replacement therapy, shock liver secondary to hypoperfusion, acute respiratory failure secondary to aspiration, and sepsis). On hospital day 3, the patient was taken to the OR for a wound vacuum change. On hospital day 4, the patient expired after withdrawal of life-sustaining care.

Lesson 1: Abdominal Compartment Syndrome (ACS)

In the early 1980s, physicians began to investigate the significance of increased abdominal pressure. Much of our current understanding of the underlying pathophysiology of abdominal compartment syndrome emanates from research done in the 1980s and 1990s [1].

Founded in 2004, a physician/researcher society now called "World Society of the Abdominal Compartment Syndrome" (WSACS) was formed, comprised of the world's leading experts on abdominal compartment syndrome (ACS), which is also commonly referred to as intra-abdominal hypertension (IAH). The Society has a comprehensive website and is dedicated to promoting research and education and developing guidelines/recommendations for the treatment of ACS/IAH (http://www.wsacs.org).

Definition and Diagnosis

The term "abdominal compartment syndrome" was first coined in 1989 by Dr. Fietsam and his colleagues [2]. ACS is defined as a sustained increase in intra-abdominal pressure from normal baseline pressures of 0–7 mmHg in relatively healthy adults to greater than 20 mmHg in conjunction with new organ failure [3]. The rise in pressure is often rapid, potentially within hours, and organ systems are unable to quickly adapt and compensate. This is distinct from chronic conditions that are associated with increases in abdominal pressure such as morbid obesity, where the rise in pressure is insidious and organ systems are able to adapt and adjust over time [4].

Another term used, "intra-abdominal hypertension" (IAH), while carrying its own somewhat distinct definition, is often used interchangeably with ACS. IAH is defined by "sustained or repeated pathological elevation in intra-abdominal pressure (IAP) greater than or equal to 12 mmHg" [3] (Table 4.1).

The primary clinical finding of ACS is a severely tense, distended abdomen. This edematous state, when caused by injury to or disease originating in the abdomino-pelvic region, is referred to as primary ACS. Primary ACS can also be caused by

Table 4.1 Grading the severity of intra-abdominal hypertension (IAH) according to intra-abdominal pressure (IAP)

Grades of IAH	IAP (mmHg)
I	12–15
II	16–20
III	21–25
IV	>25

intra-abdominal hemorrhage. Alternatively, pressurized inflammation of abdominal contents can be caused by factors not originating in the abdominopelvic region such as from aggressive fluid resuscitation or septic-shock-induced inflammation, which is referred to as secondary ACS [3].

ACS may be diagnosed by measuring intra-vesical pressure. A method first devised by Dr. Kron from the University of Virginia in 1984 measures intravesical pressure using a bladder catheter as a surrogate for intra-abdominal pressure [5]. While some have challenged the reliability of bladder pressure measurements and shown that bladder pressure tends to overestimate true intra-abdominal pressure, this is nonetheless still an easy and safe method to minimally invasively measure the trend in intra-abdominal pressure in the intensive care unit [6]. WSACS recommends serial measurements of intra-abdominal pressure every 4 h in critically ill patients.

Derangements in Organ Function

The derangements in organ function seen in patients with ACS stem from the abdominal contents directly compressing the vena cava, other vessels, and the viscera, thereby impeding blood flow to all vital organs. With decreased perfusion of the kidneys, the glomerular filtration rate is decreased, and clinically patients often present with oliguria. Splanchnic perfusion is also restricted, which leads to decreases in gastric mucosal pH [7, 8]. An increase in intracranial pressure (ICP) may occur, which stems from the obstruction of venous blood flow from the cranium. Animal and human studies suggest that elevated ICP in ACS is the result of cerebral venous outflow obstruction [9, 10] (Fig. 4.1).

Effects on Ventilatory Mechanics and Gas Exchange

Of keen interest to the anesthesiologist are the changes in respiratory mechanics seen in patients with ACS. In this case, the anesthesiologist encountered considerable difficulty ventilating the patient. Several diagnostic and therapeutic steps were taken, including auscultating the lungs, checking the anesthesia circuit for leaks, hand ventilating to assess resistance and compliance, administering muscle

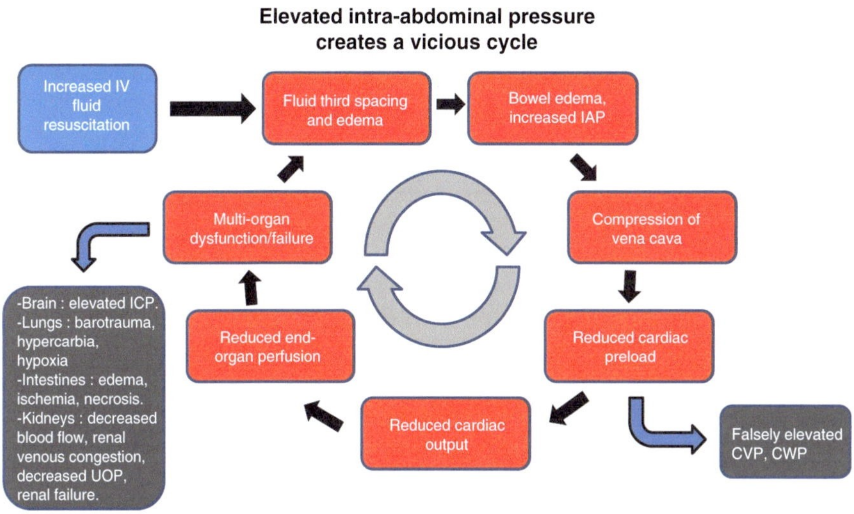

Fig. 4.1 The effects of abdominal compartment syndrome on the organs of the body

relaxants, repositioning and suctioning the ETT, and positioning the patient in slight reverse Trendelenburg position. While all of these actions were important and necessary steps, it wasn't until the surgeons opened the abdomen that the respiratory function (oxygenation and ventilation) dramatically improved and adequate tidal volumes could finally be delivered.

With the abdominal contents elevating the diaphragm cephalad, pleural and intrathoracic pressures increase. This causes a decrease in lung volumes and dramatically decreases lung compliance, which in turn produces increased peak inspiratory airway pressures (PIP) and low tidal volumes during mechanical ventilation [11]. Similar to patients with morbid obesity, ACS decreases a patient's functional residual capacity (FRC), defined as the lung volume remaining at the end of normal exhalation, leading to increased collapse of alveoli upon end exhalation. With decreased FRC, atelectasis, a normal occurrence during anesthesia, is magnified. These under-ventilated atelectatic areas of the lung may continue to receive blood flow, which leads to ventilation-perfusion mismatch. As a result, and as was seen in this patient case, hypercapnia (elevated $PaCO_2$) and hypoxemia/hypoxia (low PaO_2 and SpO_2) can be severe.

Elevation of the diaphragm in patients with ACS can affect positioning of the ETT. With the abdomen pressing upward against the lungs and impeding the ability of the lungs to expand caudally, the ETT may advance beyond the carina into the right mainstem bronchus. The result is unintended one-lung ventilation, during which hypoxia is a common complication. Even if not advanced into the right mainstem bronchus, an ETT resting against the carina may affect ventilation. As was done in this case, auscultation of the lungs and confirmation of tube placement above the carina with a fiber-optic bronchoscope may be necessary.

Effects on Hemodynamics

In ACS, direct compression of the inferior vena cava (IVC), in conjunction with increased intrathoracic pressure, results in decreased blood return to the heart (decreased preload) and reduced cardiac output [11]. Pressure against the diaphragm can cause direct cardiac compression causing tamponade-like physiology and compression of the abdominal vascular beds resulting in increased cardiac afterload [12]. Hypovolemia exacerbates the decreased cardiac output seen in ACS. Fluid resuscitation in these patients, especially in the presence of comorbid conditions such as liver failure (as in this case), is challenging. Because of the formation of edema, ACS patients are often total-body fluid overloaded while paradoxically being intravascularly depleted. Their severe intravascular volume depletion with excessive fluid in the abdominal cavity and bowel wall causes a shock state. Colloids are likely a better choice under such circumstances in order to increase oncotic pressure. Administration of crystalloids should be limited.

Changes in the patient's hemodynamics significantly impact renal function, hepatic blood flow, and the perfusion of the kidneys and bowel. Not infrequently, patients with ACS will present with severe hypotension and oliguria secondary to renal failure. They can also suffer complications of bowel ischemia and shock liver from hypoperfusion [11]. In this case, multiple vasoactive medications were required to maintain adequate preload, contractility, and afterload in an attempt to improve perfusion of vital organs.

Treatment and Intraoperative Management

Decompressive laparotomy is the definitive therapy for ACS. It has been shown to reliably lower abdominal pressures [13]. Nonsurgical approaches to abdominal decompression were previously thought to be ineffective, but there are now medical treatments considered potentially useful in ACS [14].WSACS has made recommendations, some of which may help guide patient management decisions in the operating room [3]:

1. Strategic body positioning (e.g. reverse Trendelenburg) may be used to relieve pressure against the diaphragm and facilitate improved respiratory mechanics. In this case, this maneuver was insufficient to improve ease of ventilation.
2. As was done in this patient case, neuromuscular blockade (NMB) can be used to eliminate any muscle tone. NMB is thought to improve abdominal wall compliance.
3. Controlled and closely monitored fluid resuscitation in these patients is essential. Colloids are likely a better choice under such circumstances in order to attempt to increase oncotic pressure. Administration of crystalloids should be limited. In this case, the patient's severe hypotension, hemodynamic instability, and septic

shock physiology required administration of both crystalloids and colloids in an attempt to maintain perfusion to vital organs.

4. Organ support with vasoactive medications may be necessary.
5. There is inadequate data to support the use of nasogastric decompression, GI prokinetic medications, or diuretics.

Currently there is insufficient data to make specific recommendations regarding intraoperative sedation and analgesia for patients with ACS. Myocardial depressant and vasodilating anesthetics should be used with great caution. In this case, a volatile anesthetic was used sparingly due to the patient's hemodynamic instability.

Patient Outcome

As an anesthesiologist, it can be quite dramatic when surgeons open a tense abdomen and respiratory mechanics improve almost instantly. However, despite our best efforts, greater than one third of patients presenting with severe ACS ultimately die, often from multi-organ failure [15].

De Waele et al. pooled data from 18 different studies including 250 patients who underwent decompressive laparotomy. This review revealed that despite abdominal pressure being consistently lower after decompressive laparotomy (34.6 mmHg → 15.5 mmHg), the pressures tend to remain abnormally high and recuperation of organ function is variable. Mortality in the whole group was extremely high at 49% (123/250 patients) [13].

Lesson 2: Difficulty Ventilating and Oxygenating

Hypoxia Troubleshooting

In situations in which it is difficult to ventilate a patient with a secured airway, the differential diagnosis can be divided broadly into mechanical issues with the breathing circuit versus problems with the patient's respiratory physiology. When troubleshooting in the operating room, it is valuable to distinguish between these two, but it is important to keep in mind that factors from both categories can simultaneously contribute to the clinical picture [16]. Whichever approach is taken, it is essential to be expeditious. Most of these maneuvers should be performed simultaneously.

1. **Do not hesitate to call for help** if the situation is rapidly deteriorating.
2. Increase the inspired oxygen fraction to 100% if the patient is not already receiving 100% oxygen.

3. Check the pulse oximeter waveform and evaluate whether the pulse oximetry readings are reliable. If there is a poor signal, consider switching to a new probe and/or switching to a different location (fingers, toes, ears, nose).
4. Switch off the ventilator and hand-ventilate the patient to assess lung compliance. Evaluate the ease with which breaths can be delivered to determine whether there might be bronchoconstriction or bronchospasm. Severe bronchospasm may prevent sufficient oxygen from reaching the alveoli and prevent carbon dioxide removal and must be treated immediately.
5. Auscultate the patient's lungs, listening for wheezing or stridor which may indicate airway obstruction, crackles consistent with pulmonary edema, unilateral breath sounds consistent with mainstem intubation or pneumothorax, or complete absence of breath sounds consistent with esophageal intubation. Mainstem intubation causes intrapulmonary shunt, where the alveoli are perfused, but not ventilated, resulting in more deoxygenated blood returning to systemic circulation.
6. Check the endotracheal tube to assess whether it has been dislodged (right mainstem intubation) or kinked or whether the patient might be biting down and obstructing it, and make sure the cuff is properly inflated. If available, consider using a fiber-optic bronchoscope to evaluate the proper placement of the ETT since clinical inspection of the ETT sometimes fails to identify malpositioning.
7. Consider suctioning the ETT and lower airway with a suction catheter to rule out mucus plugs, excessive secretions, or aspirated gastric contents.
8. Check the anesthesia circuit components including inspiratory and expiratory valves, bellows, pipeline, and cylinder pressures to make sure nothing is loose or disconnected. Consider disconnecting the patient from the anesthesia circuit entirely and connecting to a Mapleson circuit or self-inflating "ambu" bag with an oxygen tank. If the patient remains hypoxic and difficult to ventilate, this points toward the breathing tube/airway and the patient's physiology as the genesis of ventilation problems rather than the anesthesia machine or breathing circuit.
9. Check the ventilator settings and fresh gas flow settings. Rule out mechanical hypoventilation if the ventilator respiratory rate and tidal volume settings were inadequate.
10. Attempt a recruitment maneuver. If the patient has atelectasis, recruitment breaths will open collapsed alveoli. External compression of the lung from Trendelenburg positioning, ascites, or obesity can also cause shunt from atelectasis. Abnormal abdominal and chest wall mechanics such as those seen in patients with ACS cause atelectasis because of low functional residual capacity. Parenchymal and bronchial diseases such as asthma, chronic obstructive pulmonary disease, pneumonia, or acute respiratory distress syndrome (ARDS) can also lead to ventilation-perfusion mismatch and problems with ventilatory mechanics.
11. Assess hemodynamics. Circulatory failure impacts the delivery of oxygen to the tissues, which may result in low oxyhemoglobin saturation. Start inotropes and vasopressors if necessary (Fig. 4.2).

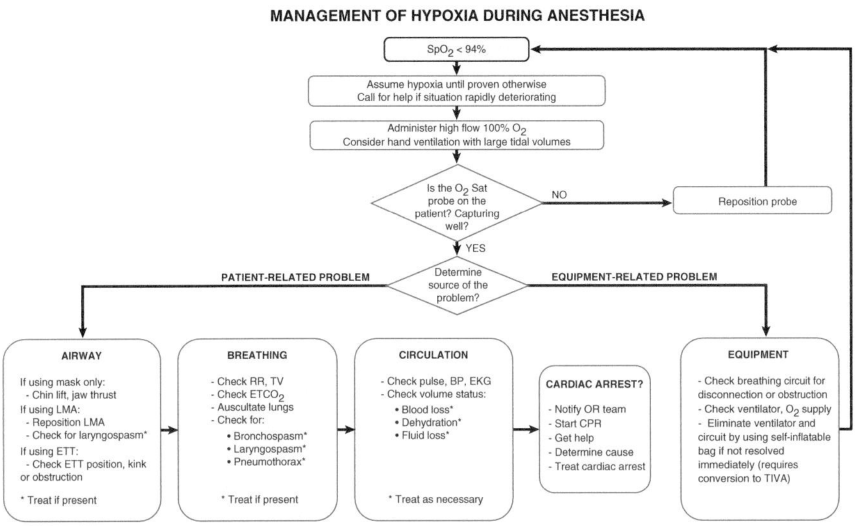

Fig. 4.2 Management of acute intraoperative hypoxia

Elevated Peak Inspiratory Pressures (PIP)

Whereas higher than normal initial PIPs may be due to a number of reasons, a sudden intraoperative increase in PIP is reason for alarm. Therefore, it is important to commit to memory a patient's initial PIP in order to be able to differentiate expected increases in PIP (insufflation of the abdomen, increase in tidal volumes, decrease in I:E ratio, application of PEEP, etc.) from problematic ones.

Sudden increases in peak airway pressures in the operating room are important as they may indicate an equipment problem or an issue with the patient's condition. All anesthesia ventilators display the peak inspiratory pressure (PIP), and generally a maximum acceptable PIP intraoperatively is <40 cmH_2O [17]. Peak pressures are a reflection of the resistance and compliance in the breathing circuit/system when a breath is delivered from the machine to the patient's lungs. In the operating room, the most common causes of high peak inspiratory airway pressures (PIP) include high airway resistance scenarios such as bronchospasm, kinking of the ETT, and airway secretions. Elevated PIP is also often seen when chest wall or lung compliance is decreased, such as in morbid obesity, endobronchial intubation, and during insufflation in laparoscopic or thoracoscopic surgery.

A way to troubleshoot elevated peak inspiratory pressures is to assess a plateau pressure [17]. Plateau pressure can be thought of as a reflection of respiratory system compliance (lungs, chest wall, and abdomen). A maneuver called "inspiratory pause" can be used to assess the pressure seen by the alveoli during a pause in inspiration. In our patient, due to his hemodynamic instability and rapid deterioration of respiratory parameters, we were unable to measure whether the plateau pressure was elevated or not. However, ventilation by hand seemed to be consistent with decreased overall compliance. In general, if PIP and plateau are increased, the etiology is most likely related to decreased pulmonary compliance. If, however, the PIP is elevated and the plateau is normal, then increased airway resistance is more likely. More specifically:

Increased PIP + normal plateau indicates increased airway resistance usually resulting from the following:

- **Mechanical** (kinked circuit, faulty inspiratory valve, scavenging failure).
- **Endotracheal tube** (kinked, secretions, depth, esophagus).
- **Conducting airways** (bronchospasm, external compression).

Increased PIP + elevated plateau indicates decreased compliance usually resulting from the following:

- **Alveolus** (atelectasis, edema, aspiration).
- **Pleural space** (tension pneumothorax, pleural thickening, pleural effusion).
- **Chest wall** (narcotic-induced rigidity, obesity, ascites, ACS).
- **Abdominal compartment** (ascites, blood, abdominal insufflation, Trendelenburg position).

When obtaining a plateau pressure in the operating room is not feasible, then physically disconnecting the patient from the ventilator and attaching the patient to a Mapleson circuit or ambu bag connected to an oxygen tank (or even turning the ventilator off and ventilating by hand, as it was done in this case due to the urgency of the situation) will help to distinguish between problems with the ventilator and circuit and an issue with the patient's respiratory system or the ETT. If hand ventilation of the patient using the Mapleson or ambu bag is easy, then there is most likely a mechanical problem with the ventilator or circuit. However, if hand ventilation continues to be difficult, the issue is most likely the ETT or the patient's clinical condition/physiology.

Diagnosis of Hypoxia and High Airway Pressures

Respiratory mechanics are profoundly impacted by increases in intra-abdominal pressure and likely played a role in our patient's initial presentation. Upon arrival to the emergency department, the patient had venous blood gas findings consistent with severe acute hypercarbic respiratory failure (pH 7.07, pCO_2 116 torr, pO_2 49 torr, HCO_3 33 mEq/L), for which he was emergently intubated.

Once in the operating room, already intubated and mechanically ventilated, the patient remained hypoxic with low SpO_2 70–80% with elevated peak inspiratory pressures of 35–45 mm H_2O. External compression of the lungs from the tense ascites combined with the abnormal abdominal and chest wall mechanics common in patients with ACS was undoubtedly preventing adequate delivery of oxygen to the alveoli and impeding removal of carbon dioxide from the lungs. Because the patient had aspirated, the alveoli may have been flooded with acidic gastric contents or fluid from the acute onset of ARDS, which further impaired proper gas exchange. The aspirated gastric contents were also potentially obstructing the airway and ETT, although none were suctioned from the upper airways. Furthermore, the patient's hemodynamic instability contributed to his hypoxia by reducing perfusion of his lungs.

Lesson 3: The Absence of End-Tidal CO_2

Differential Diagnosis

Sustained $ETCO_2$ is the routine standard by which anesthesiologists confirm ventilation with proper endotracheal tube or laryngeal mask airway (LMA) placement. End-tidal CO_2 is also used during spontaneous ventilation without airway instrumentation during monitored anesthesia care with sedation. An indicator of effective circulation (pulmonary blood flow), waveform capnography is now routinely used to ascertain the effectiveness of chest compressions during cardiopulmonary resuscitation (CPR), as recommended by the advanced cardiac life support (ACLS) guidelines. Capnographs utilized in typical anesthesia circuits sample small amounts of gas from the breathing circuit and use infrared light absorption technology to determine the concentration of exhaled CO_2 [18].

A precipitous drop in or absence of $ETCO_2$ could indicate a technical disturbance in the breathing circuit, esophageal intubation, or significant decrease in pulmonary blood flow from decreased cardiac output. Pulmonary embolism, in particular, cuts off pulmonary blood flow and decreases cardiac output, resulting in a sudden decrease in expired CO_2. Some of the very same steps that were important for troubleshooting hypoxia are also important steps to troubleshoot absent $ETCO_2$.

Disturbances in the Breathing Circuit: Leaks and Obstructions

The anesthesia circuit should be checked for leaks if there is no $ETCO_2$. The ETT should be checked for kinks or obstruction from secretions and mucus plugs.

Since the capnograph is constantly sampling exhaled gas from the anesthesia circuit, the tubing and sample chamber can become saturated with condensation, resulting in erroneous or absent $ETCO_2$. Conversely, the CO_2 analyzer could be defective, in which case the sample chamber and tubing should be changed.

In our clinical scenario, the patient was intubated in the emergency department, and records indicated that proper $ETCO_2$ color change was noted after intubation. However, when the patient was switched from the transport ventilator which did not display end-tidal CO_2 to the anesthesia circuit and there was no $ETCO_2$, the capnograph line and moisture trap were immediately replaced.

Esophageal Intubation

In the case of an esophageal intubation, the typical finding is either absent $ETCO_2$ or a steadily declining $ETCO_2$ after several breaths are delivered. Intraoperative migration of an ETT into the esophagus is exceedingly rare, but it may occur when the ETT is placed insufficiently deep and the cuff herniates above the vocal cords, expelling the ETT from the trachea. More commonly, an esophageal intubation may occur during initial placement of the ETT when visualization of the trachea is obscured (e.g., blood, emesis, anatomical features).

Decreased Cardiac Output and Pulmonary Embolism

In contrast to the respiratory issues that have been discussed above, circulatory changes may also cause profound changes in $ETCO_2$. For instance, circulatory arrest, pulmonary embolism, and a sudden severe decrease in blood pressure can all result in decreased pulmonary perfusion, which will be reflected as an acute drop in $ETCO_2$. Changes in patient hemodynamics may result in direction reversal of any intracardial shunts, also affecting $ETCO_2$.

Decreased CO_2 Production

Hypothermia, decreased metabolic rate states, and other conditions may also cause decreases in $ETCO_2$.

Lesson 4: Aspiration of Gastric Contents

Inhalation anesthetics, propofol, barbiturates, opiates, ketamine, and other sedative-hypnotics, muscle relaxants, and lidocaine are some of the agents used by anesthesiologists that depress airway reflexes (e.g., coughing and swallowing), placing patients at risk of aspiration. In addition to airway reflexes, the tone of the upper and lower esophageal sphincters plays an important role in preventing regurgitation of stomach contents. The incidence of aspiration of gastric contents is about 1/2000–3000 for elective surgical cases and higher at 1/600 for emergency surgeries, and often results in significant changes in respiratory function and hemodynamics [19].

There are specific conditions that predispose patients to greater risk of aspiration, including bowel obstruction, gastroesophageal reflux disease (GERD), hiatal hernia, obesity, ascites, pregnancy, recent meal, gastroparesis, and emergency surgery [19].

Historical Underpinnings to the Anesthesiologist's Approach to Aspiration

In 1946, an obstetrician by the name of Dr. Mendelson was the first physician to rigorously study the aspiration of gastric contents during anesthesia and the respiratory distress and hypoxemia that followed [20]. His early work was the basis for much of what anesthesiologists do today to prevent and treat aspiration.

After witnessing poor outcomes for his obstetric patients who aspirated, Mendelson was one of the first proponents of withholding oral feedings. By the 1960s, most anesthesia textbooks advocated nil per os (NPO) status at midnight

[21]. The American Society of Anesthesiologists now has an evidence-based set of NPO guidelines for surgical patients, which was originally established in 1998 and has since been updated to reflect new research findings [22]. NPO at midnight is now widely thought to be obsolete, though many health organizations continue to use this as a hospital nursing order.

Mendelson was also a proponent of the alkalinization and emptying of stomach content. While anesthesiologists routinely pharmacologically manipulate gastric pH, some argue that pharmacologic manipulation of gastric pH has not been proven effective [22]. Emptying of stomach contents is controversial, as nasogastric tubes may not remove particulate matter and may serve as a conduit for regurgitation by interfering with the lower esophageal sphincter (LES) tone [23].

Anesthesiologists often perform rapid sequence intravenous induction and intubation with apnea and cricoid pressure. The theory behind apnea is reducing the risk of insufflating the stomach with air during the delivery of breaths. Cricoid pressure is thought to occlude the esophagus, thereby preventing regurgitation of gastric contents into the trachea. However, there is much controversy over whether clinicians perform cricoid pressure optimally with the appropriate amount of pressure (40 N, equal to 9 lbs of pressure when using the English system of measures). Although the efficacy of applying cricoid pressure, even when done properly, has been questioned, it continues to be routine practice in patients thought to be at increased risk of regurgitation of gastric contents [24].

If regurgitation occurs, some physicians advocate placing the patient in Trendelenburg position to prevent flow of gastric contents into the trachea, while others argue that Trendelenburg positioning actually promotes further regurgitation. A less contentious approach involves turning the patient's head to the side and suctioning the airway. Most would recommend monitoring the patient for 24–48 h for signs and symptoms of aspiration pneumonitis (see pathophysiology timeline for details about clinical presentation). Immediate diagnostic bronchoscopy may also be useful in making the early diagnosis.

Pharmacologic Manipulation of Gastric pH and Volume (Table 4.2)

Table 4.2 Maneuvers to manipulate gastric pH and volume

Metoclopramide	10 mg IV pre-op	Increases LES tone, decreases gastric volume by speeding gastric emptying, weak antiemetic
H_2 receptor blockers (ranitidine/famotidine)	50 mg IV/20 mg IV	Inhibit gastric secretions and raise pH of new secretions but do not alter the volume or pH of gastric secretions already present in the GI system. Therefore of no use immediately preceding a rapid sequence intubation
Sodium citrate/potassium citrate/citric acid	15–30 mL PO immediately prior to induction	Non-particulate, immediate decrease in gastric fluid pH, but minor increase in intragastric volume

Pneumonitis Versus Pneumonia

We distinguish between aspiration or chemical pneumonitis and aspiration pneumonia. The former refers to a noninfectious chemically mediated inflammation of lung tissues after exposure to acidic gastric contents. Clinically, symptoms may include bronchospasm, hypoxia, and atelectasis [25]. The latter refers to an infectious process that may develop after an initial chemical insult to the fragile lung tissues, especially when foreign matter such as food particles enter airways and serve as a nidus for infection. Unless chemical pneumonitis evolves into bacterial pneumonia, it does not necessitate treatment with antibiotics. On the other hand, aspiration pneumonia requires antibiotic treatment of the most commonly encountered organisms: *E. coli*, *Pseudomonas*, *Klebsiella*, *S. aureus*, *Bacteroides fragilis*, and other gram-negative rod and anaerobes. When available, antibiotic therapy should be tailored to respiratory cultures. Steroids for the treatment of aspiration pneumonia have not been shown to improve outcome.

A widespread, unvalidated dogma in anesthesiology is that >25 mL of aspirate and a pH of <2.5 are necessary for an aspiration event. The origins of this belief date back to 1974, when two researchers directly introduced acid into the lungs of a single rhesus monkey and then extrapolated to humans and arbitrarily came up with the critical numbers of 25 mL of aspirate and a pH of 2.5 as being necessary for an aspiration event [26]. There have since been studies on healthy, fasting patients indicating that many patients routinely have greater than 25 mL of gastric contents at a pH of less than 2.5, and there is no evidence that they are at increased risk of an aspiration event [27].

In reality, many surgical patients likely aspirate small quantities of clear secretions during induction and emergence of anesthesia, which may cause coughing or brief laryngospasm. The lungs have protective mechanisms to deal with a certain degree of foreign material employing mucociliary transport and phagocytosis to clear the airways. Undoubtedly, as research experiments on animals have repeatedly shown, acid is destructive to delicate lung tissues, and larger volumes of aspirate involving food particles, blood, or blood clots can cause airway obstruction and interfere with oxygenation, resulting in significant morbidity.

Pathophysiology Timeline

As early as 3 min after the aspiration of gastric contents, critical changes occur in pulmonary function:

- Hypercarbia.
- Elevated PIP can be seen if the patient is mechanically ventilated.
- Hypoxia that does not improve with increased FiO_2 due to flooding of alveoli with gastric contents or the acute onset of ARDS.
- Atelectasis.
- Interstitial and alveolar edema.

- Peribronchial hemorrhage.
- Desquamation of the bronchial epithelium.

At 4–6 h:

- Neutrophils and fibrin can be seen in the alveoli.
- Persistent hypoxia/hypoxemia.
- Cough.
- Wheezing.
- Radiographic abnormalities (edema/consolidation/fluffy infiltrates) may appear anytime within 24 h.
- Fever.
- Leukocytosis.
- Destruction of pneumocytes and microvasculature.
- Decreased surfactant production.

At 48 h:

- The formation of hyaline membranes can be seen.

Lesson 5: Operating Team Dynamics

The operating room, being a "high-stakes environment," requires a group of health-care professionals and technicians with varied training, skill sets, and experience to come together to seamlessly care for a surgical patient. Most of us who have spent time in the operating room have undoubtedly witnessed examples of both successful, harmonious teamwork and dysfunctional team dynamics. The factors contributing to optimal teamwork are multifaceted and are often not under the control of any one individual in the group.

Teams themselves are often temporary and dynamic throughout the day in a given operating room suite. Nurses and anesthesiologists are at various times throughout the day relieved for breaks, radiology technicians and neuromonitoring staff may change during the course of an operation, and the surgeons and surgeon's assistants may also switch out from one surgery to the next. Individuals are expected to adapt to a constantly changing team. In large teaching institutions, all members of a team may not necessarily know one another by name, and at times there may be confusion as to the role of each individual (e.g., a surgical fellow may be confused with the surgeon's physician assistant, or the medical student may be confused with the anesthesia resident) in the operating room.

Training on effective communication and basic teamwork skills are infrequently a part of the formal education of the technicians, nurses, and physicians comprising a particular team caring for a surgical patient but are doubtless essential for optimal patient care. Furthermore, the traditionally hierarchical nature of medicine and the power relationships that exist in the operating room can affect team performance and lead to conflict and miscommunication.

Leadership is an essential component of effective teamwork. By default, the leader of the operating room team has historically been the surgeon. However, in this patient scenario, it was critical for the anesthesiologist to assume a leadership role and quickly diagnose, treat, delegate tasks, and communicate effectively with all members of the surgical team. The anesthesiologist was facing severe difficulty in ventilating the patient. Although several maneuvers were done to attempt to improve ventilation, resolution of the problem required the surgeons to quickly open the abdomen in order to relieve pressure against the diaphragm. This required full attention from the entire operating room team and clear communication on the part of the anesthesiologist.

It is important for both the anesthesiologist and the surgeon to understand the physiologic challenges in delivering anesthesia and ventilating a patient with ACS. While the surgeon is often focused on safely performing the surgical procedure at hand, the anesthesiologist is working to deliver favorable surgical conditions while simultaneously keeping the patient safe and supporting all vital organs. ACS presents a rare instance where the surgeon's procedure may actually make the conditions for delivering anesthesia and adequate ventilatory support more favorable. In fact, in cases of severe ACS, it might be nearly impossible, despite deploying an array of maneuvers, to deliver sufficient, life-sustaining ventilation until surgical decompression occurs. With a sound understanding of the physiologic challenges of ACS, working in cooperation with clear communication, anesthesiologists and surgeons can implement safe and effective decompressive laparotomies.

References

1. De Waele JJ, Malbrain ML, Kirkpatrick AW. The abdominal compartment syndrome: evolving concepts and future directions. Crit Care. 2015;19(1):211.
2. Fietsam R Jr, Villalba M, Glover JL, Clark K. Intra-abdominal compartment syndrome as a complication of ruptured abdominal aortic aneurysm repair. Am Surg. 1989;55(6):396–402.
3. Kirkpatrick AW. Intra-abdominal hypertension and the abdominal compartment syndrome: updates consensus definitions and clinical practice guidelines from the World Society of the Abdominal Compartment Syndrome. Intensive Care Med. 2013;39(7):1190–206.
4. Malbrain ML, De Keulenaer BL, Oda J, De Laet I, De Waele JJ, Roberts DJ, et al. Intra-abdominal hypertension and abdominal compartment syndrome in burns, obesity, pregnancy, and general medicine. Anaesthesiol Intensiv Ther. 2015;47(3):228–40.
5. Kron IL, Harman PK, Nolan SP. The measurement of intra-abdominal pressure as a criterion for abdominal re-exploration. Ann Surg. 1984;199:28–30.
6. Al-Abassi AA, Al Saadi AS, Ahmed F. Is intra-bladder pressure measurement a reliable indicator for raised intra-abdominal pressure? A prospective comparative study. BMC Anesthesiol. 2018;18:69.
7. Sugrue M, Jones F, Lee A, et al. Intra-abdominal pressure and gastric intramucosal pH: is there an association? World J Surg. 1996;20:988–91.
8. Ivatury RR, Porter JM, Simon RJ, et al. Intra-abdominal hypertension after life-threatening penetrating abdominal trauma: prophylaxis, incidence, and clinical relevance to gastric mucosal pH. J Trauma. 1998;44:1016–21.

9. Bloomfield GL, Dalton JM, Sugerman HJ, et al. Treatment of increasing intracranial pressure secondary to the acute abdominal compartment syndrome in a patient with combined abdominal and head trauma. J Trauma. 1995;39(6):1168–70.
10. Citerio G, Vascotto E, Villa F, Celotti S, Pesenti A. Induced abdominal compartment syndrome increases intracranial pressure in neurotrauma patients: a prospective study. Crit Care Med. 2001;29:1466–71.
11. Saggi BH, Sugerman HJ, Ivatury RR, Bloomfield GL. Abdominal compartment syndrome. J Trauma Inj Infect Crit Care. 1998;45:597–609.
12. Kashtan J, Green JF, Parsons EQ, Holcroft JW. Hemodynamic effects of increased abdominal pressure. J Surg Res. 1981;30(3):249–55.
13. de Waele JJ, Hoste EA, Malbrain ML. Decompressive laparotomy for abdominal compartment syndrome-a critical analysis. Crit Care. 2006;10(2):R51.
14. De Keulenaer B. What's new in medical management strategies for raised intra-abdominal pressure: evacuating intra-abdominal contents, improving abdominal wall compliance, pharmacotherapy, and continuous negative extra-abdominal pressure. Anaesthesiol Intensiv Ther. 2015;47(1):54–62.
15. Malbrain MLNG, Chiumello D, Cesana BM, Reintam Blaser A, Starkopf J, Sugrue M, et al. A systematic review and individual patient data meta-analysis on intraabdominal hypertension in critically ill patients: the wake-up project. World Initiative on Abdominal Hypertension Epidemiology, a Unifying Project (WAKE-Up!). Minerva Anestesiol. 2013;80(3):293–306.
16. Wilson IH. Management of hypoxia during anaesthesia: update in anesthesia. 2009.
17. Covert T, Niu NT. Differential diagnosis of peak airway pressures. Dimens Crit Care Nurs. 2015;34(1):19–23.
18. Siobal MS. Monitoring exhaled carbon dioxide. Respir Care. 2016;61(10):1397–416.
19. Nason KS. Acute intraoperative pulmonary aspiration. Thorac Surg Clin. 2015;25(3):301–7.
20. Mendelson CL. The aspiration of stomach contents into the lung during obstetric anesthesia. Am J Obstet Gynecol. 1946;52(2):191–205.
21. Maltby JR. Preoperative fasting guidelines. Can J Surg. 2006;49(2):138–9.
22. American Society of Anesthesiologists. Practice guidelines for preoperative fasting and the use of pharmacologic agents to reduce the risk of pulmonary aspiration: an updated report. Anesthesiology. 2011;114:495–511.
23. Salem MR, Khorasani A, Saatee S, Crystal GJ, El-Orbany M. Gastric tubes and airway management in patients at risk of aspiration: history, current concepts, and proposal of an algorithm. Anesth Analg. 2014;118:569–79.
24. Stewart JC, Bhananker S, Ramaiah R. Rapid-sequence intubation and cricoid pressure. Int J Crit Illn Inj Sci. 2014;4(1):42–9.
25. Marik PE. Aspiration pneumonitis and aspiration pneumonia. N Engl J Med. 2001;344(9):665–71.
26. Roberts RB, Shirley MA. Reducing the risk of acid aspiration during cesarean section. Anesth Analg. 1974;53:859–68.
27. Sutherland AD, Stock JG, Davies JM. Effects of preoperative fasting on morbidity and gastric contents in patients undergoing day-stay surgery. Br J Anaesth. 1986;58:876–8.

Chapter 5
Massive Pulmonary Hemorrhage During Pulmonary Thromboendarterectomy

Ryan Suda and Gerard R. Manecke

Introduction

Pulmonary hemorrhage is rare, but it does occur during certain surgeries, and severe cases can be life-threatening. The management of pulmonary hemorrhage is challenging, often requiring advanced techniques and equipment. In this chapter, a case of massive pulmonary hemorrhage following cardiopulmonary bypass in a patient undergoing pulmonary thromboendarterectomy is presented. Diagnosis, physiologic perturbations, management of coagulopathy, and therapies, ranging from non-invasive to invasive, will be discussed.

Case Presentation

The patient is a 60-year-old man with past medical history of chronic thromboembolic pulmonary hypertension with NYHA class 3, chronic obstructive pulmonary disease, and hypercoagulable state secondary to a prothrombin gene mutation. He was scheduled for an elective pulmonary thromboendarterectomy. The patient had an inferior vena cava filter and was chronically receiving warfarin since his initial diagnosis of hypercoagulability but was appropriately bridged with enoxaparin in anticipation of his surgery. The patient's preoperative evaluation included an echocardiogram, right heart catheterization, and pulmonary angiogram. Pertinent findings included signs of right heart failure with a severely enlarged right ventricle

R. Suda (✉)
Department of Anesthesiology, University of California, San Diego, San Diego, CA, USA
e-mail: rsuda@ucsd.edu

G. R. Manecke
Department of Anesthesiology, University of California, UCSD Medical Center, UCSD School of Medicine, San Diego, CA, USA

J. L. Benumof, G. R. Manecke (eds.), *Clinical Anesthesiology II*,
https://doi.org/10.1007/978-3-030-12365-9_5

with severely depressed function, abnormal septal motion with elevated right ventricular systolic and diastolic pressures, mild tricuspid regurgitation, and severe pulmonary hypertension with evidence of proximal and distal thromboembolic disease in the pulmonary vessels bilaterally. Laboratory studies were notable for a platelet count of 119,000, international normalized ratio (INR) of 1.3, and activated partial thromboplastin time (aPTT) of 39.8 s. On physical examination, the patient was 6’4”, 310 lbs, with a body mass index (BMI) of 38, favorable airway, and 2+ pitting edema bilaterally in the lower extremities.

On the morning of surgery, a pre-induction radial arterial line was placed, anesthesia was induced, and the trachea was intubated uneventfully with an 8.0 endotracheal tube (ETT). A Cordis and pulmonary artery catheter were placed easily under ultrasound guidance in the right internal jugular vein. Additionally, a transesophageal echocardiography probe was inserted. The pre-cardiopulmonary bypass (CPB) course was uneventful, and bypass was initiated smoothly. The patient was cooled to 18 °C. Deep hypothermic circulatory arrest was first instituted for 20 min for the endarterectomy of the left pulmonary arterial tree. This was followed by 5 min for endarterectomy on the right, with 10 min of CPB between the two arrests. The patient was then gradually rewarmed to 36 °C, and perfusion machine flows were reduced in preparation to separate from CPB. However, after initial separation from bypass, blood was seen coming out of the ETT and persisted despite suction via ETT suction catheter. CPB was immediately reinstituted, and diagnostic flexible fiberoptic bronchoscopy revealed steady hemorrhage in the bronchus intermedius, likely originating from the right middle or lower lobe (**Lesson I**). The 8.0 ETT was exchanged over an airway exchange catheter under direct laryngoscopy for a 9.0 ETT, in anticipation of bronchial blocker placement, and positive end-expiration pressure (PEEP) was increased to 10 cm H_2O (**Lesson IV**). A 9 Fr Fuji Uniblocker (Fuji Systems Corporation, Tokyo, Japan) was placed into the bronchus intermedius with successful isolation of the pulmonary hemorrhage (**Lesson V**). Protamine was given after successful separation from CPB to reverse systemic heparinization. Platelets were administered to treat any functional thrombocytopenia, and fresh frozen plasma was given for any clotting factor deficiency, while the surgeons closed the chest (**Lesson III**). However, despite aggressive ventilation strategies and therapeutic bronchoscopy to clear patent airways, oxygenation and ventilation were still inadequate, likely secondary to significant intrapulmonary shunt (**Lesson II**). Inhaled nitric oxide was trialed without success. A coordinated decision with the cardiothoracic surgeon was made to initiate veno-venous extracorporeal membrane oxygenation (ECMO) due to the worsening oxygenation, respiratory acidosis, and pulmonary hypertension (**Lesson VI**). A Cordis and triple-lumen catheter were placed in the left internal jugular vein under ultrasound guidance for administration of inotropic and vasoactive infusions. The right Cordis was exchanged over a wire for a 27 Fr Avalon Elite ® bicaval dual-lumen ECMO cannula (Maquet, Wayne, N.J.) under transesophageal echocardiography guidance. Oxygenation and respiratory acidosis improved on minimal ECMO settings. The patient was transported successfully to the cardiovascular intensive care unit (ICU). The ICU course was complicated by multi-organ failure requiring escalating vasopressor and inotropic support, continuous renal replacement therapy, and blood product transfusions. The patient expired on post-op day 2.

Lesson I: How Do You Diagnose the Etiology and Source of Pulmonary Hemorrhage?

Lesson I-A: What Are the Causes of Pulmonary Hemorrhage?

Massive pulmonary hemorrhage is a life-threatening emergency defined by severe, acute bleeding from the lung. Pulmonary hemorrhage may present as a medical emergency where an anesthesia provider is consulted to assist in airway management or occur during a procedure where they are the primary provider (surgery, pulmonary artery catheterization, airway management). There are numerous etiologies of pulmonary hemorrhage (Table 5.1). However, the incidence is quite rare, occurring in less than 1% of anesthetics. Ongoing pulmonary hemorrhage is very rare because it either resolves spontaneously, it is treated successfully, or the patient expires [1].

The patient undergoing pulmonary thromboendarterectomy is at greatest risk for direct vessel trauma from disruption/perforation of the pulmonary artery during a challenging endarterectomy. The cardiothoracic surgeon must identify the optimal plane to dissect the pulmonary artery. If the surgeon dissects too deeply into the vessel wall, there is a greater risk of pulmonary hemorrhage; if dissection is too superficial, the clot will break proximally, leaving distally compromised pulmonary blood flow and risk for recurrence of chronic thromboembolic pulmonary hypertension. Friability of the vessels, advanced age, and presence of residual pulmonary hypertension likely exacerbate the risk for bleeding [2].

Lesson I-B: What Is the Anatomy of the Tracheobronchial Tree?

A thorough understanding of tracheobronchial tree anatomy is essential in diagnosing and treating pulmonary hemorrhage. Complete knowledge of tracheobronchial anatomy is a key factor in determining optimal position of lung isolation devices [3], which will be discussed in Lesson V. The trachea is a fibromuscular tube on average 10–12 cm in length with an average outer diameter of 19–22 mm. The adult trachea is lined with 16–22 C-shaped cartilaginous rings, which reinforce the

Table 5.1 Causes of massive pulmonary hemorrhage

Bronchiectasis
Bronchogenic carcinoma (large, centrally located, squamous cell carcinoma)
Hydrostatic gradient bleeding (negative pressure in airway obstruction, severe acute pulmonary hypertension)
Idiopathic pneumonia syndrome after bone marrow transplantation
Immunologic lung disease (Goodpasture's syndrome, granulomatosis with polyangiitis, systemic lupus erythematosus)
Pulmonary arteriovenous malformations
Pulmonary emboli (septic, post-anticoagulant, or thrombolytic agent)
Pulmonary infection (tuberculosis [Rasmussen's aneurysm], fungal infection, abscesses)
Pulmonary vessel trauma (thoracic trauma, pulmonary artery rupture)

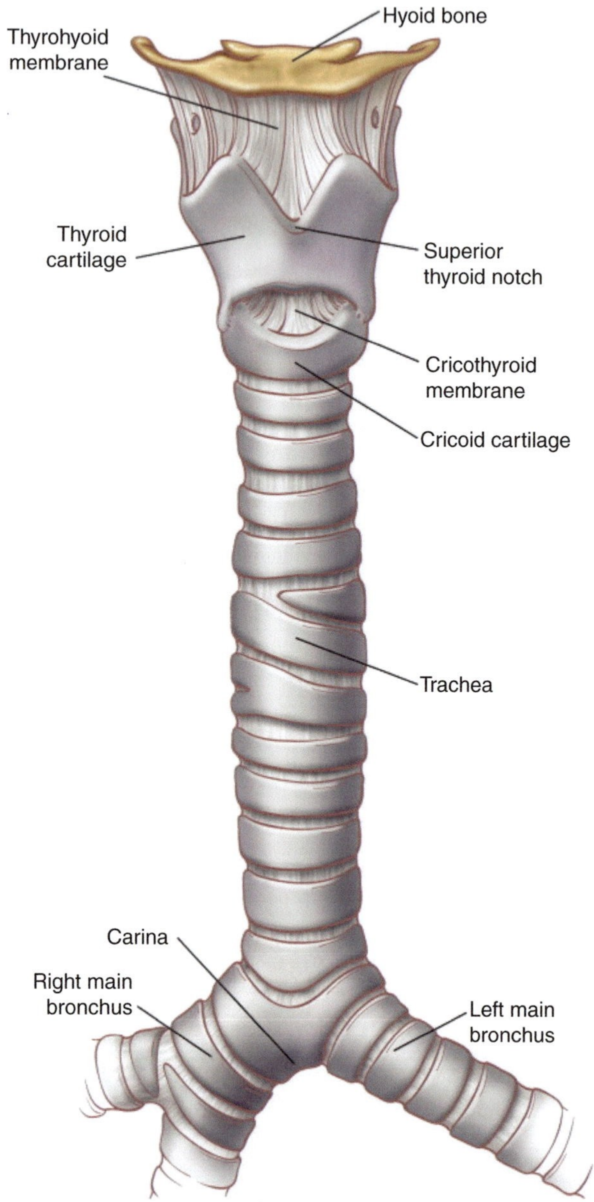

Fig. 5.1 Tracheal anatomy for 170 cm individual. (Modified from Minnich et al. [6]. With permission from Elsevier)

anterior and lateral walls to prevent airway collapse. The trachea terminates at the carina where it gives rise to the right and left mainstem bronchi. The right main bronchus is 1.5–2 cm in length, has a larger diameter (14–17 mm), and branches from the trachea at a more vertical (~25°) angle compared to the left main bronchus, which is longer (4.5–5 cm), is smaller in diameter (~12 mm), and leaves the trachea at a ~45° angle. After the posterior takeoff of the right upper lobe bronchus, the airway continues as the bronchus intermedius, it gives off the right middle lobe bronchus anteriorly and continues as the right lower lobe bronchus [4] (Fig. 5.1).

Each lung is divided into ten bronchopulmonary segments (Fig. 5.2a), each with a tertiary bronchus supplying a portion of the lung (Fig. 5.2b). The right upper lobe is comprised of the apical, posterior, and anterior segments (numbered 1–3). The right middle lobe is comprised of lateral and medial segments (numbered 4–5). The right lower lobe is comprised of the superior, medial basal, anterior basal, lateral basal, and posterior basal segments (numbered 6–10). The left upper lobe is comprised of the apico-posterior, anterior, superior lingular, and inferior lingular segments (numbered 1+2, 3–5). The left lower lobe is comprised of the superior basal, anteromedial basal, lateral basal, and posterior basal segments (numbered 6, 7+8, 9–10) [4].

Knowledge of the bronchopulmonary segments allows for clear, concise communication of the hemorrhage location between the anesthesia provider and consultant. Familiarity with tracheobronchial anatomy hastens lung isolation strategies to maximize preservation of healthy lung areas.

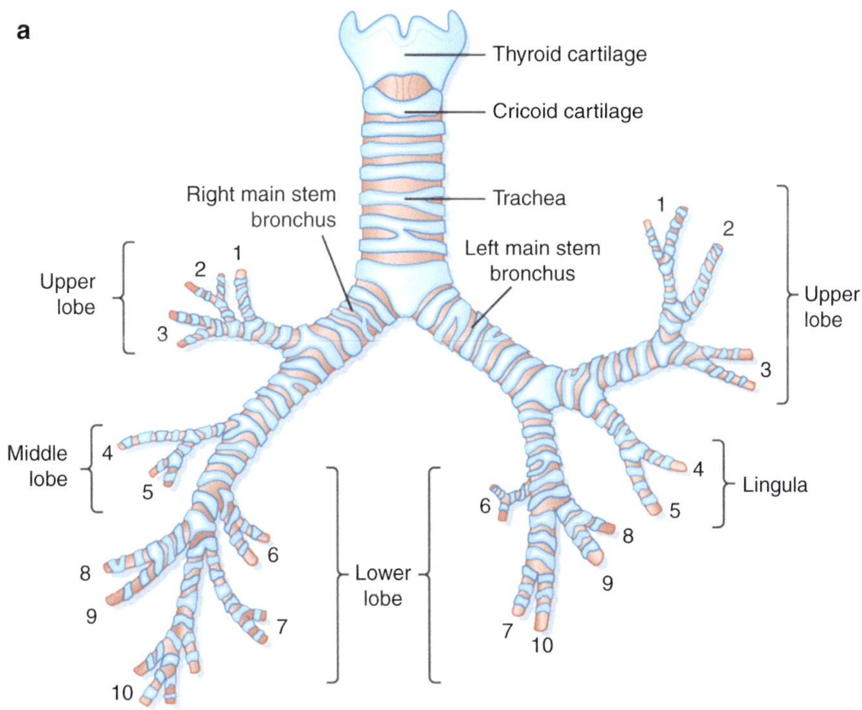

Fig. 5.2 (**a**) Bronchopulmonary segments, anterior view. The numbers correspond to specific segmental bronchi. Right side: 1 = apical, 2 = posterior, 3 = anterior, 4 = lateral, 5 = medial, 6 = superior, medial basal, 7 = anterior basal, 8 = lateral basal, and 9 = posterior basal. Left side: 1+2 = apico-posterior, 3 = anterior, 4 = superior lingular, 5 = inferior lingular, 6 = superior basal, 7+8 = antero-medial basal, 9 = lateral basal, and 10 = posterior basal. (**b**) Topography of the lung demonstrating the lobes, segments, and fissures. (Reprinted from Cloutier and Thrall [47]. With permission from Elsevier)

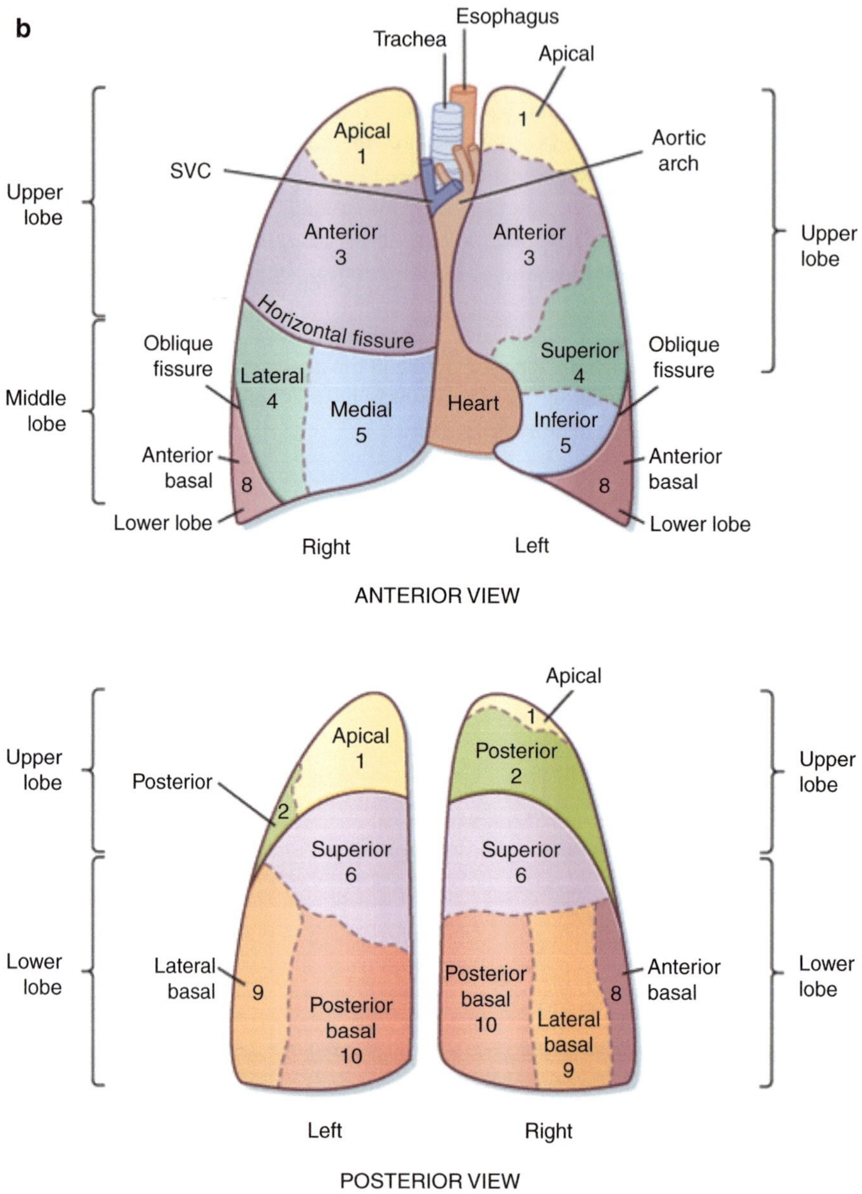

Fig. 5.2 (continued)

Lesson I-C: What Is the Blood Supply to the Lungs?

A thorough understanding of the blood supply to the lungs is essential in diagnosing and treating pulmonary hemorrhage. The lung is supplied by blood from the pulmonary and bronchial arteries. The pulmonary circulation facilitates gas exchange of mixed venous blood to provide metabolic and oxygen requirements for the alveolar parenchyma and systemic circulation. The bronchial arteries supply oxygenated blood to the conductive airways and connective tissues of the lung [5]. There are typically three bronchial arteries consisting of the superior, middle, and inferior (Fig. 5.3). While there is great variation in bronchial arterial anatomy, one right-sided aortic branch most often supplies the right mainstem bronchus, and the two left-sided aortic branches most often supply the left mainstem bronchus (Fig. 5.4) [6]. The bronchial arteries travel and divide with the branching bronchi down to the respiratory bronchioles where they anastomose with the pulmonary arteries. Each bronchopulmonary segment has its own pulmonary and bronchial artery blood supply (Fig. 5.5).

During pulmonary hemorrhage, blood is first apparent in the airway or endotracheal tube (ETT). Dark blood usually indicates bleeding from the pulmonary artery, while bright red blood usually indicates bronchial (systemic) arterial bleeding [1]. Knowledge of the blood supply to the lungs and airways can expedite the location and treatment of pulmonary hemorrhage.

Lesson I-D: How Do You Perform a Complete Flexible Fiberoptic Bronchoscopy Exam?

Flexible fiberoptic bronchoscopy is an invaluable skill required for the management of pulmonary hemorrhage. The standard adult fiberoptic bronchoscope has a 5.7 mm external diameter with a 2 mm suction channel and requires a 7 mm or greater ETT if such tube is to be used as a conduit [7]. The fiberoptic bronchoscope should be inserted through the largest ETT safely achievable to minimize the decreased cross-sectional area available for ventilating the patient. PEEP is created when the fiberoptic bronchoscope is passed through an ETT, so it should be discontinued prior to bronchoscope insertion. A fiberoptic bronchoscope swivel adapter with a self-sealing valve is used to facilitate simultaneous ventilation and bronchoscope manipulation.

A thorough examination of the bronchopulmonary segments will correctly identify the location of hemorrhage. A systematic and complete exam includes a clear view of the anterior wall (tracheal cartilage) and posterior wall (membranous portion) of the trachea and carina below the vocal cords. When advancing the bronchoscope through the right mainstem bronchus, there is a clear view of the bronchus intermedius with the orifice of the right upper bronchus at the 3 o'clock position. Viewing inside the right upper bronchus reveals the only structure in the tracheobronchial tree with three orifices: apical, anterior, and posterior segments. Viewing the bronchus intermedius distally exposes the right middle and lower lobe bronchi. The bronchoscope is then withdrawn until the tracheal carina is visualized and then advanced into the left mainstem bronchus. The left mainstem bronchus bifurcates into the left upper lobe and lingula superiorly and lower lobe inferiorly [4].

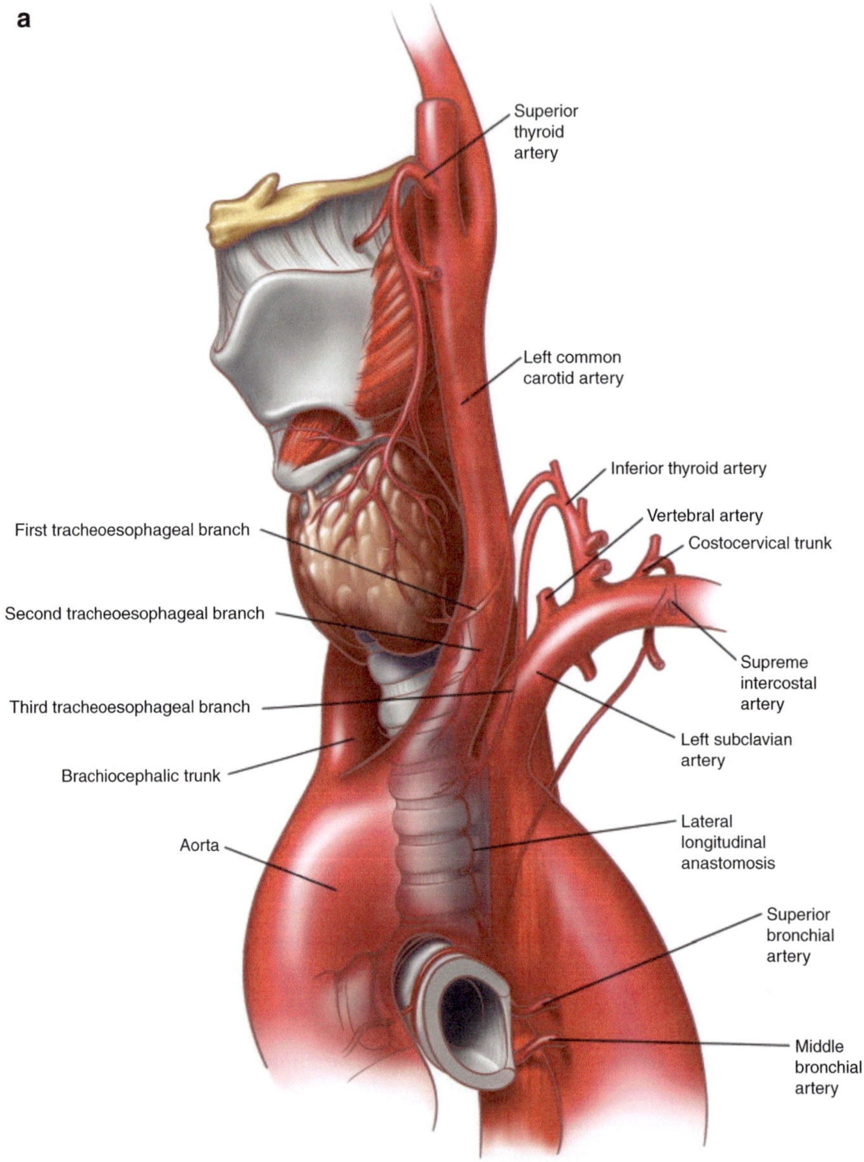

Fig. 5.3 (**a**) Tracheal and bronchial blood supply, left anterior view. (**b**) Tracheal and bronchial blood supply, right anterior view. (Modified from Minnich et al. [6]. With permission from Elsevier)

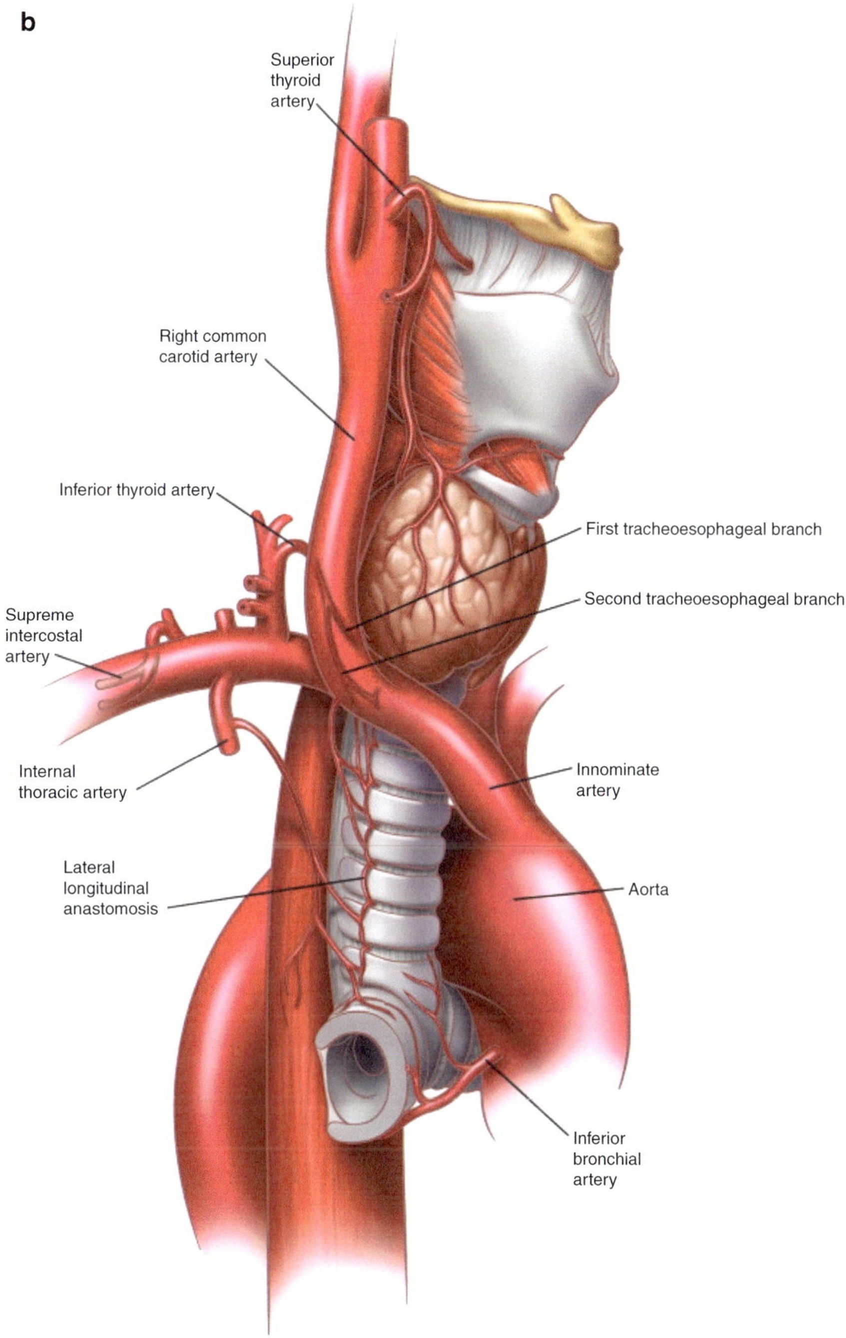

Fig. 5.3 (continued)

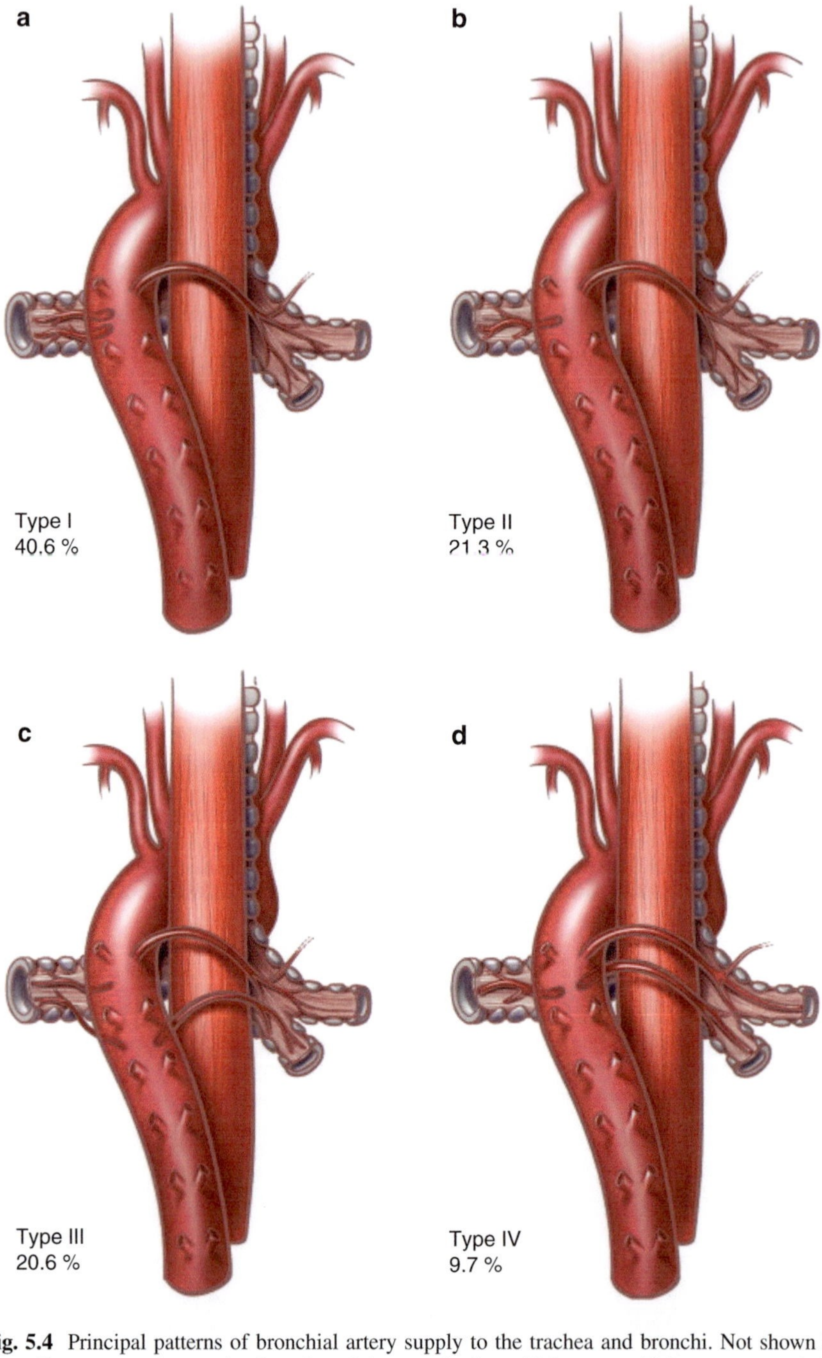

Fig. 5.4 Principal patterns of bronchial artery supply to the trachea and bronchi. Not shown in these diagrams are the proximal portion of the superior bronchial artery, which courses anteriorly over the left main bronchus to carina, and the middle bronchial branch passing beneath the left main bronchus to carinal anastomosis. (Modified from Minnich et al. [6]. With permission from Elsevier)

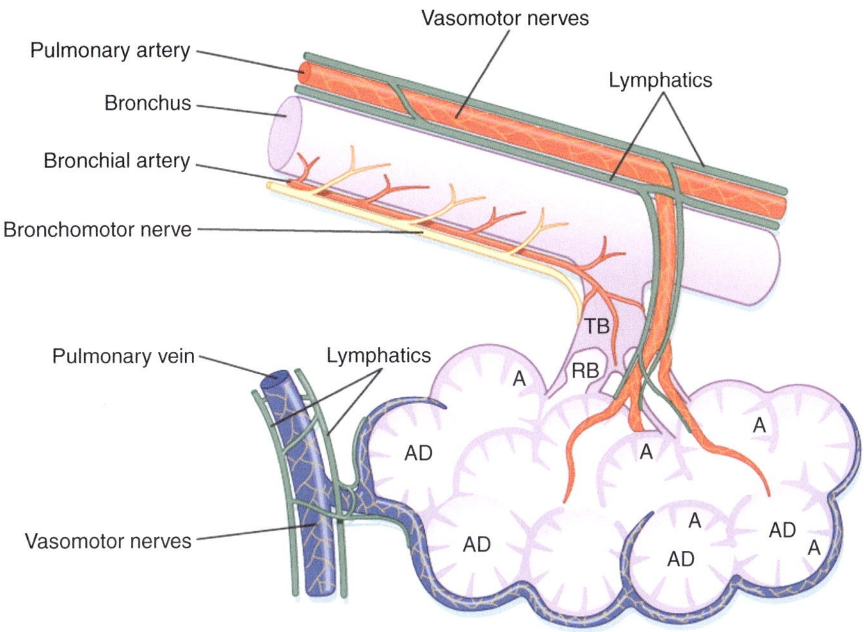

Fig. 5.5 Anatomic relationship between the airways, blood vessels, and lymphatics. TB terminal bronchioles, RB respiratory bronchioles, A alveoli, AD alveolar ducts. (Reprinted from Cloutier and Thrall [47]. With permission from Elsevier)

If bleeding is recognized before separation from cardiopulmonary bypass, allowing the heart to briefly eject with the bleeding area under direct visualization with fiberoptic bronchoscopy can establish the hemorrhagic location. The type of lung isolation technique will depend on the level and number of segmental involvement. The goal is to isolate the affected segment(s) to prevent spilling of blood into other segments, which will cause further impairment of ventilation and gas exchange [8]. The choice between bronchial blockade and double-lumen tube placement will be discussed in Lesson V.

Lesson II: What Are the Physiologic Perturbations Due to Pulmonary Hemorrhage?

Lesson II-A: How Is Ventilation Affected by Pulmonary Hemorrhage?

Ventilation is the movement of gas between the environment and the lungs via inhalation and exhalation. Pulmonary hemorrhage fills the airways with blood, making the movement of gas more difficult and sometimes impossible. As blood fills the airways, the functional diameter of the airway decreases causing a dramatic increase in airway resistance. Pulmonary hemorrhage in the upper airways is not tolerated as well compared to distal airways, which increase in total parallel pathways and total cross-sectional area with each generation toward the periphery. As the airway resistance increases, ventilation becomes more difficult, requiring increasing positive pressures to achieve the same tidal volumes. Prolonged exposure to high inspiratory pressures can cause exacerbated lung injury, worsening ventilation and oxygenation. If enough blood is introduced into the airway, the airway becomes occluded, with resulting distal atelectasis and intrapulmonary shunt. A pulmonary shunt occurs when alveoli of the lungs are perfused with blood but are unable to participate in gas exchange. Elimination of carbon dioxide is usually not affected until the physiologic shunt fraction exceeds 75–80% of the cardiac output [5], but oxygenation is dramatically affected by shunt (Lesson II-B). The extent of hypercapnia depends on the site and degree of obstruction and coexisting native lung pathology.

Isolating bleeding bronchopulmonary segments to prevent further lung contamination is crucial to successful ventilation and oxygenation. Suctioning blood from contaminated segments should be aggressively attempted to maximize airway patency and prevent pulmonary shunting due to atelectasis. The extent of lung involved in the pulmonary hemorrhage will dictate the type of isolation device, which will be discussed in Lesson V. If there is bilateral pulmonary hemorrhage, ventilation strategies are aimed at minimizing inspiratory pressures and utilizing PEEP to slow bleeding and maximize airway patency, which is discussed in Lesson IV.

Lesson II-B: How Is Oxygenation Affected by Pulmonary Hemorrhage?

Oxygenation is the process by which oxygen is added to the body. Pulmonary hemorrhage impairs oxygenation primarily through atelectasis by decreasing the total number of available alveoli for gas exchange. Blood fills the airways impairing distal ventilation and transport of oxygen. Pulmonary shunting occurs due to poor ventilation despite adequate perfusion. The more proximal the hemorrhage, the greater the pulmonary shunt since all distal branching airways and alveoli will not be ventilated. Hypoxic pulmonary vasoconstriction is stimulated by hypoxia and can decrease flow to hypoventilated areas, but this response can be overwhelmed during massive pulmonary hemorrhage [5]. If there is bleeding into alveoli, there are added diffusion perturbations, which impair gas exchange.

Lesson II-C: How Much Blood Can Be Lost During Pulmonary Hemorrhage?

Pulmonary hemorrhage can range in severity from minor (scant) to massive (liters) [2, 9]. The severity of bleeding into the airway seems to be independent of whether blood enters the airway via a direct communication between a branch of the pulmonary or bronchial artery and its bronchus or via the parenchyma [9]. Bronchovascular fistulas can present as small herald bleeds, while massive bleeding can occur in the absence of a demonstrable lesion in either the airway or pulmonary vessels. Additionally, blood can enter the pleural space or be contained in the lung parenchyma. The location and speed of the bleed will determine the overall blood loss. A very brisk hemorrhage in a location difficult to access for therapeutic measures can lead to massive blood loss, with the patient left to exsanguinate if untreated [1, 9]. A concomitant coagulopathy can worsen the blood loss and make treatment more difficult. Diagnosis and treatment of a coagulopathy are discussed in Lesson III.

Large bore intravenous (IV) access should be obtained if not already in place. Administration of appropriate IV fluids or blood products should be given to treat hypotension as inadequate pulmonary perfusion can impair oxygenation. Rapid infusion devices can be useful for administration of large volumes of IV fluids and blood products. Cardiopulmonary bypass may provide time necessary to locate the bleeding source but requires systemic anticoagulation.

Lesson II-D: What Are the Effects of Blood Clots in the Airways?

Blood clots in the airways can minimally impact respiratory function or result in life-threatening ventilation impairment. The most notable finding among ventilated patients is an acute rise in peak inspiratory pressure and a concomitant decrease in tidal volume. With major atelectasis, the plateau pressure is also elevated. However, if partial obstruction of the airways occurs without atelectasis, the plateau pressure may be normal. The extent of hypoxemia and hypercapnia depends on the site and degree of obstruction, associated pulmonary hemorrhage, and underlying condition of the lungs.

Hemodynamic compromise from airway obstruction depends upon the severity and location of the obstruction. In distal obstruction patent airways with normal lung compliance transmit elevated airway pressures to extraparenchymal intrathoracic regions, resulting in decreased venous return and cardiac output. In proximal airway obstruction, the distal pressures are normal with a distinct absence of hemodynamic alterations. A notable difference in presentation may occur with a ball valve clot. A ball valve clot may lead to hyperinflation with risk of pneumothorax and hemodynamic compromise [10].

Lesson III: How Do You Diagnose and Treat a Perioperative Coagulopathy?

Lesson III-A: What Diagnostic Tests Are Useful in Treating a Coagulopathy?

Perioperative bleeding results from a localized pathologic process or a disorder of the hemostatic process, involving a complex interplay among vascular integrity, platelets, coagulation factors, and fibrinolysis. A cell-based model with three overlapping stages (initiation, amplification, propagation) (Fig. 5.6) has replaced the

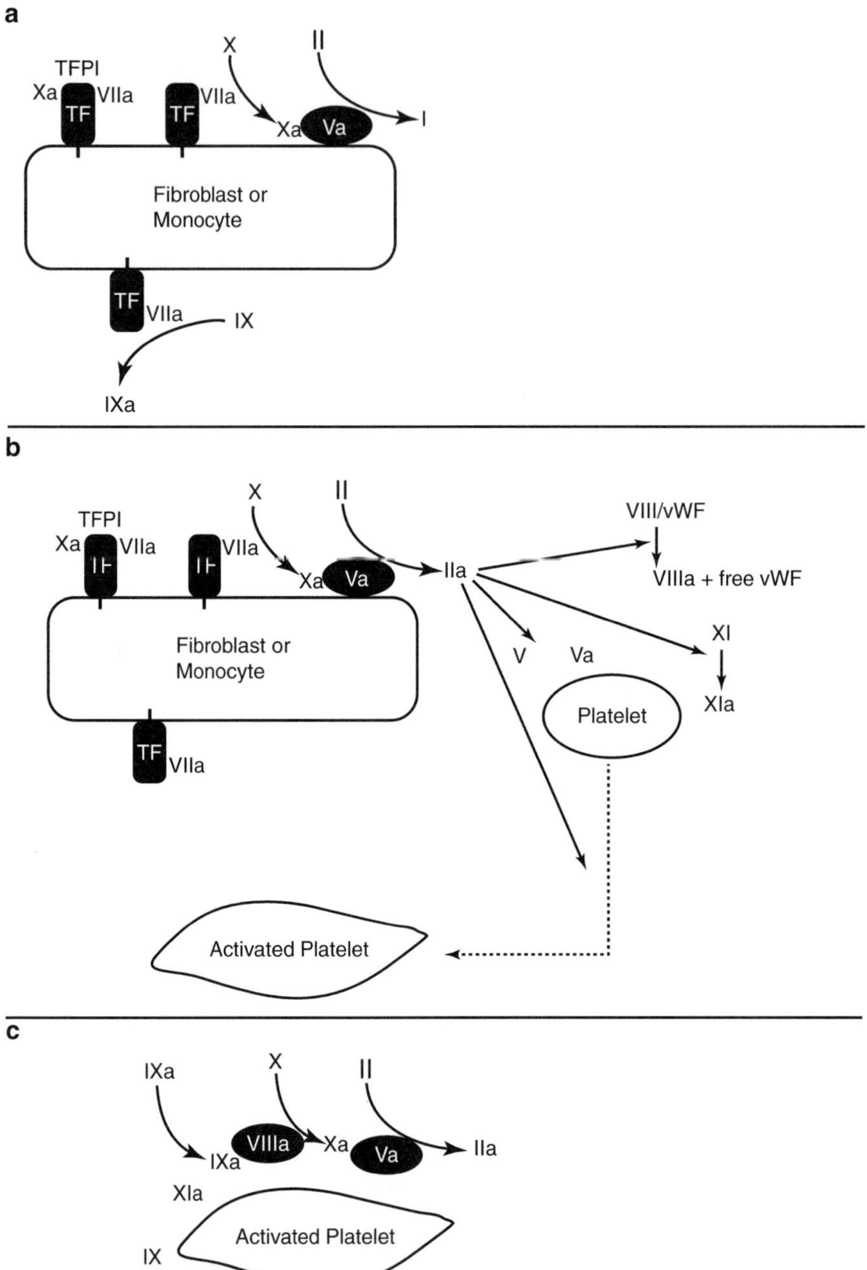

Fig. 5.6 Steps in a cell-based model of coagulation. (**a**) Initiation occurs on the tissue factor (TF)-bearing cell as activated factor X (FXa) combines with its cofactor, FVa, to activate small amounts of thrombin. (**b**) The small amount of thrombin generated on the TF-bearing cell amplifies the procoagulant response by activating cofactors, factor XI, and platelets. (**c**) The large burst of thrombin required for effective hemostasis is formed on the platelet surface during the propagation phase. TFPI tissue factor pathway inhibitor, vWF von Willebrand factor. (Reprinted from Hoffman and Monroe [11]. With permission from Elsevier)

classical coagulation cascade model (Fig. 5.7) to better represent in vivo hemostasis [11, 12]. However, the cascade model is still useful for understanding the in vitro coagulation tests (Fig. 5.8). There are numerous inherited disorders of hemostasis; however, this discussion will focus on the diagnostic workup of acquired disorders of hemostasis. Coagulation dysfunction can be broadly divided into disorders of hemostasis and disorders of thrombosis, although there is a small intermediate group that involves both [13]. It is not uncommon for patients to be on antiplatelet or anticoagulant medications in the perioperative period.

The plasma prothrombin time (PT) measures the functioning of the extrinsic and final common coagulation pathway (Figs. 5.7 and 5.8). The factors specific to the extrinsic pathway are tissue factor and factor VII. The factors specific to the common pathway are factors X and V, prothrombin (factor II), and fibrinogen. The PT is more sensitive than aPTT to deficiencies in the common pathway. The INR is a standardization to correct for different PT instrument reagent systems. INR is calculated as a ratio of the patient's PT to a control PT. PT and INR are useful in monitoring warfarin therapy and assessment of liver synthetic function.

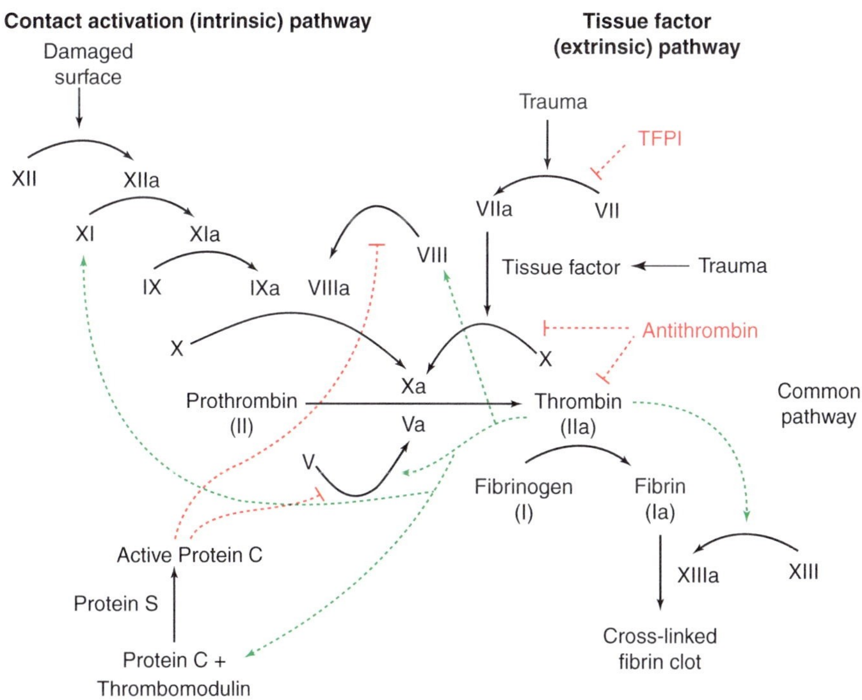

Fig. 5.7 Classical coagulation cascade. Each coagulation factor is represented by its Roman numeral designation with the activated form illustrated with an (**a**). TFPI tissue factor pathway inhibitor

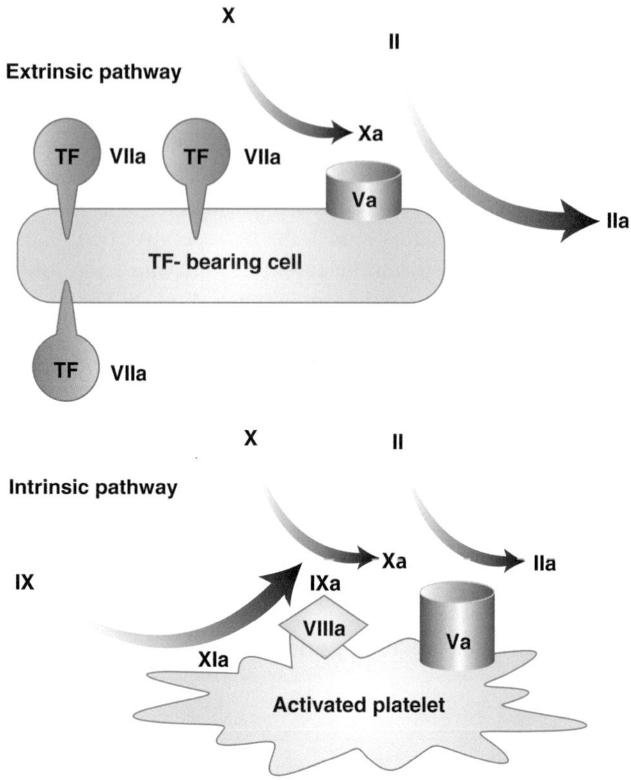

Fig. 5.8 Cell-based intrinsic and extrinsic pathways. Each coagulation factor is represented by its Roman numeral designation with the activated form illustrated with an (**a**). TF tissue factor. (Reprinted from Hoffman and Monroe [11]. With permission from Elsevier)

The aPTT measures the functioning of the intrinsic and common pathways of coagulation (Figs. 5.7 and 5.8). The factors specific to the intrinsic pathway are factors XI, XII, VIII, and IX. The aPTT is sensitive to inhibitors such as heparin and to deficiencies of all coagulation factors except factors VII and XIII. However, high levels of a single factor can shorten the aPTT. It is used to monitor therapy with unfractionated heparin and direct thrombin inhibitors.

The thrombin time (TT) measures the final step in the common pathway, the conversion of fibrinogen to fibrin monomers, and the formation of an initial clot by thrombin (Fig. 5.7). It is used to evaluate a patient with a prolonged PT and aPTT and for detection of heparin in a sample. Fibrin cross-linking, mediated by factor XIII, is not measured by this assay. The reptilase time (RT) is similar to the TT but uses reptilase, an enzyme derived from snake venom, which is not inhibited by antithrombin or the antithrombin-heparin complex. The RT is useful for detecting abnormalities in fibrinogen and the presence of heparin. If heparin is present, the TT will be prolonged, but the RT will be normal. If fibrinogen is abnormal, both the TT and RT will be prolonged.

Table 5.2 Summary of clotting time tests

Test	Intrinsic pathway	Extrinsic pathway	Common pathway	Heparin resistant
PT		X	X	
aPTT	X		X	
ACT	X		X	
TT			X	
RT			X	X

The activated whole blood clotting time (ACT) measures the time it takes the whole blood to clot when exposed to substances that activate the ACTcontact factors. Like the aPTT, the ACT assesses the intrinsic and common coagulation pathways. The ACT is primarily used in adjusting heparin dosing during procedures where large doses of heparin are administered (Table 5.2).

Plasma concentrations of fibrinogen and D-dimer can be measured in plasma. Fibrinogen is the precursor to fibrin, the principle component of a fibrin clot. Abnormally low levels of fibrinogen (typically <50–100 mg/dL) can result in impaired clot formation and increased bleeding risk. Fibrin D-dimer is one of the major fibrin degradation products released upon cleavage of cross-linked fibrin by plasmin. Elevated concentrations of plasma D-dimer (>500 nm/mL by ELISA) indicate recent or ongoing intravascular coagulation and fibrinolysis.

Thromboelastography (TEG) and rotational thromboelastometry (RoTEM) are global tests of hemostasis performed on whole blood, unlike the previously described clotting time tests, which are performed only on plasma. TEG and RoTEM can obtain rapid assessment of the kinetics of clot formation, strength, and dissolution as they reflect platelet function and coagulation (Figs. 5.9 and 5.10). RoTEM is an adaptation of TEG, and they provide essentially identical information. Variables of interest include reaction time (R, in seconds), clot kinetics or time from R until the clot reaches 20 mm (K, in seconds), angular measurement from a tangent line drawn to the curve of the TEG tracing starting from the point of clot reaction time (α), and maximum amplitude (MA, in millimeters). R is a period of time from initiation of the test to the initial fibrin clot formation. K is a measure of time from the beginning of clot formation until the amplitude of the TEG reaches 20 mm and represents the dynamics of clot formation. α angle is an angle between the line in the middle of the TEG tracing and the line tangential to the developing "body" of the TEG tracing and represents the acceleration (kinetics) of fibrin buildup and cross-linking. MA reflects strength of a clot, which is dependent on the number and function of platelets and its interaction with fibrin. Other parameters measured include lysis at 30 min (% of clot lysed) and clot firmness (G, dynes/cm^2). Tracings TEG and RoTEM are tests best used to assess changes in global coagulative function over time where a baseline is known and are frequently used to assess the response to interventions such as transfusion therapy [14]. Specific coagulopathy treatments will be discussed in the following section, Lesson III-B. Tracings of various coagulation states are illustrated in Fig. 5.11.

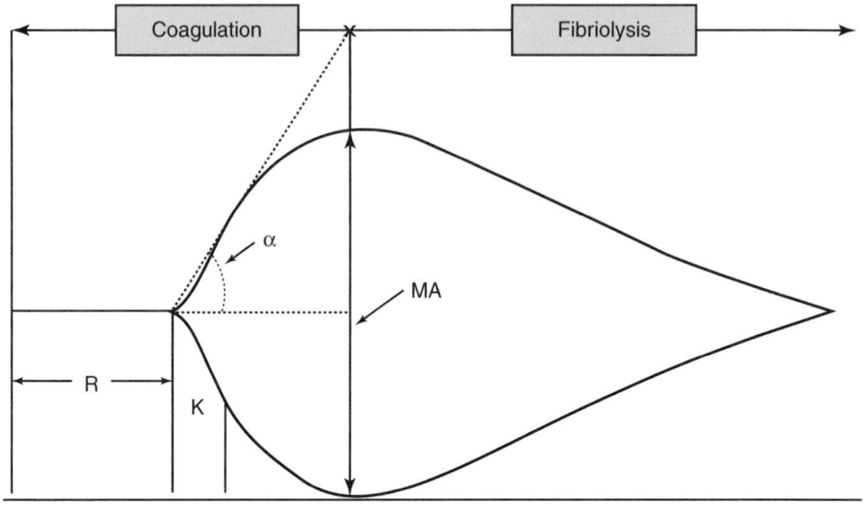

Fig. 5.9 Thromboelastography (TEG) tracing. R reaction time in seconds, K clot kinetics or time from R until the clot reaches 20 mm in seconds, α angular measurement from a tangent line drawn to the curve of the TEG tracing starting from the point of clot reaction time in degrees, MA maximum amplitude in millimeters. (Reprinted from Trapani [14]. With permission from Scientific Research)

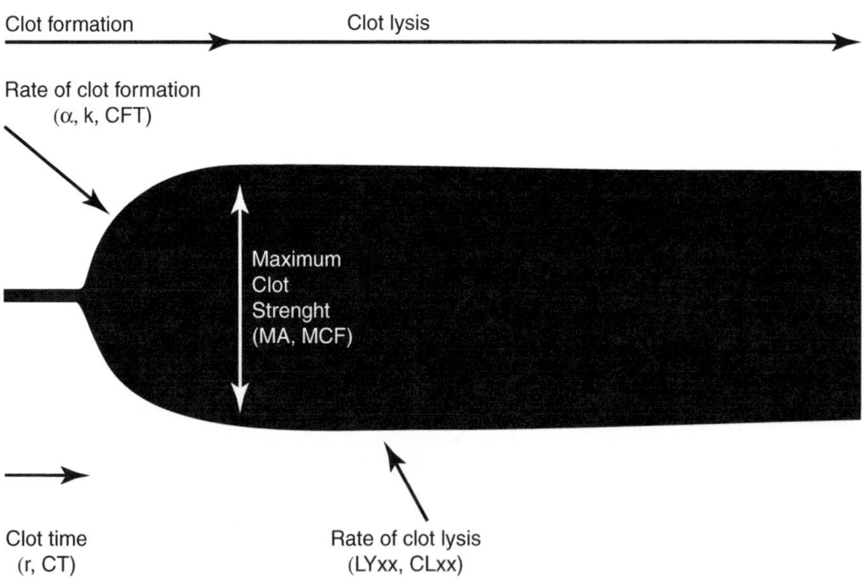

Fig. 5.10 Rotational thromboelastometry tracing. R reaction time in seconds, K clot kinetics or time from R until the clot reaches 20 mm in seconds, α angular measurement from a tangent line drawn to the curve of the TEG tracing starting from the point of clot reaction time in degrees, MA maximum amplitude in millimeters, CFT clot formation time, MCF maximal clot firmness, CT clot time. (Reprinted from Luddington [48]. With permission from Elsevier)

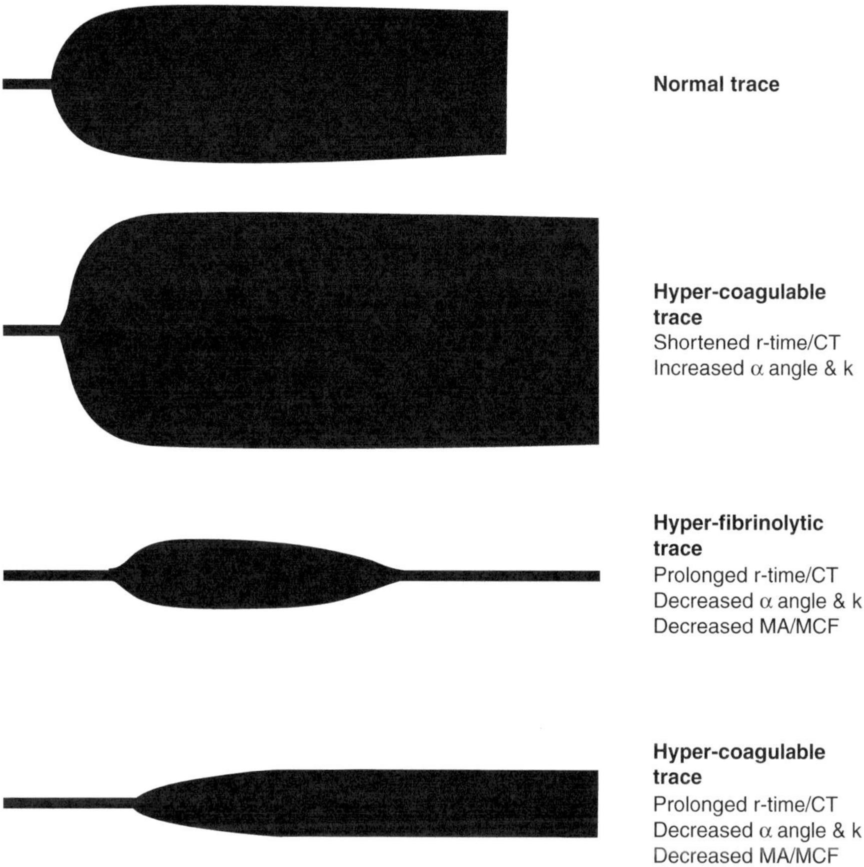

Fig. 5.11 Examples of abnormal rotational thromboelastometry tracings. R reaction time in seconds, K clot kinetics or time from R until the clot reaches 20 mm in seconds, α angular measurement from a tangent line drawn to the curve of the TEG tracing starting from the point of clot reaction time in degrees, MA maximum amplitude in millimeters, CFT clot formation time, MCF maximal clot firmness, CT clot time. (Reprinted from Luddington [48]. With permission from Elsevier)

Platelets play a key role in both hemostasis and thrombosis. An adequate number of platelets are required for hemostasis, but the minimum number is not clear. Equally important are adequately functioning platelets. A simple complete blood count (CBC) will usually give a good estimate of the number of platelets available. There are various types of platelet function tests, and they differ with regard to the underlying principle (static vs dynamic), agonists, and sample material used for testing. Dynamic tests (viscoelastic and agonist response) are more reflective of platelet function over time [15]. The first test of platelet function was the bleeding time, which was invasive, insensitive, and time-consuming but did not require expensive equipment. Platelet aggregometry is the gold standard and involves testing whole blood or platelet-rich plasma with a number of different agonists. It is still a widely used test, but it requires trained personnel, transport to a laboratory for processing, and, ideally, testing within 2 h of blood draw [16]. There are a number of newer platelet function tests with point-of-care capabilities such as the Platelet Function Analyzer (PFA-100®) (Siemens Healthcare, Marburg, Germany), VerifyNow ® system (Accriva Diagnostics, San Diego, CA), Plateletworks ® (Helena Laboratories, Beaumont, USA), TEG ® with Platelet Mapping ® Assay (TEG; Haemoscope, Niles, USA), and the Cone and Plate(let) Analyzer (Diamed, Cressier, Switzerland) [15]. The capability to perform rapid bedside platelet analysis enables the provider to initiate appropriate targeted therapy.

Lesson III-B: What Blood Products Should Be Administered?

Perioperative treatment of excessive bleeding involves the transfusion of red blood cells (RBC), fresh frozen plasma (FFP), cryoprecipitate, and platelets. In February 2015, the American Society of Anesthesiologists (ASA) Task Force on Perioperative Blood Management released guidelines for perioperative blood management [17]. A restrictive RBC transfusion strategy should be followed, but the determination of whether hemoglobin concentrations between 6 and 10 g/dl justify or require RBC transfusion should be based on potential or actual ongoing bleeding (rate and magnitude), intravascular volume status, signs of organ ischemia, and adequacy of cardiopulmonary reserve. RBC should be administered unit by unit with interval reassessment whenever possible.

FFP should be administered for correction of excessive microvascular bleeding in the presence of an INR greater than 2.0 in the absence of heparin. Transfusion of FFP is also appropriate for excessive microvascular bleeding secondary to coagulation factor deficiency in patients transfused with more than one blood volume (approximately 70 ml/kg) and when PT or INR and aPTT cannot be obtained in a timely fashion. Additionally, FFP should be transfused for urgent reversal of warfarin therapy when prothrombin complex concentrates (PCC) are not available and correction of known coagulation factor deficiencies for which specific concentrates are unavailable. FFP administration should be in doses calculated to achieve a minimum of 30% of plasma factor concentration. When possible, coagulation tests (PT, INR, aPTT) should be obtained prior to FFP transfusion.

Cryoprecipitate should be administered when a test of fibrinogen activity indicates a fibrinolysis, when the fibrinogen concentration is less than 80–100 mg/dl in the presence of excessive bleeding, and as an adjunct in massively transfused patients when fibrinogen concentrations cannot be measured in a timely fashion. Fibrinogen levels should be assessed prior to fibrinogen administration when possible.

Platelet transfusion may be indicated despite an apparently adequate platelet count or in the absence of a platelet count if there is known or suspected platelet dysfunction (presence of potent antiplatelet agents, cardiopulmonary bypass, congenital platelet dysfunction, and bleeding). When possible, a platelet count, and platelet function test if there is concern for platelet dysfunction (inherited, acquired, or drug-induced), should be obtained prior to transfusion.

Excessive bleeding may require pharmacologic treatment when blood product administration is insufficient to obtain hemostasis. Desmopressin 0.3 mcg/kg (in 50 mL of saline over 15–30 min) IV may be used in patients with excessive bleeding and platelet dysfunction. Improvement in bleeding is seen in 1 h and lasts for 4–8 h, but tachyphylaxis usually develops after the second dose. Consider topical hemostatics such as fibrin glue or thrombin gel. Use of antifibrinolytics (ε-aminocaproic acid, tranexamic acid) should be considered if fibrinolysis is documented or suspected and if these agents are not already being used. ε-Aminocaproic acid 4–5 g IV during the first hour may be used, followed by 1 g/h for 8 h or until the bleeding improves. Alternatively, tranexamic acid 1000 mg IV over 10 min may be used, followed by 1000 mg over the next 8 h. PCCs may be used in patients with excessive bleeding and increased INR. In four-factor PCC, or three-factor PCC if four-factor PCC is unavailable, 1500–2000 international units IV infused at 100 international units per minute may be given to target an INR less than 1.4. Vitamin K 10 mg IV infused at 1 mg per minute should also be given if PCC is administered for excessive bleeding with an elevated INR [18].

Lesson III-C: When Should Recombinant Factor VII Be Administered?

Recombinant factor VIIa (rFVIIa) is an initiator of thrombin generation FDA approved for use in individuals with hemophilia who have antibody inhibitors to coagulation factors VIII or IX, patients with acquired hemophilia, and those with congenital factor VII deficiency. Currently, there is no widely accepted guideline for off-label rFVIIa usage in bleeding patients. It is often used off-label as a rescue therapy when transfusion and other approaches to hemostasis have failed. There are anecdotal reports of the successful use of rFVIIa in patients with pulmonary hemorrhage following a variety of insults, including pneumonia, hematopoietic cell transplant, metastatic choriocarcinoma, and microscopic polyangiitis [19–23]. According to the ASA Task Force on Perioperative Blood Management, rFVIIa should be considered when traditional options for treating excessive bleeding due to coagulopathy have been exhausted. Dosing should be proportionate to the degree of hemostatic impairment and be given before hypothermia and acidosis impair effectiveness of the coagulation system. An initial dose of 90 mcg/kg IV may be appropriate if the patient is truly coagulopathic and the degree of impairment is severe, but few will present with the degree of impairment seen in hemophilia, and a lower dose should be considered.

Lesson IV: What Noninvasive Therapies Are Available to Treat Pulmonary Hemorrhage?

Lesson IV-A: What Ventilator Adjustments Can Be Made to Optimize Ventilation and Oxygenation?

PEEP is routinely used during mechanical ventilation to prevent end-expiratory alveolar collapse and may reduce the incidence of ventilator-associated pneumonia and lung injury. During instances of pulmonary hemorrhage, PEEP is a noninvasive treatment that can help tamponade the airway bleeding [2, 9]. The increased end-expiratory pressure can slow bleeding and prevent alveolar collapse thus improving ventilation and oxygenation. However, if airway pressure exceeds the pressure in the pulmonary vessel, air can enter the circulation leading to varying degrees of air embolism [9]. While the lung is usually a good filter for air, this function can be exhausted with increasing quantities of air. Lung protective ventilation strategies utilizing lower tidal volumes, increased PEEP, and inverse ratio ventilation can help in preventing further lung injury [24, 25].

Lesson IV-B: Should Topical Vasoconstrictors Be Administered to the Airway?

Topical vasoconstrictors can be given through the ETT or locally via the fiberoptic bronchoscope. Topical administration of vasopressin 20 mL (2 units per mL), phenylephrine 20 mL (100 mcg per mL), or epinephrine 20 mL (5 mcg per mL) may decrease blood flow to hemorrhagic blood vessels and help decrease airway bleeding [2]. Fiberoptic bronchoscopy can more precisely direct the vasoconstrictor administration and is the preferred method if available.

Lesson V: What Options Are Available for Endobronchial Lung Isolation?

Lesson V-A: What Is a Bronchial Blocker, and How Is It Useful During Pulmonary Hemorrhage?

A bronchial blocker is a device inserted through an ETT and into a mainstem or segmental bronchus to block distal ventilation. During pulmonary hemorrhage, they are used to isolate bleeding lung segments and prevent contamination of healthy lung areas. The use of bronchial blockers to provide lung isolation has grown in recent years, and it is the preferred technique for lung isolation during airway

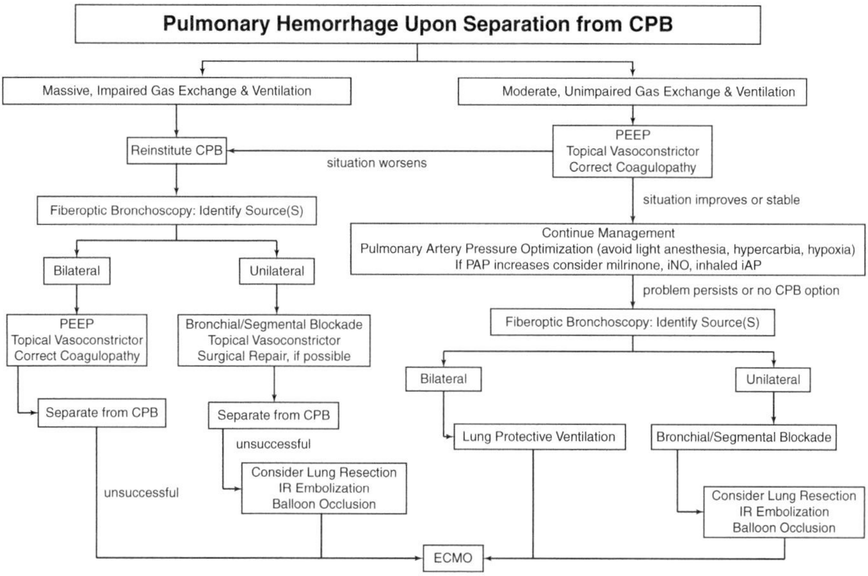

Fig. 5.12 A general algorithm for the approach to post-cardiopulmonary bypass (CPB) pulmonary hemorrhage [6]. PEEP positive end-expiratory pressure, iNO inhaled nitric oxide, iAP inhaled aerosolized prostacyclin, PAP positive airway pressure

bleeding [2, 8]. The two main goals during the management of pulmonary hemorrhage are to prevent exsanguination and to maintain adequate gas exchange. A general algorithm for the approach to post-cardiopulmonary bypass pulmonary hemorrhage is illustrated in Fig. 5.12. If adequate hemodynamic status and gas exchange can be maintained, previously discussed conservative management techniques consisting of ventilator maneuvers, topical vasoconstrictors, and correction of coagulopathies can be implemented [2]. When significant airway bleeding occurs, an attempt is made to isolate the bleeding segment to prevent spillage of blood into other segments, preserving further impairment of ventilation and oxygenation. If airway bleeding is recognized prior to separation from cardiopulmonary bypass, allowing the heart to briefly eject while directly visualizing the suspected bleeding area using fiberoptic bronchoscopy can identify the hemorrhagic location [8]. If not, cardiopulmonary bypass should be resumed, and the bleeding source must be identified via diagnostic bronchoscopy [2]. Lung isolation can be useful in unilateral bleeding, with segmental or lobar endobronchial blockade being ideal to preserve maximal lung parenchyma for gas exchange [3]. Using the largest single-lumen ETT facilitates easy passage and advancement of the blocker and flexible fiberoptic bronchoscope [26]. All bronchial blockers and the flexible fiberoptic bronchoscope need to be tested and liberally lubricated prior to insertion into the airway.

The specific features of the individual bronchial blockers in current use may impact the relative utility of using one of these devices (Table 5.3). The bronchial blockers currently receiving the greatest usage are the Arndt Endobronchial Blocker (Cook, Bloomington, IN), the Cohen Flexitip (Cook, Bloomington, IN), the Uniblocker (Fuji Systems, Tokyo, Japan), and the Rusch EZ-Blocker (Teleflex Medical Incorporated, Research Triangle Park, NC) (Fig. 5.13) [27]. The adult size is

Table 5.3 Specifications of commonly used bronchial blockers. SLET, single-lumen endotracheal tube

	Arndt blocker	Cohen blocker	Fuji uniblocker	EZ-blocker
Size	5F, 7F, and 9F	9F	4.5F, 9F	7F
Balloon shape	Spherical or elliptical	Spherical	Spherical	Spherical × 2
Guidance mechanism	Nylon wire loop that is coupled with the fiberoptic bronchoscope	Wheel device to deflect the tip	None, preshaped tip	None
Smallest recommended *SLET for coaxial use	5F (4.5 SLET), 7F (7.0 SLET), 9F (8.0 SLET)	9F (8.0 SLET)	9F (8.0 SLET)	7.5
Murphy eye	Present in 9F	Present	Not present	Not present
Central Channel	1.4 mm internal diameter	1.6 mm internal diameter	2.0 mm internal diameter	1.4 mm internal diameter

Based on data from Ref. [26]

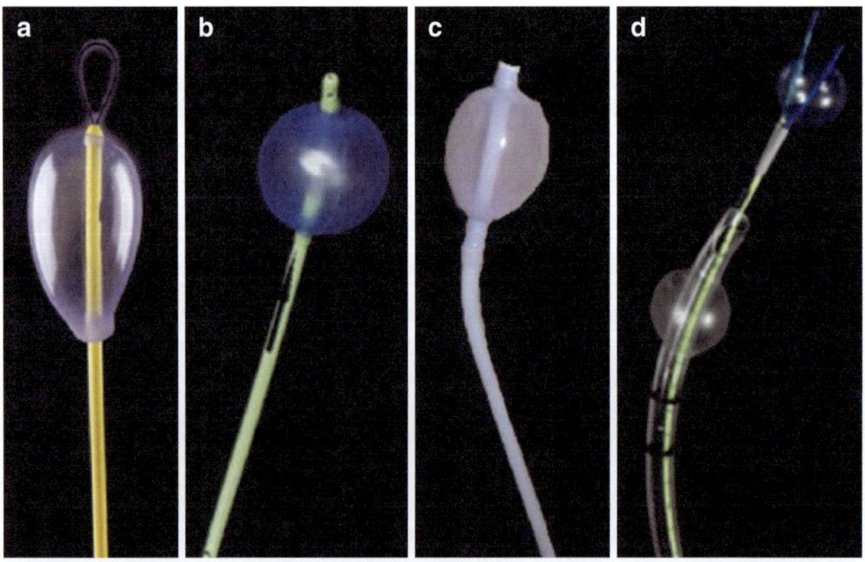

Fig. 5.13 Commonly used bronchial blockers. (**a**) The distal tip of an Arndt Blocker. (**b**) The Cohen Flexitip Blocker. (**c**) The Fuji Uniblocker. (**d**) The EZ-Blocker with a bifurcated distal tip with a balloon in each end, through a single-lumen endotracheal tube. (Reprinted from Campos [26]. With permission from Javier H. Campos)

9 Fr for all bronchial blockers, but the EZ-Blocker only comes in 7 Fr. The Arndt Blocker requires multiple steps for proper placement making it somewhat cumbersome to use. A disadvantage of the Arndt Blocker is the distal tip of the blocker is not seen when the guide wire is coupled with the fiberoptic bronchoscope because the fiberoptic bronchoscope is emerging farther than the tip of the blocker. The Cohen Flexitip has a wheel at the operator end that, when turned, flexes the tip toward an arrow inscribed near the blocker tip. The Uniblocker comes preinserted through a multiport connector and has a bent tip that is simply turned toward the side to be blocked. The EZ-Blocker has a Y-shaped distal end with one blocker for each bronchus giving it the advantage of being able to be placed blindly if a fiberoptic bronchoscope is not available or if visualization proves difficult. The tip of the Cohen, Fuji Uniblocker, and EZ-Blocker can be observed and deflected into a desired target bronchus during bronchial blocker passage through the single-lumen ETT while using the fiberoptic bronchoscope [27].

For a right mainstem bronchus blockade, all blockers can be advanced independently, and confirmation on the entrance into the right mainstem bronchus is done with fiberoptic visualization. Optimal placement in the right bronchus is achieved when the outer surface of the blocker's balloon is seen with the fiberoptic bronchoscope at least 1 cm below the tracheal carina in the right bronchus, and a proper seal is obtained when the balloon is inflated with air (Fig. 5.14). For a left-sided mainstem bronchus blockade, the Arndt Blocker has the advantage of coupling with the fiberoptic bronchoscope via the guide wire to direct the blocker into the left bronchus entrance. For the other blockers (Cohen Flexitip, Fuji Uniblocker, and EZ-Blocker), turning the patient's head to the right and twisting the torque part of the blocker facilitate insertion into the left bronchus. The optimal position in the left bronchus is achieved when the outer surface of the blocker's balloon is seen with the fiberoptic bronchoscope at least 1 cm below the tracheal carina in the left bronchus, and a proper seal is obtained when the balloon is inflated with air. Optimal position for selective segmental bronchial blockade may be accomplished using similar techniques as described above [3]. The major complication arising from bronchial blocker use during pulmonary hemorrhage pertains to malposition from dislodgement [26].

Lesson V-B: What Is a Double-Lumen Endobronchial Tube, and How Is It Useful During Pulmonary Hemorrhage?

A double-lumen endobronchial tube (DLT) is a large tube constructed with two lumens of unequal length fixed side by side. The shorter tube ends above the carina in the trachea, while the longer tube is placed in either the left or right mainstem bronchus to selectively isolate and ventilate the patient's lungs. Lung isolation is essential for the successful management of pulmonary hemorrhage. When uncontrolled unilateral airway bleeding begins to encroach on the contralateral lung, placement of a DLT may be warranted. DLTs can be safely, easily, quickly, and accurately placed to provide the necessary lung isolation to facilitate the control of pulmonary hemorrhage. The large lumens of a DLT allow either lung to be

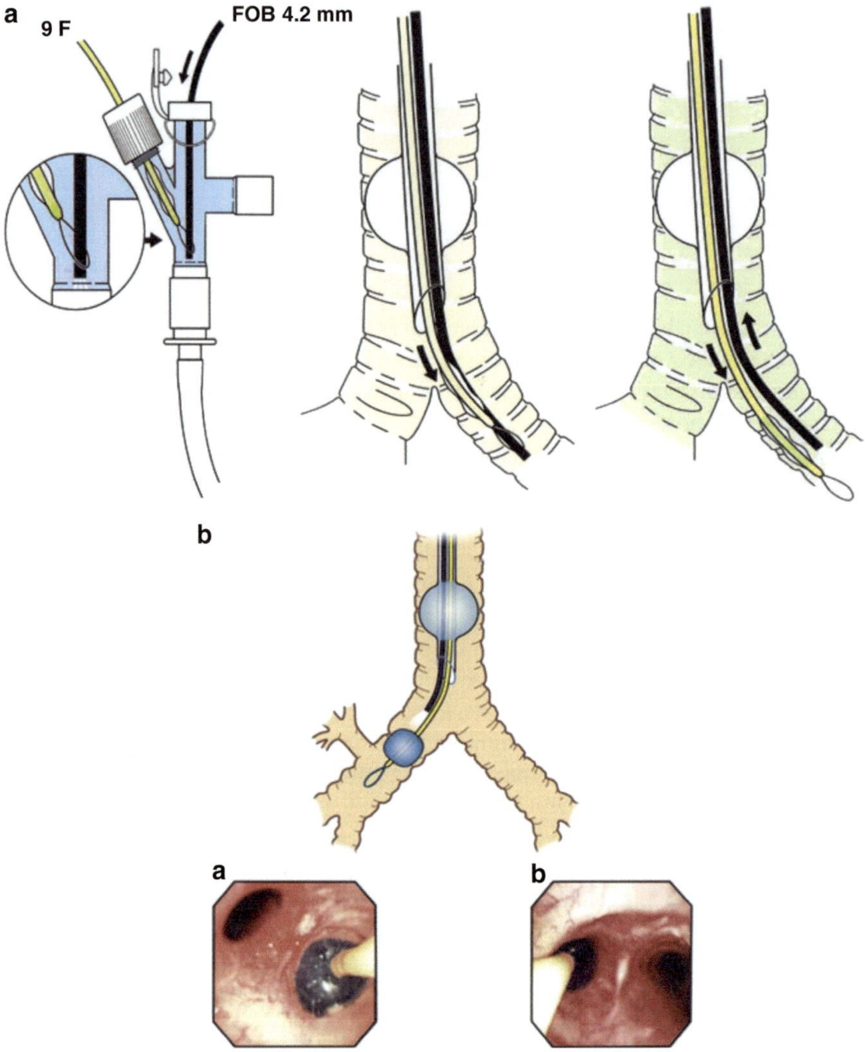

Fig. 5.14 Schematic for bronchial blockade using the Arndt Blocker. (**a**) Placement of an Arndt Blocker through a single-lumen endotracheal tube with the fiberoptic bronchoscope advanced through the guide wire loop. (**b**) Optimal position of a bronchial blocker in the right or left mainstem bronchus as seen with a fiberoptic bronchoscope. (**a**) Right mainstem blocker. (**b**) Left mainstem blocker. (Reprinted from Campos [49]. With permission from Medpharm Publications (Pty) Ltd.)

suctioned at any time during the procedure without interrupting ventilation to the nonoperated lung, albeit with a smaller (pediatric/intubating) fiberoptic bronchoscope [28]. DLTs have the disadvantages of not allowing placement of a large bronchoscope with superior suction capabilities, potential placement difficulty in the setting of a bleeding airway, and safety concerns about exchanging it with a single-lumen tube at the conclusion of the procedure [8].

Table 5.4 Selection of double-lumen tube size based on sex and height

Sex	Height (cm)	DLT size (Fr)
Male	>170	41
	160–170	39
	<160	37 or 39
Female	>160	37
	150–160	35
	<160	32 or 35

Based on data from Ref. [29]

Table 5.5 Selection of double-lumen tube size based on bronchial diameter

		Left bronchial lumen outer diameters from four manufacturers (mm)			
Measured bronchial diameter (mm)	DLT size (Fr)	Mallinckrodt (St. Louis, MO)	Rusch (Duluth, GA)	Sheridan (Argyle, NY)	Portex (Keene, NH)
≥ 12	41	10.6	11.5	10.7	12.0
12	39	10.1	10.8	9.9	11.2
11	37	10.0	10.1	9.9	10.2
10	35	9.5	9.4	9.3	9.7

Based on data from Ref. [30]

Various algorithms based on patient gender and height, or radiologically measured bronchial size, have been proposed for choosing the appropriate sized tube, but there is no consensus on the best method (Tables 5.4 and 5.5). Clinically, an appropriate size DLT should result in an air leak when the bronchial cuff is deflated but be airtight when the cuff is inflated with a volume of less than 3 mL [30].

It is more common to place a DLT into the left mainstem bronchus, as it is longer than the right mainstem bronchus, creating a greater margin of safety (Fig. 5.15) [31]. DLTs are specifically designed for use on either the right or left, and care should be taken to assure the correct "side" DLT is used for the intended endobronchial intubation. Under direct laryngoscopy, the endobronchial tip is inserted through the vocal cords, the stylet removed, and the left DLT rotated 90 degrees counterclockwise while being advanced. Fiberoptic bronchoscopy can guide initial placement of DLTs; however, a blind insertion technique is more commonly used, with fiberoptic confirmation of the proper placement following [32]. Regardless of insertion method, the routine use of fiberoptic bronchoscopy to confirm optimal left DLT placement is recommended and mandatory for right DLT placement [4]. The optimal placement for a left DLT is with the tube inserted, so the upper edge of the bronchial cuff is 1 cm beyond the carina in the left mainstem bronchus (Fig. 5.16). The optimal placement for a right DLT is with the tube inserted, so the bronchial side orifice of the DLT is aligned with the right upper lobe bronchus (Fig. 5.17) [33]. The major complications related to DLT use during pulmonary hemorrhage pertain to malposition. Traumatic laryngitis can occur, while tracheobronchial tree disruption is rare.

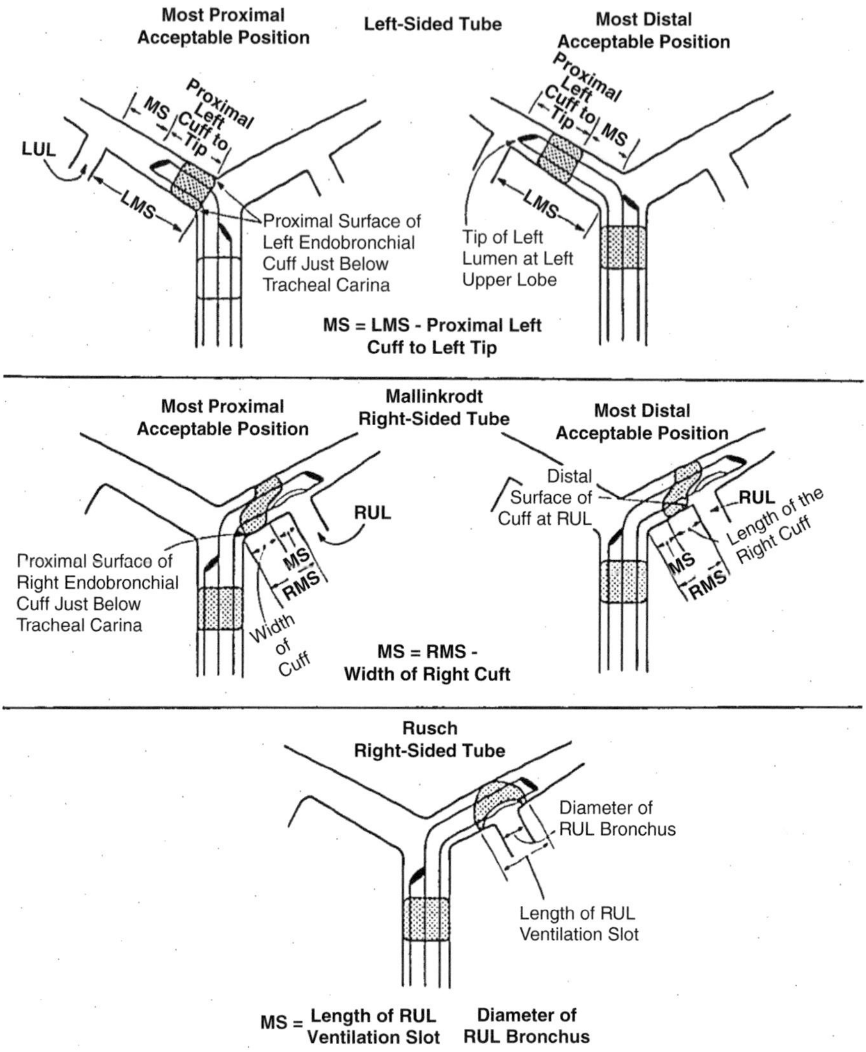

Fig. 5.15 Margin of safety in positioning left- and right-sided DLTs [8]. LMS length left mainstem bronchus, RMS length right mainstem bronchus, MS margin of safety, LUL left upper lobe, RUL right upper lobe. (Reprinted from Benumof et al. [31]. With permission from Wolters Kluwer Health)

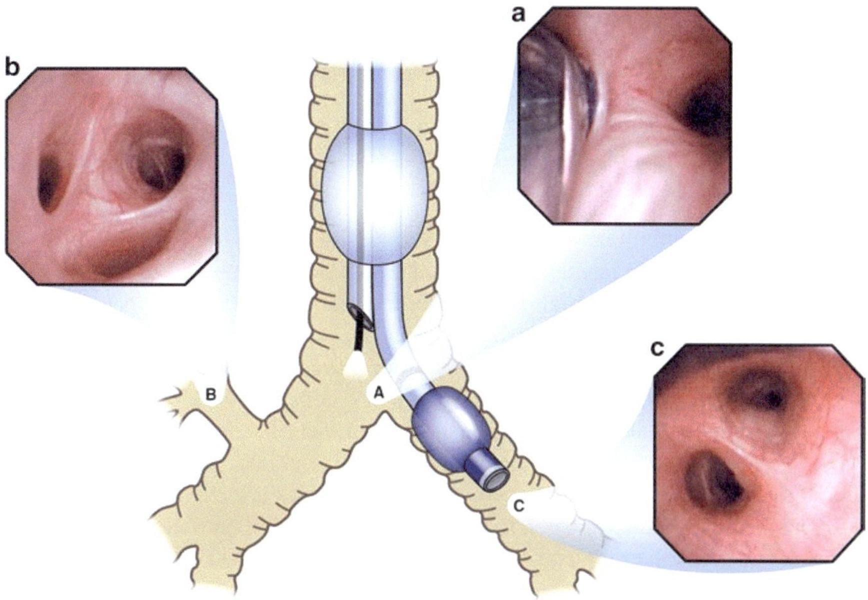

Fig. 5.16 Optimal position of left double-lumen tube in left mainstem bronchus. (**a**) View from the tracheal lumen of the unobstructed entrance of the right mainstem bronchus. (**b**) View from the tracheal lumen of the right-upper bronchus. (**c**) View from the bronchial lumen of the left-upper (above) and left-lower (below) lobe bronchi. (Modified from Campos [33]. With permission from Elsevier)

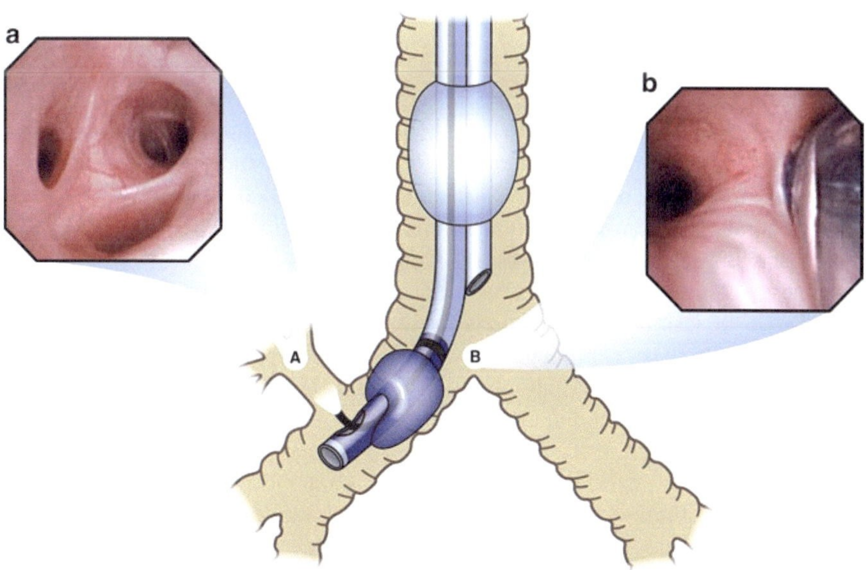

Fig. 5.17 Optimal position of right double-lumen tube in right mainstem bronchus. (**a**) The view of the right upper lobe through the ventilating side slot of the bronchial lumen. (**b**) The view from the tracheal lumen of the main carina with the bronchial lumen in the right mainstem bronchus. (Modified from Campos [33]. With permission from Elsevier)

Lesson VI: What Invasive Therapies Are Available to Treat Pulmonary Hemorrhage?

Lesson VI-A: What Catheter-Based Interventions Are Available to Treat Pulmonary Hemorrhage?

Bronchial artery embolization (BAE) is a very useful adjunct in the management of massive pulmonary hemorrhage. It is based on the principle that most massive airway bleeding is from the high-pressure bronchial arterial circulation and rarely from the low-pressure pulmonary artery circulation [34]. When unilateral pulmonary hemorrhage becomes uncontrolled despite sufficient attempts at lung isolation with a bronchial blocker or DLT, BAE should be considered. BAE offers a minimally invasive procedure serving as first-line treatment for hemorrhage as well as providing a bridge to more definitive medical or surgical intervention focused upon the etiology of the hemorrhage [35]. Various materials are capable of achieving vascular occlusion such as gel foams, polyvinyl alcohol particles, and microspheres. Coil embolization can be utilized for large, high-flow bronchial arteries. Lesson I-C discusses the pulmonary and bronchial circulation in detail. Complications from BAE are rare and minor. They include complications at femoral access sites (pseudoaneurysms, intimal dissection), small risk of stroke caused by embolization (this has become less common with super-selective embolization), and the risk of rebleeding [34]. The risk of rebleeding is dependent on the airway bleeding etiology and the extent of embolization. Rebleeding is thought to occur due to the development of collaterals, perfusing distributaries, or continuing inflammation.

Selective, temporary balloon occlusion of a pulmonary artery is another catheter-based technique used during the management of massive pulmonary hemorrhage. Temporary balloon occlusion can be employed if surgical resection is too risky or as an adjunct to other therapies. Pulmonary infarction rarely occurs after complete obstruction of a major pulmonary artery branch, as the lung receives dual blood supply from the pulmonary artery and from the descending aorta via the bronchial arteries, which is discussed in Lesson I-C. Advantages of an intravascular technique include concurrently being able to perform a diagnostic angiography (if the lesion is not positively localized by bronchoscopy) and avoidance of reopening the chest, if bronchoscopy reveals no recurrence of hemorrhage after careful reestablishment of pulmonary circulation to the affected lung [36]. A potential catastrophic complication is the potential pulmonary artery rupture, and the risk for this is high in the immediate postoperative setting [9, 37]. The use of selective, temporary balloon occlusion of a pulmonary artery requires one-lung ventilation to minimize ventilation of dead space. If one-lung ventilation is unable to sustain adequate oxygenation and ventilation, another therapy must be investigated.

Lesson VI-B: What Surgical Interventions Are Available to Treat Massive Pulmonary Hemorrhage?

Surgical interventions for the treatment of massive pulmonary hemorrhage include banding, temporary clamping, embolization of a branch pulmonary artery, and lung resection. Banding requires circumferential dissection and looping of the vessel. The vascular supply is cut off leading to an area of dead space ventilation. Absorbable pulmonary artery banding is a useful technique that can be used when high pulmonary blood flow must be limited, such as in cases of massive pulmonary hemorrhage, but when the natural history of the underlying lesion is one of resolution [38]. The band is gradually absorbed with time so the pulmonary artery constriction either resolves spontaneously or can be easily treated by balloon angioplasty. The bands lose their tensile strength after only a few weeks, although the materials themselves may remain present in a weakened form for up to 3 months. A potential complication of the absorbable pulmonary artery band is it may act as a nidus for scar formation and the scar tissue could maintain the hemodynamic effect of the band, long after the material itself has been absorbed.

Temporary clamping creates a quickly reversible hemostatic environment similar to banding. A clamp is placed over a branch pulmonary artery supplying the area of hemorrhage. The temporary clamping provides hemostasis, allowing time for further interventions, and itself can be therapeutic [39]. The only potential disadvantage of temporary clamping is the chance of acute lung infarction and PA branch stenosis. A downside to this technique is that it requires the chest to be surgically open for it to be utilized.

Direct surgical embolization is a novel technique for management of massive pulmonary hemorrhage. A selective pulmonary artery branch can be sealed with a hemostatic agent (Surgicel) [40]. Surgicel is a bioabsorbable hemostatic mesh believed to promote coagulation physically, rather than by altering the physiological clotting mechanism. Absorption commences within 24 h, and the rate depends on the amount of material used, the degree of local blood flow, and the tissue bed itself. There were no reported complications with the described technique but also no reported long-term follow-up.

Lung resection is a curative treatment for massive pulmonary hemorrhage but results in permanent loss of the pulmonary bronchovascular bed. Historically, pulmonary resection has been the most effective method to control and prevent recurrent bleeding [41]. The criteria of eligibility for surgery differ among institutions and seem to be subject to surgical or institutional bias. Relative contraindications to surgery include severe underlying pulmonary disease, active TB, diffuse underlying lung disease (cystic fibrosis, multiple arteriovenous malformations, multifocal bronchiectasis), and diffuse alveolar hemorrhage. Bronchopleural fistulas and infection are the primary complications associated with lung resections for pulmonary hemorrhage.

Lesson VI-C: What Is Extracorporeal Membrane Oxygenation, and How Is It Useful During Pulmonary Hemorrhage?

Extracorporeal membrane oxygenation (ECMO) is an extracorporeal technique providing respiratory and cardiac support to facilitate adequate gas exchange during a potentially reversible acute, severe cardiac or pulmonary failure unresponsive to conventional management. Intraoperative thoracic surgical catastrophes, such as massive pulmonary hemorrhage, may require extracorporeal circulation modes to support the patient, while the appropriate repair is made. Regardless of the physical environment where the emergency occurs, a multidisciplinary team approach is crucial for the successful management of pulmonary hemorrhage [42].

There are several forms of ECMO, the two most common being veno-venous (VV) and venoarterial (VA). Being knowledgeable about the capabilities and differences between cardiopulmonary bypass, VA ECMO, and VV ECMO can guide rapid intraoperative decisions under stressful conditions and greatly benefit patients [37, 43, 44]. In both VV and VA ECMO, blood is drained from the venous system and oxygenated outside the body (Figs. 5.18 and 5.19) [42]. Anticoagulation is required but less than what is necessary for cardiopulmonary bypass. In VV ECMO, blood is returned to the venous side of the heart, usually via the internal jugular vein or right atrium. A single-site, dual-lumen catheter, such as the Avalon Elite ® bicaval dual-lumen ECMO cannula, is available for insertion into the right internal jugular vein, for drainage via the superior and inferior vena cava and return to the right atrium (Fig. 5.18a) [45]. A dual-site, utilizing single-lumen catheter such as in Fig. 5.18b is also possible. VV ECMO is an invaluable tool in cases of massive pulmonary hemorrhage with oxygenation and ventilation disturbances refractory to the previously mentioned techniques [34]. VV ECMO has been successfully used without anticoagulation, which is beneficial during a pulmonary hemorrhage given heparin can impair hemostasis, contributing to airway bleeding [46]. In VA ECMO, blood is returned to the arterial system via the femoral artery or ascending aorta if cardiopulmonary bypass has already been established (Figs. 5.19 and 5.20). Active venting of the pulmonary vascular bed during VA ECMO can improve the surgical field and minimize airway bleeding during placement of lung isolation devices (Fig. 5.20) [42]. If the oxygenation and ventilatory issues are combined with a concurrent hemodynamic impairment, VA ECMO can provide assistance to both problems simultaneously.

Relative contraindications for ECMO pertain to medical futility, conditions incompatible with a meaningful life after recovery, and pre-existing conditions severely affecting quality of life. Complications from ECMO include neurologic injury (ischemic, hemorrhagic, and embolic), bleeding, hemolysis, infection, systemic and pulmonary thromboembolism, heparin-induced thrombocytopenia, and vascular injury from cannula insertion [34].

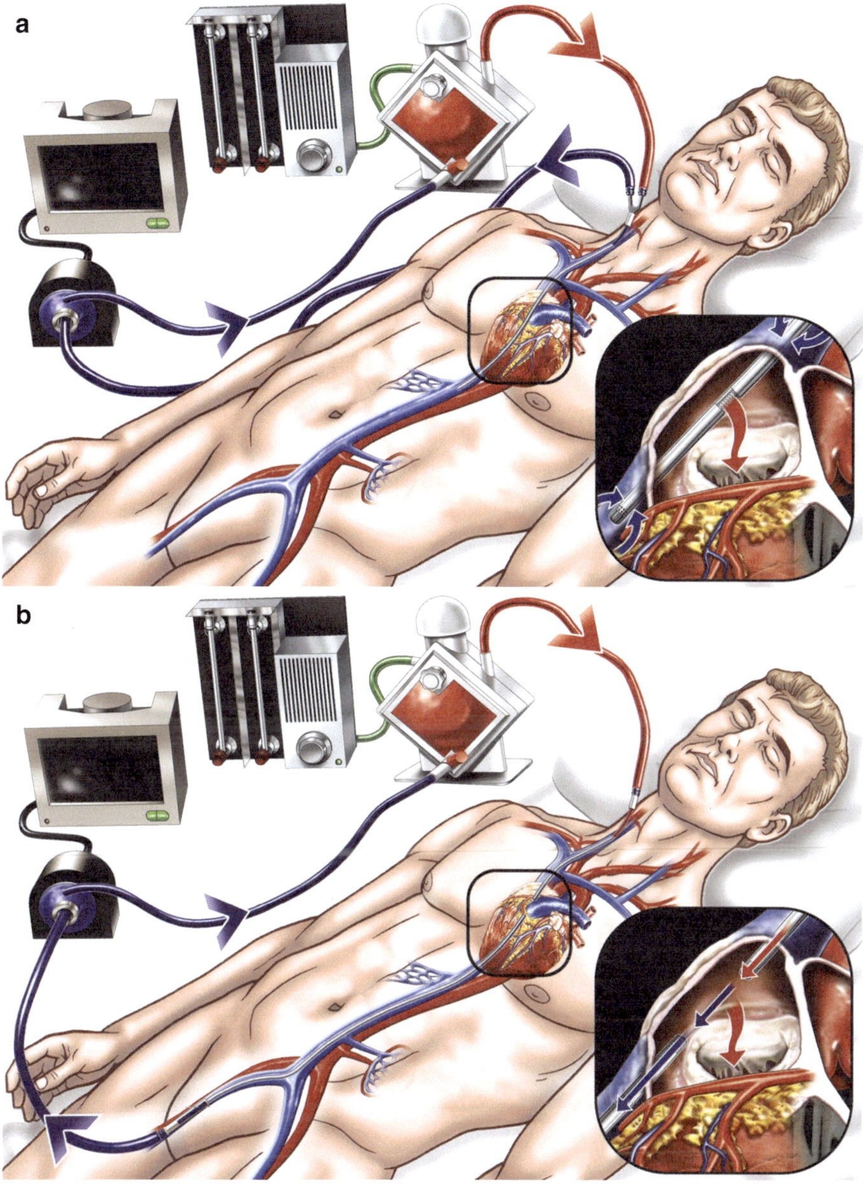

Fig. 5.18 Veno-venous extracorporeal membrane oxygenation (VV-ECMO) circuit. (**a**) Single-site setup with single dual-lumen bicaval cannula. (**b**) Dual-site setup using two single-lumen cannulas. (Reprinted from Abrams et al. [45]. With permission from Elsevier)

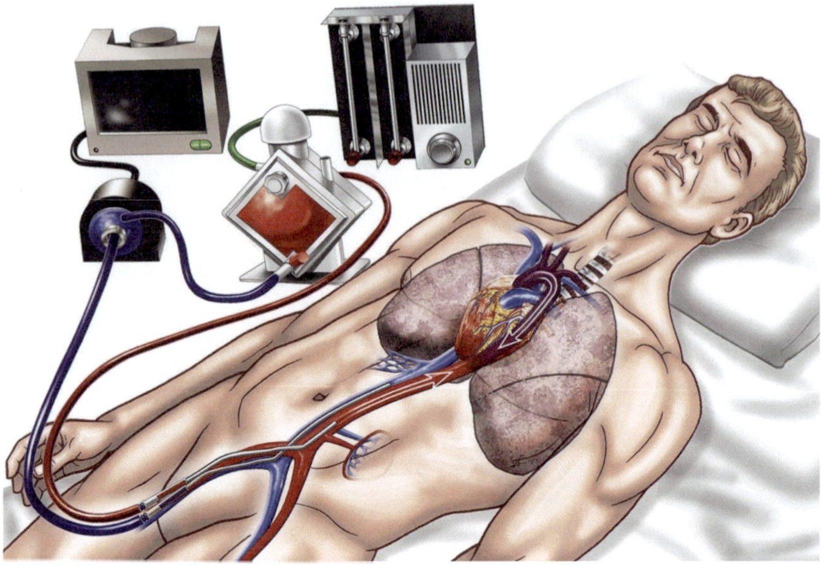

Fig. 5.19 Femoral venoarterial extracorporeal membrane oxygenation. (Reprinted from Abrams et al. [45]. With permission from Elsevier)

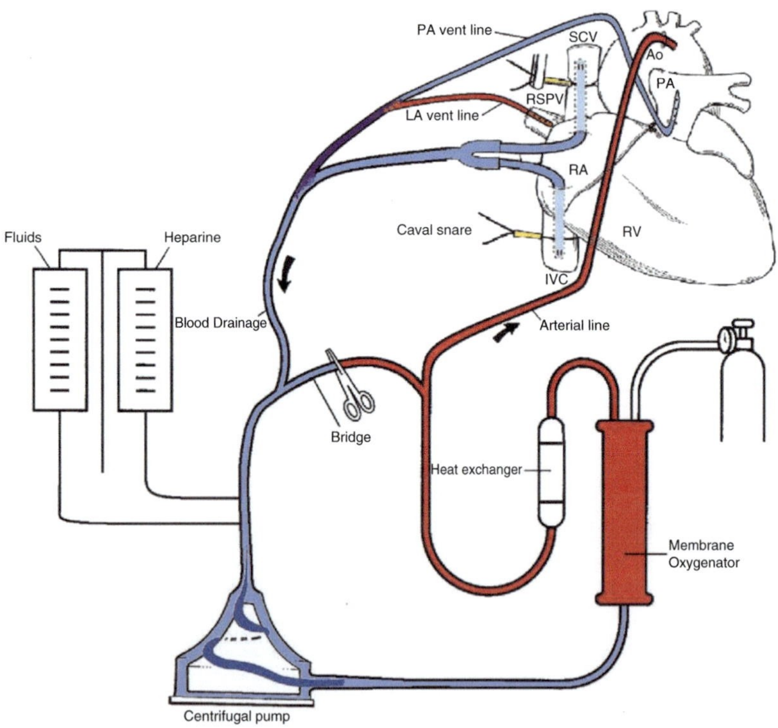

Fig. 5.20 Venoarterial extracorporeal membrane oxygenation circuit with active venting of pulmonary vascular bed. (Reprinted from Pretorius et al. [42]. With permission from Elsevier)

Conclusion

Pulmonary hemorrhage is rare, but it does occur during certain surgeries, and severe cases can be life-threatening. The management of pulmonary hemorrhage is challenging, often requiring advanced techniques and equipment. This chapter discussed a case of massive pulmonary hemorrhage following cardiopulmonary bypass in a patient undergoing pulmonary thromboendarterectomy. Rapid diagnosis and identification of the bleeding source are crucial to successful management of pulmonary hemorrhage. Physiologic perturbations can create a challenging situation where immediate action is required in multiple domains. Management of a coagulopathy is often critical during treatment of pulmonary hemorrhage. Various therapies, ranging from noninvasive to invasive, may be required to successfully and safely manage a patient with pulmonary hemorrhage.

References

1. Manecke GR Jr. Pulmonary hemorrhage. In: Nina Singh-Radcliff M, editor. The 5-minute anesthesia consult. Philadelphia: Lippincott Williams & Wilkins; 2012. p. 742–51.
2. Manecke GR Jr, Kotzur A, Atkins G, Fedullo PF, Auger WR, Kapelanski DP, Jamieson SW. Massive pulmonary hemorrhage after pulmonary thromboendarterectomy. Anesth Analg. 2004;99:672–5.
3. Campos JH. Update on selective lobar blockade during pulmonary resections. Curr Opin Anaesthesiol. 2009;22:18–22.
4. Campos JH. Update on tracheobronchial anatomy and flexible fiberoptic bronchoscopy in thoracic anesthesia. Curr Opin Anaesthesiol. 2009;22:4–10.
5. Tamul PC, Ault ML. Respiratory function in anesthesia. In: Barash PG, editor. Clinical anesthesia. 7th ed. Philadelphia: Wolters Kluwer Health/Lippincott Williams & Wilkins; 2013. p. 264–85.
6. Minnich DJ, Mathisen DJ. Anatomy of the trachea, carina, and bronchi. Thorac Surg Clin. 2007;17:571–85.
7. Eisenkraft JB, Cohen E, Neustein SM. Anesthesia for thoracic surgery. In: Barash PG, editor. Clinical anesthesia. 7 ed. Philadelphia: Wolters Kluwer Health/Lippincott Williams & Wilkins; 2013. p. 1030–71.
8. Banks DA, Pretorius GV, Kerr KM, Manecke GR. Pulmonary endarterectomy: part II. Operation, anesthetic management, and postoperative care. Semin Cardiothorac Vasc Anesth. 2014;18:331 40.
9. Stratmann G, Benumof JL. Endobronchial hemorrhage due to pulmonary circulation tear: separating the lungs and the air from the blood. Anesth Analg. 2004;99:1276–9.
10. Arney KL, Judson MA, Sahn SA. Airway obstruction arising from blood clot: three reports and a review of the literature. Chest. 1999;115:293–300.
11. Hoffman M, Monroe DM. Coagulation 2006: a modern view of hemostasis. Hematol Oncol Clin North Am. 2007;21:1–11.
12. Hoffman M, Monroe DM 3rd. A cell-based model of hemostasis. Thromb Haemost. 2001;85:958–65.
13. Martlew VJ. Peri-operative management of patients with coagulation disorders. Br J Anaesth. 2000;85:446–55.
14. Trapani LM. Thromboelastography: current applications, future directions. Open J Anesthesiol. 2013;03:23–7.
15. Enriquez LJ, Shore-Lesserson L. Point-of-care coagulation testing and transfusion algorithms. Br J Anaesth. 2009;103(Suppl 1):i14–22.

16. Smart S, Aragola S, Hutton P. Antiplatelet agents and anaesthesia. Contin Educ Anaesth, Crit Care Pain. 2007;7:157–61.
17. Practice guidelines for perioperative blood management an updated report by the American Society of Anesthesiologists Task Force on Perioperative Blood Management. Anesthesiology 2015;122:241–75.
18. Ageno W, Gallus AS, Wittkowsky A, Crowther M, Hylek EM, Palareti G. Oral anticoagulant therapy: antithrombotic therapy and prevention of thrombosis, 9th ed: American College of Chest Physicians evidence-based clinical practice guidelines. Chest. 2012;141:e44S–88S.
19. Betensley AD, Yankaskas JR. Factor viia for alveolar hemorrhage in microscopic polyangiitis. Am J Respir Crit Care Med. 2002;166:1291–2.
20. Macdonald JA, Fraser JF, Foot CL, Tran K. Successful use of recombinant factor VII in massive hemoptysis due to community-acquired pneumonia. Chest. 2006;130:577–9.
21. Pastores SM, Papadopoulos E, Voigt L, Halpern NA. Diffuse alveolar hemorrhage after allogeneic hematopoietic stem-cell transplantation: treatment with recombinant factor VIIa. Chest. 2003;124:2400–3.
22. Shenoy A, Savani BN, Barrett AJ. Recombinant factor VIIa to treat diffuse alveolar hemorrhage following allogeneic stem cell transplantation. Biol Blood Marrow Transplant: J Am Soc Blood Marrow Transplant. 2007;13:622–3.
23. Wheater MJ, Mead GM, Bhandari S, Fennell J. Recombinant factor VIIa in the management of pulmonary hemorrhage associated with metastatic choriocarcinoma. J Clin Oncol Off J Am Soc Clin Oncol. 2008;26:1008–10.
24. Gajic O, Dara SI, Mendez JL, Adesanya AO, Festic E, Caples SM, Rana R, St Sauver JL, Lymp JF, Afessa B, Hubmayr RD. Ventilator-associated lung injury in patients without acute lung injury at the onset of mechanical ventilation. Crit Care Med. 2004;32:1817–24.
25. Manecke G, Banks D, Madani M, Jamieson S. Anesthesia for pulmonary thromboendarterectomy. In: Slinger MDFP, editor. Principles and practice of anesthesia for thoracic surgery. New York: Springer; 2011. p. 537–48.
26. Campos JH. An update on the use of bronchial blockers. Paper presented at the Society of Cardiovascular Anesthesiologists Conference on thoracic anesthesia Miami Beach, FL. 2013.
27. Neustein SM. Pro: bronchial blockers should be used routinely for providing one-lung ventilation. J Cardiothorac Vasc Anesth. 2015;29:234–6.
28. Brodsky JB. Con: a bronchial blocker is not a substitute for a double-lumen endobronchial tube. J Cardiothorac Vasc Anesth. 2015;29:237–9.
29. Slinger P. Con: the new bronchial blockers are not preferable to double-lumen tubes for lung isolation. J Cardiothorac Vasc Anesth. 2008;22:925–9.
30. Hannallah M, Benumof JL, Silverman PM, Kelly LC, Lea D. Evaluation of an approach to choosing a left double-lumen tube size based on chest computed tomographic scan measurement of left mainstem bronchial diameter. J Cardiothorac Vasc Anesth. 1997;11:168–71.
31. Benumof JL, Partridge BL, Salvatierra C, Keating J. Margin of safety in positioning modern double-lumen endotracheal tubes. Anesthesiology. 1987;67:729–38.
32. Russell WJ. A logical approach to the selection and insertion of double-lumen tubes. Curr Opin Anaesthesiol. 2008;21:37–40.
33. Campos JH. Progress in lung separation. Thorac Surg Clin. 2005;15:71–83.
34. Yendamuri S. Massive airway hemorrhage. Thorac Surg Clin. 2015;25:255–60.
35. Sopko DR, Smith TP. Bronchial artery embolization for hemoptysis. Semin Interv Radiol. 2011;28:48–62.
36. Dopfmer UR, Braun JP, Grosse J, Hotz H, Duveneck K, Schneider MB. Treatment of severe pulmonary hemorrhage after cardiopulmonary bypass by selective, temporary balloon occlusion. Anesth Analg. 2004;99:1280–2.
37. Yildizeli B, Arslan O, Tas S, Eldem B, Aksoy E, Kocak T, Sunar H. Management of massive pulmonary hemorrhage following pulmonary endarterectomy. Thorac Cardiovasc Surg. 2014;62:89–91.
38. Peek GJ, Arsiwala SS, Chan KC, Hickey MSJ. Absorbable pulmonary artery band. Ann Thorac Surg. 1997;64:539–41.

39. Reddy S, Rajanbabu BB, Kumar NK, Rajani I. Temporary clamping of branch pulmonary artery for pulmonary hemorrhage after endarterectomy. Ann Thorac Surg. 2013;96:1459–61.
40. Shetty DP, Nair HC, Shetty V, Punnen J. A novel treatment for pulmonary hemorrhage during thromboendarterectomy surgery. Ann Thorac Surg. 2015;99:e77–8.
41. Bussières JS. Massive hemoptysis. In: Slinger P, editor. Principles and practice of anesthesia for thoracic surgery. New York: Springer; 2011. p. 485–96.
42. Pretorius V, Alayadhi W, Modry D. Extracorporeal life support for the control of life-threatening pulmonary hemorrhage. Ann Thorac Surg. 2009;88:649–50.
43. Machuca TN, Cypel M, Keshavjee S. Cardiopulmonary bypass and extracorporeal life support for emergent intraoperative thoracic situations. Thorac Surg Clin. 2015;25:325–34.
44. Kim NH, Delcroix M, Jenkins DP, Channick R, Dartevelle P, Jansa P, Lang I, Madani MM, Ogino H, Pengo V, Mayer E. Chronic thromboembolic pulmonary hypertension. J Am Coll Cardiol. 2013;62:D92–9.
45. Abrams D, Combes A, Brodie D. Extracorporeal membrane oxygenation in cardiopulmonary disease in adults. J Am Coll Cardiol. 2014;63:2769–78.
46. Cronin B, Maus T, Pretorius V, Nguyen L, Johnson D, Ovando J, Auger W, Madani M, Jamieson S, Banks D, Minhaj M, Esper SA, Welsby IJ. Case 13—2014: management of pulmonary hemorrhage after pulmonary endarterectomy with venovenous extracorporeal membrane oxygenation without systemic anticoagulation. J Cardiothorac Vasc Anesth. 2014;28:1667–76.
47. Cloutier MM, Thrall RS. Structure and function of the respiratory system. In: Koeppen BM, Stanton BA, editors. Berne and Levy physiology. 6th ed. Philadelphia: Mosby; 2010. p. 417–29.
48. Luddington RJ. Thrombelastography/thromboelastometry. Clin Lab Haematol. 2005;27:81–90.
49. Campos JH. How to achieve successful lung separation. South Afr J Anaesth Analg. 2014;14:22–6.

Part II
Cases Resulting in Perioperative Near Death or Very Serious Complications

Chapter 6
A Case of CHARGE Syndrome and Hypoxemia

Asheen Rama, Jonathan L. Benumof, and Alyssa Brzenski

A Case of CHARGE Syndrome and Hypoxemia

A 3-year-old male, with a history of CHARGE syndrome (L1), was scheduled for dental examination under general anesthesia. The patient met criteria for CHARGE syndrome having colobomas, retardation of growth and development, deafness, and gastroesophageal reflux. However, there was no history of cardiac or nasal cavity defects (L2). The patient also had a history of frequent, daily, breath-holding spells (L3) associated with perioral cyanosis and was recovering from a recent upper respiratory infection (URI) (L4–L6) that developed approximately 2 weeks prior to day of surgery. On arrival to the children's hospital, his vital signs were stable, and the physical exam was unremarkable.

The patient was brought back to the operating room with his parent at his side and underwent an inhalational induction with 8% sevoflurane and 100% oxygen. A 24 gauge intravenous catheter was placed in a hand, and induction was completed with propofol. Oxymetazoline was administered into the nares to prepare for nasal intubation. Using a red rubber catheter (L7–L9), a nasal 4.5 internal diameter (ID) cuffed, endotracheal tube (ETT), McGill forceps, and a #2 Miller laryngoscope blade, the patient was intubated uneventfully without any complications. Dexamethasone was administered for nausea prophylaxis. The patient was maintained under general anesthesia with sevoflurane. Once the dental exam and placement of tooth caps were completed, the patient was given ketorolac, and he was transported to the post anesthesia care unit (PACU) with the endotracheal tube in place while spontaneously ventilating.

In the PACU while emerging from anesthesia and with the ETT still in place, the patient became apneic and cyanotic. The pulse oximeter saturation reached a nadir

A. Rama (✉) · A. Brzenski
Department of Anesthesiology, University of California, San Diego, CA, USA

J. L. Benumof
Department of Anesthesiology, University of California, UCSD Medical Center, UCSD School of Medicine, San Diego, CA, USA

J. L. Benumof, G. R. Manecke (eds.), *Clinical Anesthesiology II*,
https://doi.org/10.1007/978-3-030-12365-9_6

of 84%. Continuous positive airway pressure (CPAP) was administered using a Mapleson circuit, and the patient resumed spontaneous ventilation. After several minutes, the patient displayed several signs of readiness for extubation (L10) including hip flexion, attempting to grasp the endotracheal tube, and spontaneous eye opening with the eyes conjugate and midline. The nursing staff suctioned his oral and nasal cavities, deflated the ETT cuff, and extubated the patient. The patient maintained a patent airway following extubation and was breathing spontaneously and unlabored with blow-by supplemental oxygen. After several minutes, the patient became apneic. A face mask with the Mapleson circuit was used to apply CPAP while the patient was apneic, and then the patient resumed spontaneous ventilation (L11, 12). Approximately 1–2 min later, the patient once again appeared to have another episode of apnea. However, CPAP did not assist oxygenation. The heart rate and oxygen saturation continued to decrease rapidly, with the heart rate reaching a nadir in the 40s. A "code blue" was called. Ten chest compressions were initiated according to the Pediatric Advanced Life Support Algorithm (PALS) along with mask ventilation (L13). No medications were given. After these ten compressions, the patient regained spontaneous ventilation with the heart rate returning to the 90s and oxygen saturation normalizing. A decision was made to reintubate the patient due to these multiple apneic episodes. The patient was induced with propofol and intubated with a 4.5 mm ID oral, endotracheal tube.

Later in the PACU, the patient met extubation criteria, and the decision was made to reattempt extubation. Within several seconds following extubation, the patient became cyanotic and desaturated to mid 80s on pulse oximetry, and the anesthesiologist applied aggressive CPAP which successfully treated the hypoxemia. The patient was monitored for several hours in the PACU and had intermittent desaturation to the mid 80s. The patient was admitted for observation and was discharged in the morning having been noted to be at baseline level of activity by parents.

L1: What Is CHARGE Syndrome?

CHARGE syndrome is a rare congenital condition that is estimated to occur in 1 in 10,000–12,000 live births. The acronym CHARGE stands for the following clinical signs that are frequently found in patients with CHARGE syndrome: coloboma, heart defects, choanal atresia, retardation of growth and development, genitourinary problems, and ear abnormalities. Although these signs and symptoms are found in many individuals with CHARGE syndrome, they are not the sole criteria for diagnosis. Diagnosis is primarily clinical with confirmation by genetic testing. Blake et al. [1] created a system where patients are diagnosed with CHARGE syndrome if they have at least four major features or three major features plus at least three minor features (see Table 6.1).

Over 90% of patients with CHARGE syndrome have a mutation in the CHD7 gene. Although the exact function of CHD7 is unknown, the gene is expressed in the

Table 6.1 Chart of major and minor criteria: major criteria are commonly seen in CHARGE syndrome but are rare in other syndromes, and minor criteria are less specific to CHARGE

	Includes	Frequency (%)
Major criterion		
C = Coloboma	Coloboma of iris, retina, choroid, disc; microphthalmia	80–90
C = Choanal atresia	Unilateral/bilateral, membranous/bony, stenosis/atresia	50–60
C = Characteristic ear abnormalities	External ear, middle ear, (ossicular malformations, chronic serous otitis), mixed deafness, cochlear defects	90
C = Cranial nerve dysfunction	I, anosmia; VII, facial palsy (unilateral or bilateral); VIII, sensorineural deafness and vestibular problems; IX and/or X, swallowing problems	70–90
Minor criterion		
Genital hypoplasia	Males: micropenis, cryptorchidism	70–80
	Females: hypoplastic labia	
	Both: delayed, incomplete pubertal development	
Developmental delay	Delayed motor milestones, hypotonia, cognitive delay	100
Cardiovascular malformations	All types: specially conotruncal defects (e.g., tetralogy of Fallot), atrioventricular (AV) canal defects, and aortic arch anomalies	75–85
Growth deficiency	Short stature	70
Orofacial cleft	Cleft lip and/or palate	15–20
Tracheoesophageal anomalies	Tracheoesophageal fistula	20
Distinctive face	Characteristic facial features including broad forehead with facial asymmetry and full nasal tip	70–80

Reprinted from Blake et al. [1]. With permission from Sage Publications

central nervous system and the neural crests of the pharyngeal arches—both of which involve organs affected by CHARGE. However, even if a patient does not have a mutation in the CHD7 gene, but meets clinical criteria, the patient is diagnosed with CHARGE syndrome. Given the wide spectrum of phenotypic features seen in CHARGE, there is overlap with other genetic abnormalities, most notably for chromosome 22q11.2 deletion syndrome. Despite CHARGE syndrome having a clinical diagnosis, genetic testing is important as it provides insight into the patient's clinical course and aids in management decisions. In addition, testing can provide genetic counseling for parents. For example, CHD7 mutations are usually sporadic, whereas 22a11.2 deletions can be familial [2].

One of the challenges in providing anesthesia to patients with CHARGE syndrome is congenital heart disease (CHD). Cardiac defects can be found in 75–85% of CHARGE patients [1]. An epidemiological analysis of CHARGE syndrome by Issekutz et al. found a wide variety of cardiac malformations in CHARGE patients with many patients having more than one defect [3]. Issekutz et al. compared their data to several other epidemiological studies and found that conotruncal defects were the most commonly observed congenital heart anomaly with an incidence ranging from 17% to 42% across several studies [3–6]. In addition, aortic arch

Table 6.2 Issekutz et al. reviewed several papers and found the following epidemiological data on cardiovascular malformations in CHARGE

	Issekutz et al. [3]	Lin et al. [4]	Wyse et al. [5]	Tellier et al. [6]
Number of patients	65	53	59	47
Conotruncal defects (involve malformations related to the cardiac outflow tracts)	11 (17%)	22 (42%)	17 (29%)	11 (27.5%)
Aortic arch anomalies (abnormal anatomy of the aortic arch)	7 (11%)	9 (36%)	10 (17%)	2 (5%)
ASD	18 (28%)	2 (4%)	9 (15%)	3 (7.5%)
VSD	21 (32%)	2 (4%)	12 (20%)	5 (12.5%)
PDA	28 (43%)	12 (23%)	12 (20%)	8 (20%)
SVC anomalies	5 (8%)	0	0	0
AVSD	7 (11%)	3 (6%)	5 (8%)	N/A

Based on data from Ref. [3]
ASD atrial septal defect, *VSD* ventricular septal defect, *PDA* patent ductus arteriosus, *SVC* superior vena cava, *AVSD* atrioventricular defect

anomalies were commonly observed and had an incidence of 5–36% across several epidemiological studies [3–6]. These conotruncal and aortic arch defects include tetralogy of Fallot, double outlet right ventricle, aberrant subclavian artery, right aortic arch, truncus arteriosus, interrupted aortic arch, and conoventricular VSD [4]. Of note, superior vena cava anomalies were very infrequently observed [3–6] (see Table 6.2). Depending on the type of congenital heart defect, severe cyanosis can result in addition to restrictions to pulmonary or systemic blood flow. The maintenance of a patent ductus arteriosus may be required to provide systemic cardiac output prior to repair. For all of these patients, it is important to review and obtain an electrocardiogram, echocardiogram, as well as consider a cardiology consult before proceeding with intraoperative care.

L2: What Are the Airway Abnormalities Associated with CHARGE Syndrome and Describe Management Strategies That Can Be Considered for Treating These Abnormalities?

Choanal atresia involves a unilateral or bilateral congenital blockage of the nasal passages. Approximately 50% of children with CHARGE have choanal atresia [1]. In about 70% of choanal atresia, blockage will be secondary to both membranous and bony components; the remaining 30% involve only bony blockage [7]. Since infants are obligate nasal breathers, bilateral atresia can present as respiratory distress at birth and even lead to death from asphyxia. Momentary relief occurs when the infant cries and breathes through the mouth. Accordingly, newborns with bilateral atresia undergo definitive surgical treatment as soon as the newborn is stable. Symptoms associated with unilateral atresia often present later during infancy as the child is able to breathe through one of the nasal passages without obstruction.

Micrognathia, sometimes referred to as mandibular hypoplasia, can lead to significant challenges with intubation. Several anatomic changes, which occur during early fetal development, can be highlighted and illustrate the underlying difficulties with laryngoscopy. During fetal development in the eighth week of gestation, the tongue is normally pulled downward and forward into a rapidly growing mandible. If the mandible remains hypoplastic during the early stages of fetal life, the tongue will be unable to descend into the oral cavity and will remain posteriorly displaced, resulting in glossoptosis [8]. Laryngoscopy is made more difficult by difficulty in moving the posteriorly displaced tongue. In addition, the laryngeal inlet may appear to be more anterior and thus difficult to visualize as the line of site is "sharply curved" (see Fig. 6.1). Moreover, in patients with micrognathia, the oral aperture may not open as widely [9]. The combination of these factors can lead to the inability to visualize the glottis during direct laryngoscopy, resulting in a grade 4 view. A careful preoperative assessment of the patient's anesthetic history and previous airway management can be helpful in anticipating difficulty with intubation. In a study investigating the incidence of airway abnormalities in CHARGE patients, Stack et al. found that in a cohort of 50 patients, 40% of patients with CHARGE had micrognathia [10].

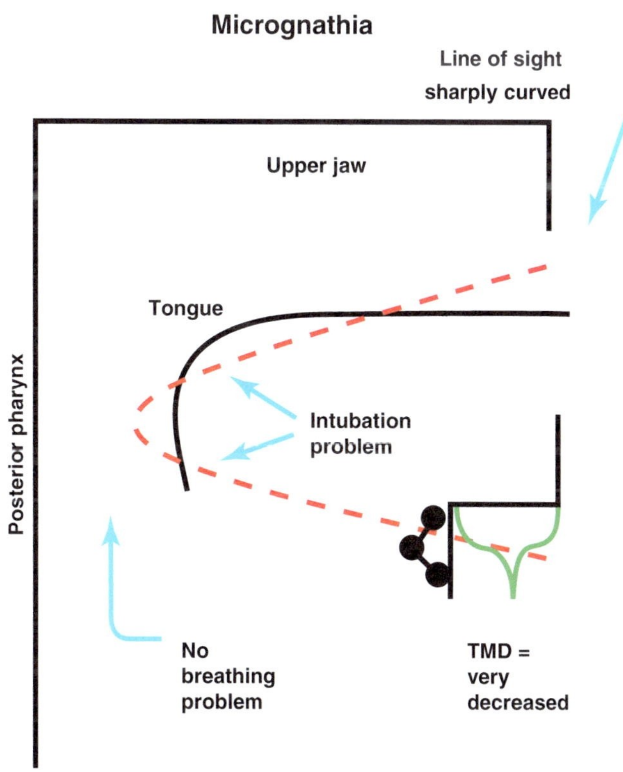

Fig. 6.1 Schematic illustrating challenges associated with glottis visualization with micrognathic patient. The dotted red line illustrates the sharp angle that the line of site has to navigate given the decreased thyromental distance (TMD). (Courtesy of Dr. Jonathan L. Benumof)

Given the difficulty with intubation, an induction technique that allows for continued spontaneous ventilation, such as a volatile induction with 8% sevoflurane and 100% oxygen, is optimal. With careful consideration of patient head position and attempt at alignment of oral, pharyngeal, and laryngeal axis, the author would attempt a gentle direct laryngoscopy to visualize the glottis. External glottic manipulation can be used to displace the cricoid cartilage and glottis, posteriorly and cephalad in an attempt to optimize line of site. If this does not bring the glottis into view, the author would consider the use of indirect laryngoscopy with video-assisted laryngoscopy such as a GlideScope as this may provide a more anterior line of site to the glottis or consider a fiber-optic intubation through an intubating laryngeal mask airway (LMA).

Laryngomalacia is an airway abnormality in which there is an inward collapse of supraglottic structures during inspiration and can result in stridor. Stack et al. studied the incidence of airway abnormalities in CHARGE patients and found, in their cohort of 50 patients, 8% had laryngomalacia [11]. Various anatomic abnormalities can contribute to laryngomalacia, including inward collapse of shorter aryepiglottic folds, a long tubular epiglottis, anterior and medial collapse of the arytenoid cartilage, and posterior inspiratory displacement of the epiglottis against the posterior pharyngeal wall [12]. Defective neuromuscular control is also thought to play a role in the collapse of supraglottic structures. Under general anesthesia, maintaining spontaneous ventilation may be challenging as the laryngeal cartilage may collapse with inspiration, and as such, continuous positive airway pressure may be helpful to splint open the airway. Placing the child in a lateral position may also help as it can shift the pressure of the chest wall from directly pushing downward on the larynx. For long-term airway management, tracheostomy may be required [11].

Subglottic stenosis can be either acquired or congenital. In patients with CHARGE Syndrome, both acquired and congenital forms may be present; patients may be born with mild congenital subglottic stenosis that is worsened by prolonged or repeated intubations during operative procedures or intensive care. Compared to other airway abnormalities, the incidence of subglottic stenosis in CHARGE patients is relatively low having been reported to be 6–8% [10, 11]. Patients are at risk for developing subglottic stenosis if they have a history of previous endotracheal intubation whether for respiratory distress as a newborn or for operative management. Direct laryngoscopy is the means by which this is diagnosed, and patients may require a smaller endotracheal tube diameter [11].

Laryngeal clefts are a developmental failure of the posterior cricoid lamina or the septa between the esophagus and trachea and can involve intrathoracic extension (see Fig. 6.2). In comparison to the previous airway abnormalities described, laryngeal clefts are rarely seen in patients in CHARGE syndrome [10, 11]. Clinically, patients will have stridor as well as difficulty with feeding, leading to pulmonary aspiration and frequent chest infections [10]. One chief concern during the performance of an anesthetic is the placement of the endotracheal tube. If the tube and cuff are not placed beyond the cleft, insufflation of the stomach may occur [10]. During the operative repair for type I–III lesions, these are often completed with a spontaneously ventilating patient under suspension laryngoscopy. With this technique, the patient maintains spontaneous ventilation. This has been accomplished with volatile

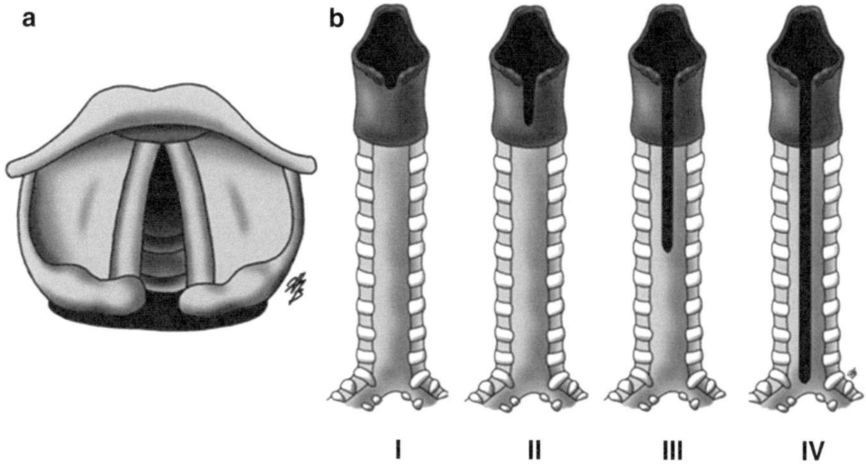

Fig. 6.2 Drawings of incomplete fusion of the posterior glottis: note the classification scheme where the laryngeal cleft can be above (I), at (II), or below (III) the cricoid or extend to inside the thorax (IV). (Reprinted from Campisi and Busato [13]. With permission from Springer Science + Business Media)

agents and total intravenous anesthetic techniques including propofol and remifentanil infusions. Type IV lesions may require repair with the patient on cardiopulmonary bypass [14].

Congenital laryngeal webs are membrane-like structures that extend across the laryngeal lumen and are located at or near the laryngeal opening (see Fig. 6.3). Rarely seen in patients with CHARGE, they are associated with respiratory distress and inspiratory stridor. The webs are the result of incomplete recanalization of the larynx during the tenth week of life [12]. The anesthetic management of a child with congenital laryngeal webs undergoing laryngeal reconstruction requires careful preoperative preparation including imaging which may require chest CT or MRI in addition to chest X-ray. An otorhinolaryngologist can be consulted to perform a bedside flexible bronchoscopy to evaluate the glottis and determine the degree of airway narrowing and the severity of the web. Intraoperatively, an inhalational induction followed by the maintenance of spontaneous ventilation using either volatiles or intravenous agents should be considered. In addition, topical lidocaine can be used to reduce the minumum alveolar concentration (MAC) requirement.

L3: What Is Breath Holding, and How Can You Tell the Difference Between Laryngospasm and Breath Holding? Also, How Would You Manage Breath Holding in the PACU?

Breath-holding spells (BHS) are a relatively common childhood disorder with an autosomal dominant inheritance pattern [15]. They constitute a nonepileptic event that is paroxysmal in nature and is triggered by an external emotional stimulus

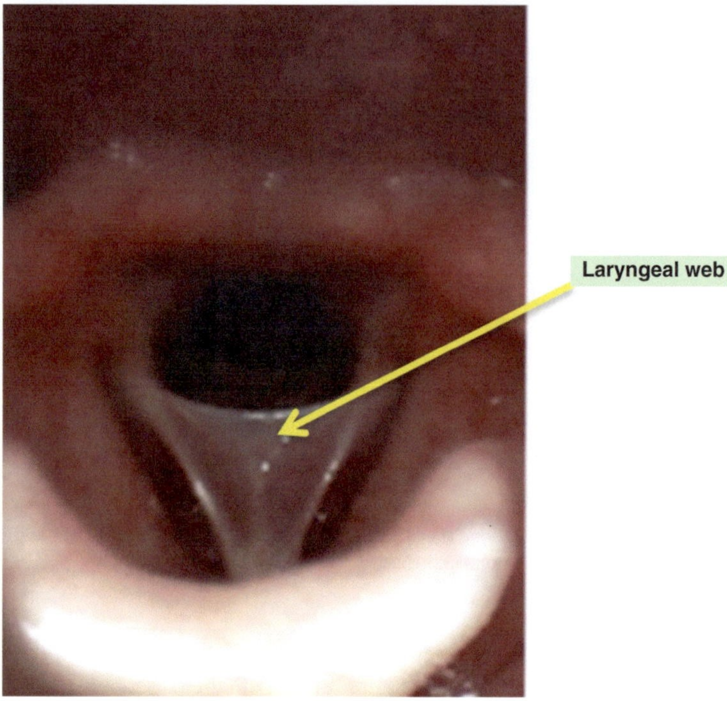

Fig. 6.3 Congenital laryngeal web. (Adapted from Campisi and Busato [13]. With permission from Springer Science + Business Media)

including fear, pain, and minor trauma [16, 17]. The spells can present before 1 year of age and are more common between 6 months and 4 years of age [18]. A BHS presents when the child is vigorously crying. At the end of expiration, they will hold their breath. Apnea is accompanied by concomitant pallor or cyanosis which may progress to a loss of consciousness. Following this loss of consciousness, some patients may exhibit convulsive movements. This condition is classified into a cyanotic, pallid, or mixed type. The underlying pathophysiology of the disorder has been postulated to be a dysregulation of the autonomic nervous system and can result in complications that include bradycardia and asystole [19]. In particular, pallid breath-holding spells may involve a rapid loss of consciousness and are concerning as they are preceded by a short period (one or a few seconds) of asystole [20]. Following an event, parents are reassured and educated about the condition. However, the periods of apnea and cyanosis can still be very difficult and frightening for parents to witness. A thorough preoperative history from the parent in determining patient triggers as well as reviewing the assessment and plans of the patient's neurologist can aid in the perioperative management of these patients.

The diagnosis of breath holding post emergence is challenging. Taking into account patient history and observing the patient's pattern of breathing can help discern laryngospasm from breath holding. Sternal retractions and paradoxical abdominal chest movement are classic for laryngospasm as the patient will continue to attempt to ventilate against a closed glottis. A similar pattern can be observed with airway obstruction from the tongue or soft tissue. Discerning between laryngospasm and a BHS may be challenging; however, the apnea and desaturation that follows may be rapid and necessitate immediate intervention regardless of etiology.

By understanding the pathophysiology, one can be prepared for the acute management of a perioperative BHS as well as develop an optimal anesthetic plan to mitigate the risk of having a BHS. During a BHS, one must consider the rapidity at which decompensation can occur as a result of hypoxemia and decreased apnea time in children. Thus, it may be prudent to temporarily re-anesthetize the patient with a sub-hypnotic dose of propofol if one is concerned about oxygenation. Providing continuous positive airway pressure followed by positive pressure ventilation with face mask if the patient becomes apneic is the next step in management. When considering pharmacological treatment, glycopyrrolate may be helpful in the acute, perioperative management of children with breath-holding spells as well as a prophylactic agent. Glycopyrrolate has been studied in a limited number of patients and appears to significantly decrease the incidence of breath-holding spells [17]. Furthermore, optimal pain control and anxiolysis are paramount in a patient with a history of breath-holding spells, as these prevent whatever stimulus that is present from triggering an event [19].

As parents will attest, when a child is having a BHS, it can be extremely anxiety-provoking to witness in addition to presenting a challenge for any member of the perioperative care team to manage. Knowledge of a patient's triggers, appropriate and timely airway management, and utilizing pharmacological agents including anticholinergics, hypnotics, anxiolytics, and analgesics are critical to safe management.

L4: What Are the Common Respiratory Events That Occur in Patients with Upper Respiratory Tract Infections (URIs), and How Can They Be Ameliorated?

Several respiratory events may occur in patients with URIs, and prompt management is critical as they can lead to significant morbidity and mortality (Table 6.3). Laryngospasm may be managed by deepening the patient's depth of anesthesia or providing muscle relaxation (see Lesson 11 for further details). Bronchospasm can be treated with the administration of beta 2 agonists, anticholinergic agents, deepening the alveolar concentration of volatile anesthetic, administering ketamine to allow for bronchodilation, and optimizing ventilatory settings by allowing for increased expiratory time. Breath holding can also occur in patients with URIs and may be prevented by optimal perioperative management of anxiety and pain. Perioperative strategies to reduce breath holding may include

Table 6.3 Respiratory events and URIs

Respiratory events	Management
Laryngospasm	Deepen anesthetic versus muscle relaxation
Bronchospasm	Pharmacotherapy with bronchodilators including albuterol, ketamine, and epinephrine or increasing depth of volatile anesthetic and optimizing ventilation to allow for increased expiratory time
Breath holding	Premedication and clear fluid intake 2 h prior to surgery may reduce risk as well as providing optimal analgesia and anxiolysis
Post-intubation croup	Racemic epinephrine, steroids, and prolonged observation

premedication, considering a parental induction, and clear liquid intake 2 h prior to surgery to reduce irritability [20]. In addition, post-intubation croup can also occur in patients with URIs. Racemic epinephrine and steroids can be used for treatment. Racemic epinephrine, however, may lead to rebound edema, and prolonged observation may be necessary along with overnight admission to a closely monitored setting [21].

L5: What Additional Factors Can Increase the Risk for Adverse Respiratory Events (Table 6.4)?

Respiratory complications are a major cause of morbidity and mortality during the perioperative period in pediatric patients. Upper respiratory tract infections lead to respiratory complications in these pediatric patients and remain a major concern for pediatric anesthesiologists caring for children. However, laryngospasm, bronchospasm, coughing, breath holding, and need for postoperative oxygen can result from several additional factors related to the patient's medical history, anesthetic management, and surgical procedure.

During the preoperative evaluation, specific focus should remain on factors related to the patient that may increase respiratory complications: medical history of asthma, history of prematurity with bronchopulmonary dysplasia, and exposure to tobacco smoke in the household. Asthma is one of the most common respiratory illnesses that is encountered with an incidence of 9.5% in children between the ages of 0 and 17 years living in the United States [27]. Symptoms of asthma including nocturnal cough, frequent wheezing (>3 times in the last 12 months), and wheezing during exercise are predictive of bronchospasm and laryngospasm during the perioperative period [22]. Nocturnal cough conferred the highest risk of perioperative respiratory complications, with a relative risk of 10.5 for bronchospasm in patients with these symptoms. Frequent wheezing (>3 episodes over 12 months) or wheezing with exercise also increased the risk of bronchospasm (RR = 7.17, 7.73, respectively) and laryngospasm (RR = 2.64, 3.28, respectively). In one large study from Perth, Australia, respiratory complications were more frequent in these asthmatic

Table 6.4 Risk factors for adverse respiratory events

Risk factors	Salient points
Preoperative evaluation	
Asthma	Symptoms include nocturnal cough, frequent wheezing, and wheezing during exercise and increases risk of perioperative laryngospasm and bronchospasm [22]
Passive exposure to tobacco smoke	Increases the risk of asthma and high risk of perioperative respiratory event [23]
Preterm and bronchopulmonary dysplasia	May have a high level of bronchoreactivity secondary to bronchopulmonary dysplasia [24]
Anesthetic technique	
Choice of volatile for maintenance	Sevoflurane shown to have less rate of perioperative respiratory adverse events than isoflurane and desflurane [22]
Propofol vs sevoflurane for maintenance	Lower rates of laryngospasm with propofol than sevoflurane [22]
Anesthesia delivered via endotracheal tube versus face mask only	Face mask only technique has significantly reduced risk for respiratory complications [22]
Regional anesthesia in neonates undergoing inguinal hernia repair	May decrease risk of perioperative adverse respiratory events [25]
Surgical considerations	
Type of surgery	Higher risk with ear, nose, and throat surgery likely due to airway instrumentation and secretions and bleeding in airway [26]

patients than in patients with upper respiratory tract infection during the past 2 weeks [22].

Bronchopulmonary dysplasia (BPD), a chronic lung disease in preterm neonates, is also associated with high levels of bronchoreactivity [24, 28]. Although the rate of BPD varied greatly among different institutions in the United States, BPD can occur in over 50% of preterm infants with birth weights less than 750 g [24]. Children that are diagnosed with BPD not only have respiratory complications during the neonatal period but also demonstrate increased obstructive lung function associated with increased airway hyperreactivity that may last throughout childhood and into adolescence [29, 30]. Although there are no studies comparing children with BPD who are undergoing an anesthetic compared to similar peers without BPD, the increase in airway bronchoconstriction frequently makes respiratory complications common. In addition, passive exposure to tobacco smoke leads to increased rates of bronchoreactivity and asthma in pediatric patients. Exposure to tobacco smoke is a major risk factor for perioperative respiratory adverse events [23]. The risk is greatest when both parents smoke (RR = 2.09, $p < 0.0001$), but if only one parent smokes, maternal smoking results in a 1.87 higher rate of perioperative respiratory complications. It is unclear why maternal smoking confers a greater risk than paternal smoking, but it could be postulated that the primary caregiver may provide the greatest risk to these children [22].

The technique used for the intraoperative anesthetic can affect the rate of perioperative complications. In many surgeries in pediatric patients, regional anesthetics as the sole anesthetic are not an option due to lack of psychological maturity. However, for neonates undergoing inguinal hernia repair, regional anesthesia may be associated with lower rates of perioperative pulmonary complications compared to general anesthesia [25]. For surgical procedures that require general anesthesia, maintenance of anesthesia with a less irritating volatile anesthetic (sevoflurane > isoflurane > desflurane) results in lower rates of perioperative respiratory adverse events (laryngospasm RR 6.15 in desflurane compared to sevoflurane; laryngospasm RR = 2.17 in desflurane compared to sevoflurane). There is an increased rate of laryngospasm when sevoflurane is used for maintenance of anesthesia compared with propofol (RR = 2.6, $p < 0.0001$). However, there is no difference in the rate in bronchospasm when propofol is used for maintenance of anesthesia when compared to sevoflurane [22].

In children without upper respiratory infections, Morabia et al. demonstrated that endotracheal intubation with muscle relaxants resulted in the lowest rates of respiratory complications. This study however was small which may have had an effect on the results [26]. The larger study by Habre et al. demonstrated that an endotracheal tube was associated with a fivefold increase in respiratory complications compared with anesthesia by face mask [22]. There was no difference between maintenance of anesthesia with the use of a laryngeal mask and a face mask. Finally, ear, nose, and throat surgery is associated with a 1.77 risk increase of complications compared to other elective surgical procedures [26]. These ear, nose, and throat procedures may increase the complications due to high rates of airway instrumentation, as well as the potential for secretions and bleeding following the operation.

Together the preoperative and surgical risk factors can be used to determine which patients should be postponed prior to anesthesia. The intraoperative factors can be incorporated into an anesthesiologist's armamentarium. Techniques that are associated with lower perioperative respiratory events can be used by the anesthesiologist to ameliorate the potential for these perioperative respiratory events.

L6: A Child with URI Presents for Elective Surgery, and the Decision Is Made to Cancel the Case. How Long Must the Child Wait Before Rescheduling Their Surgery?

URIs create a significant conundrum for the pediatric anesthesiologists. The risk of proceeding with an anesthetic must be weighed against the impact that canceling a case has on the parents before making a decision. Historically any URI would result in the cancelation of an anesthetic based on a case series by McGill et al. [31] that reported respiratory complications following anesthesia. Perioperative events such as bronchospasm, laryngospasm, desaturations, breath holding, and post-intubation croup occur commonly following general anesthesia in children with URIs [32]. Tait et al. [33] studied risk factors that led to complications and determined that preoperative presence of copious sputum and secretions, nasal congestion, recent URI (less than 2 weeks), and history of reactive airway disease increased the risk of perioperative adverse respiratory events. Despite these perioperative events, in the experienced hands of a pediatric anesthesiologist [34], there is not a risk for substantial morbidity or mortality in these patients. A pediatric anesthesiologist, who is experienced with managing respiratory events in younger patients, will have increased familiarity with complications and be better equipped to recognize, manage, and treat them in a timely manner. Two large studies [32, 35] examined the risk of general anesthesia in children with URI revealed 3 out of 1078 children had a significant adverse events requiring hospitalization. There are a handful of case reports of deaths in children who underwent general anesthesia during an URI each which may have had complicating factors such as viral myocarditis [36–38] as a major contributor to the ultimate death. Although significant morbidity and mortality is not seen in this patient population with an experienced anesthesiologist, care should be taken to individually evaluate all patients with URIs.

The risk of increased perioperative respiratory events must be weighed against the impact on each family. Tait et al. [39] examined the impact canceling a case in a child with a URI has on the family. There was significant socioeconomic burden placed on the parents who may be missing work to bring their child to the hospital, and this should also be considered when making the decision to reschedule a surgical procedure. This burden was manifested in parents being required to take additional time off work and in the cost of travel for the families. This socioeconomic burden is not insignificant and should be weighed against the potential for resulting complications. Ultimately, these points illustrate the importance of weighing all risks and benefits when deciding to cancel elective surgery. Using clinical judgment on each individual patient undergoing a specific surgery and recognizing modifiable risk factors that contribute to adverse respiratory events (see Table 6.4) will aid in clinical decision-making. With a thoughtfully planned anesthetic, one can reduce the risk of airway reactivity and thus consider moving forward with elective surgery. Such considerations potentially include using a laryngeal mask airway instead of an endotracheal tube, avoiding desflurane, and using prophylactic bronchodilators.

If a decision is made to postpone a surgical procedure and anesthetic, the question that arises is when should the surgery be rescheduled (see Table 6.5). Most preschool age children will have at least 6–8 colds a year with 95% of the URIs caused by viral infections. Most of these URIs are self-limiting and will resolve quickly. However, studies have shown that airway reactivity remains for several weeks following an URI [40, 41]. Reviews of clinical patients demonstrate that this hyperreactivity may remain for 4–6 weeks after resolution of their URI. However, it is likely that the child may have another URI by the time the case is rescheduled [34]. Given the frequency of URIs, 4 weeks is typically deemed sufficient time to postpone prior to rescheduling a procedure in a child with a URI.

Table 6.5 Considerations of canceling elective surgery in setting of URI

Considerations	Salient points
Socioeconomic status of family	Parent(s) may be missing work to bring child to hospital, financial burden to take additional time off, and travel expenses [39]
After URI symptoms resolve	Airway hyperreactivity will remain for 4–6 weeks [34]
Frequency of preschool age children developing URIs	At least 6–8 colds per year [34]
Postponement of elective surgery	Balance between likelihood of another URI developing and hyperactivity of airway from initial URI deems at least 4 weeks postponement

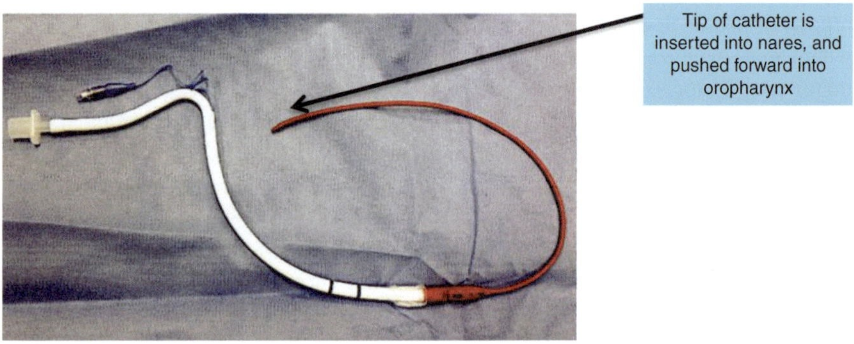

Fig. 6.4 Red rubber catheter is loaded onto the end of a nasal endotracheal tube. (Adapted from Garside and Hatfield [43]. With permission from John Wiley & Sons)

L7: Discuss Techniques Used in Nasotracheal Intubation. Are There Any Techniques Which Have Been Shown to Reduce Complication Rates?

One of the first steps in successfully performing a nasotracheal intubation is proper preparation of the nares. A topical vasoconstrictor, such as phenylephrine 0.25% or oxymetazoline, may be applied judiciously along the nasal mucosa and can aid both in increasing the patency of the nasal passage and in preventing bleeding secondary to mucosal injury caused by introduction of the tube [21]. Injury can be further minimized via dilation of the nares with nasal trumpets and softening the nasotracheal tubes via soaking in warm water prior to insertion. Watt et al. found that by guiding a nasotracheal tube through the nasopharynx using a red rubber catheter, the incidence bleeding could be reduced by two- to threefold in comparison to using a warmed tube [42]. With this technique, the nasal mucosa does not make direct contact with the sharp, beveled tip of a nasotracheal tube because it is fitted into the trailing end of the red rubber catheter (Fig. 6.4). Both the nasotracheal tube and the red rubber catheter are advanced together into the nare. The catheter is retrieved from the oropharynx using Magill forceps, and the nasotracheal tube is positioned in the glottis with the aid of direct laryngoscopy and the use of Magill forceps.

L8: What Are the Contraindications to Nasotracheal Intubation (Table 6.6)?

Nasotracheal tubes may cause complications in certain patients. Clinical judgment can be used, and further safety measures can be considered when performing nasal intubation. Prior to the procedure, a nasal speculum examination to inspect the nares for patency as well as relative size of turbinates should be considered. In addition, the anesthesiologist can guide the endotracheal tube through the nasopharynx with the aid of fiber-optic bronchoscopy. This may help to reduce the chance of directing the nasal tube through a false passage (i.e., in the case of a patient with a base of skull fracture) and minimize the chance of trauma. Table 6.6 lists the absolute and relative contraindications to nasotracheal intubation and why the contraindicated items are contraindicated.

Table 6.6 Table of absolute and relative contraindications to nasotracheal intubation

Absolute contraindications	
Choanal atresia	Boney or mucosal narrowing of nasal passage will obstruct nasotracheal tube
Transsphenoidal procedures	Nares need to be available for surgical access to sphenoid sinus
Sinusitis	Can lead to bacteremia
Thrombocytopenia/ coagulopathy [44]	High risk of bleeding
Basilar skull fracture [44]	Tube can enter a false passage and cause CNS trauma
Relative contraindications [44]	
Large nasal polyps	Injury to nasal mucosa and obstruction to passage of nasotracheal tube
Suspected nasal foreign bodies	Can cause trauma and push foreign body into oropharynx
History of recent nasal surgery	Trauma to surgical repair and bleeding
Upper neck hematoma	Nasal mucosal swelling from impairment of venous drainage can be present and lead to significant bleeding
Upper neck infection	Swelling can lead to displacement of anatomy, and if there is an abscess which ruptures, contents can be aspirated
History of frequent epistaxis	Risk of bleeding

Table 6.7 Complications associated with nasotracheal intubation

Complications	Salient points
Epistaxis	Nasotracheal tube can serve to tamponade bleeding or provide manual compression, or one can pinch the nostrils
Systemic hypertension	From absorption of topical vasoconstrictors, thus dose appropriately
Laryngospasm	Can be triggered by topical vasoconstrictor application if patient is not in a deep enough plane of anesthesia
Turbinectomy, polypectomy, and adenoidectomy	Topical vasoconstrictors can increase patency of nares, and red rubber catheter technique may reduce trauma [42, 45–48]
Bacteremia	Sinusitis is a relative contraindication to nasal intubation, and bacteremia is a potential complication [49]

L9: Describe the Complications That Can Be Associated with Nasotracheal Intubation

Several complications with nasotracheal intubation have been described (Table 6.7). The most common complication is epistaxis secondary to abrasions of the nasal mucosa. If bleeding is noticed during a successful intubation, the endotracheal tube can serve to tamponade the bleeding. If the tube cannot be passed successfully, one can consider removing the endotracheal tube and pinching the nostrils to provide manual compression to control bleeding [44]. Topicalization of the nasal mucosa with vasoconstrictors prior to the passage of the nasotracheal tube may aid in passage of the tube and limit bleeding. However, large doses of topical vasoconstrictors can lead to systemic hypertension, and thus it is important to consider the dose applied. In addition, care should be taken with respect to the timing of topical vasoconstrictor application as laryngospasm can occur if the child is in stage two of anesthesia during an inhaled induction. Furthermore, traumatic nasal intubations leading to several complications including turbinectomy, polypectomy, and adenoidectomy have all also been described in the literature [45–48]. In addition to trauma, bacteremia has been reported in nontraumatic nasal intubations [49].

L10: What Are the Important Considerations Prior to Extubating a Pediatric Patient, and When Is It Safe to Extubate a Child in a "Deep" Plane of Anesthesia?

The successful and safe extubation of a pediatric patient requires careful planning and preparation. All necessary airway equipment for ventilation and intubation such as a face mask, endotracheal tube, appropriately sized blade for direct laryngoscopy, and airway adjuncts including appropriately sized oral and nasopharyngeal airways should be readily accessible. Induction agents and muscle relaxants should also be available as the child emerges from anesthesia in the event that re-intubation becomes necessary.

Extubation can be performed when the patient is fully awake or in a relatively deep plane of anesthesia. The primary goal is to avoid extubation during stage II and allow for the return of laryngeal reflexes including a cough and gag. Prior to performing a "deep" versus an awake extubation, one must weigh the advantages and disadvantages of this clinical decision with respect to the patient, type of surgery, and postoperative care resources such as availability and training of PACU personnel. For example, in children undergoing eye surgery, a deep extubation may be less likely to produce cough or strain and thus prevent disruption of the surgical repair. However, the disadvantages of a deep extubation include the risk of aspiration, as an anesthetized patient's airway reflexes have yet to fully return, as well as the potential for obstruction or laryngospasm as the patient emerges through stage II of anesthesia without an airway in place. It is noteworthy that in a study with a relatively large cohort of 880 pediatric patients undergoing tonsillectomy and adenoidectomy, Baijal et al. observed the incidence of respiratory complications following awake versus deep extubation and found no statistical difference between these two methods [50].

If a decision is made to extubate deep, several complications may occur including ventilatory compromise related to residual anesthesia and sedation. This can be assessed by evaluating the presence of any obstruction from the tongue or upper airway soft tissue. Additionally the practitioner should be aware of the possibility and presence of laryngospasm, bronchospasm or wheezing related to airway hyperactivity or aspiration, and alveolar edema related to negative pressure pulmonary edema if significant laryngospasm develops. Inadequate reversal of muscle relaxant or excess narcotization should also be assessed if the patient is hypoventilatory.

If a child is extubated when fully awake, judgment of the child's readiness is based on several parameters. As children may be too young to follow commands, it is important to note the following physical exam features (Table 6.8):

Table 6.8 Physical exam signs and readiness for extubation

Physical exam signs	Comments
Eyes	Spontaneous eye opening, along with midline, non-divergent location
Brow furrow	Furrowing of brow can be physical exam of crying
Limbs	Movement of all limbs and attempt to grab endotracheal tube can demonstrate motor strength
Swallowing and gag reflex	Return of reflex arc and evidence that patient is capable of protecting airway against aspiration
Breathing pattern	Breathing pattern without pauses or breath holding
Oxygenation and ventilation	With minimum to no ventilatory support, patient maintains saturation and has adequate, age-corrected, tidal volumes – listening to bilateral lung fields and trachea can reveal the need for suctioning or bronchospasm

L11: How Do You Treat Laryngospasm (Fig. 6.5)?

The first step in treating laryngospasm involves distinguishing "partial laryngospasm" from "complete laryngospasm." Partial laryngospasm exists when there is evidence of turbulent airflow accompanied by high-pitched stridulous breathing and minimal chest rise. "Complete laryngospasm," which is a life-threatening emergency, often involves paradoxical chest wall movement and the complete lack of airflow and is associated with tracheal tug and intercostal retractions.

For both partial and complete laryngospasm, a useful first step involves jaw thrust followed by continuous positive airway pressure with 100% oxygen via face mask and increasing the depth of anesthesia, such as with an increased concentration of volatile agent. If the patient has partial laryngospasm, the volatile agent may be able to break the laryngospasm. Simultaneously, one can utilize a technique involving pressure placed in the "laryngospasm notch." This anatomic location is located behind the lobule of the pinna, in front of the mastoid process, and behind the ascending ramus of the mandible. This technique involves using the thumb and index fingers to provide a seal with the face mask and using the middle finger of each hand to press inward toward the base of the skull, at the most cephalad portion

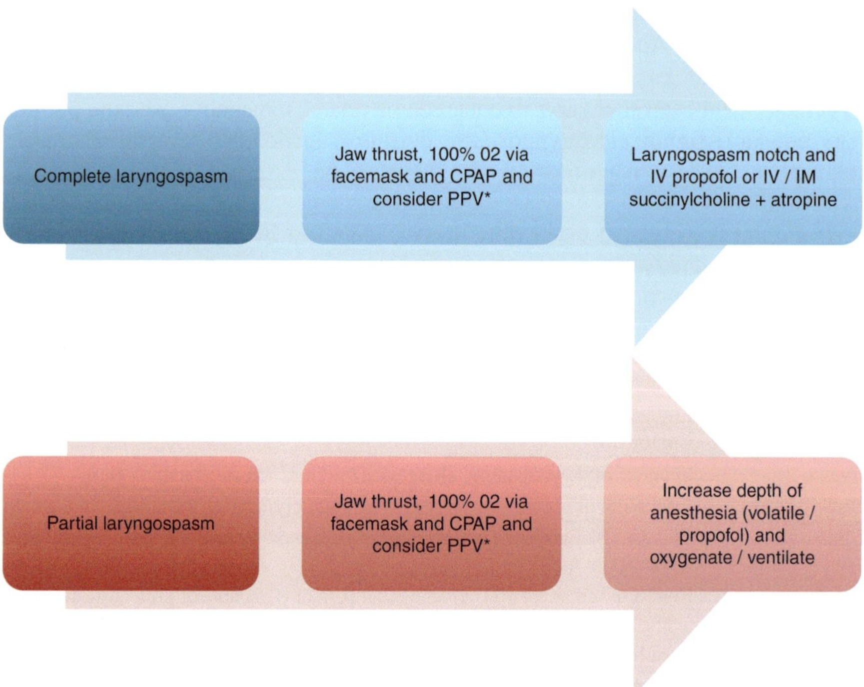

Fig. 6.5 Basic overview of laryngospasm management *If, after these maneuvers, the left upper quadrant appears distended, a nasogastric tube should be passed to suction the stomach

of the "notch." The technique has been described anecdotally; however, further studies need to be conducted regarding its efficacy [51].

Administering propofol or muscle relaxants will abduct the vocal cords. If propofol fails to treat laryngospasm, or if there is no intravenous access, a muscle relaxant can be administered. Barring any contraindications, succinylcholine can be administered intravenously at 1 mg/kg or intramuscularly at a dose of 4 mg/kg [21]. Before treating the patient with succinylcholine, atropine can be administered at 20 mcg/kg to prevent bradycardia associated with succinylcholine and the hypoxemia that may be present in the face of severe laryngospasm [21]. If there is a contraindication to succinylcholine and no IV access is available, rocuronium can be administered via intravenous or intramuscular route. If succinylcholine is used, the practitioner can likely mask ventilate until the succinylcholine wears off. If the patient receives rocuronium, it may be best to intubate the patient because of the long-acting effects of rocuronium. In addition, if mask ventilation is used, one should consider passing a nasogastric tube, especially if the left upper quadrant is protuberant or distended as prolonged mask ventilation can inflate the stomach. Finally, despite the potential for laryngospasm to break with hypoxemia, bradycardia followed by cardiac arrest can occur, and, thus, treatment should not be delayed.

After laryngospasm is treated, it is important to assess the patient for pulmonary aspiration or negative pressure pulmonary edema as well as to reassess the cause of the laryngospasm, treating the cause to prevent a reoccurrence of laryngospasm when the patient subsequently re-emerges. Oropharyngeal suctioning of secretions and blood may have been the initial stimulus. It is important to reassess and remove any offending agents that can retrigger laryngospasm upon re-emergence, and if there is impairment in the patient's ability to oxygenate or ventilate, the patient may require re-intubation in order to provide adequate ventilator support.

L12: What Techniques Have Been Studied That May Be Useful in Decreasing the Incidence of Laryngospasm During Extubation (Table 6.9)?

Several researchers have studied methods to prevent laryngospasm upon extubation in intubated patients. The research has primarily focused on extubation of children undergoing tonsillectomy and adenoidectomy. The contribution of depth of anesthesia upon extubation, the degree of stimulation during emergence, and the pharmacological interventions to prevent laryngospasm have all been investigated.

Lidocaine has been investigated and is often used in clinical practice. The studies examining the use of lidocaine have some contradictory results, depending on the timing and route of administration of the lidocaine. In a study by Baraka, the children post tonsillectomy and adenoidectomy were given an intravenous bolus of 2% lidocaine at 2 mg/kg, 1 min prior to extubation. None of the 20 patients who received

Table 6.9 Techniques to reduce the incidence of laryngospasm studied in patients presenting for tonsillectomy and adenoidectomy

Technique	Comments
Intravenous lidocaine	2% lidocaine at 2 mg/kg, 1 min prior to extubation reduced incidence [52]
Glottic topicalization	4 mg/kg of 2% lidocaine as glottic topicalization prior to intubation [53]
Subhypnotic propofol dose	Administering 0.5 mg/kg, 1 min prior to tracheal extubation [54]
Magnesium infusion	Post-intubation, providing magnesium infusion at 15 mg/kg of magnesium sulfate over 20 min [55]
"No-touch technique"	Suctioning the oropharynx while the patient is still anesthetized and then allowing the child to fully emerge in the lateral position without any stimulation [56]

intravenous lidocaine had laryngospasm, while 5 of the 20 patients in the control group did have observed laryngospasm [52]. In another study, lower doses of lidocaine (1.5 mg/kg) given closer to awakening, such as when the patient is already swallowing, did not result in a decreased incidence of laryngospasm [57]. Topicalization of the vocal cords with lidocaine may also be an effective means to reduce the incidence of laryngospasm. Koc et al. found that "spraying" the cords with topical lidocaine during induction or giving an intravenous lidocaine bolus at the end of surgery prior to emergence was effective in reducing the incidence of laryngospasm by approximately 50% compared to their control groups [53]. However, they did find that an intravenous lidocaine bolus at the end of surgery was associated with a greater degree of early postoperative sedation. Koc et al. used intravenous boluses of 2% lidocaine at 1 mg/kg given 5 min prior to extubation or 4 mg/kg of 2% lidocaine as glottic topicalization prior to intubation. It should be noted that the average duration of surgery in this study was approximately 40 min, and as such, their findings related to topical lidocaine during induction may not be applicable to longer surgeries.

In addition to lidocaine, propofol has also been investigated and found to be a useful medication to prevent laryngospasm. Propofol is not associated with an increase in airway reactivity, making it an ideal option in patients that are at high risk for laryngospasm. Batra et al. investigated the effects of sub-hypnotic doses of propofol on the incidence of emergence laryngospasm and found that by administering 0.5 mg/kg, 1 min prior to tracheal extubation, they were able to decrease the risk of emergence laryngospasm. In their study, they observed a 20% incidence of laryngospasm in their control group and a 6.6% incidence in those receiving propofol [54].

The role of magnesium in preventing laryngospasm has also been studied in children presenting for tonsillectomy and adenoidectomy. In a small study, Gulhas et al. found that magnesium infused intraoperatively to children undergoing tonsillectomy and adenoidectomy decreased the incidence of laryngospasm during awake extubation. Their intervention involved infusing a dilution of 15 mg/kg of magnesium sulfate over 20 min after intubation. In their control group, 5 of the 20 patients had laryngospasm, while in the group receiving magnesium, none of the patients had laryngospasm. In their paper, the researchers postulated that magnesium may contribute to increased depth of anesthesia and increased muscle paralysis as mechanisms by which it reduces the incidence of laryngospasm [55].

In addition to pharmacological interventions, the depth of anesthesia during tracheal extubation has been studied, but it remains unclear whether awake versus deep extubation is more effective at reducing the risk of laryngospasm. However, it is clear that a patient should not be extubated while they are in an intermediate or light plane of anesthesia. In addition, the so called, "no-touch" technique has been studied, albeit in a relatively small cohort of 20 children presenting for tonsillectomy and adenoidectomy. None of the 20 patients who were observed developed laryngospasm [56]. The "no-touch" technique involves suctioning the oropharynx while the patient is still anesthetized and then allowing the child to fully emerge in the lateral position without any stimulation. Once the patient's eyes start to open, he or she is extubated. Another technique that has been utilized during extubation involves extubating while the lungs are inflated by positive pressure. The technique may reduce laryngospasm by decreasing adductor muscle response [58].

L13: At What Point Should Chest Compressions Be Initiated in a Patient Who Becomes Acutely Hypoxemic, Appears Cyanotic, and Has Sinus Bradycardia on Telemetry?

According to the American Heart Association cardiopulmonary resuscitation guidelines (Fig. 6.6), a pediatric patient who displays clinical signs of symptomatic bradycardia despite oxygenation and ventilation should have chest compressions initiated if the heart rate is below 60 beats per minute (bpm). If the bradycardia continues, the patient may need treatment with epinephrine or atropine (refer to Fig. 6.6). In our patient, despite attempts at mask ventilation, the child continued to have desaturation on pulse oximetry and appeared increasingly cyanotic as the heart rate decreased to the 40s, down from this patient's baseline of approximately 100 bpm. Chest compressions were initiated to essentially provide external cardiac massage and assist in maintaining systemic perfusion and augmenting venous return as well as providing coronary perfusion. In order to perform high-quality chest compressions, it is recommended that the compressions be delivered at a rate of 100 bpm with a compression depth of 2 in. in children and with minimal interruptions [59].

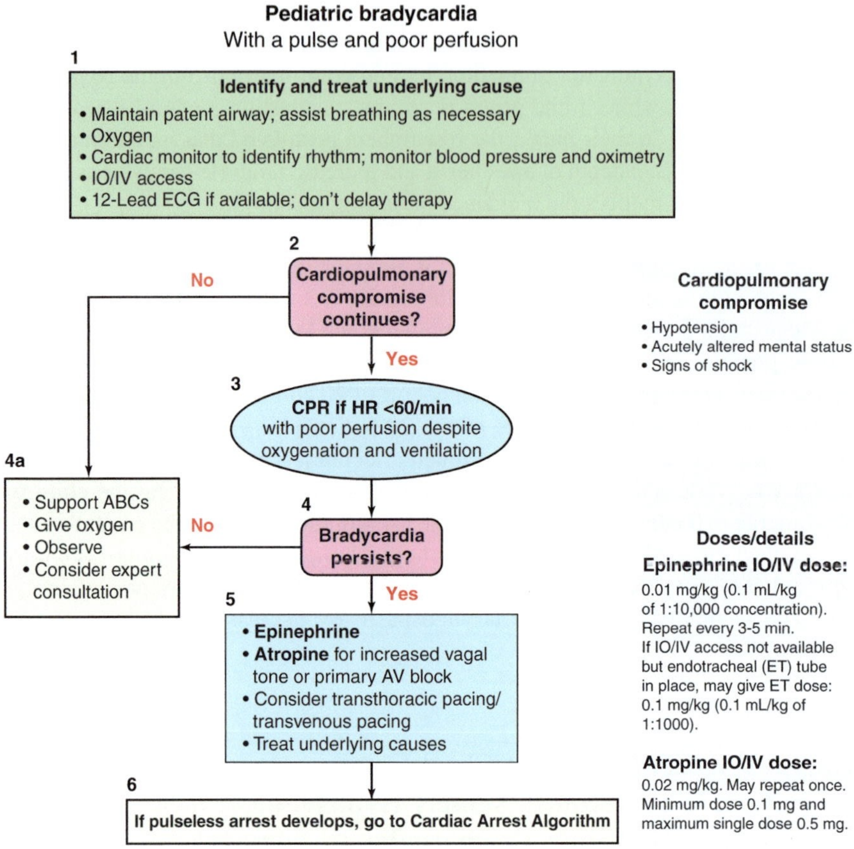

Fig. 6.6 The 2010 American Heart Association algorithm (unchanged on 2015 algorithm) for symptomatic bradycardia recommends initiating cardiopulmonary resuscitation for a heart rate less than 60 beats per minute. (Reprinted from Kleinman et al. [59]. With permission from Wolters Kluwer Health)

References

1. Blake KD, Davenport SL, Hall BD, et al. CHARGE association: an update and review for the primary pediatrician. Clin Pediatr (Phila). 1998;37(3):159–73.
2. Jyonouchi S, Mcdonald-mcginn DM, Bale S, Zackai EH, Sullivan KE. CHARGE (coloboma, heart defect, atresia choanae, retarded growth and development, genital hypoplasia, ear anomalies/deafness) syndrome and chromosome 22q11.2 deletion syndrome: a comparison of immunologic and nonimmunologic phenotypic features. Pediatrics. 2009;123(5):e871–7.
3. Issekutz KA, Graham JM, Prasad C, Smith IM, Blake KD. An epidemiological analysis of CHARGE syndrome: preliminary results from a Canadian study. Am J Med Genet A. 2005;133A(3):309–17.
4. Lin AE, Chin AJ, Devine W, Park SC, Zackai E. The pattern of cardiovascular malformation in the CHARGE association. Am J Dis Child. 1987;141(9):1010–3.

5. Wyse RK, Al-mahdawi S, Burn J, Blake K. Congenital heart disease in CHARGE association. Pediatr Cardiol. 1993;14(2):75–81.
6. Tellier AL, Cormier-daire V, Abadie V, et al. CHARGE syndrome: report of 47 cases and review. Am J Med Genet. 1998;76(5):402–9.
7. "Choanal Atresia." Children's Hospital of Philadelphia, Center for Pediatric Airway Disorders Home. http://www.chop.edu/conditions-diseases/choanal-atresia." 29 Sep 2017.
8. Bianchi DW, Crombleholme TM, D'Alton ME. Chapter 29: Micrognathia. In: Fetology, diagnosis & management of the fetal patient. New York: McGraw Hill Professional; 2000.
9. Benumof J, Hagberg CA. Benumof's airway management, principles and practice. St. Louis: Elsevier Health Sciences; 2007. p. 801.
10. Morgan D, Bailey M, Phelps P, Bellman S, Grace A, Wyse R. Ear-nose-throat abnormalities in the CHARGE association. Arch Otolaryngol Head Neck Surg. 1993;119(1):49–54.
11. Stack CG, Wyse RK. Incidence and management of airway problems in the CHARGE Association. Anaesthesia. 1991;46(7):582–5.
12. Lioy J, Sobol SE. Disorders of the neonatal airway, fundamentals for practice. New York: Springer; 2015.
13. Campisi P, Busato GM. Embryology of congenital airway disorders. In: Lioy J, Sobol S, editors. Disorders of the neonatal airway. New York: Springer; 2015. p. 3–13.
14. Ferrari LR, Zurakowski D, Solari J, Rahbar R. Laryngeal cleft repair: the anesthetic perspective. Paediatr Anaesth. 2013;23(4):334–41.
15. Dimario FJ, Sarfarazi M. Family pedigree analysis of children with severe breath-holding spells. J Pediatr. 1997;130(4):647–51.
16. Lombroso CT, Lerman P. Breathholding spells (cyanotic and pallid infantile syncope). Pediatrics. 1967;39(4):563–81.
17. Williams J, Cain N. Case report of successful treatment of pallid breath-holding spells with glycopyrrolate. Pediatrics. 2015;135(5):e1308–11.
18. Ergul Y, Otar G, Nisli K, Dindar A. Permanent cardiac pacing in a 2.5 month-old infant with severe cyanotic breath-holding spells and prolonged asystole. Cardiol J. 2011;18(6):704–6.
19. Rathore G, Larsen P, Fernandez C, Parakh M. Diverse presentation of breath holding spells: two case reports with literature review. Case Rep Neurol Med. 2013;2013:603190, 3 pages. https://doi.org/10.1155/2013/603190.
20. Crowley KL, Rehman M, Schwartz RE. Anesthetic management of a patient with asystolic spells. J Clin Anesth. 2004;16(3):207–9.
21. Lerman J, Coté CJ, Steward DJ. Manual of pediatric anesthesia. Cham: Springer; 2016.
22. Von Ungern-Sternberg BS, Boda K, Chambers NA, Rebmann C, Johnson C, Sly P, Habre W. Risk assessment for respiratory complications in paediatric anaesthesia: a prospective cohort study. Lancet. 2010;376(9743):773–83.
23. Vo P, Bair-merritt M, Camargo CA, Eisenberg S, Long W. Individual factors, neighborhood social context and asthma at age 5 years. J Asthma. 2017;54(3):265–72.
24. Van Marter LJ. Epidemiology of bronchopulmonary dysplasia. Semin Fetal Neonatal Med. 2009;14:358–66.
25. Jones LJ, Craven PD, Lakkundi A, Foster JP, Badawi N. Regional (spinal, epidural, caudal) versus general anaesthesia in preterm infants undergoing inguinal herniorrhaphy in early infancy. Cochrane Database Syst Rev. 2015;6:CD003669.
26. Mamie C, Habre W, Delhumeau C, Argiroffo CB, Morabia A. Incidence and risk factors of perioperative respiratory adverse events in children undergoing elective surgery. Paediatr Anaesth. 2004;14(3):218–24.
27. Akinbami LJ, Moorman JE, Bailey C, et al. Trends in asthma prevalence, health care use, and mortality in the United States, 2001–2010. NCHS Data Brief. 2012;94:1–8.
28. Robin B, Yim YJ, Huth J, et al. Pulmonary function in bronchopulmonary dysplasia, Pulmonary function in bronchopulmonary dysplasia. Pediatr Pulmonol. 2004;37:236–42.
29. Sj G, Iannuzzi DM, Kveselis DA, Anbar RD. Effect of preterm birth on pulmonary function at school age: a prospective controlled study. J Pediatr. 1998;133:188–92.

30. Vrijlandt EJ, Gerritsen J, Boezen HM, Grevink RG, Duiverman EJ. Lung function and exercise capacity in young adults born prematurely. Am J Respir Crit Care Med. 2006;173:890–6.
31. Mcgill WA, Coveler LA, Epstein BS. Subacute upper respiratory infection in small children. Anesth Analg. 1979;58(4):331–3.
32. Parnis SJ, Barker DS, Van der Walt JH. Clinical predictors of anaesthetic complications in children with respiratory tract infections. Paediatr Anaesth. 2001;11(1):29–40.
33. Tait AR, Knight PR. The effects of general anesthesia on upper respiratory tract infections in children. Anesthesiology. 1987;67(6):930–5.
34. Coté CJ. The upper respiratory tract infection (URI) dilemma: fear of a complication or litigation? Anesthesiology. 2001;95(2):283–5.
35. Tait AR, Malviya S, Voepel-lewis T, Munro HM, Seiwert M, Pandit UA. Risk factors for perioperative adverse respiratory events in children with upper respiratory tract infections. Anesthesiology. 2001;95(2):299–306.
36. Konarzewski WH, Ravindran N, Findlow D, Timmis PK. Anaesthetic death of a child with a cold. Anaesthesia. 1992;47(7):624.
37. Jones A. Anesthetic death of a child with a cold. Anesthesia. 1992;47:624.
38. Bloch EC. Anaesthetic death of a child with a cold. Anaesthesia. 1993;48(2):171.
39. Tait AR, Voepel-lewis T, Munro HM, Gutstein HB, Reynolds PI. Cancellation of pediatric outpatient surgery: economic and emotional implications for patients and their families. J Clin Anesth. 1997;9(3):213–9.
40. Empey DW, Laitinen LA, Jacobs L, et al. Mechanism of bronchial hyperreactivity in normal subjects after upper respiratory tract infection. Am Rev Respir Dis. 1976;113:131–9.
41. Aquillana AT, Hall WJ, Douglas RG Jr, Utell MJ. Airway reactivity in subjects with viral upper respiratory tract infections: the effects of exercise and cold air. Am Rev Respir Dis. 1980;122:3–10.
42. Watt S, Pickhardt D, Lerman J, Armstrong J, Creighton PR, Feldman L. Telescoping tracheal tubes into catheters minimizes epistaxis during nasotracheal intubation in children. Anesthesiology. 2007;106(2):238–42.
43. Garside A, Hatfield A. Using Jaques Nelaton catheter as an introducer for nasotracheal intubation. Anaesthesia. 2014;69(12):1399–401.
44. Shindell M. Nasotracheal intubation. 2015. Retrieved from http://emedicine.medscape.com/article/1663655-overview#a3.
45. Dost P, Armbruster W. Nasal turbinate dislocation caused by nasotracheal intubation. Acta Anaesthesiol Scand. 1997;41:795–6.
46. Wilkinson JA, Mathis RD, Dire DJ. Turbinate destruction—a rare complication of nasotracheal intubation. J Emerg Med. 1986;4:209–12.
47. Binning R. A hazard of blind nasal intubation. Anaesthesia. 1974;29:366–7.
48. Harvey DC, Amorosa P. Traumatic nasotracheal intubation. Anaesthesia. 1986;41:442.
49. Onçağ O, Cökmez B, Aydemir S, Balcioğlu T. Investigation of bacteremia following nasotracheal intubation. Paediatr Anaesth. 2005;15(3):194–8.
50. Baijal RG, Bidani SA, Minard CG, Watcha MF. Perioperative respiratory complications following awake and deep extubation in children undergoing adenotonsillectomy. Paediatr Anaesth. 2015;25(4):392–9.
51. Abelson D. Laryngospasm notch pressure ("Larson's maneuver") may have a role in laryngospasm management in children: highlighting a so far unproven technique. Paediatr Anaesth. 2015;25(11):1175–6.
52. Baraka A. Intravenous lidocaine controls extubation laryngospasm in children. Anesth Analg. 1978;57(4):506–7.
53. Koc C, Kocaman F, Aygenc E, et al. The use of perioperative lidocaine to prevent stridor and laryngospasm after tonsillectomy and adenoidectomy. Otolaryngol Head Neck Surg. 1998;118:880–2.
54. Batra YK, Ivanova M, Ali SS, et al. The efficacy of a subhypnotic dose of propofol in preventing laryngospasm following tonsillectomy and adenoidectomy in children. Pediatr Anesth. 2005;15:1094–7.

55. Gulhas N, Durmus N, Demirbileks S, et al. The use of magnesium to prevent laryngospasm after tonsillectomy and adenoidectomy: a preliminary study. Paediatr Anaesth. 2003;13:43–7.
56. Tsui BCH, Wagner A, Cave D, et al. The incidence of laryngospasm with a "No Touch" extubation technique after tonsillectomy and adenoidectomy. Anesth Analg. 2004;98:327–9.
57. Leicht P, Wisborg T, Chraemmer-Jorgensen B. Does intravenous lidocaine prevent laryngospasm after extubation in children? Anesth Analg. 1985;64:1193–6.
58. Landsman IS. Mechanisms and treatment of laryngospasm. Int Anesthesiol Clin. 1997;35(3):67–73.
59. Kleinman ME, Chameides L, Schexnayder SM, et al. Part 14: pediatric advanced life support: 2010 American Heart Association Guidelines for Cardiopulmonary Resuscitation and Emergency Cardiovascular Care. Circulation. 2010;122(18 Suppl 3):S876–908.

Chapter 7
A Patient with ALS Requiring Intubation

James Phillips, Seth Herway, and Alyssa Brzenski

A 39-year-old man with advancing sporadic amyotrophic lateral sclerosis **(L-1)** was admitted to an intensive care unit (ICU) service because of 2 days of worsening shortness of breath and an inability to clear secretions. The patient was wheelchair bound and used continuous positive airway pressure therapy while sleeping. On arrival to the emergency department, he was diagnosed with acute on chronic hypercarbic respiratory failure secondary to worsening muscle weakness because of an initial arterial blood gas (ABG) which showed a pH 7.17/pCO2 133 mmHg/HCO_3 30 mEq/L/paO2 187 mmHg/O_2 saturation 100%. The patient and his mother had never discussed his code status; however, the patient's mother was inclined to allow him to be intubated. Multiple physicians agreed that the patient did not have the capacity to make decisions at the time of admission to the hospital due to severe hypercarbia, and it was decided to allow for endotracheal intubation if the patient had any further respiratory decline.

Upon admission to the ICU, the BiPAP settings were incrementally increased for worsening respiratory failure over the next 4 h. Eventually, the on-call anesthesiologist was called by the ICU fellow for intubation. On the anesthesiologist's arrival to the bedside, the ICU fellow expressed a desire to intubate the patient. It was decided the ICU fellow would intubate under the direct supervision of the attending anesthesiologist. While obtaining the appropriate equipment for intubation, the patient was preoxygenated. Unbeknownst to the attending anesthesiologist, the ICU fellow had

J. Phillips
Department of Anesthesia, Community Anesthesia Providers, Clovis, CA, USA

S. Herway
Department of Anesthesia, Mountain West Anesthesia, St. George, UT, USA

Department of Anesthesiology, University of California, San Diego, CA, USA

A. Brzenski (✉)
Department of Anesthesiology, University of California, San Diego, CA, USA
e-mail: abrzenski@ucsd.edu

J. L. Benumof, G. R. Manecke (eds.), *Clinical Anesthesiology II*,
https://doi.org/10.1007/978-3-030-12365-9_7

already ordered etomidate and succinylcholine induction medications for the bedside nurse to give. Etomidate 16 mg followed by 120 mg succinylcholine **(L-2)** were pushed intravenously by the bedside nurse, due to the previous order by the ICU fellow, without notifying the anesthesiologist. The bedside nurse announced that etomidate and succinylcholine had been administered. At the instruction of the attending anesthesiologist, the nurse attempted to withdraw the medications through the IV; however, they had already been flushed in.

Immediately after administration of the induction agents, the patient's heart rate rapidly dropped from 110 to 70 bpm. As the ICU fellow inserted the laryngoscope, the patient developed ventricular tachycardia **(L-3)**. The laryngoscope was removed, chest compressions were initiated, and a code blue was called. The attending anesthesiologist, without difficulty, then intubated the patient while compressions were continued. A colorimetric carbon dioxide detector and bilateral breath sounds confirmed tracheal intubation. Epinephrine, bicarbonate, and calcium chloride were given **(L-4)**. Within a minute the patient was found to have palpable pulses, and the ventricular tachycardia subsequently spontaneously converted to sinus rhythm. Cardiopulmonary resuscitation (CPR) was stopped, while mechanical ventilation was continued. The initial ABG, obtained during CPR, showed a potassium level of 6.5 meq/L, which decreased to 4.1 meq/L on the follow-up ABG. Following the pulseless ventricular tachycardia, the patient required intravenous pressors to maintain hemodynamic stability. A right internal jugular central venous catheter and left radial arterial line were placed for hemodynamic monitoring. An emergent bronchoscopy post-intubation found a large mucus plug that was suctioned with improvements in oxygenation and ventilation.

The patient underwent several therapeutic bronchoscopies over the next few days for a diagnosed septic pneumonia. At a family meeting several days later, the patient confirmed his desire to undergo tracheostomy placement, recognizing that long-term ventilation and long-term skilled care would be required. A percutaneous tracheostomy tube and an interventional radiology-guided gastric tube were placed. The patient was eventually discharged to a long-term care facility.

L-1: Amyotrophic Lateral Sclerosis and Anesthetic Considerations

Amyotrophic lateral sclerosis (ALS-Lou Gehrig's disease) is a degenerative motor neuron disease that is characterized by muscle wasting and spasticity and typically sporadic in nature. This degeneration involves both upper and lower motor neuron death. Typical symptoms include difficulty with swallowing, speaking, and breathing. The onset of symptoms for sporadic cases typically occurs around age 60, while symptoms in inherited cases (5–10%) typically start around age 50 [1]. Patients on average survive 3–4 years after the onset of symptoms [2]. The death rate throughout the world is 2 deaths per 100,000 people per year [3]. Riluzole, an antiglutaminergic, is currently the only available medication proven to slow the progression of ALS [4]. However, the majority of treatment is symptomatic including antispasmodics, antisialogues, breathing support, physical/occupational/speech therapy, nutrition, and palliative care.

Table 7.1 Anesthesia considerations for amyotrophic lateral sclerosis

System	Anesthetic consideration
Cardiovascular	Orthostatic hypotension and tachycardia may be a sign of autonomic dysfunction
Pulmonary	Exaggerated respiratory depression with general anesthesia and other respiratory depressants (i.e., narcotics)
	High risk of pulmonary aspiration, especially when bulbar signs/symptoms are present
Neuromuscular	Susceptible to hyperkalemia with succinylcholine administration
	Increased sensitivity to and prolonged action of nondepolarizing muscle relaxants
	Regional anesthesia is not contraindicated
	No increased risk for malignant hyperthermia
Positioning	Care must be taken to document and protect all known ulcerations and skin breakdown
	Muscular atrophy predisposes peripheral nerves to positioning injuries
Temperature	Decreased muscle bulk predisposes to intra- and postoperative hypothermia

There are a number of anesthetic considerations in a patient with ALS (see Table 7.1). Avoidance of succinylcholine is imperative due to its association with hyperkalemic arrest/arrhythmias in patients with denervation and immobility. ALS, along with any state that causes denervation, induces the body to produce extrajunctional acetylcholine receptors. It's these receptors that have the potential to greatly add to the efflux of potassium from the cell when activated by succinylcholine.

Likewise, the use of acetylcholinesterase inhibitors should also be used with caution. Nondepolarizing paralytics may have a prolonged effect. The combination of bulbar dysfunction and decreased pulmonary control puts ALS patients at an increased risk of aspiration. These patients may also be overly sensitive to respiratory depressants, such as narcotics [5]. The muscular atrophy in ALS patients puts peripheral nerves at an increased risk of injury. Areas that were previously protected by muscle tone and bulk may now be exposed, depending upon the patient's extent of disease. Careful documentation of all current skin breakdown and injuries is advised. Autonomic dysfunction may be seen in ALS patients. Orthostatic hypotension with tachycardia merits further workup.

L-2: Contraindication to Succinylcholine

Succinylcholine is contraindicated in the setting of multiple medical conditions (see Table 7.2). First, patients with acute hyperkalemia, motor neuron diseases, myopathies associated with an increase in creatinine kinase levels, and multiple/severe traumas have an increased risk of precipitating clinically significant hyperkalemia if succinylcholine is administered. Second, succinylcholine increases intraocular pressure; therefore, patients with closed-angle glaucoma or penetrating eye trauma

Table 7.2 Contraindications to succinylcholine

Contraindication	Why
Acute hyperkalemia	Increases risk of clinically significant acute hyperkalemia
Closed-angle glaucoma	Raises intraocular pressure in closed space-> direct pressure on optic nerve-> nerve damage/blindness
Penetrating eye trauma	Raises intraocular pressure in open space-> extrusion of eye contents through penetrating injury
Malignant hyperthermia	MH-triggering agent
Disorders of pseudocholinesterase	Unpredictable drug metabolism
Motor neuron diseases, skeletal denervation	Increases risk of clinically significant acute hyperkalemia
Multiple traumas (burns, crush injuries)	Increases risk of clinically significant acute hyperkalemia

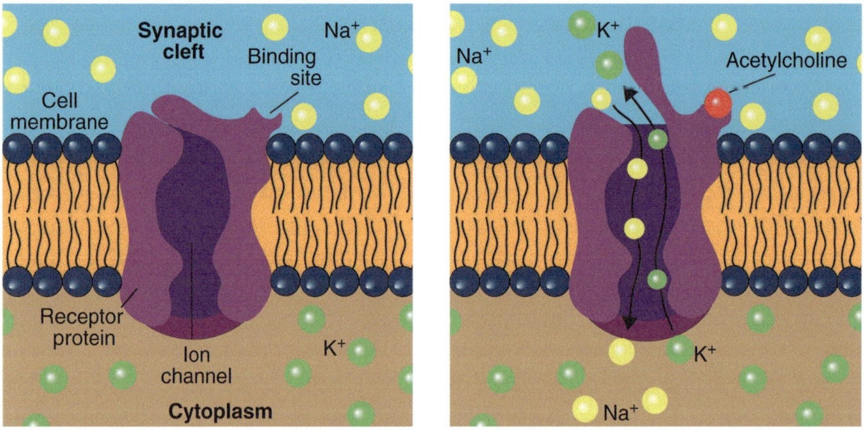

Fig. 7.1 Effect of acetylcholine. Showing the binding of acetylcholine to its receptor. This allows for sodium (Na) to enter the cell and potassium (K) to exit the cell

have an increased risk for optic nerve damage by severely increasing pressure on the nerve. Third, succinylcholine is a triggering agent for those at risk of having malignant hyperthermia. Fourth, disorders of pseudocholinesterase can cause unpredictable metabolism of succinylcholine. In addition, succinylcholine should be avoided in any disease state causing extensive denervation of skeletal muscle, especially those associated with muscle atrophy because of the risk of hyperkalemia [6].

Hyperkalemia occurs due to the extracellular migration of potassium while the acetylcholine receptor is activated and opened (see Fig. 7.1). The more acetylcholine receptors that are present, the higher the serum potassium can potentially rise when depolarization occurs. A typical rise of serum potassium in a healthy person is 0.5–1 mmol/L. This number can be increased severely by the appearance of extrajunctional acetylcholine receptors, as in crush injury, burns, and denervation diseases and injuries. It is these extrajunctional receptors that are responsible for the large-scale efflux of potassium into the extracellular and intravascular space.

This patient had ALS and was acidotic likely due to acute on chronic respiratory failure resulting in an increase in serum potassium. The patient's serum potassium increased further due to depolarization of an increased number of extrajunctional acetylcholine receptors. In this setting, considering the patient's likely need for prolonged intubation, administration of a rapid sequence dose of nondepolarizing neuromuscular-blocking agent (e.g., 1.2 mg/kg of rocuronium) would be the most appropriate medication to achieve muscle relaxation during endotracheal intubation.

L-3: Treatment of Ventricular Tachycardia

Ventricular tachycardia secondary to hyperkalemia is treated with the same advanced cardiac life support (ACLS) protocol as with all other causes of ventricular tachycardia; however there are a few points that deserve extra emphasis. Cardiopulmonary resuscitation (CPR), immediate defibrillation, and blood pressure support are the foundation of treatment (see Fig. 7.2). An emphasis on acutely decreasing serum potassium should be made (see L-4). If acute and temporary potassium-lowering measures are ineffective, emergent hemodialysis should be considered.

L-4: Treatment of Hyperkalemia

Treatment of hyperkalemia involves three separate tenants (see Table 7.3):

1. *Decreasing myocardial excitability.* Administering intravenous calcium (typically calcium chloride 1 g IV) helps decrease the myocardial excitability. Calcium is a cation that increases the voltage difference (membrane potential) between intracellular and extracellular voltage, thus stabilizing the myocardium and decreasing the likelihood to reach the threshold potential.
2. *Temporarily decreasing serum potassium levels.* Interventions *that* temporarily decrease serum potassium include insulin treatment, beta-2 agonist administration, hyperventilation, and bicarbonate administration. Insulin (typically 10U IV) shifts extracellular potassium inside the cell via sodium-potassium (Na-K) ATPase activity [7]. Effects last on the order of a few hours. Glucose must be given in order to avoid hypoglycemia. Glucose 25 g IV can also be given independently resulting in release of endogenous insulin. Intracellular potassium is important for sympathetic activity and neuron excitability. Beta-2 agonists (albuterol 4 puffs via ETT, epinephrine 10–100 MCG IV) promote the intracellular movement of potassium. Hyperventilation promotes a respiratory alkalosis, which shifts potassium intracellularly. As a rule of thumb, an increased pH of 0.1 units will result in a decrease of

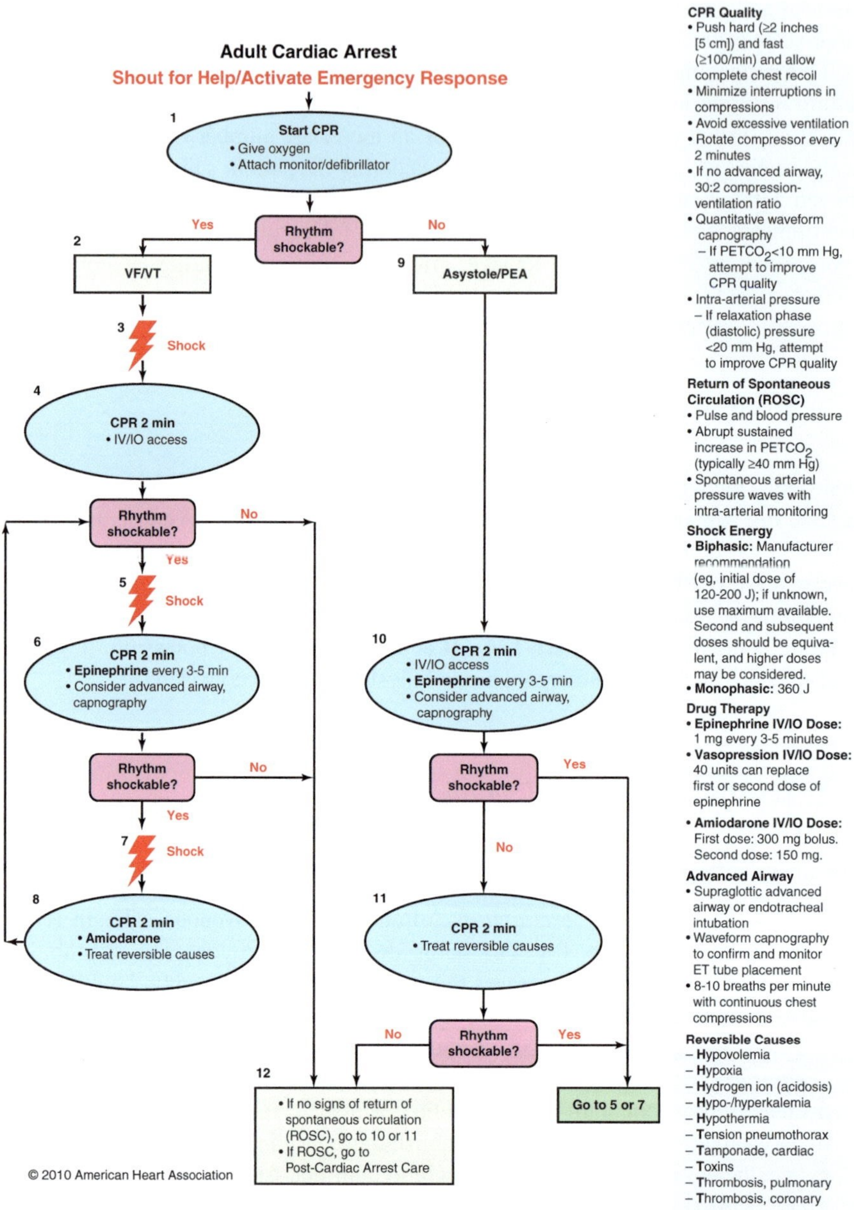

Fig. 7.2 ACLS cardiac arrest algorithm. The American Heart Association Advanced Cardiac Life Support algorithm for tachyarrhythmias. Special attention should be paid to synchronized cardioversion. (Reprinted from Neumar et al. [8]. With permission from Wolters Kluwer Health Inc.)

Table 7.3 Treatment of hyperkalemia

Tenant	Treatment
↓ Myocardial excitability	CaCl 0.1 mg–1 mgIV
↓ K+ levels (temporize)	Insulin 10 units IV with glucose 25 g, albuterol 4 puffs via endotracheal tube, hyperventilation (EtCO_2 goal 30), sodium bicarbonate 1 ampule or 44.6 mEq IV, epinephrine 10–25 mcg IV
↑ K+ elimination	Hemodialysis, binding agents (kayexalate 15–60 g PO), loop diuretics IV (furosemide 20–100 mg IV), mineralocorticoid IV (fludrocortisone 50 mg IV)

0.5–1.5 mEq change in serum potassium. Bicarbonate (1 ampule or 44.6 mEq IV) shifts potassium intracellularly via its effect on serum pH. However, administration of bicarbonate during hyperkalemic ventricular tachycardia is controversial due to the concomitant decrease in serum calcium levels (and a concomitant increase in myocardial excitability) with bicarbonate administration. It is important to note that these temporary measures to reduce serum potassium all have unpredictable short-lived effect. Measurement of serum potassium with regular arterial blood gases (ABG) is of utmost importance.

3. *Extracellular potassium elimination.* This is accomplished via hemodialysis, oral binding agents (e.g. kayexalate 15–60 g PO), loop diuretics (furosemide 20–100 mg IV), and mineralocorticoid medications (e.g. fludrocortisone 50 mg IV). Hemodialysis should be considered when the underlying cause of hyperkalemia cannot be corrected with other measures. It should be noted that hemodialysis can be time-intensive to start and cause large fluid shifts which may not be tolerated in many hyperkalemic patients.

References

1. Kiernan MC, Vucic S, Cheah BC, et al. Amyotrophic lateral sclerosis. Lancet. 2011;377:942–55.
2. Malamut. In: Sirven JI, Barbara L, editors. Clinical neurology of the older adult. 2nd ed. Philadelphia: Wolters Kluwer Health/Lippincott Williams & Wilkins; 2008. p. 421.
3. ALS Association. Quick facts about ALS & the ALS association.
4. Carlesi C, Pasquali L, Piazza S, Lo Gerfo A, Caldarazzo Ienco E, Alessi R, Fornai F, Siciliano G. Strategies for clinical approach to neurodegeneration in amyotrophic lateral sclerosis. Arch Ital Biol. 2011;149:151–67.
5. Miller R, et al. Miller's anesthesia. 7th ed. Philadelphia: Elsevier Health Sciences; 2009. p. 1172–3.
6. Flower RJ. Rang and Dale's pharmacology. London, UK: Elsevier Science Health Science Division; 2011.
7. Allon M, Shanklin N. Effect of bicarbonate administration on plasma potassium in dialysis patients: interactions with insulin and albuterol. Am J Kidney Dis. 1996;28:508–14.
8. Neumar RW, Otto CW, Link MS, et al. Part 8: adult advanced cardiovascular life support. Circulation. 2010;122(18suppl 3):S729–67.

Chapter 8
Blowtorch Airway Fire

Kimberly A. Pollock and Jonathan L. Benumof

Case Summary

This is a case of a patient with a vocal cord lesion presenting for CO_2 laser ablation of the lesion, which resulted in a blowtorch fire of the patient's airway. The patient is now ventilator dependent and will never breathe, speak, or eat again on his own. In order to understand airway fires, a general knowledge of the three components needed to start a fire (ignition source, oxidizer, fuel) is necessary (see **Lesson 1** [**L-1**]).

Case Specifics

The specifics of the case are as follows: A 64-year-old male, 6′0″, 110 kg with a body mass index (BMI) of 34 was undergoing left vocal cord ablation by CO_2 laser. The patient had undergone a right upper lobectomy for carcinoma and was placed on a ventilator for 1 week postoperatively. He was successfully weaned from the ventilator but suffered from hoarseness and was found to have a left vocal cord lesion. The patient was scheduled for a CO_2 laser resection of the left vocal cord lesion. Patient's medical history, physical exam, and airway exam were normal other than a room air saturation of 92% on room air (likely due to COPD).

The patient was taken to the operating room, routine monitors were placed, and the patient underwent an intravenous induction of anesthesia. The patient

K. A. Pollock (✉)
Department of Anesthesiology, University of California, San Diego, CA, USA

J. L. Benumof
Department of Anesthesiology, University of California, UCSD Medical Center, UCSD School of Medicine, San Diego, CA, USA

J. L. Benumof, G. R. Manecke (eds.), *Clinical Anesthesiology II*,
https://doi.org/10.1007/978-3-030-12365-9_8

was adequately ventilated via mask with a fraction of inspired oxygen (FIO_2) of 1.0. The patient was then appropriately paralyzed and ready for intubation (see **Lesson 2** [**L-2**]).

The patient was intubated with a 5.0 mm internal diameter (I.D.) Medtronic laser-resistant (L-R) endotracheal tube (ETT) (see **Lesson 3** [**L-3**]). The ETT was placed so that the 21 cm mark was at the upper incisor and the cuff was filled with saline from a 5 cc syringe (see **Lesson 4** [**L-4**] and **Lesson 5** [**L-5**]). An FIO_2 of 1.0 was used due to patient's obesity, long smoking history, COPD, and a room air saturation of 92% (see **Lesson 6** [**L-6**]). An attempt was made to block the cuff with saline-soaked pledgets (see **Lesson 7** [**L-7**] and **Lesson 8** [**L-8**]). The laser beam went medial to the vocal cords, hitting the L-R ETT cuff so that the distal high O_2 concentration gas spilled out into the laser beam and surgical field (see green area in Fig. 8.1) and so that the non L-R part of the ETT was exposed to the laser beam. The next laser beam hit the non L-R part of the ETT in the 100% O_2 environment resulting in a blowtorch fire (see Fig. 8.2). Smoke then billowed up out of the patient's mouth (see Fig. 8.3). The laser beam energy used in this case was unclear (see **Lesson 9** [**L-9**]).

The operating room table was first turned 180° so that the head of bed was near the anesthesiologist. The L-R ETT was then removed; however, approximately 1–2 min more of the ETT burning within the oropharynx (OP), laryngopharynx (LP),

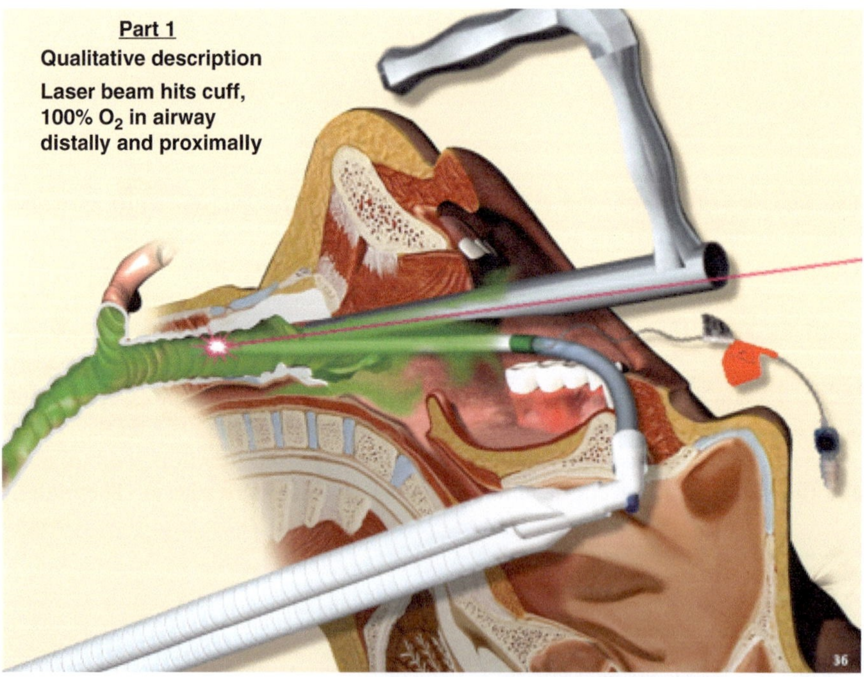

Fig. 8.1 Sagittal view of the airway with the laser beam striking the cuff thereby allowing 100% oxygen (represented in green) to spill out into the laser beam and surgical field

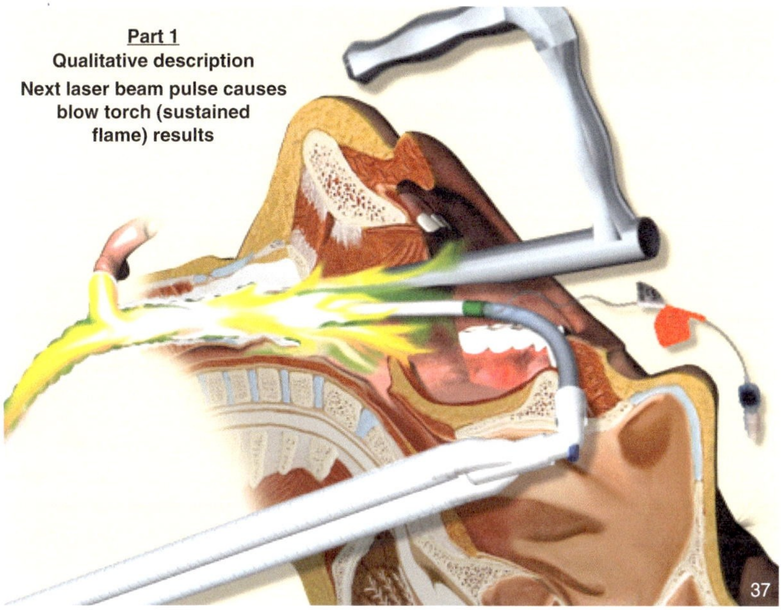

Fig. 8.2 Sagittal view of the airway after the laser beam has ruptured the cuff in the presence of 100% oxygen, causing ignition of the airway and blowtorch fire (represented in yellow)

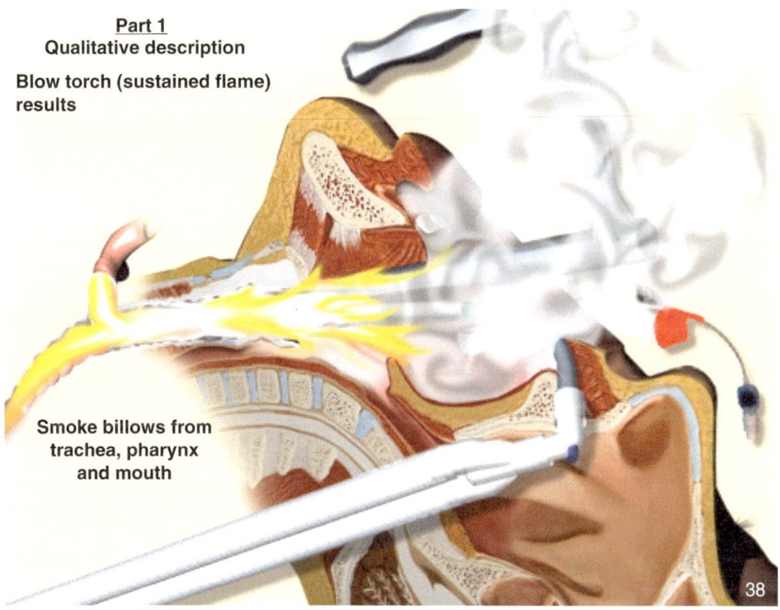

Fig. 8.3 Sagittal view of the airway after the laser beam has ignited the ETT resulting in a blowtorch fire and smoke (represented in white/gray) billowing from the trachea, laryngopharynx, and oropharynx

and tracheobronchial tree (TBT) occurred, while the OR table was being turned. A new ETT was placed, and fiber-optic bronchoscopy was performed which revealed extensive damage to the OP, LP, proximal esophagus, trachea, main stem bronchi, and even lobar bronchi (see **Lesson 10 [L-10]**). The patient remains ventilator dependent, never able to breathe, cough, speak, or eat again on his own.

Lessons Learned

L-1: What Are the Components Needed to Start and Maintain a Fire?

Components needed to start a fire include an ignition source, an oxidizer, as well as fuel for the fire (see Fig. 8.4). In this particular case, the ignition source was the laser, the oxidizer was 100% oxygen, and the fuel was the ETT and airway tissues. Examples of different components required to start a fire are outlined in Table 8.1.

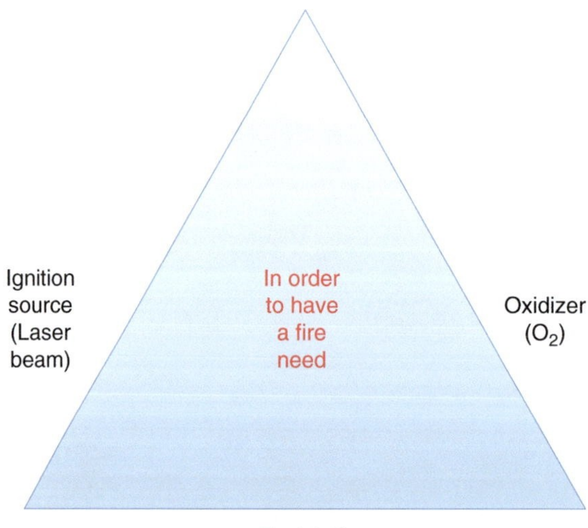

Fig. 8.4 The fire triangle: components necessary in starting and maintaining a fire. Ignition source includes things like a laser beam, a spark, and electrocautery; in this case it was a laser beam. Oxidizer includes oxygen and nitrous oxide; in this case it was high O2 concentration. Fuel includes items such as an endotracheal tube, tissue, blood, secretions, dry pledgets, operating room drapes, and blankets; in this case the major source of fuel, by far, was the ETT

Table 8.1 Commonplace examples of ignition sources, oxidizers, and fuel sources in creating a fire

Ignition sources	Oxidizer	Fuel sources
Laser[a]	Oxygen[a]	Tracheal tubes[a]
Electro-surgical or electro-cautery devices	Nitrous oxide	Sponges
Heated probes	An oxidizer-enriched atmosphere commonly exists within closed or semi-closed breathing systems	Drapes
Drills and burrs		Gauze
Argon beam coagulators		Alcohol containing solutions
Fiber-optic light cables		Ether
Defibrillator paddles or pads		Acetone
		Oxygen masks
		Nasal cannulae
		Patient's hair
		Dressings
		Ointments
		Gowns
		GI tract gases
		Blankets
		Suction catheters
		Flexible endoscopes
		Fiberoptic cable coverings
		Gloves
		Packaging materials

Based on data from Ref. [2]
[a]Components of the fire in this case in red

L-2: What Types of CO_2 Laser Resistant (L-R) Endotracheal Tubes Are Available?

There are various laser-resistant (L-R) endotracheal tubes (ETT) available for use. The two most common endotracheal tubes in use at UCSD are the Medtronic Xomed Laser-Shield II and Mallinckrodt Laser-Flex, and therefore these tubes will be discussed in more detail. The Rusch Lasertubus is a third ETT that is used at the Veterans Association Medical Center and will also be addressed here. Saline should be used to fill all cuffs of all L-R ETTs; saline acts as a laser beam heat/energy absorbent, which is the principle mode of action of the saline. An indicator dye in the saline is highly desired when using the Medtronic and Mallinckrodt L-R ETTs. The purpose of the dye is to indicate whether or not the laser has damaged the cuff. In theory, if the cuff is damaged, the released dye should be visible either in the surgical field or on the pledgets. When using the Medtronic Xomed Laser-Shield II (see Figs. 8.5a and 8.6), methylene blue indicator powder is already present in the

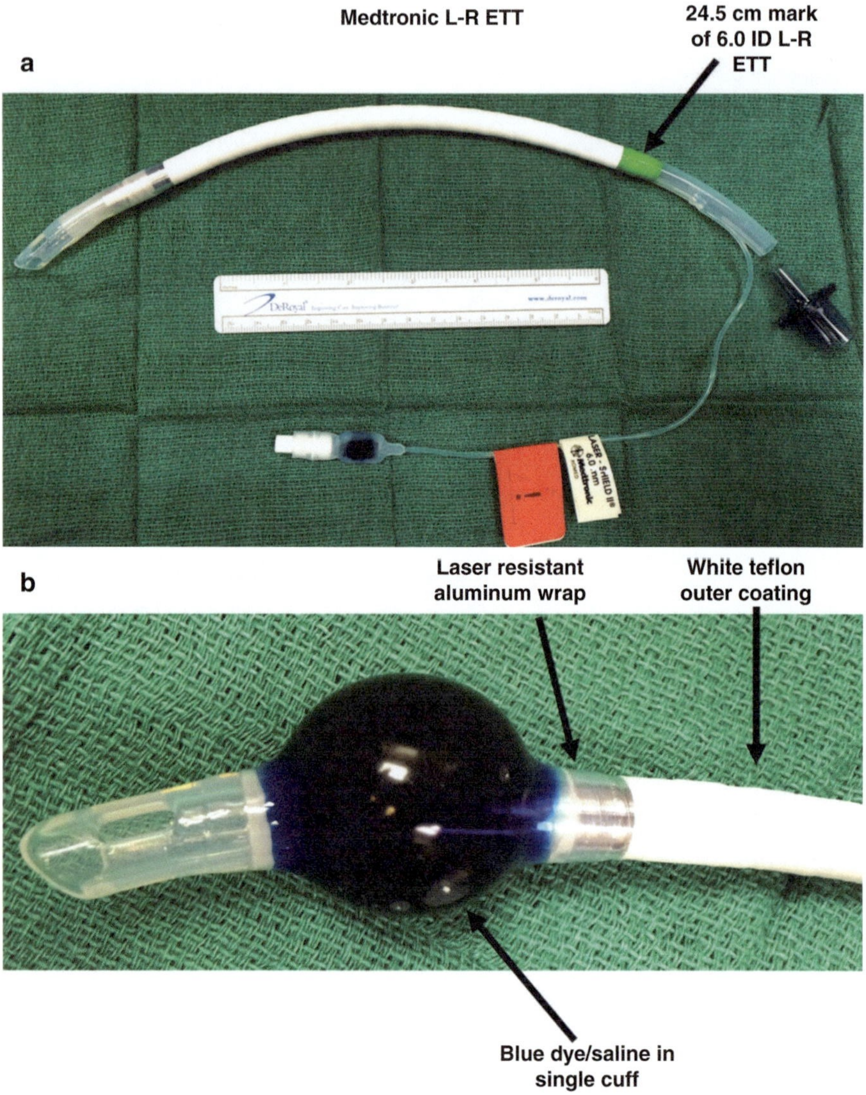

Fig. 8.5 (**a**) Medtronic L-R ETT with dried methylene blue indicator in pilot balloon. (**b**) Medtronic L-R ETT with saline mixed methylene blue indicator dye in cuff

pilot balloon so that saline can be easily injected to inflate the cuff while at the same time filling the cuff with indicator dye (see Fig. 8.5b). Advantages of the Medtronic L-R ETT include indicator dye already present in the pilot balloon, and the Teflon L-R coating on the ETT is soft; however, disadvantages include the fact that there is only one cuff, causing potential for an airway fire if this cuff does not fully seal or is ruptured by the laser beam (see Fig. 8.7). When using the Mallinckrodt Laser-Flex L-R ETT, there are two cuffs present (see Figs. 8.8a and 8.9). The proximal

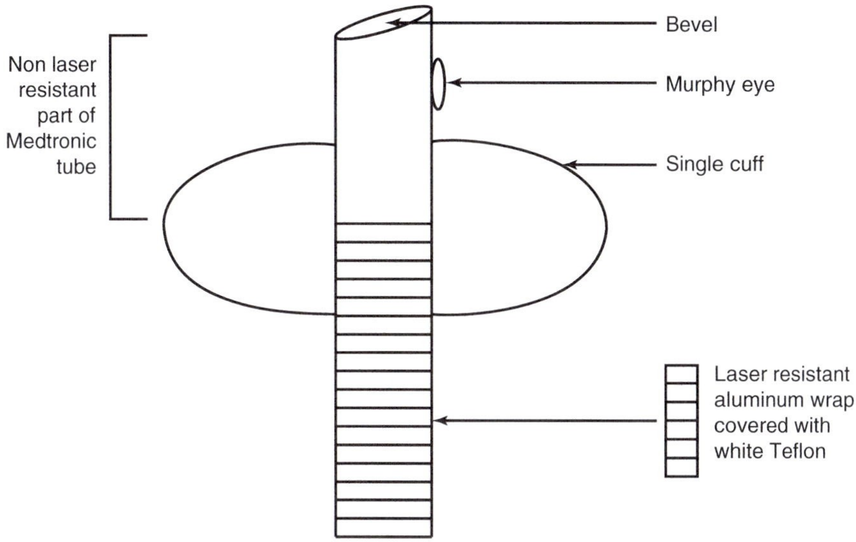

Fig. 8.6 Schematic of the Medtronic Xomed Laser-Shield II Endotracheal Tube

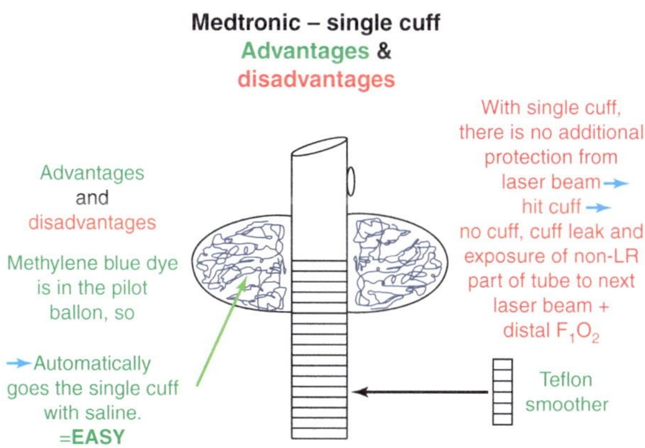

Fig. 8.7 Schematic displaying the advantage and disadvantages of the Medtronic Xomed Laser-Shield II ETT. Advantages are shown in green; disadvantages are shown in red

cuff is filled with indicator fluid (0.2–0.4 cc of methylene blue or indigo carmine dye is diluted into 10 cc of normal saline), while the distal cuff is inflated with clear saline (see Fig. 8.8b). If there is a breach in the cuff, caused by the laser beam, it will insult the proximal cuff first, spilling dye into the surgical field or onto the pledgets. If this is recognized, there is still a distal cuff that is inflated with saline, which continues to prevent the oxygen in the lungs from mixing with the laser beam ignition source and ETT and starting an airway fire. The double cuff design of the

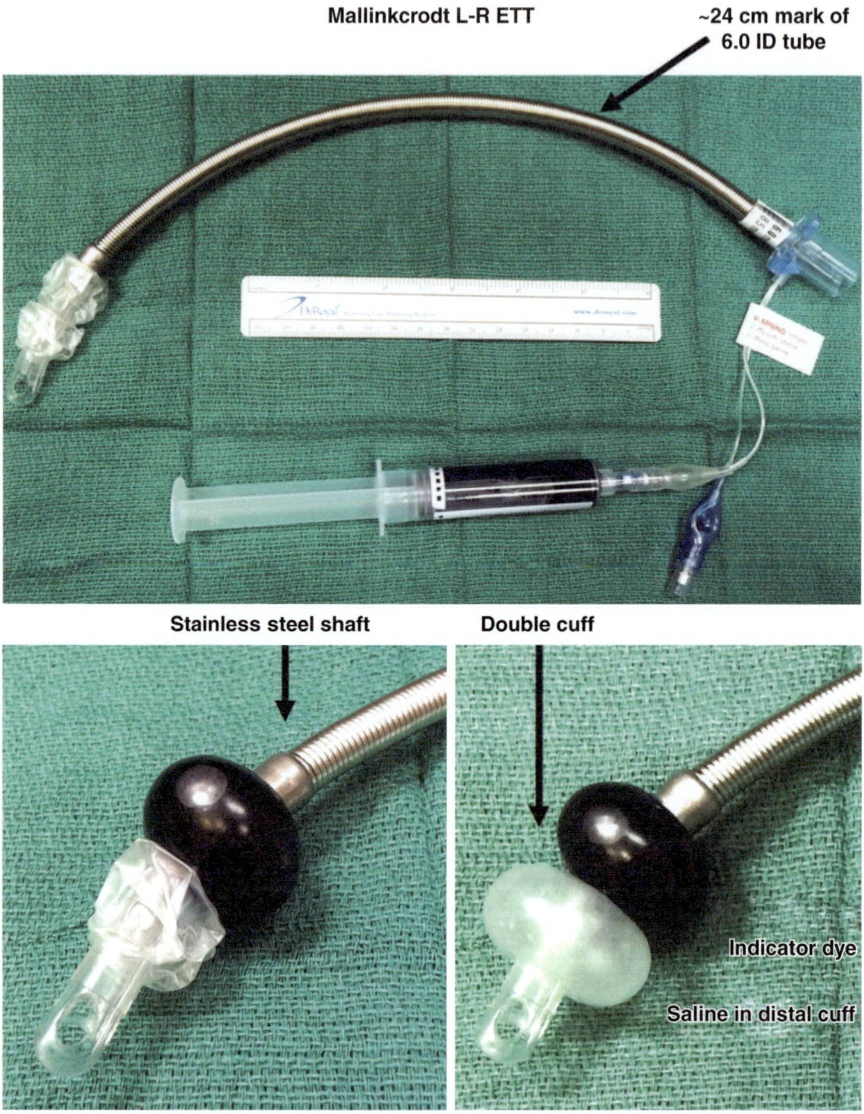

Fig. 8.8 (**a**) Mallinckrodt L-R ETT with 0.4 cc methylene blue mixed with 9.6 cc saline in a 10 cc syringe attached to pilot balloon. (**b**) Left: Proximal cuff inflated with 10 cc of indicator/saline mixture. Right: Distal cuff inflated with 10 cc saline, in addition to proximal cuff containing indicator

Mallinckrodt L-R ETT is advantageous because the proximal cuff protects the distal cuff from the laser beam and the distal cuff protects the proximal cuff from a leak if the laser beam ruptures the proximal cuff (see Fig. 8.10). Disadvantages of this ETT include the fact that indicator dye is not already present in the pilot balloon and must

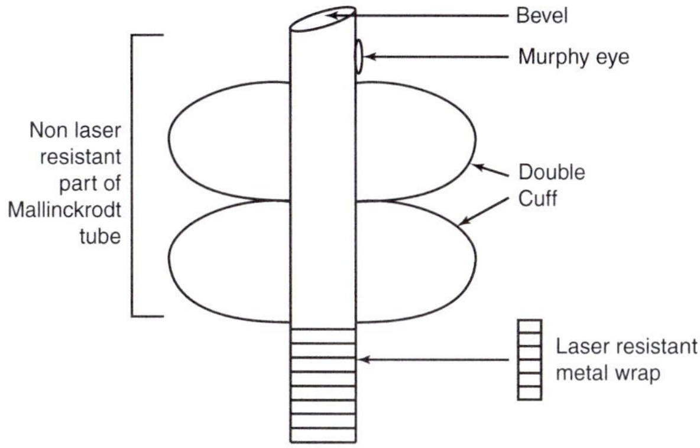

Fig. 8.9 Schematic of the Mallinckrodt Laser-Flex Endotracheal Tube

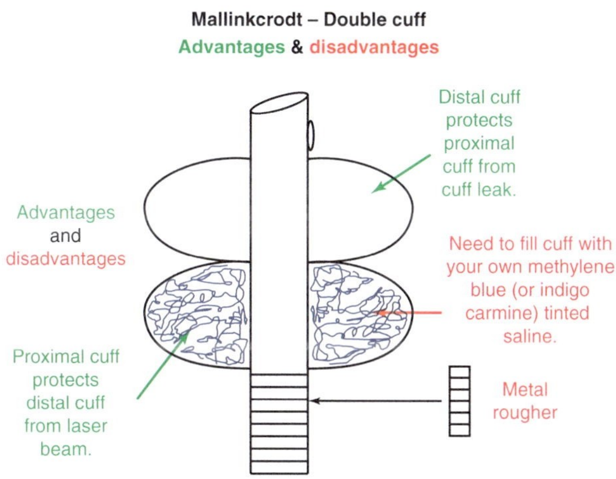

Fig. 8.10 Schematic displaying the advantage and disadvantages of the Mallinckrodt Laser-Flex ETT. Advantages are shown in green; disadvantages are shown in red

be injected by the anesthesiologist. Furthermore, the L-R metal coating is rougher than the Teflon of the Medtronic L-R ETT, and there is potential for damage to the airway (see Fig. 8.10). The third type of laser-resistant tube available to UCSD anesthesiologists is the Rusch Lasertubus. This L-R ETT is made of soft white rubber, reinforced with corrugated copper foil and an absorbent sponge. The absorbent sponge must be heavily wetted with normal saline in order to offer laser resistance. It is fitted with a double cuff design that offers protection against airway fires (see Figs. 8.11, 8.12, and 8.13). The double cuff design of the Lasertubus offers an advantage similar to that of the Mallinckrodt L-R ETT in that if the outer cuff is ruptured, the inner cuff protects against oxygen mixing with the laser beam; however, this L-R ETT has an extremely larger outer diameter not desirable for airway

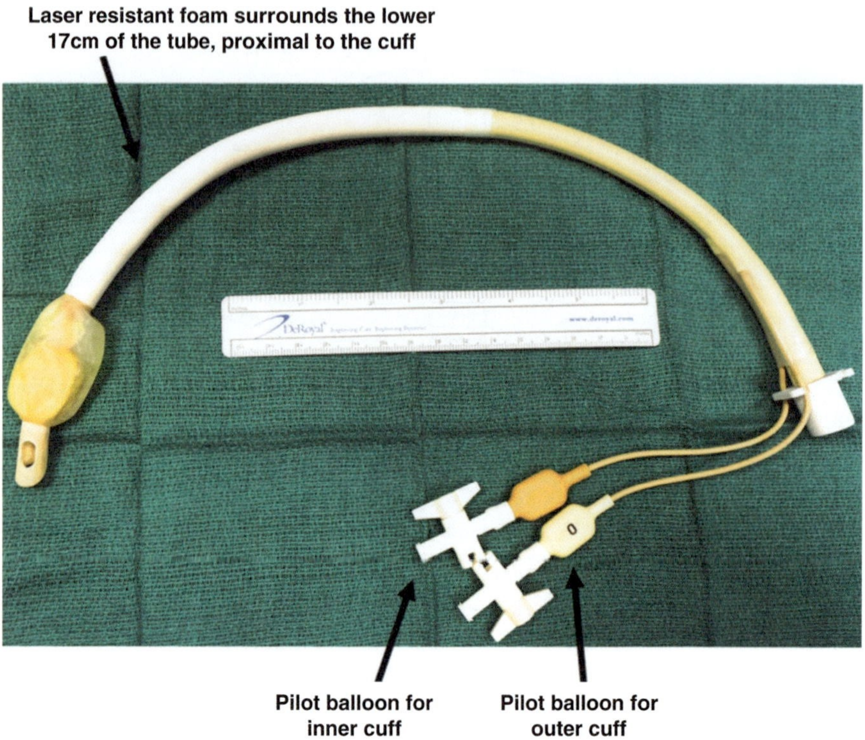

Fig. 8.11 Rusch Lasertubus ETT

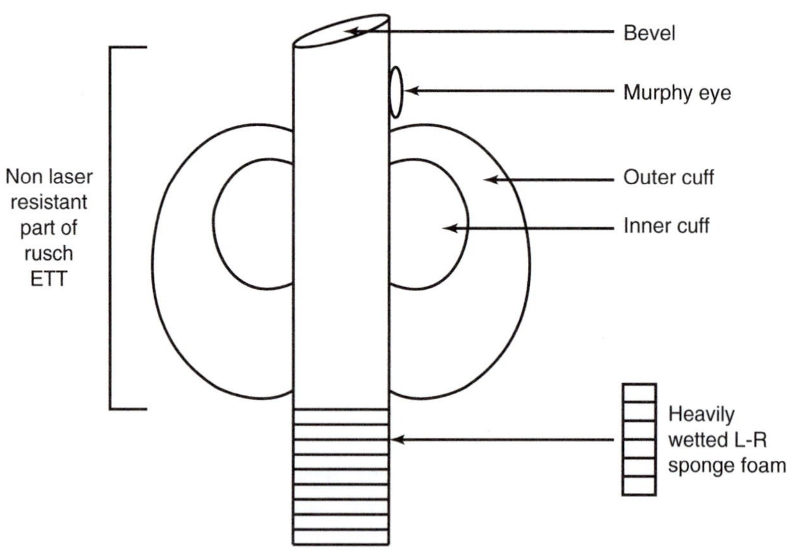

Fig. 8.12 Schematic of the Rusch Lasertubus Endotracheal Tube

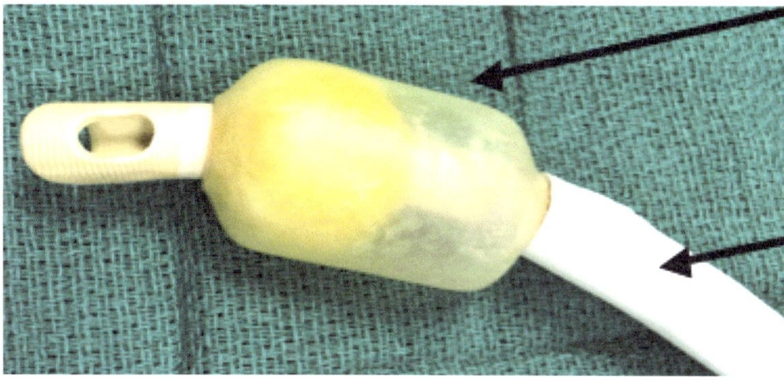

Fig. 8.13 Rusch Lasertubus ETT with both inner and outer cuffs inflated with saline

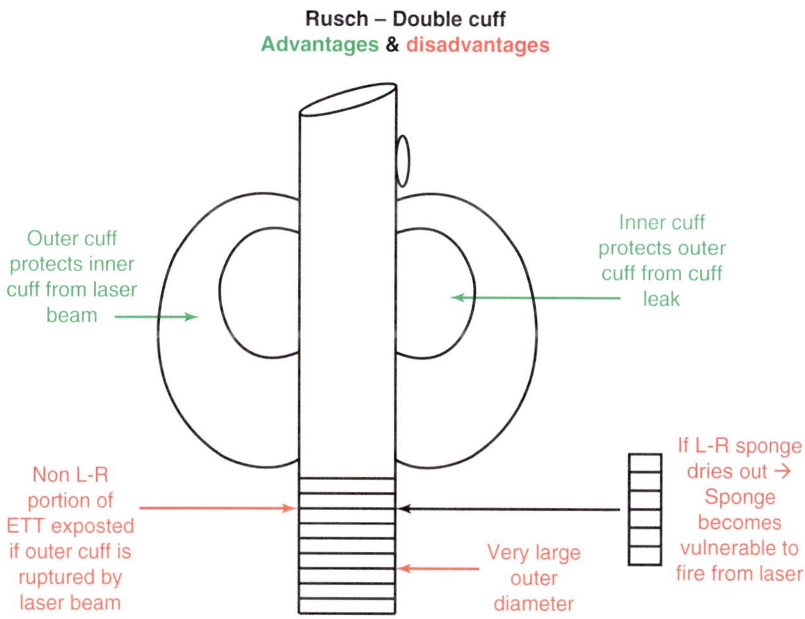

Fig. 8.14 Schematic displaying the advantage and disadvantages of the Rusch Lasertubus ETT. Advantages are shown in green; disadvantages are shown in red

cases in which the surgeons need room in their surgical field (see Fig. 8.14). Some physical characteristics and a concise summary of the advantages and disadvantages of all three endotracheal tubes are displayed in Table 8.2. Other L-R ETTs include the Norton Laser ETT, the Binona Laser ETT, and the Sheridan Laser-Trach ETT. Descriptions of these ETTs and their advantages and disadvantages can be found in Benumof and Hagberg's book, *Airway Management* [1].

Table 8.2 Summary of advantages and disadvantages of the various L-R ETTs

Laser-resistant ETT	Inner diameter (mm)/outer diameter (mm)	Compatible laser types	Advantages	Disadvantages
Medtronic Xomed Laser-Shield II	6.0/9.0	CO_2	Dried methylene blue already present in pilot balloon	Only single cuff
		KTP		
Mallinckrodt Laser-Flex	6.0/8.5	CO_2	Double cuff	Need to inject indicator
		KTP		
Rusch Lasertubus	6.0/10.8	CO2	Double cuff	Large outer diameter
		Nd:YAG		
		Ar		Made of latex

CO2 carbon dioxide, *KTP* potassium titanyl phosphate, *Nd:YAG* neodymium/yttrium-aluminum-garnet

L-3: What Size L-R ETT Should Be Used for Laser Surgery of the Airway?

This is an important issue because ETT size dictates the quality of surgical exposure, how big a target for the laser beam the cuff is, the contact area of the cuff with the trachea (determining quality of cuff seal), and the resistance and pressure related to airflow through the ETT. All of these clinical concerns must be considered when choosing a tube size. Advantages and disadvantages of using a both too small and too large a tube are illustrated in Figs. 8.15, 8.16, and 8.17. In general, a size 5.5 I.D. L-R ETT is a good compromise between anesthesia and surgical goals (at odds with one another in several of the aforementioned respects) in an averaged-sized adult (see advantages and disadvantages in Figs. 8.15, 8.16, and 8.17).

L-4: At What Depth Should the ETT Be Placed?

It is important to note the distance of the green marking on the Medtronic L-R ETT so that you have a reference point for depth of intubation. The green mark on a 6.0 Medtronic ETT is approximately 24.5 cm from the distal tip (see Fig. 8.6a). When using the Mallinckrodt L-R ETT, it is a good idea to first mark a distance, for example, 24 cm, from the distal end of the ETT with pink tape so that, again, you have a reference point for depth of insertion after direct laryngoscopy and L-R ETT placement. If the ETT cuff is too close to the vocal cords, you run the risk of cuff rupture caused by the laser beam (left side of Fig. 8.18). However, placing the ETT too deep runs the risk of causing a main stem bronchial intubation. Ideally, the L-R cuff should be positioned so that the tip of the L-R ETT is just above the carina (i.e., 1–2 cm) so that the cuff is far away from the vocal cords (see right side of Fig. 8.18) and difficult to hit with the laser beam.

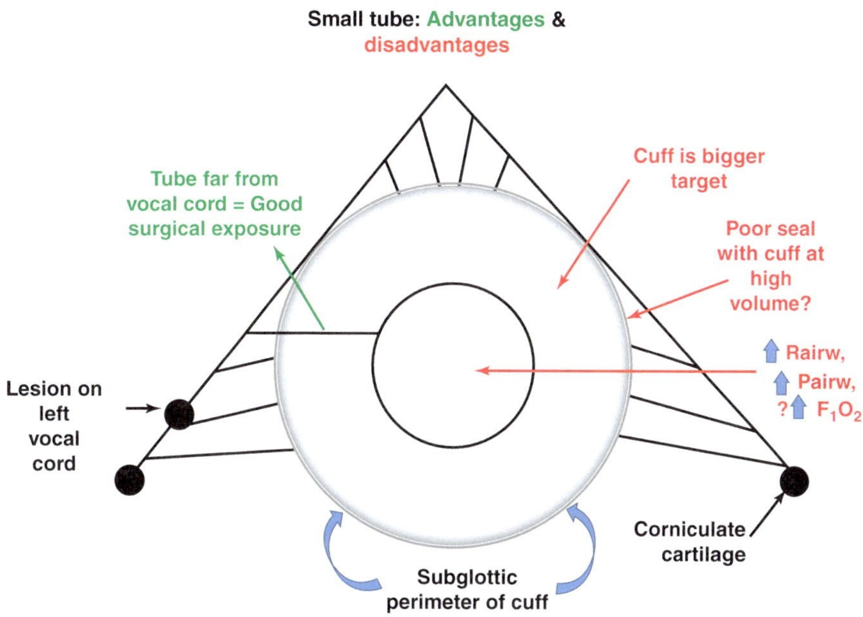

Fig. 8.15 Schematic displaying advantages and disadvantages of using a smaller L-R ETT. Advantages are shown in green; disadvantages are shown in red

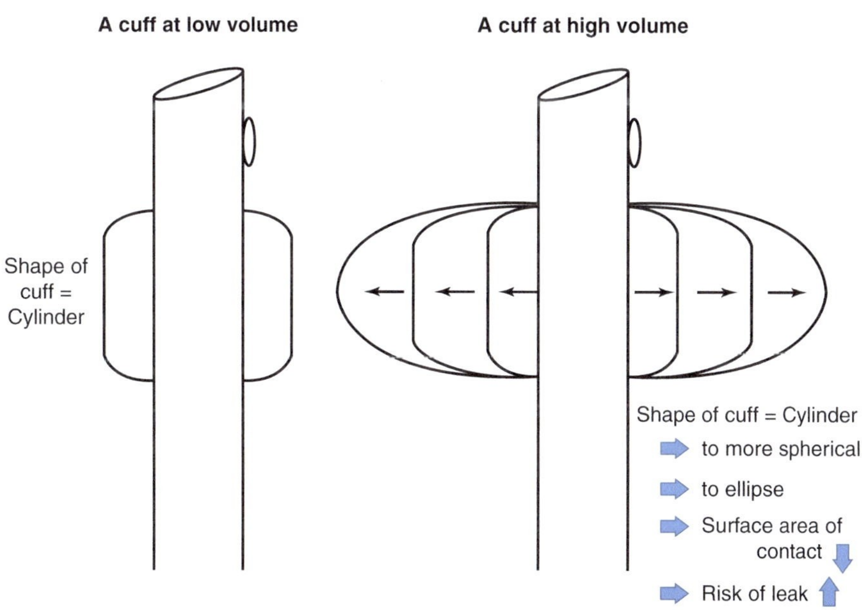

Fig. 8.16 Schematic displaying what happens to the shape of the cuff as more volume is used for inflation

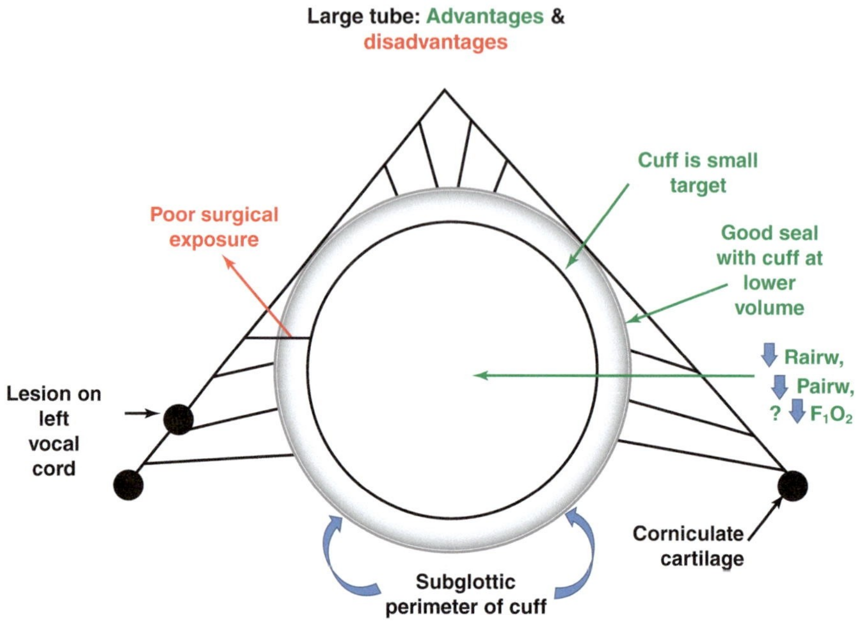

Fig. 8.17 Schematic displaying advantages and disadvantages of using a larger L-R ETT. Advantages are shown in green; disadvantages are shown in red

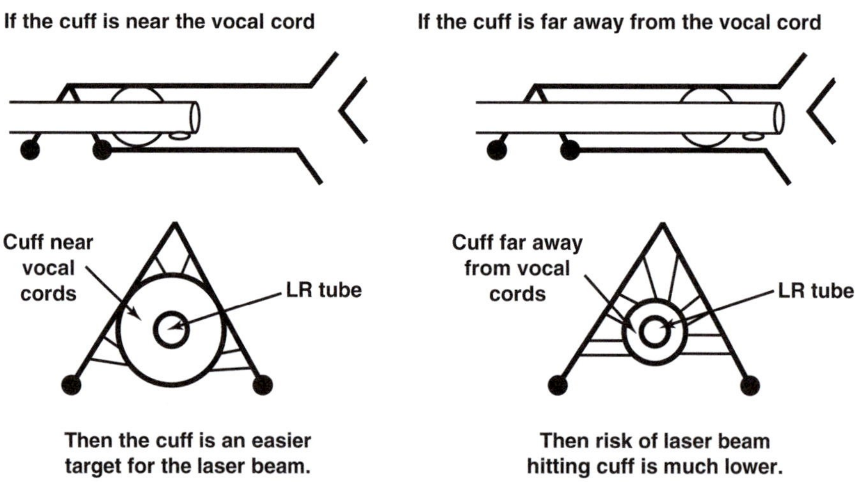

Fig. 8.18 Schematic displaying the cuff's proximity to the vocal cords (and therefore laser beam) when the L-R ETT is placed at a more shallow depth (Left) vs. when the L-R ETT is advanced more deeply and sits closer to the carina (Right)

L-5: How Much Saline with Dye Indicator Should Be Placed in Cuff?

Leakage of any increased percentage of FIO_2 around the cuff and into the surgical and laser beam field could result in a blowtorch fire disaster; therefore, there is no benefit in a "just seal" volume of saline/dye in the cuff. The benefit of avoiding mucosal damage in these short cases is near zero, and the risk is infinite. According to the package insert for the Medtronic Laser-Shield II, a minimum of 3 cc of normal saline put into the pilot balloon in order to inflate the cuff is necessary to obtain maximal amount of indicator mixing and color in the cuff. Ten cubic centimetre of normal saline was used for the above photographs. A reasonable and appropriate end point for inflation of the L-R ETT cuff would be a somewhat more tense feel of the pilot balloon on palpation with the fingertip, keeping in mind the risks/benefits of under filling the cuff.

L-6: What FIO_2 Should Be Used?

Oftentimes, patients undergoing procedures involving their airways do not have oxygen saturations that are within normal limits (WNL). It is important to note the patient's preoperative oxygen saturation (SpO_2), but it is not imperative for these patients to maintain an SpO_2 that is within normal limits when their baseline SpO_2 values are less than WNL. In this case, the patient's baseline room air saturation was 92%; however, an FIO_2 of 1.0 was used during the laser ablation case in an attempt to raise the patient's intraoperative O_2 saturations. In hindsight, the risk of airway fire greatly outweighs the risk of desaturation, even to a value of less than 92%. According to the 2013 Practice Advisory for Prevention and Management of Operating Room Fires, one should "reduce the oxygen concentrations to the minimum required to avoid hypoxia. For oxygen dependent patients, reduce supplemental oxygen delivery to the minimum required to avoid hypoxia. Monitor oxygenation with pulse oximetry, and if feasible, inspired, exhaled, and/or delivered oxygen concentration" [2]. We recommend decreasing FIO_2 to 0.21 or until SpO_2 is $90 \pm 2\%$, whichever occurs first. Any FIO_2 above 0.21 progressively causes (with ignition source and fuel) a fire that starts faster and more easily, will have an increased surface area, and burns hotter therefore causing more damage at the site of burn. Thus, the severity of injury due to a fire, in every respect, is directly related to FIO_2. If 100% O_2 is intermittently used between laser firings, it is important to understand that when the FIO_2 is decreased from one level to another, the FIO_2 and end tidal O_2 ($FETO_2$) decrease exponentially, and the FEN_2 increases

Table 8.3 End tidal O2% after set number of delivered breaths with fixed FRC and TV

After breath (number)	End tidal O2 (%)
1	73
2	55
3	43
4	33
5	28
6	25

Assume functional residual capacity = 2 l and tidal volume = 1.0 l. Suddenly switch 100% O2 to 21% O2 (room air)
FRC functional residual capacity, *TV* tidal volume

exponentially, and to have an understanding of the number of breaths, it takes to get the patient's FIO_2 and $FETO_2$ to decrease toward 0.21 and 0.16, respectively, when changing the FIO_2 from 1.0 to 0.21 (see Table 8.3). Both the FIO_2 and $FETO_2$ are relevant to this discussion. If the laser beam hits the cuff during inspiration, then the O_2 that spills out is the FIO_2. If the laser beam hits the cuff during exhalation, then the O_2 concentration that spills out is the $FETO_2$. In general, with a small functional residual capacity (FRC) and large tidal volumes (TV), it takes approximately eight breaths to get FIO_2 to decrease from 1.0 to 0.21 and $FETO_2$ to decrease from 0.95 to 0.16. With a large FRC and small TV, it takes more than eight breaths to reach an FIO_2 of 0.21 and $FETO_2$ of 0.16. The more breaths you administer and the longer you wait, the safer the situation is, especially if nitrous was being used (nitrous oxide, being more soluble in blood than O_2, takes longer to wash out). It is important to communicate with the surgeons that the change in FIO_2 and $FETO_2$ is not immediate and some patience must be exercised (e.g., a minute) in order to continue safely.

L-7: Should Nitrous Oxide Be Used?

The answer to the **L-7** question is "NO." Nitrous oxide is almost as good an oxidizer as oxygen and also supports combustion almost as well as oxygen. The package inserts for these laser-resistant endotracheal tubes warn against the use of nitrous oxide for the dilution of oxygen and state that, "nitrous oxide is a flammable gas and may result in ignition and serious patient injury" [3].

L-8: What Is the Purpose of Saline-Soaked Blocking Pledgets?

Saline-soaked blocking pledgets are placed by the surgeon proximal to the ETT cuff in order to serve as a heat sink (main mechanism of action) as well as a mechanical barrier (minor mechanism of action) to absorb the laser beam (see Fig. 8.19). The utility of moistened pledgets in preventing or delaying cuff ignition from CO_2 laser exposure has been confirmed [4].

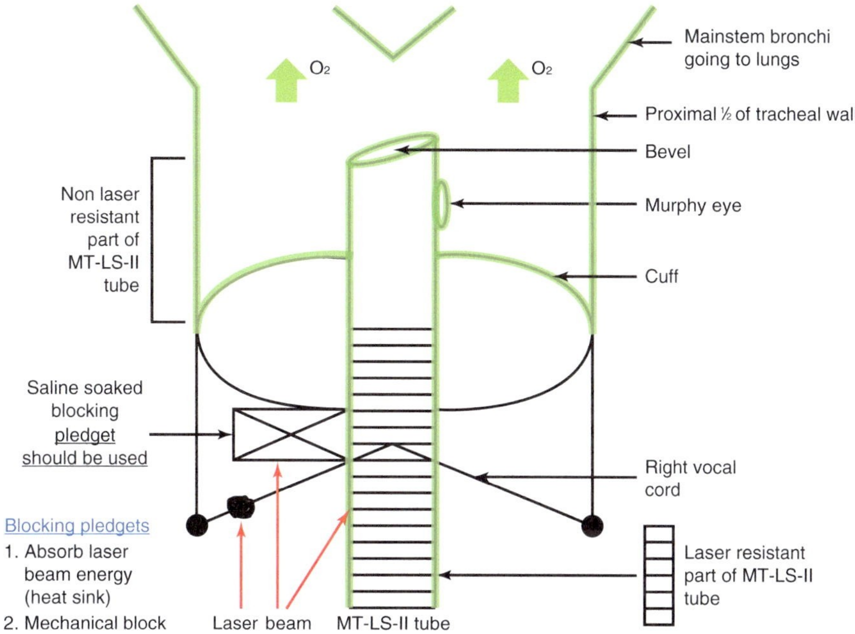

Fig. 8.19 Schematic displaying the Medtronic Xomed Laser-Shield II (MT-LS-II) with saline-soaked blocking pledget in place proximal to the ETT cuff. The red arrows represent the laser beam striking the vocal cord lesion, the pledget, as well as the L-R part of the ETT

Fig. 8.20 Watts vs. time representation of laser beam energy (joules) when administered in a continuous mode (left) and pulsed mode (right)

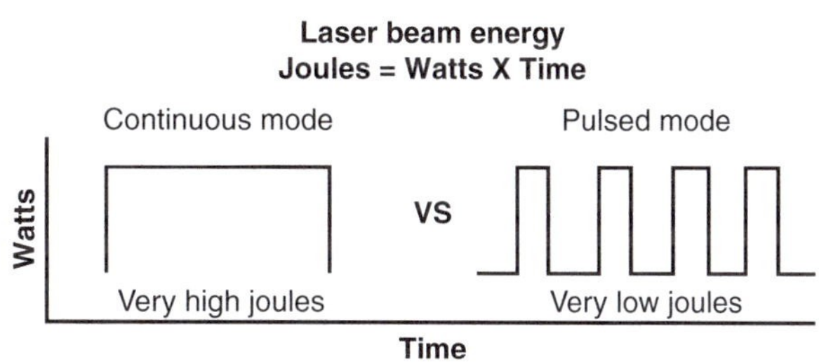

L-9: What Should the Laser Beam Be Set at to Provide Maximum Safety?

Laser beam energy is measured in joules. Joules are calculated by multiplying wattage by time (Joules = Watts X Time). It takes 2 J of energy to rupture an ETT cuff. Therefore, a laser beam firing at 20 W for 0.1 s has an energy level of 2 J. In order to minimize the ignition source, the laser beam should be in short-pulsed mode and ≤18 W. Figure 8.20 demonstrates the difference in joules when a laser is fired continuously vs. pulsed; obviously, the area under the square wave of a long pulse (i.e., the joules/energy of the pulse) (left side of Fig. 8.20) is much greater than the area under the square wave of any given short pulse (right side of Fig. 8.20).

L-10: What to Do If an Airway Fire Occurs?

The practice advisory for the prevention and management of operating room fires outlines what to do in the case of an airway fire (see Fig. 8.21). Upon realization that an airway fire has occurred (see Figs. 8.1, 8.2, and 8.3), the surgeon must first turn off the laser (remove ignition source, Fig. 8.4). Next, the L-R ETT must be removed from the patient's airway (remove fuel; see Fig. 8.4). This can be a difficult maneuver for an anesthesiologist who may feel hesitant to remove a secured airway in a patient who may be difficult to re-intubate; however, the ETT is serving as fuel for the airway fire and must be removed promptly. The surgeon, or whoever is at the head of the bed, should pull the ETT if appropriate. Simultaneous with ignition source and laser beam removal, any O_2 above room air should be shut off, thereby removing the oxidizing source. Turning the bed 180° should immediately follow ignition, fuel, and O_2 removal. If possible, put or spray saline on any remaining burning site and re-intubate the patient. A flexible bronchoscopy should then be performed to assess airway damage (see Figs. 8.1, 8.2, and 8.3 as well).

The mandate to remove the L-R ETT is not absolutely inviolate. There is one case report in which the ETT was not removed upon discovery of an airway fire. Chee and Benumof describe a patient scheduled for an elective tracheostomy whose airway evaluation revealed "an in situ 8-mm-ID polyvinyl chloride (PVC) ETT, swollen lips, an edematous tongue protruding out of the mouth, and an oropharynx filled with secretions." General anesthesia was induced, and the patient was administered 100% oxygen immediately before insertion of the tracheostomy tube. Shortly thereafter, surgeons noted a blue flame emerging from the patient's neck. The breathing circuit was disconnected from the ETT, and saline was flushed in the ETT. The fire was extinguished promptly. The ETT was not removed because the ability to re-intubate was uncertain. Despite a leak around the perforated cuff, the seal was sufficient to generate a peak inspiratory pressure of 20 cm H_2O. Meanwhile, the surgeons were able to insert a tracheostomy tube into the trachea [5].

In the case being reported herein, the operating room table was turned first, thus leading to delay in removing the ETT. Furthermore, 100% O_2 was being used which resulted in an airway fire that was larger, hotter, and more sustained than if a lower FIO_2 had been used. The extent of damage to the airway was catastrophic (see Figs. 8.22, 8.23, and 8.24).

Fig. 8.21 Steps to take if an airway fire occurs

What to do if an Airway Fire Occurs

1. Turn off laser (Remove ignition source)
2. Remove endotracheal tube (Eliminate fuel source)
3. Switch to room air (Turn off oxidizer)
4. Douse with saline over any burning area
5. Place new endotracheal tube
6. Perform fiberoptic bronchoscopy of airway to assess damage

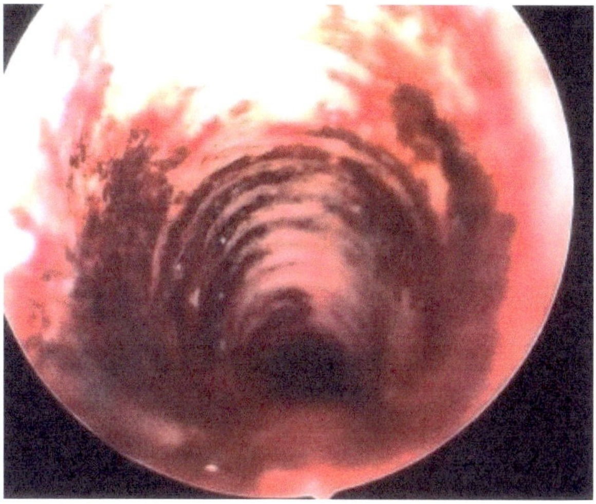

Fig. 8.22 Fiber-optic view of proximal trachea through new ETT following airway fire

Fig. 8.23 Fiber-optic view showing foreign body (ETT tip) lodged in the left main stem bronchus

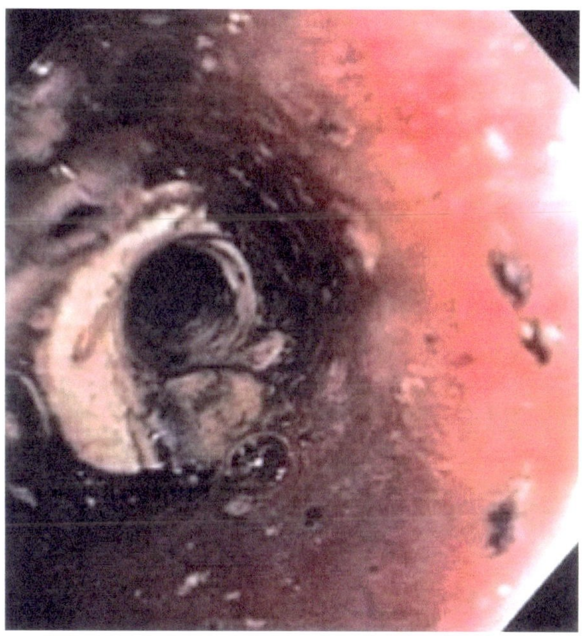

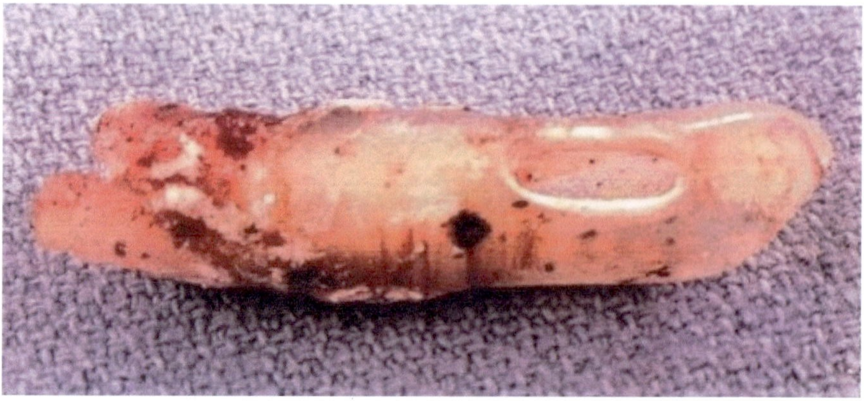

Fig. 8.24 Photograph of retrieved tip of L-R ETT from the left main stem bronchus

References

1. Benumof JL, Hagberg CA. Airway management. 3rd ed. Philadelphia: Elsevier Saunders; 2013. p. 837–41.
2. Jacoby WG. Practice advisory for the prevention and management of operating room fires. Anesthesiology. 2013;118:271–90.
3. Medtronic Laser-Shield II package insert, page 2. 68E1503B 12/06.
4. Miller RD, Eriksson LI, Fleisher L, Wiener-Kronish JP, Young WL. Miller's anesthesia, vol. 1. 7th ed. Philadelphia: Churchill Livingstone Elsevier; 2009. p. 2414.
5. Chee WK, Benumof JL. Airway fire during tracheostomy: extubation may be contraindicated. Anesthesiology. 1998;89(6):1576–8.

Chapter 9
Anesthetic Implications of Duchenne Muscular Dystrophy and the Surgical Repair of Scoliosis

Sonya M. Seshadri, Karim T. Rafaat, and Alyssa Brzenski

Case Presentation

A 9-year-old boy (Wt 20 kg, Ht 44 in.) with Duchenne muscular dystrophy **(Lesson I, a–b)** presented for posterior spinal fusion and instrumentation of T6-L3 **(Lesson IV and V)**. His medical history was remarkable for progressive muscle weakness which had left him wheelchair-bound, progressively declining pulmonary function, and thoracolumbar kyphoscoliosis **(Lesson III)**. Preoperative forced vital capacity (FVC) was 40% of predicted. An echocardiogram performed 2 months prior to the day of surgery showed an ejection fraction of 56%, no valvular abnormalities, and some mild-moderate left ventricular diastolic dysfunction **(Lesson Ic)**.

Induction of anesthesia and intubation proceeded uneventfully and were followed by placement of a radial arterial line, two 20 gauge peripheral intravenous catheters, and a triple lumen central venous catheter. The patient was then positioned prone. Anesthesia and analgesia were maintained with propofol and remifentanil infusions **(Lesson II)**. Somatosensory evoked potentials (SSEPs) were monitored during the case **(Lesson Va)**.

Due to ongoing surgical blood loss, the hematocrit (Hct) decreased to 25% from a preoperative Hct of 32%. One unit packed red blood cells (pRBCs) was then transfused. Later during the dissection, mean arterial pressures (MAPs) fell from above 70 to 40 mmHg over 7–10 min **(Lesson Vb, Vc)**. This was associated with loss of SSEPs in the patient's bilateral lower extremities. Over the next 15 min, multiple boluses of ephedrine and Neo-Synephrine were given, and a dopamine infusion was started. A second unit of blood and 400 mL 5% albumin were also given. Both the

S. M. Seshadri
Department of Anesthesiology, Southern California Permanente Medical Group, San Diego, CA, USA

K. T. Rafaat (✉) · A. Brzenski
Department of Anesthesiology, University of California, San Diego, CA, USA
e-mail: krafaat@ucsd.edu

J. L. Benumof, G. R. Manecke (eds.), *Clinical Anesthesiology II*,
https://doi.org/10.1007/978-3-030-12365-9_9

MAPs and SSEPs returned to baseline. The final hematocrit was approximately 30%. The surgery was completed without further issue, and the patient was transported to the pediatric intensive care unit intubated and sedated. Upon recovery, the patient exhibited no neurological deficits.

Lesson I: What Is Duchenne Muscular Dystrophy?

Epidemiology

Duchenne muscular dystrophy (DMD) is the most common hereditary neuromuscular disease worldwide. It has an incidence of 1:3600 male births and affects all races and ethnic groups [1, 2]. The disease is inherited as an X-linked recessive trait; however, 30% of mutations are caused by spontaneous mutations, and therefore the mother is not a carrier [1]. The onset of muscle weakness occurs around 2–3 years of age and then progresses to a wheelchair-bound state before the early teen years. Definitive diagnosis is made with a combination of elevated creatinine kinase levels, genetic testing, and muscle biopsy. There is currently no cure for DMD, and the mean age of death is 19 in the absence of supportive interventions. However, with appropriate glucocorticoid therapy, focused surgical management, and significant cardiac, respiratory, and physical rehabilitation, patients may survive into the fourth decade of life [2].

Pathophysiology

Muscular dystrophy is a progressive, inherited disease of muscle tissue characterized by degeneration or death of muscle fibers. The mutation responsible for DMD (usually a deletion) occurs at the p21 locus on the X chromosome, which carries a large gene that codes for the protein *dystrophin*. *Dystrophin* is a critical protein that maintains the integrity of both the sarcolemma (cell membrane) and cytoskeleton in skeletal, brain, retinal, and cardiac muscle cells [1].

Clinically, DMD is usually asymptomatic at birth and infancy. Gross motor skills and walking typically develop normally. Poor head control may be an early sign of the disease. Subtle signs of hip girdle weakness and Gowers' sign (a patient using his arms to assist with standing from a sitting or squatting position to compensate for weak hip and thigh muscles) may be present by 2–3 years of age. Common presentations in toddlers and younger children include trouble walking up and down stairs or running, falling, and developmental delay. One of the hallmark clinical findings is pseudohypertrophy of the calves due to replacement of muscle tissue with connective tissue such as fat and collagen. As muscle weakness progresses, most patients are wheelchair-bound by ages 7–10. Patients may remain fully or partially ambulatory in the early teen years with bracing, physical therapy, and minor orthopedic surgery [1, 2].

Medical Conditions Associated with Duchenne Muscular Dystrophy

Because *dystrophin* is an important protein in cells of multiple organ systems, patients with DMD have many conditions associated with their clinical presentation (Fig. 9.1). *Dystrophin* deficiency in cardiac myocytes leads to muscle fiber degeneration, accumulation of intracellular calcium, and microvascular changes. These changes cause ischemia and render the myocardium metabolically and structurally abnormal [3]. Cardiomyopathy is seen in 50–80% of patients with DMD, leading to persistent tachycardia and heart failure. Notably, cardiomyopathy does not correlate well to the degree of skeletal muscle weakness [1]. Once a patient is no longer ambulatory, joint contractures and scoliosis rapidly progress. Without glucocorticoid therapy, a patient with DMD has a 90% chance of developing progressive scoliosis [4]. As it progresses in severity, thoracic scoliosis can cause significant compression of the heart and lungs [1]. Pulmonary and pharyngeal muscle dysfunction can also be present and lead to ineffective cough, nocturnal hypoventilation, and frequent respiratory infections [5]. Other medical problems common in DMD include intellectual impairment, retinal disease, gastroesophageal reflux, obesity, and osteoporosis [1] (Table 9.1).

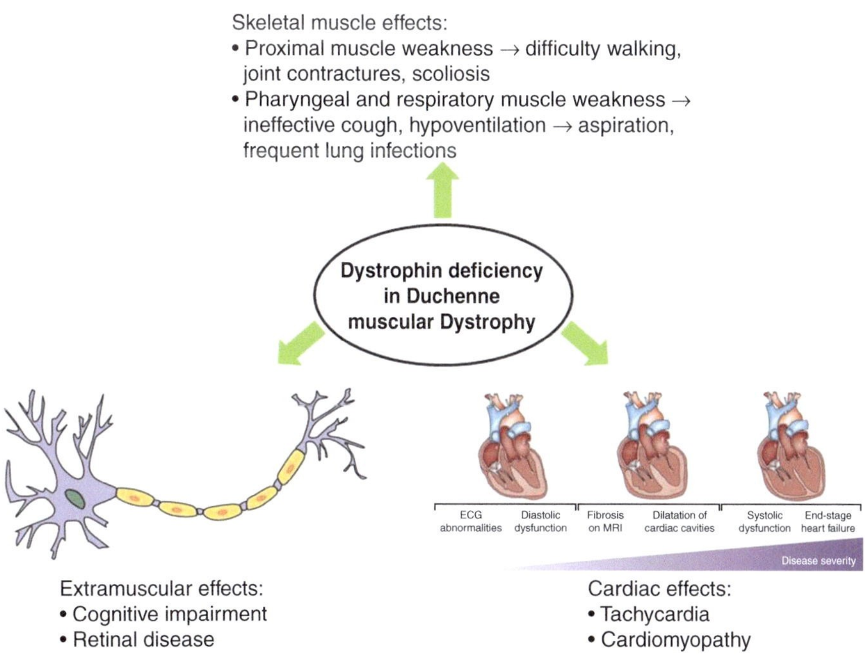

Fig. 9.1 Various organ systems affected by dystrophin deficiency in DMD. (Adapted from Finsterer and Cripe [85]. With permission from Nature Publishing Group)

Table 9.1 Anesthesia for patients with Duchenne muscular dystrophy

Organ system	Consideration	Preparation
Airway	Possible difficult airway due to tongue hypertrophy and limited neck and back mobility	Immediate availability of advanced airway equipment
Pulmonary	Decreased pulmonary reserve and lung volumes due to compression of lungs from thoracic scoliosis	Preoxygenation, backup airway plan formulated in advance, careful awake extubation
	Weak cough and inspiratory effort due to muscle weakness	Proactive management of secretions, use of cough assist devices and NIPPV after extubation
Cardiac	Cardiomyopathy from metabolically and structurally abnormal cardiac myocytes	ECHO and EKG within 1 year of surgery to evaluate for tachycardia, arrhythmias, and depressed ventricular function; TEE can be used for intraoperative evaluation
Gastrointestinal	Aspiration risk from gastroesophageal reflux and abnormal gastrointestinal motility	NPO guidelines, decompress stomach with NG or OG tube
Endocrine	Adrenal suppression from chronic steroid therapy	Stress dose steroids may be needed
	Obesity from physical inactivity	Medication dosing based on ideal body weight
Musculoskeletal	Contractures	Careful positioning, padding of pressure points
	Osteoporosis	Secure patient well to operating table, gentle patient movement and positioning
Other	Anesthesia-induced reactions: hyperkalemia, cardiac arrest, rhabdomyolysis	No succinylcholine
		TIVA anesthetic
		Flush anesthesia machine for at least 10 min to remove inhaled anesthetics
		Dantrolene of no clear benefit

NIPPV noninvasive positive pressure ventilation, *ECHO* echocardiogram, *EKG* electrocardiogram, *TEE* transesophageal echocardiography, *NPO* nil per os, *NG* nasogastric, *OG* orogastric, *TIVA* total intravenous anesthetic

Lesson II: What Are the Anesthetic Implications of Duchenne Muscular Dystrophy?

Airway Management

Patients with DMD may have a difficult airway due to a large tongue from muscle tissue hypertrophy, craniofacial abnormalities from muscle degeneration, and difficulty with supine positioning due to severe spinal deformities [1, 5]. Furthermore, these patients suffer rapid arterial oxygen desaturation on induction due to decreased pulmonary reserve from physical compression of the lungs caused by scoliosis and chest wall weakness. Finally, their gastroesophageal reflux and abnormal gastrointestinal motility place them at risk for aspiration. Therefore, immediate availability of advanced airway equipment is imperative.

Pulmonary Considerations

Respiratory muscle weakness from DMD leads to a weak cough and poor inspiratory effort. Also, thoracic compression from scoliosis can lead to a restrictive lung pattern with decreased lung volumes. This puts patients at risk for postoperative atelectasis, extubation failure, and pneumonia [5]. Patients with an FVC <30–50% of predicted should have proactive respiratory management after extubation with cough assist devices and noninvasive positive pressure ventilation [6].

Cardiac Considerations

Symptoms of cardiomyopathy in DMD may be difficult to illicit on preoperative evaluation due to the physical inactivity of a wheelchair-bound patient. An electrocardiogram (EKG) and an echocardiogram (ECHO) should be done if the last cardiac evaluations were more than 1 year prior to surgery or if there was an abnormal result in the last 7–12 months [5]. EKG changes characteristic of cardiomyopathy from DMD include increased R-to-S ratio in right precordial leads, deep Q wave in lateral leads, conduction abnormalities, and arrhythmias. Abnormal ECHO findings include decreased ejection fraction and increased left ventricular volumes and mass [3].

Anesthesia-Induced Rhabdomyolysis: Hyperkalemia and Cardiac Arrest

Succinylcholine is known to cause acute rhabdomyolysis in patients with progressive myopathies such as DMD. The resultant hyperkalemia can then progress to ventricular dysrhythmias, cardiac arrest, and death [7]. Succinylcholine is therefore contraindicated in the setting of a known myopathy. Furthermore, given the difficulty of diagnosing a myopathy in very young patients, the FDA has issued a black box warning against the use of succinylcholine (Anectine) in all children, especially males, under the age of 8 [8].

Independent of the effects of succinylcholine, halogenated inhaled anesthetics (Halothane, Isofluorane, Sevofluorane, Enfluorane) have been associated with a number of adverse clinical presentations in patients with DMD during and after anesthesia.

In a review of such cases, Hayes et al. identified three distinct presentations: (1) hyperkalemic cardiac arrest with rhabdomyolysis, (2) gradual rise in temperature and heart rate, and (3) isolated postoperative rhabdomyolysis without cardiac arrest. Despite sharing some similarities with the presentation of malignant hyperthermia (MH), these reactions did not occur with other signs of a systemic hypermetabolic state (rapidly rising end tidal CO_2, metabolic acidosis, body temperature >38.8 °C). Furthermore, these reactions did not respond to dantrolene and often occurred in DMD patients who had negative halothane-caffeine contracture tests [9].

These findings led the authors to suggest that a reaction distinct from MH, called "anesthesia-induced rhabdomyolysis" (AIR), can occur in patients with myopathies due to stress on structurally abnormal muscle tissue [9]. Given the potential for these reactions, many experts have advocated total intravenous anesthetic (TIVA) and complete flushing of the anesthesia machine to remove residual inhaled anesthetics for patients with DMD [10–12]. In the event that AIR is suspected in a patient without a known diagnosis of DMD, the inhaled agents should be discontinued, and measures to reduce potassium levels (sodium bicarbonate, insulin and dextrose, hyperventilation) should be swiftly undertaken. The AHA guidelines for the treatment of hyperkalemic cardiac arrest also advocate for the immediate administration of calcium chloride [13]. There does not appear to be a clear role for dantrolene in AIR [9].

Other Anesthetic Considerations

Patient positioning in patients with DMD may be challenging due to obesity, scoliotic changes, and contractures of the ankles, knees, hips, and elbows. Careful attention should be paid to padding of pressure points and securing the patient to the operating table. If patients are on steroids for treatment of their disease, a perioperative plan including stress dose steroids should be formulated [5].

Lesson III: What Is Scoliosis?

Definition and Types

Scoliosis refers to lateral, or sideways, curvature of the spine in the frontal plane of the body. A related but distinct term is kyphosis which is a frontal, or forward, curvature of the spine in the sagittal plane of the body. Diagnosis of scoliosis is made with an index called the Cobb angle (Fig. 9.2). The apex of the curved spine, or point of maximum deviation from midline in the frontal plane, is identified. Then, one line is drawn parallel to the superior aspect of the most tilted vertebrae cephalad to the apex and another is drawn parallel to the inferior aspect of the most tilted vertebrae caudad the apex. Two additional lines are drawn, one perpendicular to each of the first two lines. The angle at the intersection of the perpendicular lines is

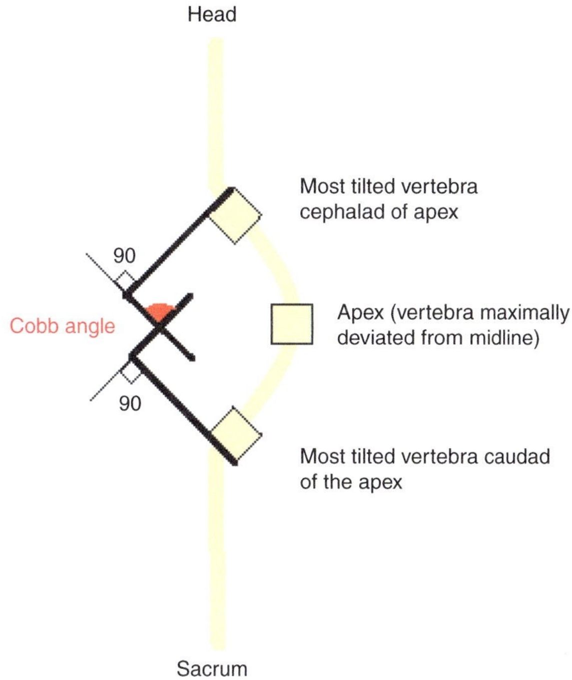

Fig. 9.2 Illustration of Cobb angle for diagnosis of scoliosis

the Cobb angle. Diagnosis of scoliosis is made when the Cobb angle is >10° on radiographic imaging [14].

The main types of scoliosis are idiopathic, neuromuscular, and congenital. Idiopathic scoliosis has both genetic and environmental causes and is further classified by the age of onset of curvature as infantile (birth to 3 years), juvenile (3–10 years), or adolescent (>11 years). Neuromuscular scoliosis can be neuropathic and originate from upper or lower motor neuron diseases, or myopathic, and arise as a consequence of dystrophies that lead to an imbalance of the trunk or pelvic musculature with varying degrees of spasticity. Congenital scoliosis results from failure of formation or failure of segmentation of the vertebrae during gestation. Because of its onset in utero, congenital scoliosis is often associated with underlying spinal cord, renal, and cardiac anomalies. Differing degrees of scoliosis can also be caused by neurofibromatosis, mesenchymal diseases, tumors, infection, trauma, and compensatory changes for other orthopedic problems [14, 15] (Fig. 9.3).

Epidemiology

Two to 3% of all children will be affected by scoliosis at some point in their lives, and 70% of these are idiopathic [14, 15]. The prevalence of severe scoliosis (Cobb angle >30°) is 0.3% in the general population, and girls are ten times more likely

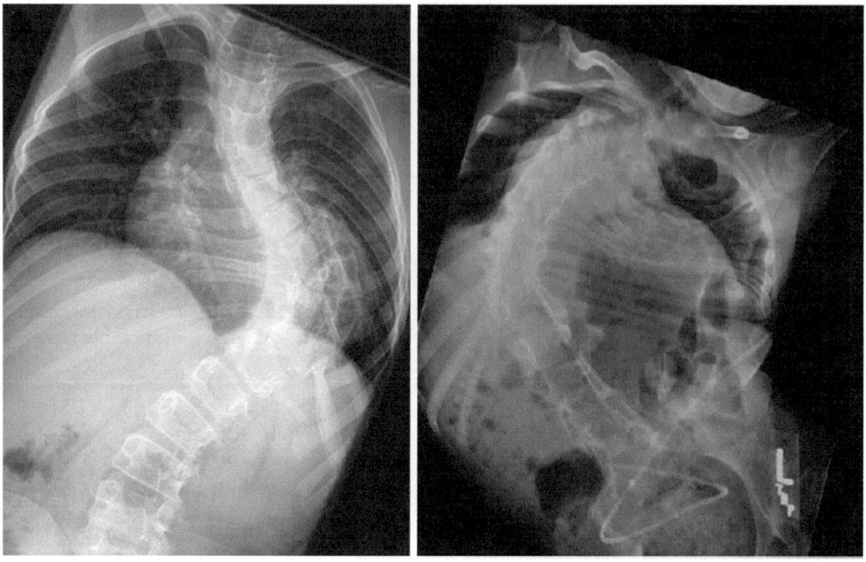

Fig. 9.3 Severe idiopathic scoliosis of the thoracic spine (left). Severe scoliosis of thoracic spine due to Duchenne muscular dystrophy (right). Left panel. (Reprinted from Musson et al. [87]. With permission from BMJ Publishing Group Ltd.). Right panel (Courtesy of Dr. Karim Rafaat)

than boys to develop a curvature of >30° in idiopathic scoliosis. After skeletal maturity, idiopathic scoliotic curves <30° typically do not progress. However, more severe curves or curves due to neuromuscular disease can continue to progress independent of skeletal maturity. Curvatures with angles >80° can result in restrictive pulmonary disease with ventilation-perfusion mismatch, and angles >100° can lead to cor pulmonale and cardiorespiratory failure [14].

Lesson IV: How Is Scoliosis Surgically Treated?

Indications and Timing for Surgery

In general, factors that are considered when planning surgical management of scoliosis include magnitude of curvature and associated medical conditions [14]. For idiopathic scoliosis, Cobb angles >40°, poor response to nonoperative treatment (i.e., external bracing of the spine), and a significant amount of time until skeletal maturity are indications for surgical correction [16, 17]. For idiopathic scoliosis, the progression of the disease will significantly slow once skeletal maturity is achieved obviating the need for surgical correction. For neuromuscular scoliosis (such as that caused by DMD), surgery is considered when the Cobb angle is >20° because disease progression will not slow with skeletal maturity and progression of pulmonary and cardiac disease may make later surgery high risk. In neuromuscular scoliosis, surgical intervention can slow the progression of restrictive lung disease in those who already have compromised pulmonary status due to muscle weakness. Surgical correction also alleviates pain from vertebral compression fractures and costo-pelvic impingement [1, 18]. For congenital scoliosis, surgical intervention is variable depending on the underlying anomaly and expected course [16].

Surgical Process and Complications

Posterior instrumented fusion is the most common procedure for the surgical correction of scoliosis (Fig. 9.4), although a combination of anterior and posterior approaches may be necessary. Generally, hardware consisting of two rods attached by hooks or wires to stabilizing pedicle screws are implanted. The surgical dissection for this procedure can be very extensive. In a posterior approach, the skin, supraspinous ligament, and paraspinal muscles are reflected, and the spinous processes, the interspinous ligaments, and the facet joints are all sacrificed. After stabilization and implantation of hardware, bone graft is placed all along the area to be fused. The anterior approach involves retroperitoneal dissection through thoracoabdominal or flank incisions [15].

Complications that can occur after spinal fusion include neurological injury, bleeding (both independent of and secondary to coagulopathy), and infection.

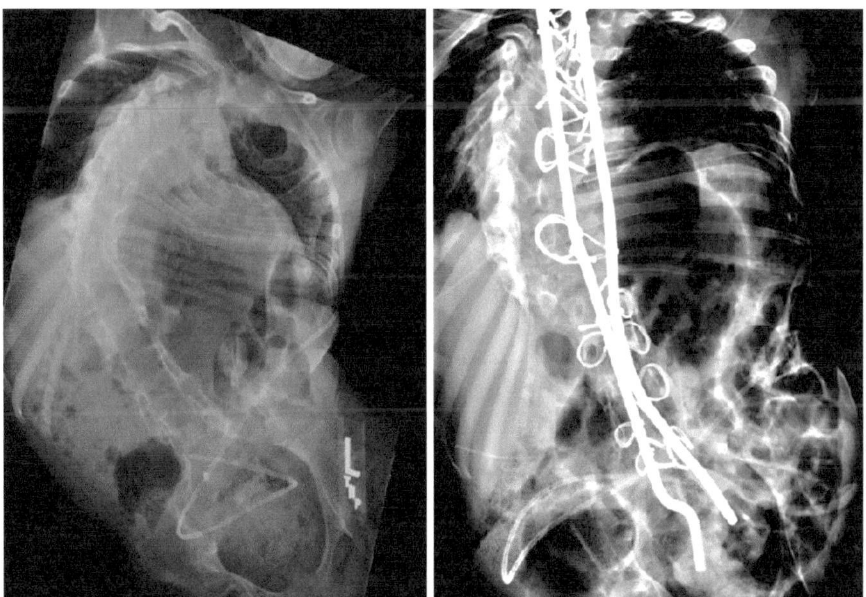

Fig. 9.4 A patient with thoracic scoliosis from Duchenne muscular dystrophy before (left) and after (right) posterior spinal fusion with instrumentation. (Courtesy of Dr. Karim Rafaat)

Studies of morbidity and mortality after spinal fusion for various underlying pathologies have shown that overall complication rates are about equal in posterior spinal fusion and anterior spinal fusion. However, the overall complication rates are higher – twice as high in one study – with combined anterior-posterior fusion as compared to posterior spinal fusion or anterior spinal fusion alone [19, 20]. For scoliosis repair, patients with neuromuscular scoliosis experience a higher overall rate of complications. In a literature review, Weiss and Goodall found that the incidence of all complications for patients with neuromuscular scoliosis (NS) correction was 17.4% versus 8.6% for patients with idiopathic scoliosis (IS). They also found that death from these complications was 6.5% for NS versus 0.03% for IS [21]. A similar trend was shown by Reames et al. who found the surgical complication rate of patients with NS correction to be 17.9% versus 6.3% for patients with IS. These authors reported a 0.34% overall mortality rate for NS patients compared with only 0.02% among IS patients [22]. The leading causes of postoperative mortality among patients with NS included respiratory failure or aspiration, excessive blood loss, sepsis, cardiac, pulmonary embolus, brain stem herniation, transfusion-related acquired lung injury, and fluid overload [22].

A specific complication of concern in scoliosis correction is neurological injury. In a 5-year British national review of corrective surgeries all types of scoliosis showed incomplete neurological deficit with resolution in 0.65% of patients, incomplete neurological deficit without resolution in 0.32% of patients, and complete neurological deficit in 0.13% [23]. Reames et al. found that patients with NS experienced more postoperative neurological deficits (1.1%) than those with IS (0.8%) [22]. The specific types of neurological injury were further categorized as nerve root injury (0.4% in NS vs 0.3% in IS), cauda equina deficit (0.06% in NS), incomplete spinal cord deficit (0.4% both NS and IS), and complete spinal cord deficit (0.15% both NS and IS). Higher rates of new neurologic deficits were associated with revision procedures, the use of corrective osteotomies, and the use of certain type of hardware such as anterior screws or posterior wires [22].

Lesson V: What Are the Anesthetic Implications of Scoliosis Surgery?

Intraoperative Neurophysiologic Monitoring

Continuous neurophysiologic monitoring can be used to assess the integrity of motor and sensory neural pathways intraoperatively. On a basic level, neuromonitoring involves monitoring the central nervous system during surgery by generating an electrical stimulus at one area along a neural pathway then measuring a response (evoked potential) at a second area along the same pathway. Somatosensory evoked potentials (SSEPs) can be recorded when a peripheral nerve (typically median, ulnar, or posterior tibial) is stimulated and a response is measured with epidural or

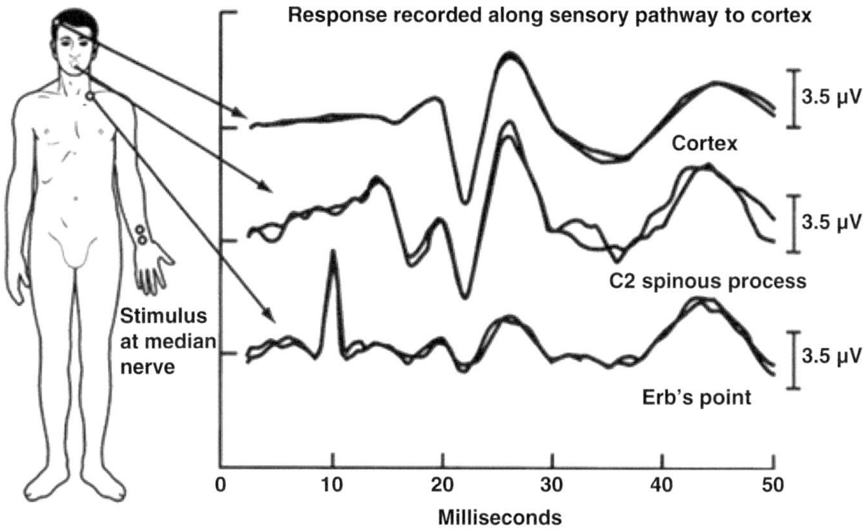

Fig. 9.5 SSEPs measure electrical activity centrally after peripheral electrical stimulus. SSEPs after stimulation to the left median nerve recorded transcutaneously from points along the somatosensory pathway: from Erb's point over the second cervical spinous process and over the somatosensory cortex. (Reprinted from Banoub et al. [88]. With permission from Wolters Kluwer Health)

cortical electrodes (Fig. 9.5). SSEPs are not very loud against background noise so, for a readable result, summation of multiple stimuli is performed. SSEPs are limited in that they only monitor the dorsal area of the spinal cord (dorsal column medial lemniscus) that is not the most at risk area for ischemia due to receiving blood supply from two posterior spinal arteries. Motor evoked potentials (MEPs) can be recorded when the motor cortex is stimulated transcranially and a response is measured at epidural or muscle belly electrodes as a compound action potential (Fig. 9.6). MEPs monitor the motor pathway in the ventral spinal cord (anterior corticospinal tracts) – which is supplied by a single anterior spinal artery. In contrast to the dorsal sensory columns, this area is only supplied by a single artery and is thus more susceptible to ischemia [15, 24].

Neurophysiologic signals are quantified by their amplitude and latency (Fig. 9.7). Latency is defined by the time required between the administered stimulus and the detection of a response. Amplitude is the magnitude of the response. Ischemia or mechanical insult to the neurological pathway being monitored appears as a decreased amplitude and an increased latency (in the case of SSEPs) or a decrease in amplitude (in the case of MEPs) [24]. If signals become altered, this can serve as a clue that the spinal cord or a nerve are being affected, usually as a result of an alteration in its oxygen supply. Possible solutions to an alteration in neuromonitoring signals depend on the suspected mechanism behind the decrease in oxygen delivery. If perfusion pressure is low, hypotension should be corrected; if oxygen saturation is low (SpO_2), ventilation should be improved; if anemia is present, oxygen carrying capacity

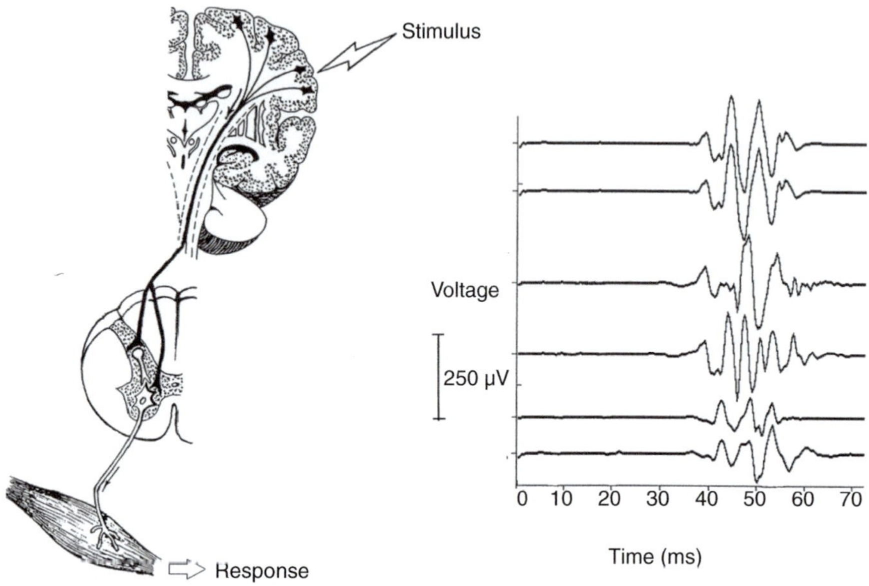

Fig. 9.6 Motor evoked potential measure the electromyographic response to brain stimulus. Schematic of the motor pathway and motor evoked potential (MEP) measurement. The stimulus at the motor cortex elicits action potentials propagating to the spinal cord activating motor neurons and producing muscle responses. (Reprinted from Zhou and Zhu [88]. With permission from Wolters Kluwer Health)

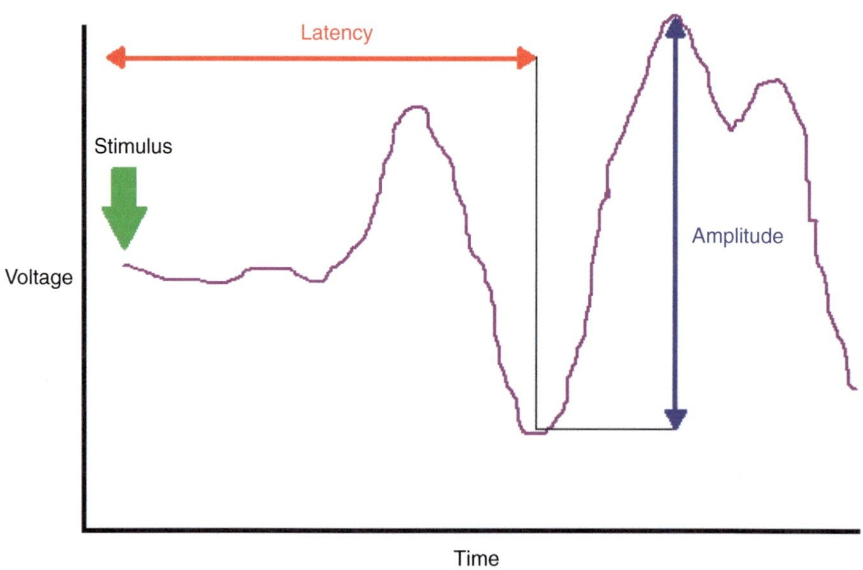

Fig. 9.7 Evoked response tracing of amplitude versus time after a stimulus

should be restored; if external surgical pressure is in excess of perfusion pressure, the last surgical intervention should be reversed [15].

Neurophysiologic signals are affected by a number of anesthetic agents. Signals are generally depressed by inhaled agents, nitrous oxide, propofol, and large boluses of opioids. Ketamine and etomidate, on the other hand, augment these signals. Additionally, paralysis may affect the consistency of MEPs; therefore neuromuscular blockade is typically omitted. Due to these effects, a typical anesthetic for surgery with neuromonitoring will combine little or no inhaled anesthetic (<0.5 MAC at most), an IV anesthetic infusion to supplement anesthesia (typically propofol), and a narcotic infusion or intermittent low-dose opioid bolus. Neuromuscular blockers and nitrous oxide are usually avoided during neuromonitoring [15, 24].

As mentioned previously, patients with scoliosis from neuromuscular disease are at greater risk for neurological complications postoperatively than patients with idiopathic scoliosis. Unfortunately, while it is possible to monitor both SSEPs and MEPs in patients with neuromuscular scoliosis, it is often difficult to obtain baseline monitoring in this subset of patients [25, 26]. MEPs are particularly difficult to monitor. Furthermore, there is limited evidence that intraoperative responses to changes in neuromonitoring reduce the rate of postoperative neurological deterioration [27]. This is possibly due in part to the fact that less than half of postoperative neurological injuries are proceeded by an intraoperative change in neuromonitoring [28]. Regardless of these limitations, neuromonitoring is the best currently available modality to detect and address neurological injury during surgery.

Managing Blood Loss in Scoliosis Repair

The surgical repair of scoliosis is associated with significant blood loss and both dilutional and consumptive coagulopathies [15]. Blood loss in scoliosis correction surgery is strongly related to the length of the procedure as well as the number of segments fused [29–31]. One retrospective review of posterior spinal fusion in the pediatric population with idiopathic scoliosis by Guay et al. concluded that patients had an average blood loss of 200 mL per level. This review also found that patients who weighed less than 30 kg were more likely to lose greater than one blood volume and require fresh frozen plasma or platelets to correct coagulopathy [30]. Patients with neuromuscular scoliosis are at a higher risk for blood loss than patients with idiopathic scoliosis likely due to the need for more segments to be fused as well as longer operation times to stabilize osteopenic bone [32–34, 31]. Furthermore, while patients with DMD do not appear to have clinically significant bleeding disorders at baseline, they can have dysfunction in platelet aggregation, poor vasoconstrictive response, increased bleeding time, and fibrinolysis when undergoing invasive surgical procedures [35–37]. Numerous techniques have been described to decrease blood loss and minimize allogenic transfusion (Table 9.2).

Table 9.2 Summary of methods to minimize blood loss and transfusion in surgery

Method	Timing	Technique
Epoetin alfa	Preoperative, 3–4 weeks before surgery	SQ weekly injection of 300 IU/kg up to 10,000 IU with iron supplementation
Autologous blood donation	Preoperative	Serial phlebotomy prior to surgery to be available for transfusion during surgery
Acute normovolemic hemodilution	After induction of anesthesia, day of surgery	Patient's blood is collected and replaced with crystalloid or colloid
Controlled hypotension	Intraoperatively	Reduction of baseline SBP or MAP with anesthetic or antihypertensive agents
Cell saver	Intraoperatively and postoperatively	Blood is collected via suction from the surgical wound, and then washed RBCs are returned to the patient
Antifibrinolytic agents	Intraoperatively and postoperatively	TXA: loading dose is 10 mg/kg; maintenance dose is 1 mg/kg/h
		Amicar: loading dose is 100 mg/kg; maintenance dose is 10 mg/kg/h
Intrathecal opioid	Prior to surgical start	Lumbar intrathecal injection of 5 mcg/kg preservative-free morphine

IU international units, *SBP* systolic blood pressure, *MAP* mean arterial pressure, *RBCs* red blood cells, *TXA* tranexamic acid, *Amicar* ε-aminocaproic acid

Preoperative

Before the day of surgery, patients can have their hematocrit augmented with epoetin alfa. Epoetin alfa (Procrit or Epogen), a recombinant form of the hormone erythropoietin, stimulates red blood cell production in the bone marrow. The typical dose is 300 IU/kg up to 10,000 IU subcutaneously weekly for 3 weeks before surgery. Protocols for preoperative epoetin alfa also include iron supplementation [31, 38, 39]. Infrequent side effects of epoetin alfa include hypertension, myocardial infarction, and thrombosis, but these do not appear to be of significant concern in the pediatric population [31, 38, 39]. In a series of retrospective analyses, Vitale et al. found that patients with idiopathic scoliosis treated with epoetin alfa had a significantly lower rate of transfusion (3.9% in the Epo treated group versus 23.5% in the untreated group) and an average of 2.5 days less in the hospital [38]. While patients undergoing surgical correction for neuromuscular scoliosis treated with epoetin had higher starting and discharge hematocrits, they had no difference in absolute risk of transfusion or hospital length of stay [31, 39]. This may be due to the fact that patients with neuromuscular scoliosis often have more complicated and lengthy surgical corrections, and these studies did not report the number of units transfused, only the ordinal variable of whether transfusion was needed.

Another preoperative measure to minimize the need for allogenic transfusion is autologous blood donation. Autologous preoperative donation involves serial phlebotomy in the weeks prior to surgery to have a quantity of the patient's own blood available for transfusion during surgery. Epoetin alfa and iron supplementation often facilitate this process. Autologous donation results in a significantly lower need for allogenic blood transfusion intraoperatively in spinal fusions, an effect more pronounced in patients with idiopathic scoliosis than those with neuromuscular scoliosis, and can be attempted in children as small as 30 kg [32, 40]. However, the utility of this technique may be limited in the pediatric population due to vasovagal reactions with phlebotomy, technical difficulties with blood collection, and poor cooperation particularly among very young or developmentally delayed patients [32, 41, 42].

Intraoperative

Intraoperative methods to decrease blood loss and minimize transfusion include acute normovolemic hemodilution, controlled hypotension, intrathecal morphine administration, cell saver, and antifibrinolytic agents. These methods will be further discussed below. Other measures that can be taken by the anesthesiologist to reduce intraoperative blood loss include maintenance of normothermia to avoid coagulopathy and prevention of increases in intrathoracic and intra-abdominal pressure that can engorge extradural veins and increase blood loss during surgical dissection. Venous engorgement can be prevented in the prone position by keeping the abdomen free of direct pressure to avoid vena caval compression [15, 35].

Acute normovolemic hemodilution (ANH) is the process by which a quantity of the patient's blood is collected via phlebotomy after induction of anesthesia and replaced with crystalloid or colloid to induce a hemodynamically stable anemia and subsequent loss of anemic blood once the surgery starts. The collected whole blood (RBCs and coagulation factors) can then be returned to the patient during or after surgery as needed [43]. ANH has been safely used in children undergoing correction of idiopathic scoliosis and has been found to reduce the need for autologous and homologous transfusions [44, 45]. One limitation of ANH is the logistics of collection and safe storage of the blood, which requires planning and experience on the part of the anesthesiologist [43].

Controlled, or induced, hypotension is defined as a reduction of the systolic blood pressure to 80–90 mmHg, a reduction of mean arterial pressure (MAP) to 50–65 mmHg, or a 30% reduction of baseline MAP [46]. This is typically accomplished by deepening anesthesia with sedatives or narcotics. An example of this approach would be a propofol infusion or inhaled anesthetic and an adjuvant such as a remifentanil infusion [42, 46]. Short-acting antihypertensives such as sodium nitroprusside, nitroglycerin, or beta-blocking medications can also be used [42, 46, 47]. This technique has been investigated retrospectively and prospectively in spinal fusion surgery for healthy patients with idiopathic scoliosis and found to decrease overall blood loss by 40–55%, reduce the need for intraoperative and postoperative transfusion, and shorten operation times [42, 47, 48]. This technique requires appropriate patient selection (excluding those with comorbidities that limit their ability to tolerate hypotension), accurate and frequent blood pressure monitoring, and careful attention to perfusion of various organ systems. The operative must also be aware that controlled hypotension may also interfere with obtaining adequate baseline SSEPs [49].

Intrathecal opioid given after induction of anesthesia may also significantly reduce intraoperative blood loss. The evidence to support this comes from studies in which intrathecal morphine (with or without sufentanil) was injected into the lumbar intrathecal space of patients undergoing surgical repair of idiopathic scoliosis [50–52]. The mechanism behind this affect is thought to be the creation of relative hypotension and maintenance of hemodynamic stability intraoperatively [50]. Patients given intrathecal morphine also have lower IV opioid requirement and better pain control when compared to IV PCA for the first 24 h postoperatively [51, 52]. The optimum dose appears to be 5 mcg/kg intrathecal morphine to achieve both reduction of blood loss and improved pain control on the first postoperative day [51, 52]. Potential limitations of the administration of intrathecal opioids include postoperative respiratory depression, creation hypotension that is not easily reversible if there is acute blood loss, and difficulty accessing the intrathecal space in patients with NMS.

Cell Saver is a process by which blood is collected via suction from the surgical wound, washed to isolated red blood cells (no coagulation factors or platelets), and then returned to the patient. Cell saver has been used in multiple prospective trials and found to decrease allogenic transfusion requirements up to 50% [53, 54]. Some limitations of cell saver include the inability of the anesthesiologist to use it for acute resuscitation due to the processing time involved before the red blood cells are available to give back to the patient and the significant quantity of blood that must be collected in order to have enough to process for return to the patient.

Numerous studies have demonstrated the efficacy of antifibrinolytic agents including ε-aminocaproic acid, tranexamic acid, and aprotinin for reducing blood loss during scoliosis surgery [17, 55–57]. Amicar (ε-aminocaproic acid) and tranexamic acid (TXA) are lysine analogs that inhibit plasmin, a key proteolytic enzyme in fibrinolysis. Aprotinin is a nonspecific serine protease inhibitor derived from bovine lung that interferes with plasmin and the kinin-kallikrein cascade. Of note, the FDA has removed aprotinin from the market due to safety concerns related to mortality from thrombotic events and renal dysfunction in adults [58, 59]. Also, TXA should be avoided in patients with known seizure disorders because TXA inhibits glycine and GABA receptors which can create an excitatory state in the central nervous system leading to seizures postoperatively [60]. A Cochrane review of the evidence behind the use of these agents showed that the use of all three resulted in less perioperative blood loss (approximately 426 mL on average). The three agents appeared to be comparable to one another in terms of efficacy for reducing blood loss [35, 59]. The risk of being transfused was not found to be lower in patients receiving antifibrinolytics, but the amount of blood transfused was 327 mL less on average in these patients. The long-term safety profile of these agents also requires more investigation due to the small number of pediatric patients who receive antifibrinolytic therapy [35]. Given currently available data, the use of amicar or tranexamic acid is appropriate during scoliosis procedures with high risk for significant blood loss. For tranexamic acid, the loading dose is 10 mg/kg infused over 15 min, while the maintenance dose is 1 mg/kg/h. For ε-aminocaproic acid, the loading dose is 100 mg/kg infused over 15 min, while the maintenance dose is 10 mg/kg/h [55–57].

Goal Directed Therapy in Pediatric Anesthesia

Scoliosis repair is often a large operation that requires the anesthesiologist to undertake significant resuscitative measures. The goal of such resuscitation is maintain adequate oxygen delivery by preserving cardiac output, perfusion pressure, and oxygen carrying capacity. From studies of sepsis, timely and appropriate volume resuscitation has been shown to improve survival [61, 62], but too much fluid resuscitation can increase mortality [63–65]. Therefore, indices to guide fluid administration are necessary for finding the right balance. Static variables alone such as heart rate, systolic arterial pressure, and central venous pressure are not reliable guides for fluid administration especially in mechanically ventilated patients undergoing anesthesia and surgery [66–69]. Dynamic measures of fluid responsiveness rely on variations in preload delivered to the heart due to positive pressure ventilation. In mechanically ventilated patients, right ventricular venous return decreases with inspiration due to vena caval compression. This decrease in preload to the right side of the heart is then transmitted to the left heart after two to three heartbeats, resulting in decreased stroke volume [70]. This ventilation-dependent variability in stroke volume can be observed as variation in aortic blood flow, arterial blood pressure, and plethysmographic waveform amplitude. This effect is more pronounced in hypovolemic states [71].

Dynamic variables, such as pulse pressure variation (PPV), stroke volume variation (SVV), and plethysmographic variability index (PVI), have been shown to have good predictive value for fluid responsiveness in adults [72, 73], but their utility in children is less clearly supported [74–77]. This finding may be due to physiologic differences in pediatric patients including increased chest wall and lung compliance, increased arterial compliance, and decreased ventricular compliance of pediatric patients [66]. A meta-analysis of multiple studies by Gan et al. investigated numerous static and dynamic hemodynamic variables in mechanically ventilated pediatric patients receiving a fluid bolus. They found that only direct transthoracic echocardiography measurement of variation in aortic blood flow was a reliable predictor of fluid responsiveness, defined in studies as a 15% increase in stroke volume within 10 min of fluid administration seen on transthoracic echocardiography [66, 78, 79].

Because variation in aortic blood flow appears to correlate with volume responsiveness, esophageal Doppler monitoring may represent a possible future direction

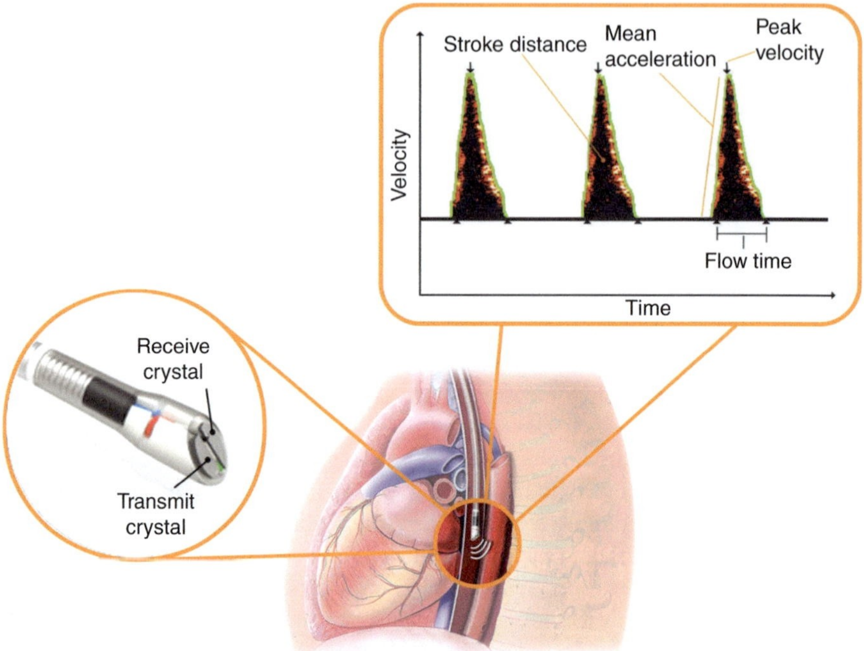

Fig. 9.8 Illustration of esophageal Doppler probe position in a patient. The waveform generated by the esophageal Doppler probe is a graph of blood velocity versus time. (Reprinted from Deltex Medical Launches E-learning Center [82]. With permission from Deltex Medical Limited)

Table 9.3 Summary of parameters measured by esophageal Doppler

Esophageal Doppler parameter	Traditional clinical correlate	Normal ranges with references
Stroke distance (SD)	Directly related to stroke volume (SV) and body surface area adjusted stroke volume index (SVI)	Varies with age and size
		Adults [82]
		SV 60–100 mL
		SVI 35–45 mL/m^2
		Pediatrics [84]
		SVI 25–45 mL/m^2
Flow time (FT_c)	Inversely related to afterload	Adults [82]
		330–360 ms
		Pediatrics
		In isolated studies, values >357 ms [34] and >394 ms [68] predicted fluid responsiveness
Peak velocity (PV)	Directly related to ventricular myocardial contractility	PV decreases with age [82]
		90–120 cm/s at age 20
		70–100 cm/s at age 50
		50–80 cm/s at age 70

for noninvasive monitoring of dynamic variables in pediatric patients [67, 68, 80, 81]. Deltex Medical™ manufactures a 5 mm pediatric esophageal probe that can be used for patients as small as 3 kg. A Doppler probe placed in the esophagus can record aortic blood flow characteristics with each heartbeat to derive stroke volume estimations. The waveform generated by esophageal Doppler is a graph of blood velocity versus time (Fig. 9.8). Key variables on this graph are stroke distance, flow time, and peak velocity (Table 9.3). Stroke distance (SD), the area under the curve, represents the distance traveled by a column of blood in the descending thoracic aorta (cm/s) and can be used to derive stroke volume. Flow time (FT), the width of the base of the curve, is the total time of systolic ejection. Because FT varies significantly with heart rate, corrected flow time (FTc) is often used instead of absolute FT. FTc is inversely related to systemic vascular resistance and therefore left ventricular afterload. Peak velocity (PV), the apex of the curve, represents the fastest speed of red blood cell ejection during the cardiac cycle and is directly related to ventricular contractility [82]. These values can be used to guide decisions about the fluid responsiveness of a patient (Fig. 9.9) [83]. Possible limitations of this monitoring tool for scoliosis surgery include limited space in a child's oropharynx for another probe, difficulty obtaining good waveform in prone position, and lack of this equipment in all centers.

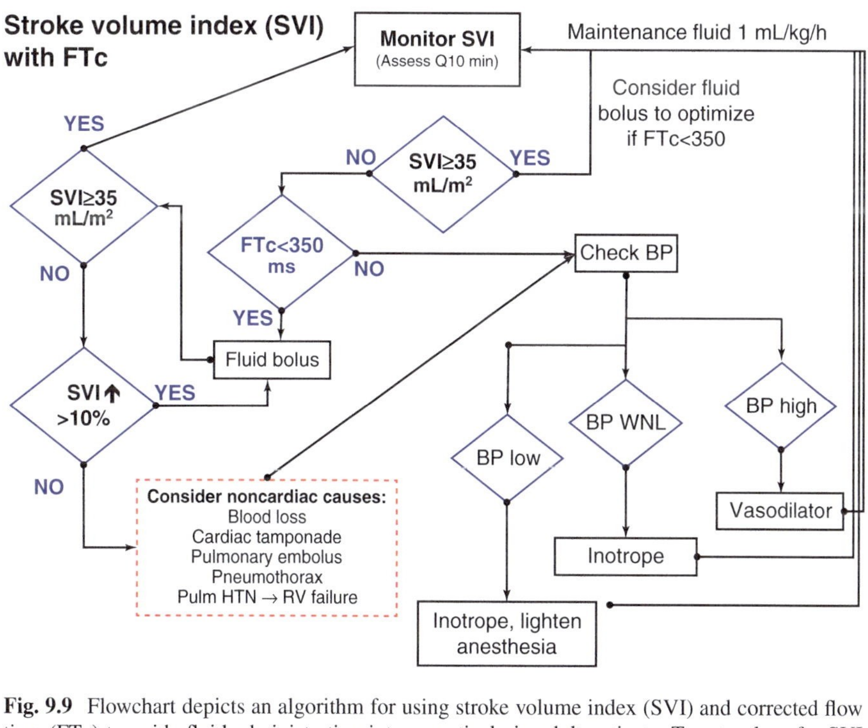

Fig. 9.9 Flowchart depicts an algorithm for using stroke volume index (SVI) and corrected flow time (FTc) to guide fluid administration intraoperatively in adult patients. Target values for SVI and FTc vary depending on the age size and physiological state of the patient. (Reprinted from Manecke [83]. With permission from Gerard Manecke)

Key Learning Points

- Duchenne muscular dystrophy (DMD) is the most common hereditary neuromuscular disease worldwide and is caused by an X-linked recessive mutation in the gene coding for *dystrophin*, an integral protein in the cell membrane and cytoskeleton of muscle cells.
- The onset of proximal skeletal muscle weakness occurs at age 2–3 and progresses rapidly to a wheelchair-bound state by the early teen years. Other medical conditions associated with DMD include cardiomyopathy, respiratory failure, restrictive lung disease, scoliosis, intellectual impairment, retinal disease, GERD, obesity, and osteoporosis.
- Anesthetic management of patients with DMD includes a thorough preoperative cardiac and pulmonary evaluation, the availability of advanced airway equipment, aspiration precautions, and careful attention to positioning.
- While patients with DMD are not at risk for malignant hyperthermia specifically, they are at risk for anesthesia-induced reactions including hyperkalemia, rhabdomyolysis, and cardiac arrest. Therefore, avoidance of succinylcholine, flushing the anesthesia machine, and a total intravenous anesthetic are recommended.
- Scoliosis refers to lateral, or sideways, curvature of the spine in the frontal plane of the body. The most common classifications of scoliosis are idiopathic, neuromuscular, and congenital. The severity of scoliosis is quantified by an index called the cobb angle, with greater angles representing more severe disease.
- Planning for surgical correction of scoliosis depends on patent age, skeletal maturity, cobb angle, and associated medical conditions. The surgery involves spinal fusion, through an anterior approach, a posterior approach, or a combination of the two.
- The risk of surgical complications such as neurological injury and blood loss is higher for patients with neuromuscular scoliosis than those with idiopathic scoliosis due to the need for longer and more complex surgeries to fuse more levels of the spine.
- To optimize neuromonitoring signals, a small concentration of inhaled anesthetic (<0.5 MAC), a supplemental anesthetic infusion, and intermittent or low-dose opioid are typically used. Neuromuscular blockers and nitrous oxide are usually avoided.
- Techniques to minimize blood loss and allogenic transfusions include administration of epoetin alfa, autologous donation, acute normovolemic hemodilution, controlled hypotension, intrathecal morphine administration, cell saver, and antifibrinolytic agents.
- Indices to guide volume resuscitation in pediatric patients include variation in aortic blood flow on echocardiography and esophageal Doppler monitoring.

References

1. Sarnat HB. 601.1 Duchenne and Becker muscular dystrophies. In: Nelson textbook of pediatrics. Philadelphia: W.B. Saunders; 2000. p. 2119–22.
2. Bushby K, Finkel R, Birnkrant DJ, Case LE, Clemens PR, Cripe L, Kaul A, Kinnett K, Mcdonald C, Pandya S, Poysky J, Shapiro F, Tomezsko J, Constantin C. Diagnosis and management of Duchenne muscular dystrophy, part 1: diagnosis, and pharmacological and psychosocial management. Lancet Neurol. 2010;9:77–93.
3. Verhaert D, Richards K, Rafael-Fortney JA, Raman SV. Cardiac involvement in patients with muscular dystrophies: magnetic resonance imaging phenotype and genotypic considerations. Circ Cardiovasc Imaging. 2011;4:67–76.
4. Sussman M. Duchenne muscular dystrophy. J Am Acad Orthop Surg. 2002;10:138–51.
5. Bushby K, Finkel R, Birnkrant DJ, Case LE, Clemens PR, Cripe L, Kaul A, Kinnett K, Mcdonald C, Pandya S, Poysky J, Shapiro F, Tomezsko J, Constantin C. Diagnosis and management of Duchenne muscular dystrophy, part 2: implementation of multidisciplinary care. Lancet Neurol. 2010;9:94–107.
6. Birnkrant DJ, Panitch HB, Benditt JO, et al. American College of Chest Physicians consensus statement on the respiratory and related management of patients with Duchenne muscular dystrophy undergoing anesthesia or sedation. Chest. 2007;132:1977–86.
7. Litman RS. Management of general anesthesia. In: Pediatric anesthesia: the requisites in anesthesia. St. Louis: Elsevier Mosby; 2004. p. 153–4.
8. Anectine, succinylcholine. Black box warnings. Epocrates, Inc. 2017. https://online.epocrates.com/drugs/198211/Anectine/Black-Box-Warnings. Web. 4 Sept 2015.
9. Hayes J, Veyckemans F, Bissonnette B. Duchenne muscular dystrophy: an old anesthesia problem revisited. Pediatr Anesth. 2007;18:100–6.
10. Brownell AK, Paasuke RT, Elash A. Malignant hyperthermia in Duchenne muscular dystrophy. Anesthesiology. 1983;58:180–2.
11. Yemen TA, McClain E. Muscular dystrophy, anesthesia and the safety of inhalational agents revisited again. Pediatr Anesth. 2006;16:105–8.
12. Goresky GV, Cox RG. Inhalation anesthetics and Duchenne's muscular dystrophy. Can J Anaesth. 1999;46:525–8.
13. American Heart Association Guidelines for Cardiopulmonary. Resuscitation and emergency cardiovascular care. Circulation. 2005;112:IV-1–IV-203.
14. Spiegel DA, Dormans JP. 671: the spine. In: Nelson textbook of pediatrics. Philadelphia: W.B. Saunders; 2000. p. 2365–73.
15. Gibson PR. Anaesthesia for correction of scoliosis in children. Anaesth Intensive Care. 2004;62:548–59.
16. Winter RB, Lonstein JR. Juvenile and adolescent scoliosis. In: Herkowitz H, Garfin SR, Balderstone RA, Eismont FJ, Bell GR, Wiesal SW, editors. Rothman-Simeone, the spine. 4th ed. Philadelphia: WB Saunders Company; 1999. p. 325–72.
17. Shiga T, Wajima Z, Inoue T, Sakamoto A. Aprotinin in major orthopedic surgery: a systematic review of randomized controlled trials. Anesth Analg. 2005;10:1602–7.
18. Vialle R, Thévenin-Lemoine C, Mary P. Neuromuscular scoliosis. Orthop Traumatol Surg Res. 2013;99:S124–39.
19. Coe JD, Arlet V, Donaldson W, Berven S, Hanson DS, Mudiyam R, Perra JH, Shaffrey CI. Complications in spinal fusion for adolescent idiopathic scoliosis in the new millennium. A report of the Scoliosis Research Society Morbidity and Mortality Committee. Spine. 2006;31:345–9.
20. Memtsoudis SG, Vougioukas VI, Ma Y, Gaber-Baylis LK, Girardi FP. Perioperative morbidity and mortality after anterior, posterior, and anterior/posterior spine fusion surgery. Spine. 2011;36:1867–77.
21. Weiss HR, Goodall D. Rate of complications in scoliosis surgery – a systematic review of the pub med literature. Scoliosis. 2008;3:9.

22. Reames DL, Smith JS, Fu KM, et al. Complications in the surgical treatment of 19,360 cases of pediatric scoliosis: a review of the Scoliosis Research Society Database. Spine. 2011;36:1484–91.
23. Divecha HM, Siddique I, Breakwell LM, Millner PA. Complications in spinal deformity surgery in the United Kingdom: 5-year results of the Annual British Scoliosis Society National Audit of Morbidity and Mortality. Euro Spine J. 2014;23:55–60.
24. Barash PG, Cullen BF, Stoelting RK. Anesthesia for neurosurgery. In: Clinical anesthesia. Philadelphia: Lippincott Williams & Wilkins; 2006. p. 996–1003.
25. Hammett TC, Boreham B, Quraishi NA, Mehdian SMH. Intraoperative spinal cord monitoring during the surgical correction of scoliosis due to cerebral palsy and other neuromuscular disorders. Eur Spine J. 2013;22:38–41.
26. Dicindio S, Theroux M, Shah S, Miller F, Dabney K, Brislin RP, Schwartz D. Multimodality monitoring of transcranial electric motor and somatosensory-evoked potentials during surgical correction of spinal deformity in patients with cerebral palsy and other neuromuscular disorders. Spine. 2003;28:1851–5.
27. Fehlings MG, Brodke DS, Norvell DC, Dettori JR. The evidence for intraoperative neurophysiological monitoring in spine surgery: does it make a difference? Spine. 2010;35:S37–46.
28. Eccher M. Intraoperative neurophysiologic monitoring: are we really that bad? J Clin Neurophysiol. 2012;29:157–9.
29. Nuttall GA, Horlocker TT, Santrach PJ, Oliver WC, Dekutoski MB, Bryant S. Predictors of blood transfusions in spinal instrumentation and fusion surgery. Spine. 2000;25:596–601.
30. Guay J, Haig M, Lortie L, Guertin MC, Poitras B. Predicting blood loss in surgery for idiopathic scoliosis. Can J Anaesth. 1994;41:775–81.
31. Vitale MG, Privitera DM, Matsumoto H, Gomez JA, Waters LM, Hyman JE, Roye DP. Efficacy of preoperative erythropoietin administration in pediatric neuromuscular scoliosis patients. Spine. 2007;32:2662–7.
32. Murray DJ, Forbes RB, Titone MB, Weinstein SL. Transfusion management in pediatric and adolescent scoliosis surgery: efficacy of autologous blood. Spine. 1997;22:2735–40.
33. Edler A, Murray DJ, Forbes RB. Blood loss during posterior spinal fusion surgery in patients with neuromuscular disease: is there an increased risk? Paediatr Anaesth. 2003;13:818–22.
34. Lee JH, Kim JT, Yoon SZ, Lim YJ, Jeon Y, Bahk JH, Kim CS. Evaluation of corrected flow time in oesophageal Doppler as a predictor of fluid responsiveness. Br J Anaesth. 2007;99:343–8.
35. Tzortzopoulou A, Cepeda MS, Schumann R, Carr DB. Antifibrinolytic agents for reducing blood loss in scoliosis surgery in children. Protoc Cochrane Database Syst Rev. 1996:1–26.
36. Forst J, Forst R, Leithe H, Maurin N. Platelet function deficiency in Duchenne muscular dystrophy. Neuromuscul Disord. 1998;8:46–9.
37. Turturro F, Rocca B, Gumina S, De Cristofaro R, Mangiola F, Maggiano N. Impaired primary hemostasis with normal platelet function in Duchenne muscular dystrophy during highly-invasive spinal surgery. Neuromuscul Disord. 2005;15:532–40.
38. Vitale MG, Stazzone EJ, Gelijns AC, et al. The effectiveness of preoperative erythropoietin in averting allogeneic blood transfusion among children undergoing scoliosis surgery. J Pediatr Ortho Surg. 1998;7:203–9.
39. Roye DP, Rothstein P, Rickert JB, et al. The use of preoperative erythropoietin in scoliosis surgery. Spine. 1992;17:S204–5.
40. MacEwen G, Bennett E, Guille J. Autologous blood transfusions in children and young adults with low body weight undergoing spinal surgery. J Pediatr Orthop. 1990;10:750–3.
41. Simpson MB, Georgopoulos G, Orsini E, et al. Autologous transfusions for orthopaedic procedures at a children's hospital. J Bone Joint Surg Am. 1992;74:652–8.
42. McNeil TW. Controlled hypotensive anesthesia in scoliosis surgery. J Bone Joint Surg. 1974;56-A:1167–72.
43. Araújo LMT, Garcia LV. Acute normovolemic hemodilution: a practical approach. OJAnes. 2013;3:38–43.

44. Copley LAB, Richards BS, Safavi FZ, Newton PO. Hemodilution as a method to reduce transfusion requirements in adolescent spine fusion surgery. Spine. 1999;24:219–22.
45. Hur S, Huizenga BA, Mjor M. Acute normovolemic hemodilution combined with hypotensive anesthesia and other techniques to avoid homologous transfusion in spinal fusion surgery. Spine. 1992;17:867–73.
46. Degoute CS. Controlled hypotension: a guide to drug choice. Drugs. 2007;67:1053–76.
47. Nigel MS, McMaster M. The use of induced hypotension to control bleeding during posterior spinal fusion for scoliosis. J Bone Joint Surg. 1983;65-A:255–8.
48. Patel NJ, Patel BS, Paskin S, Laufer S. Induced moderate hypotensive anesthesia for spinal fusion and Harrington-rod instrumentation. J Bone Joint Surg. 1985;67-A:1384–7.
49. Llndop MJ. Complications and morbidity of controlled hypotension. Br J Anaesth. 1975;47:799–803.
50. Lesniak AB, Tremblay P, Dalens BJ, Aucoin M, Mercier P. Intrathecal morphine reduces blood loss during idiopathic scoliosis surgery: retrospective study of 256 pediatric cases. Paediatr Anaesth. 2013;23:265–70.
51. Eschertzhuber S, Hohlrieder M, Keller C, Oswald E, Kuehbacher G, Innerhofer P. Comparison of high and low-dose intrathecal morphine for spinal fusion in children. Br J Anaesth. 2008;100:538–43.
52. Gall O, Aubineau JV, Bernière J, Desjeux L, Murat I. Analgesic effect of low-dose intrathecal morphine after spinal fusion in children. Anesthesiology. 2001;94:447–52.
53. Behrman MJ, Keim HA. Perioperative red blood cell salvage in spine surgery. Clin Orthop Relat Res. 1992;278:51–7.
54. Flynn JC, Metzger CR, Csencsitz TA. Intraoperative autotransfusion (IAT) in spinal surgery. Spine. 1982;7:432–5.
55. Florintino-Pineda I, Blakemore LC, Thompson GH, Poe-Kochert C, Adler P, Tripi P. The effect of EACA on perioperative blood loss in patients with idiopathic scoliosis undergoing posterior spinal fusion: a preliminary prospective study. Spine. 2001;26:1147–51.
56. Verma K, Errico T, Diefenbach C, Hoelscher C, Peters A, Dryer J, Huncke T, Boenigk K, Lonner BS. The relative efficacy of antifibrinolytics in adolescent idiopathic scoliosis: a prospective randomized trial. J Bone Joint Surg. 2014;96:e80.
57. Neilipovitz DT, Murto K, Hall L, Barrowman NJ, Splinter WM. A randomized trial of tranexamic acid to reduce blood transfusion for scoliosis surgery. Anesth Analg. 2001;93:82–7.
58. Fergusson DA, Hebert PC, Mazer CD, et al. A comparison of aprotinin and lysine analogues in high-risk cardiac surgery. N Engl J Med. 2008;358:2310–31.
59. Henry DA, Carless PA, Moxey AJ, et al. Anti-fibrinolytic use for minimising perioperative allogeneic blood transfusion. Cochrane Database Syst Rev. 2011;1:CD001886.
60. Schwinn DA, Mackensen GB, Brown EN. Understanding the TXA seizure connection. J Clin Invest. 2012;122:4339–41.
61. Rivers E, Nguyen B, Havstad S, Ressler J, Muzzin A, Knoblich B, Peterson E, Tomlanovich M. Early goal-directed therapy collaborative group. Early goal-directed therapy in the treatment of severe sepsis and septic shock. N Engl J Med. 2001;345:1368–77.
62. Han YY, Carcillo JA, Dragotta MA, Bills DM, Watson RS, Westerman ME, Orr RA. Early reversal of pediatric-neonatal septic shock by community physicians is associated with improved outcome. Pediatrics. 2003;112:793–9.
63. Rosenberg AL, Dechert RE, Park PK, Bartlett RH, NIH NHLBI ARDS Network. Review of a large clinical series: association of cumulative fluid balance on outcome in acute lung injury: a retrospective review of the ARDSnet tidal volume study cohort. J Intensive Care Med. 2009;24:35–46.
64. Murphy CV, Schramm GE, Doherty JA, Reichley RM, Gajic O, Afessa B, Micek ST, Kollef MH. The importance of fluid management in acute lung injury secondary to septic shock. Chest. 2009;136:102–9.

65. Boyd JH, Forbes J, Nakada TA, Walley KR, Russell JA. Fluid resuscitation in septic shock: a positive fluid balance and elevated central venous pressure are associated with increased mortality. Crit Care Med. 2011;39:259–65.
66. Gan H, Cannesson M, Chandler JR, Ansermino JM. Predicting fluid responsiveness in children. Anesth Analg. 2013;17:1380–92.
67. Raux O, Spencer A, Fesseau R, Mercier G, Rochette A, Bringuier S, Lakhal K, Capdevila X, Dadure C. Intraoperative use of transoesophageal Doppler to predict response to volume expansion in infants and neonates. Br J Anaesth. 2012;108:100–7.
68. Tibby SM, Hatherill M, Durward A, Murdoch IA. Are transoesophageal Doppler parameters a reliable guide to paediatric haemodynamic status and fluid management? Intensive Care Med. 2001;27:201–5.
69. Chandler JR, Cooke E, Hosking M, Froese N, Karlen W, Ansermino JM. Volume responsiveness in children, a comparison of static and dynamic variables. Proceedings of the IARS 2011 Annual Meeting; 2011. p. S–200.
70. Michard F. Changes in arterial pressure during mechanical ventilation. Anesthesiology. 2005;103:419–28.
71. Perel A, Pizov R, Cotev S. Systolic blood pressure variation is a sensitive indicator of hypovolemia in ventilated dogs subjected to graded hemorrhage. Anesthesiology. 1987;67:498–502.
72. Marik PE, Cavallazzi R, Vasu T, Hirani A. Dynamic changes in arterial waveform derived variables and fluid responsiveness in mechanically ventilated patients: a systematic review of the literature. Crit Care Med. 2009;37:2642–7.
73. Sandroni C, Cavallaro F, Marano C, Falcone C, De Santis P, Antonelli M. Accuracy of plethysmographic indices as predictors of fluid responsiveness in mechanically ventilated adults: a systematic review and meta-analysis. Intensive Care Med. 2012;38:1429–37.
74. Florence J, Hilly J, Sallah TB, Skhiri A, Michelet D, Brasher C, Varin L, Nivoche Y, Dahmani S. Plethysmographic variability index (PVI) accuracy in predicting fluid responsiveness in anesthetized children. Pediatr Anesth. 2013;23:536–46.
75. Vergnaud EC, Verchere VJ, Miatello J, Meyer P, Carli P, Orliaguet G. Stroke volume variation and indexed stroke volume measured using bioreactance predict fluid responsiveness in postoperative children. Br J Anaesth. 2014;114:103–9.
76. Pereira de Souza Neto E, Grousson S, Duflo F, Ducreux C, Joly H, Convert J, Mottolese C, Dailler F, Cannesson M. Predicting fluid responsiveness in mechanically ventilated children under general anaesthesia using dynamic parameters and transthoracic echocardiography. Br J Anaesth. 2011;106:856–64.
77. Renner J, Broch O, Gruenewald M, Scheewe J, Francksen H, Jung O, Steinfath M, Bein B. Non-invasive prediction of fluid responsiveness in infants using pleth variability index. Anaesthesia. 2011;66:582–9.
78. Byon HH, Lim CW, Lee JH, Park YH, Kim HS, Kim CS, Kim JT. Prediction of fluid responsiveness in mechanically ventilated children undergoing neurosurgery. Surv Anesthesiol. 2013;57:306–7.
79. Durand P, Chevret L, Essouri S, Haas V, Devictor D. Respiratory variations in aortic blood flow predict fluid responsiveness in ventilated children. Intensive Care Med. 2008;34:888–94.
80. Tibby, et al. Use of transoesophageal Doppler ultrasonography in ventilated pediatric patients: derivation of cardiac output. Crit Care Med. 2000;28:2045–450.
81. Murdoch IA, Marsh MJ, Tibby SM, McLuckie A. Continuous haemodynamic monitoring in children: use of transoesophageal Doppler. Acta Paediatr. 1995;84:761–4.
82. Deltex Medical Launches E-learning Center. Deltex Medical Education. Web. 29 Jan 2016.
83. Manecke G. UCSD goal directed fluid therapy algorithms. Clinical Guidelines – Department of Anesthesiology. UC San Diego Health Sciences, Oct 2015. Web. 5 July 2016.
84. Hazinski MF. Manual of pediatric critical care. St. Louis: Mosby; 1999.
85. Finsterer J, Cripe L. Treatment of dystrophin cardiomyopathies. Nat Rev Cardiol. 2014;11:168–79.

86. Musson RE, Warren DJ, Bickle I, Connolly DJ, Griffiths PD. Imaging in childhood scoliosis: a pictorial review. Postgrad Med J. 2010;86:419–27.
87. Banoub M, Tetzlaff JE, Schubert A. Pharmacologic and physiologic influences affecting sensory evoked potentials. Anesthesiology. 2003;99:716–37.
88. Zhou HH, Zhu C. Comparison of isoflurane effects on motor evoked potential and F wave. Anesthesiology. 2000;93:32–8.

Suggested Reading

1. Pathology Index. Pathology index. Washington University, St. Louis, MO. Web. 12 Jan 2016.
2. Bithal P, Ali Z. Intra-operative neurophysiological monitoring. J Neuroanaesthesiol Crit Care. 2015;2:179.

Chapter 10
Pulmonary Atresia with Intact Ventricular Septum

Daniel J. Sisti and Karim T. Rafaat

Case Narrative

A 2-day-old child is brought to the emergency department by paramedics. He is the product of a full-term, uncomplicated pregnancy and was delivered at home. The paramedics were called for fast respiratory rate and a dusky color. Upon arrival to the emergency department, the paramedic is delivering 100% O_2 via bag and mask and is gently assisting respirations. There is no intravenous access present. Heart rate is 175 bpm; blood pressure is 57/19 mmHg; respiratory rate is 45 breaths per minute; oxygen saturation is 62%.

The patient is quickly taken to the PICU where an IV is inserted, the infant is subsequently intubated, and an infusion of prostaglandin E_2 started. The child's saturations slowly increase to 82% on an FiO_2 of 100%. A transesophageal echocardiogram reveals pulmonary atresia with an intact ventricular septum (**L-1,2,3,4**). The child is later taken to the operating room where a Norwood procedure is performed (**L-5,6,7**). Following an unremarkable operative course, the patient is transported back to the PICU being ventilated by manual hand-mask bag positive pressure ventilation with an FiO_2 of 100% and infusions of dopamine of 7 mcg/kg/min, milrinone at 0.25 mcg/kg/min, and calcium chloride at 5 mg/kg/h. En route, the patient's oxygen saturations are 95%, but it is noted that the patient is dusky and grey. Invasive arterial pressures are 54/17 mmHg. Attempts are made to improve pressures via 1 mcg/kg boluses of epinephrine without success (**L-8**). The patient is rushed to the PICU, where, after being attached to the ICU ventilator, blood pressure improves over time (**L-8**).

D. J. Sisti (✉) · K. T. Rafaat
Department of Anesthesiology, University of California, San Diego, CA, USA

J. L. Benumof, G. R. Manecke (eds.), *Clinical Anesthesiology II*,
https://doi.org/10.1007/978-3-030-12365-9_10

Lesson 1: What Is Pulmonary Atresia with Intact Ventricular Septum?

Pulmonary atresia with intact ventricular septum (PA/IVS) is a rare cyanotic congenital heart defect (CHD). The structural abnormalities seen in this disease are an absent connection between the right ventricle (RV) or right ventricular outflow tract (RVOT) to the pulmonary arteries, and the RV and left ventricle (LV) are separated from one another by an intact septum. Commonly the RV is small and hypoplastic. See Lesson 2 for a detailed discussion of morphology in PA/IVS.

Estimated incidence of all types of CHD is low, ranging from 4 to 13 per 1000 live births [1–7]. This includes relatively simple defects such as atrial septal defects or patent ductus arteriosus as well as more complicated malformations such as tetralogy of Fallot. PA/IVS is a small fraction of the total cases of CHD, accounting for 0.5 per 1000 live births or less [2, 4, 5, 8, 9]. The pathogenesis of PA/IVS is unknown, but proposed etiologies include rare autosomal gene defects [10] and maternal inflammatory processes or viral infection during gestation [11].

Lesson 2: What Is the Morphology of PA/IVS?

The morphology of PA/IVS (Fig. 10.1) is extremely heterogeneous (Table 10.1). Generally, PA/IVS can be subdivided into two types: valvar and muscular atresia. Valvar atresia accounts for approximately 70% of cases and is characterized by the presence of a recognizable but imperforate membranous pulmonic valve. The remainder of patients have muscular atresia, with obliteration of the infundibular portion of the RV. Those with muscular atresia tend to have more severe RV hypoplasia and more frequent anomalous coronary connections from the RV [15, 16].

The RV and the tricuspid valve are very heterogeneous in PA/IVS. Functionally, the RV can be divided into three parts: the inlet, apex, and outlet (or infundibulum). The majority of PA/IVS patients have all three parts, i.e., they have a tripartite ventricle with inlet, body, and outlet. Some patients have a bipartite ventricle with an obliterated apex, and some patients have a unipartite, severely hypoplastic RV with an obliterated apex and outlet. RV apical sinusoids, a remnant of embryologic development, are commonly found. These often lead to fistulous connections from the RV to the coronary circulation. These fistulae can lead to proximal coronary stenoses, coronary ostial atresia, or coronary circulation that is dependent on blood flow from the RV [17, 18]. Patients with coronary anomalies are more likely to have left ventricular dysfunction and are more likely to require palliation via the Fontan procedure (see Lesson 5) rather than undergoing biventricular repair [19–21].

The tricuspid valve can be dysplastic or small and may have significant regurgitation and/or stenosis. A small subset of PA/IVS patients have Ebstein's anomaly with an inferiorly displaced tricuspid valve. This valve displacement or dysplasia may lead to a massively dilated RV [22]. Significant tricuspid regurgitation can lead to severe dilatation of the right atrium [23].

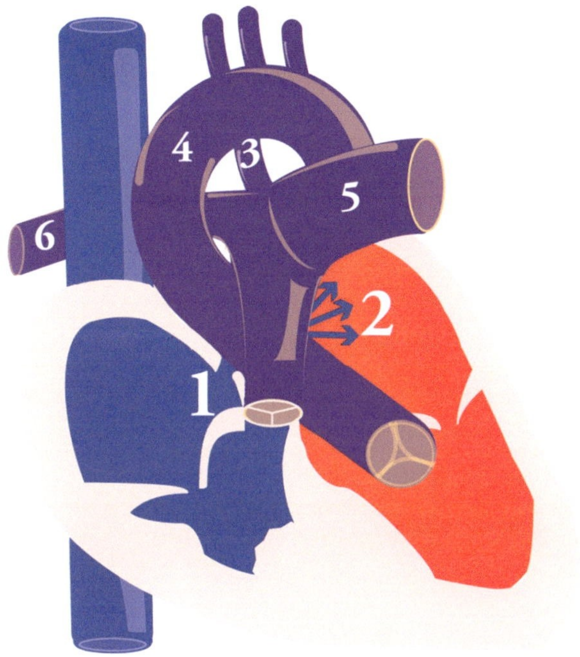

Fig. 10.1 Pulmonary atresia with intact ventricular septum. The right ventricle is hypoplastic and the pulmonic valve is imperforate. Venous ("blue") blood shunts across the patent foramen ovale, mixing with arterial ("red") blood, resulting in partially deoxygenated ("purple") blood being delivered to both systemic and pulmonary circulations via the patent ductus arteriosus. (1) Patent foramen ovale (PFO); (2) "blue" blood shunting to left atrium via PFO; (3) patent ductus arteriosus; (4) aorta; (5) left pulmonary artery; (6) right pulmonary artery

See Fig. 10.1 for an illustration of the basic morphology of PA/IVS, and refer to Table 10.1 for a summary of morphological variations that can be seen.

Lesson 3: What Is the Pathophysiology of PA/IVS?

The three main problems of PA/IVS are decreased, ductal-dependent pulmonary blood flow, hypoxemia, and right ventricular dysfunction.

Normal fetal circulation features high pulmonary vascular resistance (PVR). In fetal life, blood entering the right atrium has two possible paths: it can either shunt across the foramen ovale to the left atrium, or it can flow through the RVOT. After entering the main pulmonary artery, most of the blood will shunt across the ductus arteriosus to the aorta because of the high resistance in the pulmonary vasculature. A fetus with PA/IVS (Fig. 10.2) would be unable to survive without a patent foramen ovale or atrial septal defect because it lacks a patent RVOT (Fig. 10.3).

Table 10.1 Morphology in PA/IVS

Anatomy	Variation	Significance
Pulmonic valve	*Valvar atresia*	May be more amenable to biventricular repair
	Membranous, imperforate valve	
	Muscular atresia	Worse RV hypoplasia
	Obliteration of infundibulum	More anomalous coronary anatomy
Right ventricle	*Size*	Size and shape of RV influence surgical planning
	Often small/hypoplastic; may be massively dilated with dysplastic TV	
	Shape	
	Tri- vs bi- vs unipartite	
Tricuspid valve	Often small/dysplastic	Tricuspid valve size is an important determinant of bi- vs univentricular surgery [12, 13]
	Occasionally Ebstein's anomaly	
Coronary anomalies	RV sinusoids may contain RV-coronary fistulae	Risk of perioperative myocardial ischemia
	Coronary anomalies are common, and circulation may depend on blood from RV	Delineation of coronaries by angiography is needed for surgical planning [14]

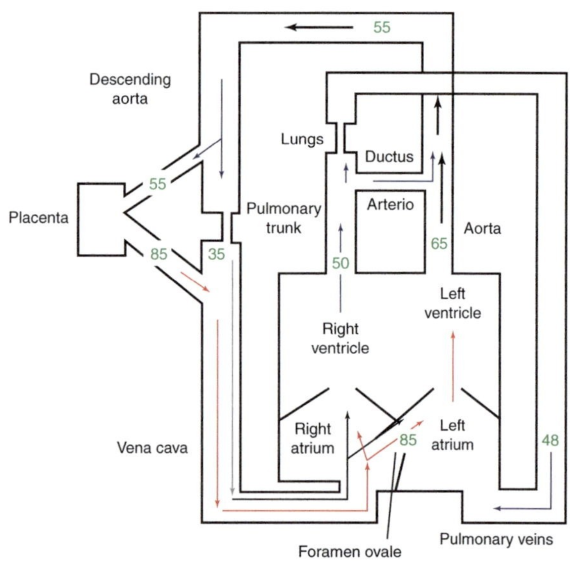

Fig. 10.2 Normal fetal circulation. Schematized depiction of circulation in the normal fetus. Note more blood flow from the pulmonary trunk goes through systemic circulation than pulmonary circulation. Green numbers depict approximate oxygenation values. (Reprinted from Rudolph [24]. With permission from BMJ Publishing Group Ltd.)

At birth, there is a drop in the PVR as the lungs expand and fill with air. With the fall in PVR, there is a greater pressure differential from the RA to the pulmonary bed, so more blood flows through the RVOT. Additionally, the foramen ovale functionally closes as right atrial pressures fall below left atrial pressures. As the PVR falls, ductal blood flow reverses, transitioning from right-to-left (ductus-to-aorta) to left-to-right (aorta-to-ductus). In PA/IVS, the blood flow through the ductus arteriosus is only left-to-right [24] and is the sole source of pulmonary blood both before and after birth.

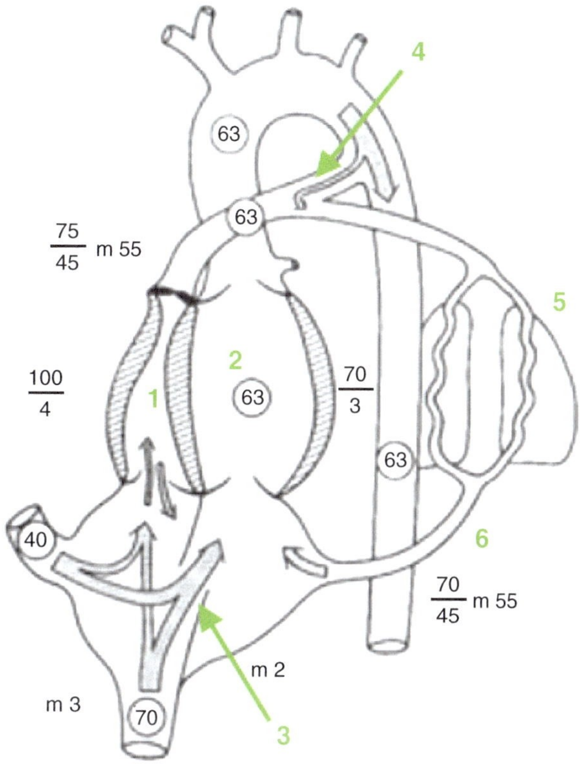

Fig. 10.3 Fetal circulation in PA/IVS. Blood can only reach the systemic circulation through a patent foramen ovale. Unlike in normal fetal circulation, flow through the ductus is left to right. Circled numbers represent oxygenation values, while non-circled numbers represent blood pressures. (1) Hypoplastic right ventricle with stenotic pulmonary valve; (2) left ventricle; (3) patent foramen ovale with venous blood shunting to left atrium; (4) patent ductus arteriosus; (5) lungs; (6) pulmonary vein. (Adapted from Rudolph [24]. With permission from BMJ Publishing Group Ltd.)

The ductus arteriosus constricts after birth and normally closes completely by 24–48 h [25, 26]. With constriction of the ductus arteriosus, the neonate with PA/IVS will inevitably become hypoxemic. The ASD or PFO will continue to allow right-to-left shunting of blood as right-sided atrial pressures remain high. While blood flow may continue, the circulating blood becomes progressively more hypoxic. This then becomes a self-perpetuating downward spiral as hypoxemia leads to acidosis, decreased cardiac output, and decreased systemic blood pressure. Hypotension further exacerbates the rapidly decreasing flow through the progressively narrowing ductus arteriosus, hastening the diminution of pulmonary blood flow even further, yet again worsening hypoxemia. The deoxygenated blood delivered to the left ventricle causes myocardial ischemia and further compromised hemodynamic status. Without intervention, closure of the ductus is a uniformly lethal event for patients with this cardiac lesion (see Lesson 4).

Lesson 4: What Caused the Child to Arrive in Extremis?

This child's catastrophic presentation is due to constriction of the ductus arteriosus. As previously discussed, the only source of blood to the pulmonary circulation is a left-to-right shunt through a patent ductus arteriosus. As the ductus constricts, the

Table 10.2 Ductal-dependent lesions

Ductal-dependent systemic blood flow	Ductal-dependent pulmonary blood flow
Hypoplastic or interrupted aortic arch	Critical pulmonic stenosis
Critical aortic coarctation	Pulmonary atresia with intact ventricular septum
Aortic stenosis	Tricuspid atresia
Hypoplastic left heart syndrome	Tetralogy of Fallot with significant RVOT obstruction
Mitral stenosis	Ebstein's anomaly

neonate becomes progressively hypoxemic and presents with respiratory distress and cardiovascular collapse.

There are several other forms of CHD that can present in a manner similar to this newborn. Any obstructive lesion will depend on a patent ductus for either systemic or pulmonary blood flow (Table 10.2). These obstructions will correspondingly be either left- or right-sided. Left-sided obstructive lesions include interrupted or hypoplastic aortic arch, critical aortic stenosis, hypoplastic left heart syndrome, critical aortic coarctation, and mitral stenosis. Right-sided obstructive lesions include PA/IVS, critical pulmonic stenosis, tricuspid atresia, and tetralogy of Fallot with significant RVOT stenosis ("blue tet"). Certain variations of Ebstein's anomaly may require a patent PDA until PVR is sufficiently low to allow the dysfunctional RV to pump blood into the pulmonary circulation.

After birth, breakdown of endogenous prostaglandin E_2 is one of the factors driving closure of the ductus arteriosus [27], and clinicians have known since the 1970s that infusions of prostaglandin E_1 or E_2 maintain patency of the ductus [28]. Clinically, E-type prostaglandin (PGE) infusions are given to neonates with known or suspected congenital heart disease to stabilize them prior to surgical correction or palliation. In the case narrative, the patient was given PGE_2, which kept the ductus open, allowing pulmonary blood flow with improvement in oxygen saturation from 62% to 82%.

Infants receiving PGE require careful monitoring, because it can cause hypotension and apnea [28, 29], and higher doses are associated with necrotizing enterocolitis [30].

Lesson 5: What Is the Norwood Procedure?

The Norwood procedure is the first surgery in a three-stage reconstruction for infants with severe CHD with a single functional ventricle (Table 10.3). The Norwood operation (Fig. 10.4) involves reconstructing a new aorta from the existing ascending aorta and main pulmonary trunk to conduct blood to the systemic circulation from the single ventricle. Pulmonary blood flow is then supplied by a shunt from the systemic circuit to the pulmonary arteries. Commonly, the Norwood procedure employs a modified Blalock-Taussig (MBT) shunt, where a synthetic

Table 10.3 Staged single-ventricle reconstruction

Stage I	Norwood operation with MBT or VPA shunt
Stage II	Bidirectional cavopulmonary anastomosis (Glenn or hemi-Fontan)
Stage III	Total cavopulmonary anastomosis (Fontan)

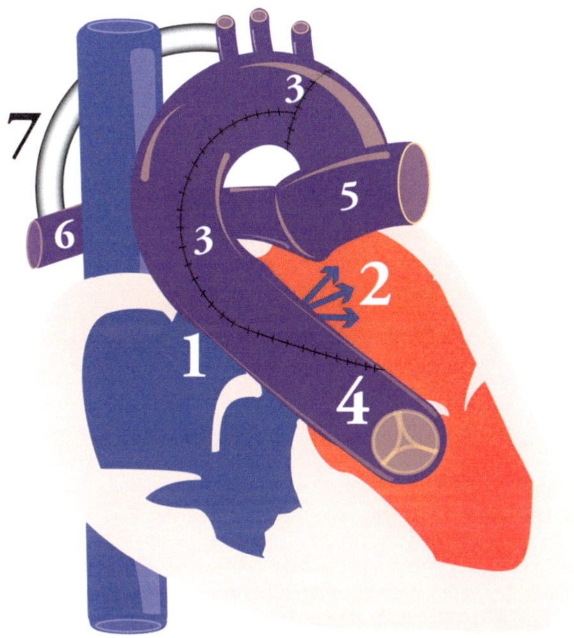

Fig. 10.4 Norwood procedure with modified Blalock-Taussig shunt. The main pulmonary artery is resected, and a neoarta is created by suturing together the ascending aorta and main pulmonary trunk. The neoarta is then connected to the single ventricle. Pulmonary blood is supplied by a shunt going from the right innominate artery to the right pulmonary artery. (1) Surgically created atrial septal defect; (2) venous blood shunting to the left atrium; (3) neoarta suture lines; (4) neoarta; (5) left pulmonary artery; (6) right pulmonary artery; (7) modified Blalock-Taussig shunt

tube graft connects the innominate or subclavian artery to the PA. Alternatively, some centers may place a ventricle to pulmonary artery (VPA) shunt.

After the first stage of reconstruction, the post-Norwood patient has adequate systemic oxygen delivery to allow growth and stabilization. The Norwood physiology is untenable long-term, however, because of cyanosis and high ventricular volume loading, causing progressively worsening dilation and dysfunction. Usually by age 3–6 months, the patient has grown enough to proceed to the second stage operation which is creation of a bidirectional cavopulmonary anastomosis [31].

The 2 s stage surgeries are either the bidirectional Glenn or the hemi-Fontan anastomoses (Figs. 10.5 and 10.6). With either surgery, the systemic-pulmonary shunt (MBT or VPA shunt) is ligated. In the Glenn operation, the superior vena cava (SVC)

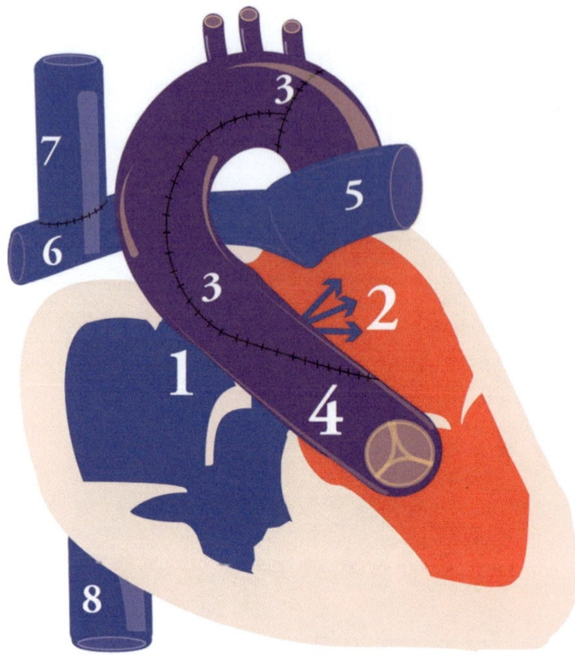

Fig. 10.5 Bidirectional Glenn. In the bidirectional Glenn operation, the superior vena cava is disconnected from the right atrium, and venous blood from the head and upper body passively drains to the right pulmonary artery. In the hemi-Fontan operation, the superior vena cava is anastomosed to the right pulmonary artery, and drainage to the right atrium is blocked by a patch. Note that in both operations, the pulmonary circulation has been separated from the systemic, and so now the pulmonary artery is "blue." (1) Surgically created atrial septal defect; (2) venous blood shunting to left atrium; (3) neoarta suture lines; (4) neoarta; (5) left pulmonary artery; (6) right pulmonary artery (RPA); (7) superior vena cava SVC, anastomosed to RPA; (8) inferior vena cava

is disconnected from the right atrium and anastomosed directly to the right pulmonary artery (RPA), allowing passive drainage of deoxygenated blood from the head to the pulmonary vessels. In the hemi-Fontan operation, an anastomosis of the proximal SVC and RPA is created, and a patch is placed between the SVC and right atrium to direct blood from the SVC directly to the pulmonary circulation. Both the Glenn and hemi-Fontan operations allow the single ventricle to experience less volume load.

Staged reconstruction culminates with total cavopulmonary anastomosis, the Fontan operation (Fig. 10.7). Completion of this step thus requires a pulmonary vascular bed with low resistance, which is one of the primary reasons that single ventricle neonates must undergo staged and prompt reconstruction. Significant delay in performing single ventricle repair can lead to pulmonary vascular remodeling. The consequent increase in PVR may be enough to make the completion of the Fontan impossible. The Fontan was originally developed for tricuspid atresia, but it has been modified and adapted for many forms of univentricular CHD including PA/IVS. It is typically performed between the

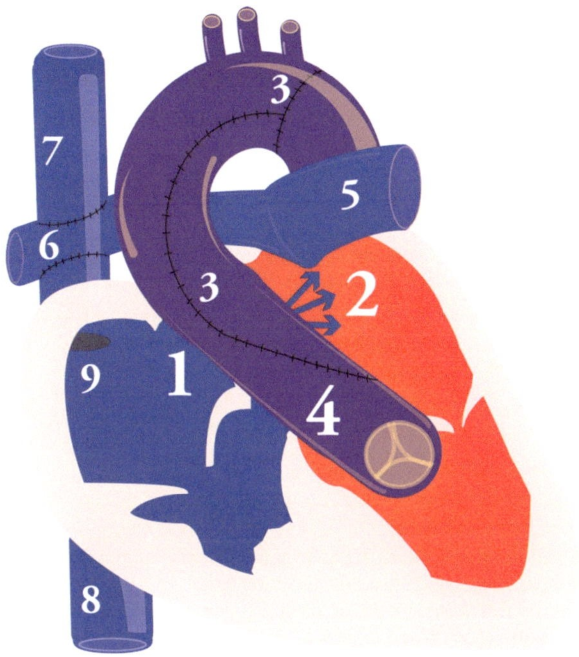

Fig. 10.6 Hemi-Fontan. In the hemi-Fontan operation, the superior vena cava is anastomosed to the right pulmonary artery, and drainage to the right atrium is blocked by a patch. The pulmonary circulation has been separated from the systemic, and so now the pulmonary artery is "blue." (1) Surgically created atrial septal defect; (2) venous blood shunting to left atrium; (3) neoarta suture lines; (4) neoarta; (5) left pulmonary artery; (6) right pulmonary artery (RPA); (7) superior vena cava SVC, anastomosed to RPA; (8) inferior vena cava; (9) patch occluding drainage from SVC to right atrium

ages of 18 and 48 months [31, 32]. Blood from the IVC is redirected to the pulmonary circuit, either through an intratrial baffle or extracardiac conduit that is connected to the right pulmonary artery. Upon completion of the Fontan, all venous blood is passively drained from the body through the pulmonary circulation. Pulmonary blood flow will thus depend on the pressure gradient from central venous to ventricular end-diastolic pressure and on pulmonary vascular resistance [33]. The ventricle exclusively pumps to the systemic circulation.

Lesson 6: What Are the Physiologic Implications of Each Stage of Single-Ventricle Reconstruction?

The key challenge of the post-Norwood patient is balancing two parallel circulatory systems. Normal cardiopulmonary physiology involves two blood flow circuits connected in series: pulmonary blood flow (Qp) and systemic blood flow (Qs). The Norwood

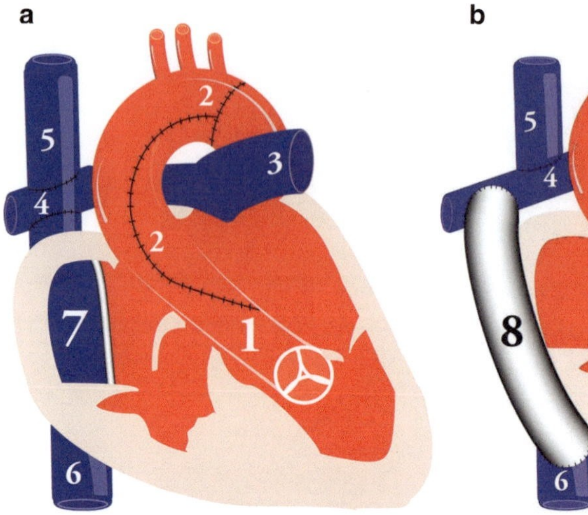

Fig. 10.7 Fontan with lateral baffle (**a**) and with extracardiac conduit (**b**). With the Fontan operation, all venous blood is returned to the pulmonary circulation. Blood from the IVC is either routed via the right atrium isolated with a baffle, or via an extracardiac conduit from the IVC to the pulmonary artery. Since all venous blood returns to the pulmonary circulation, the systemic circulation is completely "red." (1) Neoarta; (2) neoarta suture lines; (3) left pulmonary artery; (4) right pulmonary artery (RPA); (5) superior vena cava; (6) inferior vena cava (IVC); (7) right atrium isolated with synthetic baffle; (8) synthetic conduit connecting IVC to RPA

procedure connects Qp and Qs via a systemic-pulmonary shunt so that the flows are no longer in series but in parallel, each supplied by a single ventricle.

A parallel circulation palliates the newborn's critical defect, but it places the patient on a physiologic seesaw. If the ratio of Qp to Qs (Qp:Qs) is too high, implying high pulmonary blood flow, systemic hypoperfusion will ensue, leading to hypotension, acidosis, and end-organ ischemia. If Qp:Qs is too low, tissue will be perfused by poorly oxygenated blood. Ultimately, the goal is to balance the Qp:Qs in such a way so as to optimize tissue oxygen delivery (DO_2).

Properly balancing the parallel circulation will optimize DO_2. Mathematical modeling establishes that an optimally balanced Qp:Qs ratio lies between 0.5 and 1, as shown in Fig. 10.8. Note not only that total cardiac output is Qp + Qs, but the additive value of the ratio is indicative of the relative total work that the myocardium is performing (e.g., If Qp:Qs is 2:1, the single ventricle is performing three total "cardiac outputs" of work). Also note that DO_2 increases as cardiac output increases, regardless of the Qp:Qs.

There are a number of strategies available to the practitioner for optimizing DO_2 in Norwood physiology. Firstly, PVR can be manipulated to limit Qp. In the mechanically ventilated patient, increasing $PaCO_2$ via hypoventilation or mixing in CO_2 will increase PVR, lowering Qp:Qs. Blending in nitrogen to decrease FiO_2 to subatmospheric levels will raise PVR through hypoxic pulmonary vasoconstriction. Adjusting positive end-expiratory pressure (PEEP) so that end-expiratory

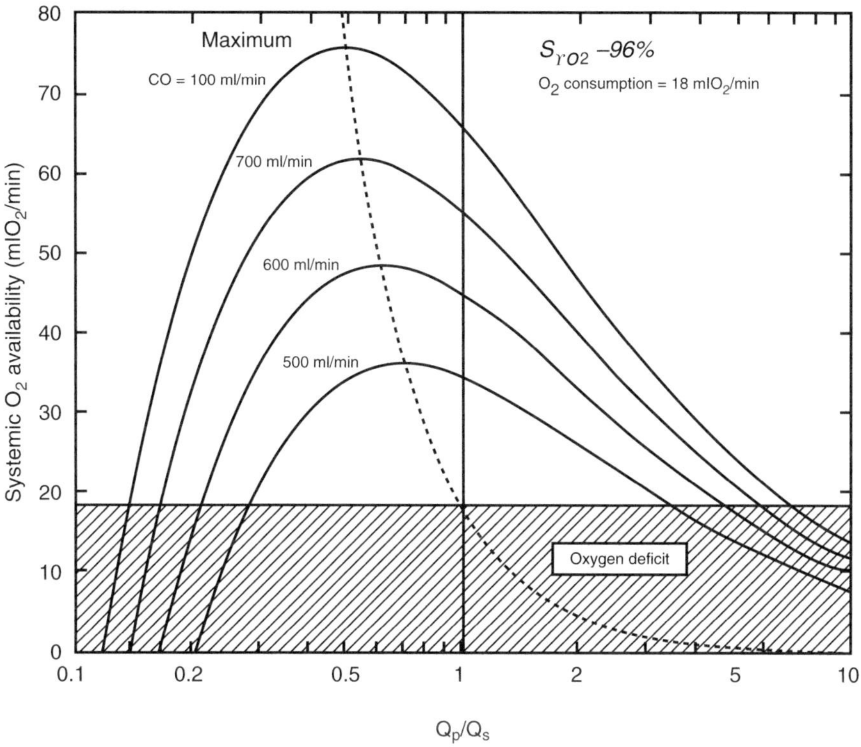

Fig. 10.8 DO_2 as a function of Qp/Qs. Mathematical model of DO_2 as a function of Qp/QS suggests that ideal oxygen delivery occurs at a Qp/QS between 0.5 and 1. Optimum oxygen delivery requires adequate cardiac output, regardless of Qp/QS. (Reprinted from Barnea et al. [34]. With permission from Elsevier)

lung volumes remain above FRC increases PVR as well. Minding acid-base status is also important as alkalosis will decrease PVR.

Secondly, lowering SVR will increase Qs, thereby increasing DO_2. For a patient that is being mechanically ventilated, adequate sedation to decrease sympathetic output will help keep SVR low. Further interventions for lowering include using vasodilators such as nitroprusside or milrinone or using alpha-antagonists [35]. Thirdly, increased cardiac output will increase DO_2, so inotropic agents such as epinephrine and dopamine are mainstays in the perioperative care of Norwood patients. The inotropy and vasodilation provided by milrinone make it an especially helpful drug for this setting [36]. Finally, blood transfusion to an appropriate hemoglobin level will ensure adequate oxygen-carrying capacity to support DO_2.

Ideally, there should be a way to assess how effective these interventions are in optimizing DO_2. From the Fick principle, a simplified mathematical expression of Qp:Qs can be stated as:

$$\frac{Qp}{Qs} = \frac{(SaoO_2 - SmvO_2)}{(SpvO_2 - SpaO_2)}$$

where SaO_2 is aortic oxygen saturation, $SmvO_2$ is mixed venous oxygen saturation, $SpvO_2$ is pulmonary vein oxygen saturation, and $SpaO_2$ is pulmonary artery oxygen saturation. This equation can be further simplified. In single ventricle patients, aortic and pulmonary artery saturations are the same. Furthermore, most babies have healthy lungs, so the $SpvO_2$ can be assumed to be 96%. Lastly, we can assume a normal systemic A-VO_2 of 25%. Thus, the equation becomes:

$$\frac{Qp}{Qs} = \frac{25}{(96 - SaO_2)}$$

Theoretically one can then estimate Qp:Qs simply by measuring the SaO_2. In practice, however, the underlying assumptions of this simplified estimation make it problematic. Investigators have shown that pulmonary venous desaturations occur frequently in the perioperative period of Norwood surgery [37]. Moreover, in the setting of abnormally high A-VO_2 (from poor systemic DO_2), a patient can have a normal SaO_2 yet have an untenably high Qp:Qs [38].

Rather than relying on just the above equation, a combined approach of measuring SaO_2, mixed venous oxygen saturation, and base deficit may be the safest approach. SaO_2 measurement will give at least some indication of what the Qp:Qs is. $SmvO_2$ (sampled from the central line) denotes oxygen utilization. Base deficit, or lactate levels, indicates anaerobic metabolism and thus insufficient DO_2.

The second stage of reconstruction, with either the bidirectional Glenn or hemi-Fontan operation, involves removal of the systemic-pulmonary shunt and has profound implications for the heart and the pulmonary circulation. Probably the greatest benefit of the second stage is volume unloading the single ventricle. Previously it had to pump both Qp and Qs, but separation of the parallel circulations means it only has to drive Qs. Over time the ventricle will remodel, have better function with lower oxygen consumption, and may thus ultimately be ready to transition to the full Fontan circulation.

Another benefit of separating the two circulations is preload now comes from the lower body, so increases in PVR will not compromise systemic cardiac output. Cyanosis is inevitable as deoxygenated blood from the lower body gets pumped back into the systemic circulation. A well-functioning Glenn or hemi-Fontan patient will live with saturations at 75–85% which is typically well tolerated until the Fontan is completed.

With the second stage physiology, a low transpulmonary gradient is necessary to maintain oxygenation and cardiac output. This goal of unobstructed pulmonary blood flow can be frustrated in three arenas: impeded venous return from the upper body, elevated atrial pressures, or high pulmonary vascular tone. Venous return can be obstructed by thrombosis in the SVC near the cavopulmonary anastomosis. It can also be obstructed by positive-pressure ventilation with high mean airway pressures. In the immediate postoperative period, however, there needs to be adequate lung recruitment to avoid atelectasis, which raises PVR. In the absence of countervailing pulmonary or airway issues, early extubation can be helpful as negative-pressure ventilation will improve Qp.

Further downstream, high atrial pressures will impede pulmonary blood flow as well. This can arise from an incompetent AV valve, from dysrhythmias, or from ventricular diastolic dysfunction. Finally, pulmonary vascular tone may still be high, because second stage patients are often not at their physiological nadir of PVR. Note, however, that attempting to lower pulmonary vascular tone with hyperventilation or alkalosis will increase cerebral vascular tone, thus impeding venous return. Inhaled nitric oxide acts selectively on the pulmonary vasculature and may be the best treatment in the setting of compromised Qp from high PVR.

The third and final stage of single ventricle construction is the Fontan operation. After completion of the Fontan, all systemic venous blood bypasses the heart and goes directly to the pulmonary circulation. There are two main approaches to achieve this. One approach is to place an extracardiac conduit connecting the IVC to the RPA. Potential advantages of the extracardiac Fontan are the need for minimal or no cardiopulmonary bypass and reduced risk of atrial arrhythmias. The major disadvantage is that the conduit cannot increase in size as the patient grows, and so will need to be changed in the future. The other approach is to place an intracardiac baffle within the right atrium, thereby redirecting blood from the IVC to RPA. If the prior operation was a hemi-Fontan, this is accomplished by removing the RA patch between the SVC and RA. The lateral tunnel approach is potentially advantageous for less thrombotic risk and the possibility of growth without severe dilatation. There is a higher risk of atrial arrhythmias due to the new suture line.

With either approach, the surgeon may create a fenestration in the extracardiac conduit or through the intracardiac baffle allowing right-to-left shunting. Well-functioning Fontan physiology will result in normal oxygen saturations, but this fenestration will cause minimal arterial desaturation. This “pop-off valve” helps maintain cardiac output in the face of elevated pulmonary vascular pressures or ventricular dysfunction, both common in the early postoperative period.

As in the bidirectional cavopulmonary anastomosis, a successful Fontan physiology requires a low transpulmonary gradient. Thus, elevated PVR, AV valve dysfunction, dysrhythmias, diastolic dysfunction, and blood flow obstructions can all lead to desaturation and low cardiac output. In the ICU, goals are to keep PVR low with minimal ventilator settings and early extubation, inotropic support as needed while avoiding increases in afterload, and treating dysrhythmias appropriately.

Lesson 7: What Are the Long-Term Implications of Single-Ventricle Physiology?

Single ventricle reconstruction is palliative, not curative. The Fontan operation has been used for over 40 years, and many patients may now survive into adulthood. Yet with increased survival comes a cost. Post-Fontan survivors have abnormal hemodynamics with chronically elevated central venous pressure, limited ability to augment preload to meet exercise demand, and chronically elevated ventricular afterload [39]. As a consequence of both the surgery itself and the postoperative hemodynamics, Fontan patients are at risk of multiple potential complications, including progressive decrease in exercise tolerance, hepatic cirrhosis, plastic bronchitis, protein-losing enteropathy, arrhythmias, and thromboembolic disease [40, 41].

There may also be long-term implications dependent on which ventricle—left or right—is available for reconstruction. With its normally thin wall and curved geometry, the right ventricle may not be particularly well suited to the work of systemic circulation. Studies have suggested that patients with single right ventricles have worse ventricular function [42], have a higher incidence of protein-losing enteropathy [43], and are at increased risk of early mortality [44, 45]. Thus, patients with PA/IVS who undergo Fontan reconstruction may fare better in the long run than patients with hypoplastic left heart syndrome.

Lesson 8: Why Did the Child Almost Die on the Way Back to the PICU?

The patient's oxygen saturation was noted to be 95% on the way back to the PICU. Per the discussion in Lesson 6, this indicates an unbalanced Qp:Qs ratio, with overcirculation of the pulmonary bed and insufficient systemic perfusion, resulting in hypotension. Boluses of epinephrine were given, but the child remained hypotensive until he recovered after some time in the PICU on the ventilator. One of the most likely culprits of this neonate's distress is inappropriate hyperventilation with manual ventilation [46], which would lower pulmonary vascular resistance and thereby create an excessively high Qp:Qs ratio. Another consideration is the inappropriate use of 100% O_2 during the transport back to the ICU. Both of these would result in a low PVR, increasing Qp:Qs, adversely affecting systemic perfusion. For this reason, neonates should always be transported with an oxygen mixer so that an appropriate oxygen percentage can be delivered. Oxygen can be referred to as a drug, with both positive and negative effects, and this scenario is an excellent example of the harmful misuse of what is usually thought to be an innocuous and universally beneficial gas.

References

1. Ferencz C, Rubin JD, Mccarter RJ, Brenner JI, Neill CA, Perry LW, Hepner SI, Downing JW. Congenital heart disease: prevalence at livebirth the Baltimore-Washington Infant Study. Am J Epidemiol. 1985;121(1):31–6.
2. Hoffman JI, Kaplan S. The incidence of congenital heart disease. J Am Coll Cardiol. 2002;39:1890–900.

3. Šamánek M, Voříšková M. Congenital heart disease among 815,569 children born between 1980 and 1990 and their 15-year survival: a prospective Bohemia survival study. Pediatr Cardiol. 1999;20(6):411–7.
4. Tanner K, Sabrine N, Wren C. Cardiovascular malformations among preterm infants. Pediatrics. 2005;116(6):e833–8.
5. Reller MD, Strickland MJ, Riehle-Colarusso T, Mahle WT, Correa A. Prevalence of congenital heart defects in metropolitan Atlanta, 1998–2005. J Pediatr. 2008;153(6):807–13.
6. Wu MH, Chen HC, Lu CW, Wang JK, Huang SC, Huang SK. Prevalence of congenital heart disease at live birth in Taiwan. J Pediatr. 2010;156(5):782–5.
7. Khoshnood B, Lelong N, Houyel L, Thieulin AC, Jouannic JM, Magnier S, Delezoide AL, Magny JF, Rambaud C, Bonnet D, Goffinet F. Prevalence, timing of diagnosis and mortality of newborns with congenital heart defects: a population-based study. Heart. 2012;98(22):1667–73.
8. Joelsson BM, Sunnegårdh J, Hanseus K, Berggren H, Jonzon A, Jögi P, Lundell B. The outcome of children born with pulmonary atresia and intact ventricular septum in Sweden from 1980 to 1999. Scand Cardiovasc J. 2001;35(3):192–8.
9. Ishikawa T, Iwashima S, Ohishi A, Nakagawa Y, Ohzeki T. Prevalence of congenital heart disease assessed by echocardiography in 2067 consecutive newborns. Acta Paediatr. 2011;100(8):e55–60.
10. Grossfeld PD, Lucas VW, Sklansky MS, Kashani IA, Rothman A. Familial occurrence of pulmonary atresia with intact ventricular septum. Am J Med Genet. 1997;72(3):294–6.
11. Kutsche LM, Van Mierop LH. Pulmonary atresia with and without ventricular septal defect: a different etiology and pathogenesis for the atresia in the 2 types? Am J Cardiol. 1983;51(6):932–5.
12. Daubeney PE, Wang D, Delany DJ, Keeton BR, Anderson RH, Slavik Z, Flather M, Webber SA. Pulmonary atresia with intact ventricular septum: predictors of early and medium-term outcome in a population-based study. J Thorac Cardiovasc Surg. 2005;130(4):1071–e1.
13. Gardiner HM, Belmar C, Tulzer G, Barlow A, Pasquini L, Carvalho JS, Daubeney PE, Rigby ML, Gordon F, Kulinskaya E, Franklin RC. Morphologic and functional predictors of eventual circulation in the fetus with pulmonary atresia or critical pulmonary stenosis with intact septum. J Am Coll Cardiol. 2008;51(13):1299–308.
14. Calder AL, Peebles CR, Occleshaw CJ. The prevalence of coronary arterial abnormalities in pulmonary atresia with intact ventricular septum and their influence on surgical results. Cardiol Young. 2007;17(04):387–96.
15. Daubeney PE, Delany DJ, Anderson RH, Sandor GG, Slavik Z, Keeton BR, Webber SA. Pulmonary atresia with intact ventricular septum: range of morphology in a population-based study. J Am Coll Cardiol. 2002;39(10):1670–9.
16. Kipps AK, Powell AJ, Levine JC. Muscular infundibular atresia is associated with coronary ostial atresia in pulmonary atresia with intact ventricular septum. Congenit Heart Dis. 2011;6(5):444–50.
17. Calder AL, Sage MD. Coronary arterial abnormalities in pulmonary atresia with intact ventricular septum. Am J Cardiol. 1987;59(5):436–42.
18. Anderson RH, Spicer D. Fistulous communications with the coronary arteries in the setting of hypoplastic ventricles. Cardiol Young. 2010;20(S3):86–91.
19. Dyamenahalli U, McCrindle BW, McDonald C, Trivedi KR, Smallhorn JF, Benson LN, Coles J, Williams WG, Freedom RM. Pulmonary atresia with intact ventricular septum: management of, and outcomes for, a cohort of 210 consecutive patients. Cardiol Young. 2004;14(03):299–308.
20. Cheung EW, Richmond ME, Turner ME, Bacha EA, Torres AJ. Pulmonary atresia/intact ventricular septum: influence of coronary anatomy on single-ventricle outcome. Ann Thorac Surg. 2014;98(4):1371–7.
21. Guleserian KJ, Armsby LB, Thiagarajan RR, Pedro J, Mayer JE. Natural history of pulmonary atresia with intact ventricular septum and right-ventricle–dependent coronary circulation managed by the single-ventricle approach. Ann Thorac Surg. 2006;81(6):2250–8.

22. Freedom RM, Jaeggi E, Perrin D, Yoo SJ, Anderson RH. The "wall-to-wall" heart in the patient with pulmonary atresia and intact ventricular septum. Cardiol Young. 2006;16(01):18–29.
23. Barr PA, Celermajer JM, Bowdler JD, Cartmill TB. Severe congenital tricuspid incompetence in the neonate. Circulation. 1974;49(5):962–7.
24. Rudolph AM. Congenital cardiovascular malformations and the fetal circulation. Arch Dis Child Fetal Neonatal Ed. 2010;95(2):F132–6.
25. Huhta JC, Cohen M, Gutgesell HP. Patency of the ductus arteriosus in normal neonates: two-dimensional echocardiography versus Doppler assessment. J Am Coll Cardiol. 1984;4(3):561–4.
26. Kiserud T. Physiology of the fetal circulation. Semin Fetal Neonatal Med. 2005;10(6):493–503.
27. Coggins KG, Latour A, Nguyen MS, Audoly L, Coffman TM, Koller BH. Metabolism of PGE2 by prostaglandin dehydrogenase is essential for remodeling the ductus arteriosus. Nat Med. 2002;8(2):91–2.
28. Lewis AB, Freed MD, Heymann MA, Roehl SL, Kensey RC. Side effects of therapy with prostaglandin E1 in infants with critical congenital heart disease. Circulation. 1981;64(5):893–8.
29. Lim DS, Kulik TJ, Kim DW, Charpie JR, Crowley DC, Maher KO. Aminophylline for the prevention of apnea during prostaglandin E1 infusion. Pediatrics. 2003;112(1):e27–9.
30. McElhinney DB, Hedrick HL, Bush DM, Pereira GR, Stafford PW, Gaynor JW, Spray TL, Wernovsky G. Necrotizing enterocolitis in neonates with congenital heart disease: risk factors and outcomes. Pediatrics. 2000;106(5):1080–7.
31. Ohye RG, Sleeper LA, Mahony L, Newburger JW, Pearson GD, Lu M, Goldberg CS, Tabbutt S, Frommelt PC, Ghanayem NS, Laussen PC. Comparison of shunt types in the Norwood procedure for single-ventricle lesions. N Engl J Med. 2010;362(21):1980–92.
32. Khairy P, Fernandes SM, Mayer JE, Triedman JK, Walsh EP, Lock JE, Landzberg MJ. Long-term survival, modes of death, and predictors of mortality in patients with Fontan surgery. Circulation. 2008;117(1):85–92.
33. Goldberg DJ, Paridon SM. Fontan circulation the search for targeted therapy. Circulation. 2014;130(23):1999–2001.
34. Barnea O, Austin EH, Richman B, Santamore WP. Balancing the circulation: theoretic optimization of pulmonary/systemic flow ratio in hypoplastic left heart syndrome. J Am Coll Cardiol. 1994;24(5):1376–81.
35. Tweddell JS, Hoffman GM, Fedderly RT, Berger S, Thomas JP, Ghanayem NS, Kessel MW, Litwin SB. Phenoxybenzamine improves systemic oxygen delivery after the Norwood procedure. Ann Thorac Surg. 1999;67(1):161–7.
36. Hoffman TM, Wernovsky G, Atz AM, Kulik TJ, Nelson DP, Chang AC, Bailey JM, Akbary A, Kocsis JF, Kaczmarek R, Spray TL. Efficacy and safety of milrinone in preventing low cardiac output syndrome in infants and children after corrective surgery for congenital heart disease. Circulation. 2003;107(7):996–1002.
37. Taeed R, Schwartz SM, Pearl JM, Raake JL, Beekman RH, Manning PB, Nelson DP. Unrecognized pulmonary venous desaturation early after Norwood palliation confounds Qp:Qs assessment and compromises oxygen delivery. Circulation. 2001;103(22):2699–704.
38. Schwartz SM, Dent CL, Musa NL, Nelson DP. Single-ventricle physiology. Crit Care Clin. 2003;19(3):393–411.
39. Davies RR, Pizarro C. Decision-making for surgery in the management of patients with univentricular heart. Front Pediatr. 2015;3:1–19.
40. Rychik J. Forty years of the Fontan operation: a failed strategy. Semin Thorac Cardiovasc Surg Pediatr Card Surg. 2010;13(1):96–100.
41. Khairy P, Poirier N, Mercier LA. Univentricular heart. Circulation. 2007;115(6):800–12.
42. Anderson PA, Sleeper LA, Mahony L, Colan SD, Atz AM, Breitbart RE, Gersony WM, Gallagher D, Geva T, Margossian R, McCrindle BW. Contemporary outcomes after the Fontan procedure: a Pediatric Heart Network multicenter study. J Am Coll Cardiol. 2008;52(2):85–98.

43. Powell AJ, Gauvreau K, Jenkins KJ, Blume ED, Mayer JE, Lock JE. Perioperative risk factors for development of protein-losing enteropathy following a Fontan procedure. Am J Cardiol. 2001;88(10):1206–9.
44. Gentles TL, Mayer JE Jr, Gauvreau K, Newburger JW, Lock JE, Kupferschmid JP, Jonas RA, Castañeda AR, Wernovsky G. Fontan operation in five hundred consecutive patients: factors influencing early and late outcome. J Thorac Cardiovasc Surg. 1997;114(3):376–91.
45. Julsrud PR, Weigel TJ, Van Son JA, Edwards WD, Mair DD, Driscoll DJ, Danielson GK, Puga FJ, Offord KP. Influence of ventricular morphology on outcome after the Fontan procedure. Am J Cardiol. 2000;86(3):319–23.
46. Tobias JD, Lynch A, Garrett J. Alterations of end-tidal carbon dioxide during the intrahospital transport of children. Pediatr Emerg Care. 1996;12(4):249–51.

Chapter 11
Necrotizing Enterocolitis in the Premature Infant

Christopher Nguyen, Karim T. Rafaat, and Jonathan L. Benumof

Case Narrative

A 37-week-old, 2.4 kg, ex-28-week premature female was scheduled for an exploratory laparotomy for suspected necrotizing enterocolitis (**L-1**). The patient's history included a small persistent muscular ventricular septal defect, chronic lung disease, and recent sepsis complicated by disseminated intravascular coagulation. Her surgical history included a previous patent ductus arteriosus ligation and a two-part omphalocele repair at 30 weeks (**L-2**). She remained intubated and ventilated in the neonatal intensive care unit (NICU), on pressure control ventilation with a peak inspiratory pressure of 25 cmH_2O and a rate of 22 breaths per minute. Her end-tidal CO_2 was 70 mmHg.

At the time of surgery, the patient was brought to the operating room in stable condition. Vital signs prior to induction were blood pressure 80/28 mmHg, heart rate 154 beats per minute, and oxygen saturation 100% on 40% inspired oxygen. Existing intravenous access included a peripherally inserted central catheter (PICC) and a 22-gauge peripheral IV. The patient was transferred to the anesthesia machine ventilator, and settings were adjusted to pressure control at 35 cmH_2O and a rate of 22–28 breaths per minute. The patient was induced with propofol and sevoflurane uneventfully (**L-3**). A femoral central line was inserted without complication.

Surgery was started and initially proceeded uneventfully. Intraoperative fluids were titrated according to hemodynamic need and totaled 200 mL of albumin 5%,

C. Nguyen · K. T. Rafaat (✉)
Department of Anesthesiology, University of California, San Diego, Orange, CA, USA
e-mail: krafaat@ucsd.edu

J. L. Benumof
Department of Anesthesiology, University of California, UCSD Medical Center, UCSD School of Medicine, San Diego, CA, USA

J. L. Benumof, G. R. Manecke (eds.), *Clinical Anesthesiology II*, https://doi.org/10.1007/978-3-030-12365-9_11

400 mL of Plasma-Lyte, 120 mL of packed red blood cells (PRBC), 60 mL of fresh frozen plasma (FFP), and 20 mL of platelets (**L-4**). Maintenance fluids of Isolyte-P in 10% dextrose were administered concurrently at a rate of 15 mL/h. Approximately 5 min after the surgeon began closing the abdominal wound, there was a sudden decrease in heart rate from 140 to 40 beats per minute. While the three-lead EKG was showing a bradycardic rhythm, there was a loss of the pulse oximeter waveform, and the noninvasive blood pressure cuff was unable to obtain a reading. The anesthesiologist hand ventilated the patient with 100% oxygen while administering code medications. The operative team began performing chest compressions, while the surgeon reopened the abdomen. Multiple doses of atropine and epinephrine were given, for a total of 120 mcg of atropine and 100 mcg of epinephrine (**L-5**). After approximately 60 s, there was return of vital signs with blood pressure 115/63 mmHg (mean arterial pressure 65 mmHg), heart rate 150 beats per minute, and oxygen saturation above 90%. Abdominal closure was abandoned, the incision was packed, and the patient was transported to the NICU.

L-1: What Is Necrotizing Enterocolitis (NEC)?

NEC is a disease of infants and is characterized by necrosis of the ileum and/or colon. The level of involvement can range from mild inflammation of the bowel wall to frank, full-thickness necrosis, leading to bowel perforation and consequent devastating morbidity. NEC is the most common gastrointestinal (GI) emergency in premature infants [1], with an overall incidence of approximately 1 in 1000 live births. This incidence increases to 3–10% in infants born at less than 1500 g. This is a highly morbid disease, with overall mortality ranging from 15% to 30% and increasing to 50% in patients going to surgery [2]. The presentation of NEC varies from mild intestinal signs to severe systemic illness, but the common underlying disorder is severe inflammation of the GI tract. This is thought to be due to an inappropriate inflammatory response to a variety of insults, including ischemia and hypoxia, with contribution from abnormalities in bacterial colonization, intestinal motility, barrier function, and immune response [1].

The etiology of NEC has not been traced to a single clear mechanism, but several risk factors have been found to have a strong association with NEC [3]. Predisposing factors to NEC can be divided into intrinsic and extrinsic categories in relationship to the neonate, as well as belonging to either the peripartum period or the neonatal period or being feeding-related (Table 11.1). A shared characteristic of many of these risk factors is that they can affect the systemic circulation and potentiate downstream ischemia. The patient in this case chapter presents with three intrinsic factors of significance: congenital heart disease, a history of respiratory distress syndrome, and sepsis.

Several extrinsic factors have also been implicated in the development of NEC. The most studied extrinsic factor is feeding practices. Initiating feeds too early and increasing feeds too rapidly are both associated with a higher risk of

Table 11.1 List of proposed risk factors for NEC. Known intrinsic risk factors affecting the patient in this are in bold italics

	Proposed risk factors for neonatal necrotizing enterocolitis	
Period	Intrinsic	Extrinsic
Peripartum events	Maternal eclampsia or preeclampsia Absent or reversed end-diastolic umbilical artery blood flow Fetal distress	Premature rupture of membranes Delivery by cesarean section Perinatal asphyxia Perinatal hypothermia
Neonatal period	*Respiratory distress syndrome* Apneic episodes *Congenital heart disease* Persistent fetal circulation *Persistent ductus arteriosus (PDA)* *Sepsis*	Umbilical catheterization Exchange transfusion Pharmacological treatment of PDA Histamine-2 blockers
Feeding regimen		Formula feed (as opposed to breast milk) High-density milk formula Early enteral feeding Rapid advancement of enteral feeding

NEC, possibly due to mucosal damage from the feeds' hyperosmolarity [3]. The use of human breast milk appears to reduce both the incidence of NEC and the incidence of surgery for NEC, likely because it contains immunologically protective components [4]. Histamine 2 blockers also appear to increase the incidence of NEC, presumably due to the effect of changes in gastric pH on the bacterial flora of the GI tract [5].

The initial diagnosis and staging is made using systemic, abdominal and radiographic criteria; it is logical to diagnose and stage NEC in terms of certainty and severity (Table 11.2). Treatment for NEC is most often medical. Initial management includes bowel rest, abdominal decompression, broad-spectrum antibiotics, IV fluid resuscitation, and parenteral nutrition [1]. Additional supportive care is dictated by the patient's clinical condition and serial examinations, and imaging should be performed to determine if surgery is necessary.

There are absolute and relative indications for surgery in NEC. The only absolute indication for surgery is frank bowel perforation [6] , which can be detected on abdominal imaging as pneumoperitoneum (Fig. 11.1) (or, less commonly, by finding the presence of stool or bile on paracentesis). Relative indications include clinical deterioration despite maximal medical therapy, radiographic findings such as portal venous gas or fixed loops on abdominal radiograph, or physical exam findings such as abdominal wall erythema and palpable abdominal mass (Table 11.3). The two primary surgical interventions are laparotomy versus primary peritoneal drainage. Although patients receiving primary peritoneal drainage often undergo laparotomy at a later time, both methods have similar 90-day outcomes [7]. The primary goals of surgical treatment are to remove necrotic bowel and control intra-abdominal sepsis. These are balanced with the consideration of preservation of as

Table 11.2 Modified bell criteria for staging NEC

Stage	Systemic criteria	Abdominal criteria	Radiographic criteria
1a: suspected NEC	Temperature instability, apnea, bradycardia	Increased pregavage residuals, mild abdominal distension, occult blood in stool	Normal or intestinal dilatation, mild ileus
1b: suspected NEC	Same as above	Grossly bloody stool	Same as above
2a: definite NEC; mildly ill	Same as above	Same as stage 1 plus lack of bowel sounds, possible abdominal tenderness	Ileus, pneumatosis intestinalis
2b: definite NEC; moderately ill	Same as stage 1 plus mild metabolic acidosis, mild thrombocytopenia	Same as above plus peritonitis, definite abdominal tenderness, possible cellulitis, right lower quadrant mass	Same as above plus possible portal venous gas
3a: advanced NEC; severely ill, intact bowel	Same as stage 2b plus hypotension, severe apnea, combined respiratory and metabolic acidosis, disseminated intravascular coagulation, and neutropenia	Same as above with marked tenderness and abdominal distension	Same as above plus ascites
3b: advanced NEC; severely ill, perforated bowel	Same as stage 3a	Same as stage 3a	Pneumoperitoneum

Adapted from Dominguez and Moss [1]. With permission from Elsevier

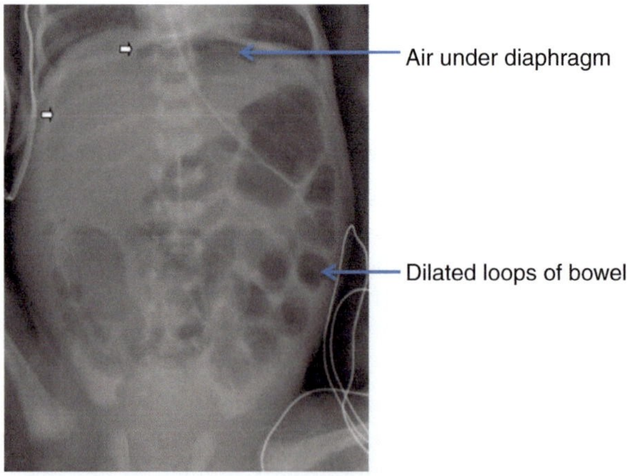

Fig. 11.1 Upright abdominal radiograph showing pneumoperitoneum in an infant with NEC. This is a sign of advanced NEC and an indication for surgical intervention. (Adapted from Hall et al. [3]. With permission from Elsevier)

Table 11.3 List of indications for surgery in acute NEC

Indications for surgery in acute NEC	
Absolute indications	Frank bowel perforation (pneumoperitoneum or evidence of stool/bile on paracentesis)
Relative indications	Clinical deterioration despite maximal medical treatment Abdominal mass with persistent intestinal obstruction Increased abdominal tenderness, distension, and/or discoloration Portal vein gas

Based on data from Ref. [3]

much intestinal length as possible. Postoperative care consists of physiologic support, which may include fluid resuscitation, vasopressor use, and ventilator support. Antibiotics are continued and gastric decompression is continued until bowel function returns. Approximately 5% of NEC cases recur, most commonly in patients with an underlying disease such as congenital heart disease. Usually recurrence can be managed nonoperatively [8].

L-2: What Is the Significance of This Infant's Comorbidities (VSD, PDA, CLD, Abdominal Wall Defects)

In addition to the expected technical issues related to performing surgery and anesthesia on a low birth weight (LBW) or very low birth weight (VLBW) infant (see L-3), this patient had several comorbidities that are commonly associated with prematurity. Each of these likely had some contribution to her course and the development of NEC, so it is important for the anesthesiologist to understand some key clinical features of each of these conditions.

Ventricular Septal Defect (VSD)

VSDs are the most common congenital heart defects, comprising 20–30% of all congenital heart defects [9], with a prevalence of 2.6/1000 in the general population. The direction and magnitude of blood flow through the VSD depends on the size of the defect and the difference between left-sided and right-sided ventricular pressures. In the fetal circulation, the right ventricle must generate high pressures in response to the relatively high resistance of the pulmonary vascular bed. Therefore, VSD flow is typically right to left. However, at birth, the transition from fetal to neonatal circulation causes a decrease in pulmonary vascular resistance and a corresponding decrease in right ventricular workload. Concurrently there is an increase in systemic vascular resistance, and the left ventricle becomes the dominant ventricle [9].

Thus, in the infant, flow through the VSD is typically left to right during systole. This results in higher right ventricular end-diastolic volumes and increased pulmonary blood flow. The left-to-right shunt can lead to a corresponding decrease in systemic blood flow and, ultimately, a decrease in mesenteric blood flow. Also, in the critically ill neonate, pulmonary vascular resistance may occasionally be higher than systemic due to the stiff lung parenchyma and the effects of positive pressure ventilation. A right-to-left shunt will result in a decrease in systemic oxygen delivery due to a lower saturation of hemoglobin. Both scenarios can result in intestinal ischemia and injury and thus produce an environment that predisposes the infant to developing NEC. In one large study, infants with VSDs had a 7.8% incidence of NEC, compared to an incidence of 6.2% in infants without septal defects [10]. Small VSDs are usually tolerated well from a hemodynamic standpoint, but infants with large VSDs are prone to ventricular dilation and ventricular dysfunction, especially if left unrepaired. In this patient the VSD was reported as small and hemodynamically insignificant and thus was likely not the most significant contributor to the development of NEC.

Patent Ductus Arteriosus (PDA)

PDA is a congenital condition in which the ductus arteriosus connecting the aorta and the pulmonary artery fails to close after birth. The ductus arteriosus exists as part of the fetal circulation, allowing blood to bypass the fluid-filled lungs. Normally, at birth, the loss of prostaglandin E2 from the placenta allows the ductus to close and become the vestigial ligamentum arteriosum. Failure of the ductus arteriosum to close is common in premature infants, with an incidence of 20–40% in infants born at less than 1000 g [11]. Delayed closure of the ductus results in continued flow through it, with direction and magnitude depending on the difference between the resistances of the pulmonary and systemic vascular beds. Typically, as systemic pressures are higher than pulmonary pressures in the infant, the PDA will result in a left-to-right shunt.

As with a VSD, a PDA with a significant amount of flow can lead to pulmonary overcirculation and a concomitant decrease in systemic and mesenteric flow. Thus, it is thought that the existence of PDA also contributes to the development of NEC. One study showed a 9.4% incidence of NEC in infants with PDAs versus a 5.5% incidence in all infants [12]. Treatment of PDA consists of either surgical ligation or medical treatment with indomethacin, a prostaglandin inhibitor. The use of indomethacin in patients at risk for NEC is controversial as indomethacin is thought to also have a vasoconstricting effect on mesenteric vessels, potentially increasing the risk of NEC. However, one systemic review did not demonstrate a difference in the incidence of NEC when looking at surgically repaired PDAs versus those treated with indomethacin [13].

Chronic Lung Disease (CLD)

CLD is seen in premature infants who have undergone prolonged mechanical ventilation, usually for treatment of respiratory failure or apnea. Multiple issues contribute to the development of CLD, including barotrauma, oxygen toxicity, and chronic inflammation. Clinically, CLD manifests as increased airway resistance and decreased lung compliance in addition to problems with gas exchange, all of which lead to ventilation/perfusion mismatch [14]. Ventilation of these patients can be challenging, requiring a balance between adequate oxygenation and ventilation without worsening barotrauma and oxygen toxicity. Lessons from the ARDSNet low tidal volume protocol have been applied to this case, with permissive hypercapnia being tolerated in order to use lower mean airway pressures during ventilation [15]. The end-tidal CO_2 of 70 mmHg in the patient is indicative of the aforementioned concerns and strategies. Ventilation that would target a normal carbon dioxide tension would have required increased mean airway pressure that would exacerbate barotrauma and volutrauma. Anesthesiologists often have a strong compulsion to optimize ventilation and oxygenation whenever possible, and this drive should be tempered in such a situation.

Gastroschisis and Omphalocele

Gastroschisis is a rare abdominal wall defect, with an incidence of 0.3–2 per 10,000 births [16]. Omphalocele is slightly more common, with an incidence of approximately 1 in 5000 births. These two conditions are similar in gross physical appearance but have some key differences in etiology and clinical associations (Fig. 11.2). An omphalocele is essentially a midline defect of the umbilical ring, with the abdominal contents extruding through the defect but contained within a sac composed of the peritoneal and amniotic membranes. Seventy-five percent of infants with an omphalocele will have other anomalies, including cardiac defects (most commonly VSDs) and cranial, urogenital, and limb abnormalities [17] (Table 11.4). Up to 40% are found to be syndromic (most commonly Beckwith-Wiedemann), with 20–30% having a chromosomal abnormality. In contrast, the defect in gastroschisis usually occurs to the right of the umbilical cord, and the extruded bowel is not covered by a sac (although it may be covered with an inflammatory exudate). Gastroschisis usually occurs as an isolated defect, although there is an association with intestinal malrotation and intestinal atresia.

Management of both defects is similar and ultimately requires surgical repair. Preoperative management includes fluid resuscitation, maintenance of normothermia, gastric decompression, and broad-spectrum antibiotics. Surgical repair is often staged, as forcing the viscera into an underdeveloped abdominal

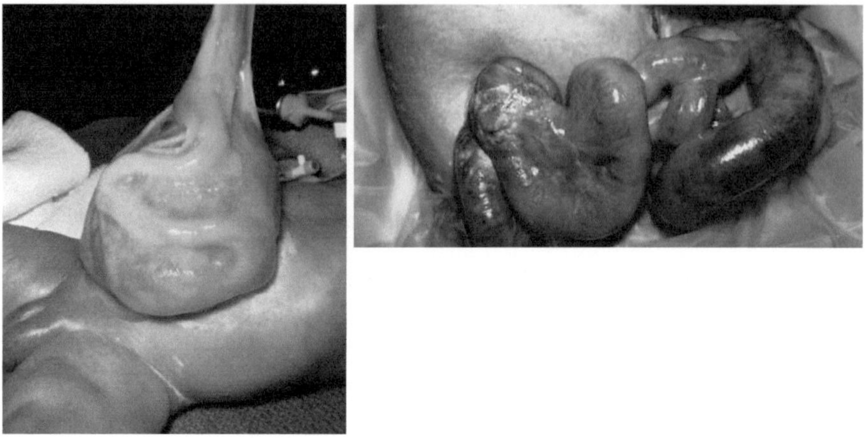

Fig. 11.2 Morphologic differences between omphalocele and gastroschisis. Omphalocele, in the left image, is characterized by a sac covering the bowel contents. Gastroschisis, seen in the above image, has no covering over the extruded bowel. (Reprinted from Langer [35]. With permission from Springer Science + Business Media)

Table 11.4 Incidence of associated comorbidities in 93 patients with omphalocele and 29 patients with gastroschisis

Abdominal wall defect	Associated comorbidity	% of patients affected
Omphalocele	Chromosomal syndrome	20
	Beckwith-Wiedemann	12
	Pentalogy of Cantrell	9
	Cardiac	24
	Cranial	11
	Urogenital	10
	Limb	10
	Umbilical	8
	Total	73
Gastroschisis	Cardiac	12
	Urogenital	7
	Limb	2
	Total	23

Based on data from Ref. [17]

cavity can impair ventilation and venous return. Although repair is usually quite efficacious and 95–97% survival is expected, it is important to note that these defects do have an association with NEC [9]. This is due to several factors, including bowel ischemia from increased abdominal pressure, an overall increased risk of sepsis, and the development of adhesions and/or bowel obstruction.

L-3: What Were the Anesthetic Issues During the Induction and Maintenance of Anesthesia (Monitoring and Vascular Access and Induction and Maintenance Medications)

Monitoring and Vascular Access

In addition to the ASA standard monitors for oxygenation, ventilation, circulation, and temperature, an important decision for this patient is the use of invasive hemodynamic monitors. Direct measurement of arterial blood pressure using a catheter is indicated when precise beat-to-beat blood pressure monitoring is required or if frequent blood samples are required (usually for measuring arterial blood gas values). Indications for serial arterial blood gases include patients with significant abnormalities in gas exchange due to pre-existing disease or related to the procedure, such as the use of lung isolation [9]. In this patient, both hemodynamic and respiratory factors point toward a need for an indwelling arterial catheter, given that she was undergoing a large abdominal surgery and also had pre-existing CLD with abnormal pulmonary function. During this case an arterial line was attempted, but the patient's prolonged NICU stay and history of previous indwelling arterial catheters made it extremely technically difficult. Given the urgent nature of the case and concern for impending decompensation, it was decided to proceed with surgery rather than to continue struggling with the arterial line. For academic interest, we will note that the anatomic sites most frequently used for arterial line placement are the radial, ulnar, dorsalis pedis, posterior tibial, and femoral arteries. The brachial artery is avoided because of the poor collateral flow around the elbow, but the axillary artery may be a favorable option because it has more collateral flow [18]. Other options include using a Doppler flow transducer to localize an artery that is difficult to palpate or using a surgical cutdown technique for patients in whom percutaneous attempts have failed.

Central venous catheter placement has three relative indications: inadequate peripheral venous access, central venous pressure (CVP) monitoring, and infusion of hyperosmolar or sclerosing substances. This patient arrived in the OR with a 22-gauge 1-in.-long peripheral IV, which has a mean flow rate of 24–26 mL/min [9]. While this would usually suffice for more minor surgery in a small infant, patients with significant fluid requirements (such as those undergoing open abdominal surgery) may require additional access. Infusion rates of at least 20 mL/kg/h are commonly maintained during surgery for NEC, with additional fluids often required [14]. Peripherally inserted central catheters, being of small gauge and long relative length, are limited by Poiseuille's law to significantly restricted flow and are thus not useful for rapid infusion. The use of central venous pressure for hemodynamic monitoring is discussed further in L-4, but it is worthwhile to mention that CVP data can be used in combination with other data to help form a fluid management plan, particularly in patients in whom large fluid shifts or blood loss are expected. CVP data is also useful for measuring visceral compression during abdominal closure [19]. Therefore the insertion of a femoral central venous catheter was very reasonable in this patient.

Induction and Maintenance Medications

An important goal of induction for premature infants is the avoidance of large hemodynamic swings. Endotracheal intubation with inadequate anesthesia may cause a sudden rise in arterial and intracranial pressure, leading to intraventricular hemorrhage [14]. Conversely, anesthesia-induced hypotension can reduce cerebral and systemic blood flow, which may lead to cerebral and systemic ischemia. An additional complication is the relative immaturity of the neonatal autonomic nervous system, where parasympathetic responses predominate due to relatively reduced myocardial sympathetic innervation [20]. As a result, profound bradycardia and even cardiac arrest can occur in response to either induction hypotension or to a vagal response during intubation with inadequate anesthesia. For patients without an endotracheal tube in place, a common induction regimen includes propofol 2–3 mg/kg with vecuronium 0.1 mg/kg, although other hypnotics and paralytics can be used as well, depending on the clinical context. In hemodynamically unstable patients, more stable options for induction can include ketamine 1.5–2 mg/kg with or without fentanyl 2–5 mcg/kg or just a non-depolarizing neuromuscular blocker. For a patient with an endotracheal tube in situ, reduced doses of induction medications can be used while transitioning to maintenance anesthesia. The use of propofol in this case was made at the discretion of the anesthesiologist but evidently indicates the patient was hemodynamically stable at the start of surgery. The patient tolerated induction without evidence of hemodynamic compromise.

Anesthesia can be maintained via several different approaches, although, classically, a combined technique using a volatile anesthetic with intravenous opioids is most often used. Sevoflurane and isoflurane are currently the most common volatile anesthetics used, although they do have dose-related cardiodepressant activity. Nitrous oxide should not be used for abdominal surgery because it will diffuse into and enlarge the intestines. Non-depolarizing muscle relaxants are also often used for abdominal surgery to relax the abdomen and facilitate surgical exposure and the abdominal closure. For this patient, maintenance was achieved with sevoflurane, along with titrated doses of fentanyl and vecuronium.

L-4: What Were the Anesthetic Issues Intraoperatively (Ventilator Management, Temperature Regulation, Fluid Management)

Several issues were present during this case that presented significant anesthetic challenges, including ventilator management, temperature regulation, and fluid management.

Ventilator Management

Ventilation and oxygenation for this patient were significant issues, requiring a careful balance between optimizing tissue oxygen delivery and blood pH versus the risk of worsening long-term sequelae of mechanical ventilation. In L-2 we discussed the challenges of managing a patient with CLD with regard to ventilating a patient with abnormal lung compliance and gas delivery. Intraoperatively during this case, ventilator settings were changed from the NICU settings, with an increase in inspired pressure from 25 to 35 cmH_2O, as well as a slight increase in respiratory rate. This was done in response to high end-tidal carbon dioxide measurements, which presents three concerns. First, as previously discussed, it is often prudent to allow a degree of hypercapnia in order to implement smaller tidal volumes and lower mean airway pressures during ventilation [15]. Second, end-tidal capnography in small infants is often inaccurate, due to air leak around the endotracheal tube and a large ratio of physical dead space to tidal volume [14]. This is another reason that an indwelling arterial catheter would be useful, as it would allow direct measurement of carbon dioxide tension and blood acid-base balance. Third, the ability of some anesthesia machines to accurately measure delivered tidal volumes in small neonates is negatively affected by the compliance of the breathing circuit. This is especially significant when using volume-control modes of ventilation, where ventilators without compliance compensation can deliver less than half of the set tidal volume [21]. Furthermore, it is important to note that any increase in mean airway pressure necessarily results in an increase in intrathoracic pressure. If significant enough, or combined with concomitant hypovolemia, venous return and thus cardiac output can be impaired.

Targeting appropriate oxygen saturation is another challenge in preterm infants. It is increasingly being recognized that hyperoxia is deleterious to premature infants, having been shown to be associated with retinopathy of prematurity (ROP), injury to the developing brain, childhood cancers, and infection [22]. Unfortunately, it is less clear what the appropriate range of oxygen saturation should be and what to target intraoperatively. One recent meta-analysis came to the conclusion that targeting SpO_2 85–89% increased mortality, whereas targeting SpO_2 91–95% was associated with higher rates of ROP [23]. Part of the challenge with both ranges was difficulty in maintaining compliance; for example, caregivers targeting 91–95% would often overlook SpO_2 above the target range. The authors suggested that wider intermediate targets, such as a range of 87–94%, would allow for easier patient care and compliance. It is stressed that even temporary exposure to hyperoxia can have deleterious effects, including during transport and intraoperatively. The takeaway message for the anesthesiologist is that oxygen is a drug, with both positive and negative effects, and the decision to use hyperoxic mixtures should be made rationally and with specific intent.

Temperature Regulation

Premature and low birth weight infants are at high risk for hypothermia during surgery, due to a combination of environmental factors and immature compensatory mechanisms. Infants have a large surface area to volume ratio and reduced subcutaneous fat, thus predisposing them to radiant and convective heat loss [9]. They also depend on non-shivering thermogenesis for heat production, which utilizes mitochondrial uncoupling in brown adipose tissue to generate heat. It has been shown that volatile anesthetics are potent inhibitors of brown adipose tissue thermogenesis [24]. In addition, during abdominal surgery there is increased exposure of the visceral surfaces, and it has been shown that evaporative heat loss in this setting may equal all other sources of intraoperative heat loss combined [25]. Hypothermia is associated with potentially severe consequences related to increased oxygen consumption, metabolic acidosis, and with severe hypothermia, dysfunction at the cellular level [9]. In a patient with pre-existing cardiovascular and respiratory disease, hypothermia can be disastrous.

Measures should be taken to keep the patient warm both during transport and intraoperatively. They should be transported in a warmed incubator to a pre-warmed operating room. It is suggested that the room be warmed to 27 °C for a full-term infant and 29 °C for a premature infant [9]. Other measures that should be used are warming mattresses, forced-air warming systems, and warmed fluids. If intraoperative lavage is being used, the solutions should also be warmed to body temperature. Finally, it is also important to keep the infant's head covered and to keep the skin and drapes dry to reduce conductive heat loss [14].

Fluid Management

Perhaps the most challenging aspect of this case was assessment of volume status and management of fluid replacement. As previously stated, this infant was dealing with high rates of evaporative fluid loss from exposed viscera, in addition to ongoing surgical blood loss. The goal with fluid resuscitation is to maintain adequate cardiac output and perfusion pressure, but excessive fluid therapy has been shown to increase mortality [26]. Thus the key is to be able to predict fluid responsiveness and titrate fluids using rational parameters. Traditional clinical assessment based on physical examination and routine monitoring is often imprecise and inadequate in children [27]. Many other variables have been studied for assessing fluid responsiveness, including CVP, pulmonary artery occlusion pressures, transesophageal Doppler measurements, inferior vena cava diameter variation, and systolic pressure variation.

Ideally, a hemodynamic variable would exist that could be used to predict whether a patient would have an increase in cardiac output in response to fluid resuscitation. A recent systematic review failed to find any studies that demonstrated predictive value of heart rate, CVP, pulmonary artery occlusion pressure, left ventricular end-diastolic area, global end-diastolic volume index, ultrasound dilution measurements, and Doppler measurements [28]. Additionally, dynamic variables that are useful predictors in adults (systolic pressure variation and pulse pressure variation) were also not found to be predictive in children in this review. Only one of the seven studies investigating the use of pulse pressure variation was able to demonstrate a positive result [29]. The authors of the review speculate that dynamic variables based on arterial pressure are less useful in children than adults because the pediatric arterial system is more compliant. Such measurements are based on the magnitude of change in arterial blood pressure induced by ventilation, which will be smaller when thoracic and arterial compliance are higher. The only variable that was identified in multiple studies to be predictive was respiratory variation in aortic blood flow peak velocity, but the requirement of Doppler echocardiography precludes this from being widely used at this time.

There are a few other modalities studied recently which show some promise. One small study investigated the use of stroke volume variation as measured by continuous noninvasive cardiac output monitoring (NICOM) to predict fluid responsiveness in children after VSD repair [30]. NICOM is a bioreactance-based modality that involves electrode placement on the thorax and then analyzes relative phase shifts of the oscillating currents that occur when an induced current travels through the thorax. They found that measurements of stroke volume variation greater than 10% using NICOM were predictive of fluid responsiveness. This is the first such study in children and will require further validation but may become a future tool for directing fluid management.

For the time being, fluid management will most often be dictated by clinical status and serial laboratory studies (Table 11.5). During surgery for NEC, maintenance fluids need to be continued to replace ongoing visceral fluid loss, both evaporative and from exudation of protein-rich extracellular fluid [14]. One starting point is to use 10 mL/kg/h of crystalloid solution in combination with 10–20 mL/kg/h of 5% albumin or fresh frozen plasma. The use of colloidal fluids is rational in this context, as a large amount of protein is lost through exudative loss from the bowel. These patients often also present with thrombocytopenia and prolonged prothrombin and partial thromboplastin times, which may progress to disseminated intravascular coagulopathy if not treated [9]. The anesthesiologist must closely track blood

Table 11.5 Suggested starting regimen for fluid maintenance and replacement during surgery for NEC

Intraoperative fluid	Suggested starting rate of infusion
Crystalloid solution (0.9% sodium chloride, lactated Ringer's solution, Plasma-Lyte)	10 mL/kg/h
Colloid solution (5% albumin, fresh frozen plasma)	10–20 mL/kg/h
Packed red blood cells	As necessary to replace blood loss
Fresh frozen plasma and platelets	As necessary to treat coagulopathy

loss and replace losses with PRBCs, FFP, and platelets as necessary to treat anemia and coagulopathy. If volume replacement does not improve perfusion, inotropic support may need to be started. As we see in this case, very large volumes were necessary to resuscitate this patient, totaling 166 mL/kg of crystalloid, 83 mL/kg of 5% albumin, 50 mL/kg of PRBCs, and similarly large volumes of FFP and platelets.

L-5: Pediatric Cardiopulmonary Resuscitation

Unfortunately, despite apparently aggressive volume resuscitation during the surgery, this patient had a cardiac arrest occur shortly after abdominal closure. The most likely explanation for this event was the increased intra-abdominal pressure after fascial closure, which resulted in decreased venous return and thus decreased cardiac output. This is supported by the patient's rapid improvement after the abdomen was reopened. While this is the most likely reason for the patient's acute decompensation, other possibilities that should be considered include venous air embolism, dysrhythmias secondary to electrolyte abnormalities, inadequate ventilation or oxygenation, and medication overdose or error.

Once cardiac arrest is recognized, the protocol for pediatric cardiopulmonary resuscitation is described in the Pediatric Advanced Life Support guideline [31] (Fig. 11.3). The basic principles are similar to those in adult resuscitation, in that the focus is on supporting ventilation and circulation. The initial response once cardiac arrest is recognized should include calling for help and immediately starting chest compressions. The patient in the operating room should already be on standard monitors, but if not already present, monitors for ventilation and circulation need to be placed. Adequate ventilation should be established, either with tracheal intubation or an airway adjunct (laryngeal mask airway) if intubation is not possible [32]. This is one case where administering 100% oxygen clearly outweighs the risk of oxygen toxicity [9] in order to maximize oxygen delivery to vital organs. Chest compressions should be delivered on the lower third of the infant's sternum, with a depth of approximately one third of the anterior-posterior diameter of the chest, at a rate of approximately 100 compressions per minute [33]. Either the two-hand encircling or two-finger technique can be used, but pressure needs to be released completely between compressions to allow the chest to fully recoil. End-tidal CO_2 can be a useful monitor of chest compression quality, with measurements greater than 15 mmHg during CPR being a predictor of return of spontaneous circulation [34].

The presence of a shockable rhythm (either ventricular fibrillation or ventricular tachycardia) calls for defibrillation. The initial defibrillating dose is 2 J/kg, to be doubled if the first shock is unsuccessful. CPR should be continued between shocks and during medication administration. If the initial rhythm is found to be an unshockable rhythm, such as asystole or pulseless electrical activity (as in this case), CPR should be continued while drug therapy is started and possible treatable causes

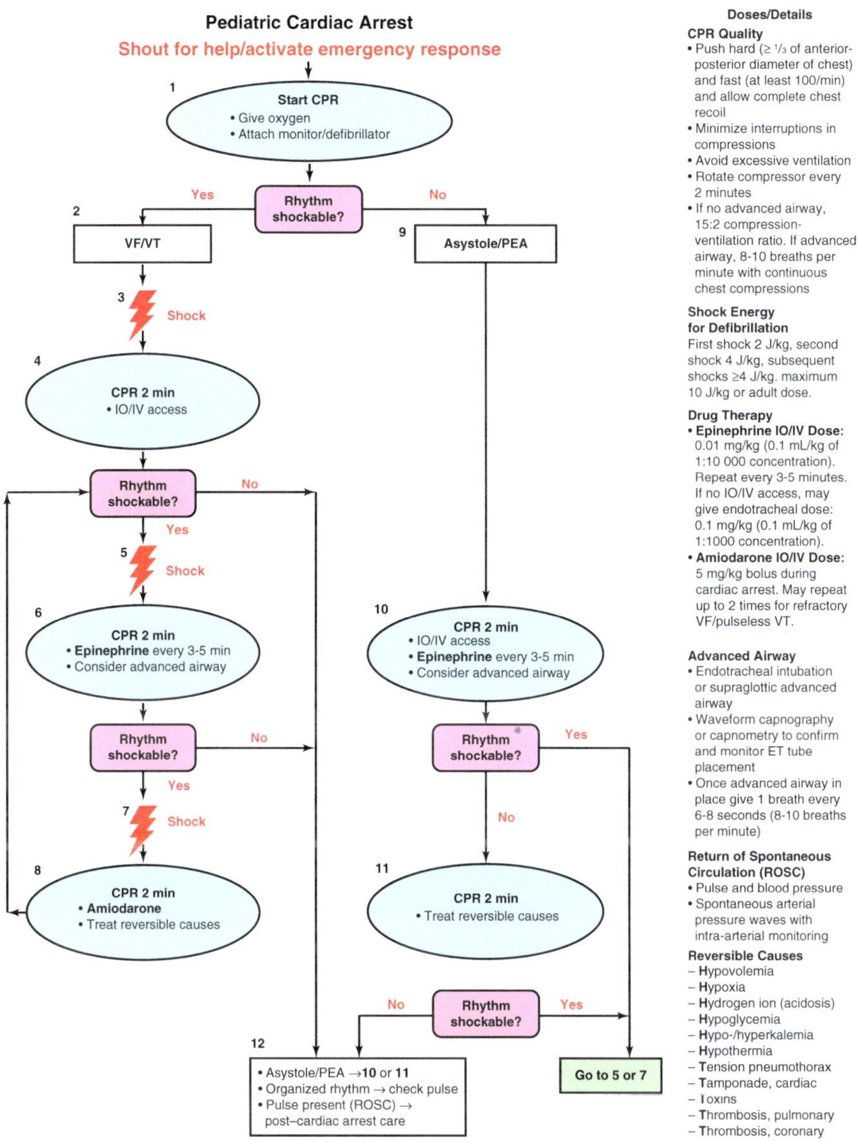

Fig. 11.3 The American Heart Association algorithm for management of pediatric cardiac arrest. (Reprinted from Kleinman et al. [31]. With permission from Wolters Kluwer Health, Inc.)

are investigated. Drug therapy should of course be individualized for the clinical situation at hand, as anesthesiologists often have a much clearer idea of the events leading up to the arrest as compared to sudden arrests that occur outside of the OR. However, it is standard to begin with intravenous epinephrine at a dose of 10 mcg/kg. This patient received a total dose of 41 mcg/kg, comprised of several divided doses. Although this dose is higher than what standardized protocols would call for, the anesthesiologist in the case adjusted the dose to treat a specific clinical situation (e.g., loss of venous preload causing decreased cardiac output and compromised myocardial perfusion). Atropine is not used in the PALS protocol, but can be given for treatment of bradycardia associated with hypotension at a dose of 0.02 mg/kg [9]. In this case, given the initial bradycardia and a possible vagal component from peritoneal stretch, the anesthesiologist gave a total of 0.05 mg/kg of atropine over divided doses.

In the case of sudden arrest with pulseless electrical activity, there is often a reversible cause, and the most important treatment is to find and correct that cause. The commonly used mnemonic for differential diagnosis is the seven H's (hypovolemia, hypoxia, hydrogen ion [acidosis], hypoglycemia, hypo-/hyperkalemia, hypothermia, and hypothermia) and five T's (tension pneumothorax, cardiac tamponade, toxins, pulmonary thrombosis, and coronary thrombosis). Recognition and treatment of these causes can often improve the chances of return of spontaneous circulation. In this case, the treating team was able to recognize the relative hypovolemia that occurred as a result of the abdominal closure. Abandoning the closure and packing the incision ultimately led to patient survival.

In retrospect, it is important to consider if there existed any actions that could have reliably prevented the cardiac arrest from occurring. Given that bradycardia did not occur until several minutes after the initiation of closure, it is reasonable to presume that there may have been some concomitant hypotension. Depending on the cycle time of the noninvasive blood pressure cuff, this may not have been noticed as expeditiously as possible. A continuous invasive monitor such as an arterial line would have allowed for quicker recognition of hypotension, and that information may have allowed the surgical team to respond faster. Similarly, CVP monitoring would have provided more rapid indication that venous return was compromised by the abdominal closure. In the setting of other abdominal surgeries, increases in CVP greater than 4 mmHg above baseline were associated with reduction in venous return and decreased cardiac output [19].

References

1. Dominguez KM, Moss RL. Necrotizing enterocolitis. Clin Perinatol. 2012;39:387–401.
2. Blakely ML, Lally KP, McDonald S, et al. Postoperative outcomes of extremely low birth-weight infants with necrotizing enterocolitis or isolated intestinal perforation: a prospective cohort study by the NICHD Neonatal Research Network. Ann Surg. 2005;241(6):984–9.
3. Hall NJ, Eaton S, Pierro A. Necrotizing enterocolitis: prevention, treatment, and outcome. J Pediatr Surg. 2013;48:2359–67.
4. Meinzen-Derr J, Poindexter B, Wrage L, et al. Role of human milk in extremely low birth weight infants' risk of necrotizing enterocolitis or death. J Perinatol. 2009;29:57–62.
5. Guillet R, Stoll BJ, Cotten CM, et al. Association of H2-blocker therapy and higher incidence of necrotizing enterocolitis in very low birth weight infants. Pediatrics. 2006;117(2):e137–42.
6. Blakely ML, Gupta H, Lally KP. Surgical management of necrotizing enterocolitis and isolated intestinal perforation in premature neonates. Semin Perinatol. 2008;32(2):122–6.

7. Rees CM, Eaton S, Kiely EM, et al. Peritoneal drainage or laparotomy for neonatal bowel perforation? A randomized controlled trial. Ann Surg. 2008;248(1):44–51.
8. Stringer MD, Brereton RJ, Drake DP, et al. Recurrent necrotizing enterocolitis. J Pediatr Surg. 1993;28(8):979–81.
9. Motoyama EK, Davis PJ, editors. Smith's anesthesia for infants and children. Philadelphia: Mosby Elsevier; 2006. Print
10. Bain J, Benjamin DK Jr, Hornik CP, et al. Risk of necrotizing enterocolitis in very-low-birth-weight infants with isolated atrial and ventricular septal defects. J Perinatol. 2014;34(4):319–21.
11. Archer N. Patent ductus arteriosus in the newborn. Arch Dis Child. 1993;69(5):529–32.
12. Dollberg S, Lusky A, Reichman B. Patent ductus arteriosus, indomethacin and necrotizing enterocolitis in very low birth weight infants: a population-based study. J Pediatr Gastroenterol Nutr. 2005;40(2):184–8.
13. Yee WH, Scotland J. Does primary surgical closure of the patent ductus arteriosus in infants <1500 g or <32 weeks' gestation reduce the incidence of necrotizing enterocolitis? Paediatr Child Health. 2012;17(3):125–8.
14. Kinouchi K. Anaesthetic considerations for the management of very low and extremely low birth weight infants. Best Pract Res Clin Anaesthesiol. 2004;18(2):273–90.
15. ARDSNet. Ventilation with lower tidal volumes as compared to traditional tidal volumes for acute lung injury and acute respiratory distress syndrome. N Engl J Med. 2000;342(18):1301–8.
16. Baird PA, MacDonald EC. An epidemiologic study of congenital malformations of the anterior abdominal wall in more than half a million consecutive live births. Am J Hum Genet. 1981;33:470–8.
17. Hwang PJ, Kousseff BG. Omphalocele and gastroschisis: an 18-year review study. Genet Med. 2004;6(4):232–6.
18. Piotrowski A, Kawczynski P. Cannulation of the axillary artery in critically ill newborn infants. Eur J Pediatr. 1995;154(1):57–9.
19. Yaster M, Buck JR, Dudgeon DL, et al. Hemodynamic effects of primary closure of omphalocele/gastroschisis in human newborns. Anesthesiology. 1988;69:84.
20. Blackburn S. Adaptions in major body systems in the pregnant woman, fetus, and neonate. In: Maternal, fetal, & neonatal physiology. St. Louis: Elsevier; 2014. p. 286.
21. Bachiller PR, McDonough JM, Feldman JM. Do anesthesia ventilators deliver small tidal volumes accurately during volume-controlled ventilation? Anesth Analg. 2008;106(5):1392–400.
22. Sola A, Rogido MR, Deulofeut R. Oxygen as a neonatal health hazard: call for détente in clinical practice. Acta Paediatr. 2007;96(6):801–12.
23. Sola A, Golombek SG, Bueno MT, et al. Safe oxygen saturation targeting and monitoring in preterm infants: can we avoid hypoxia and hyperoxia? Acta Paediatr. 2014;103:1009–18.
24. Ohlson KBE, Mohell N, Cannon B, et al. Thermogenesis in brown adipocytes is inhibited by volatile anesthetic agents. A factor contributing to hypothermia in infants? Anesthesiology. 1994;81:176–83.
25. Roe CF. Effect of bowel exposure on body temperature during surgical operations. Am J Surg. 1971;133:13.
26. Boyd JH, Forbes J, Nakada TA, et al. Fluid resuscitation in septic shock: a positive fluid balance and elevated central venous pressure are associated with increased mortality. Crit Care Med. 2011;39:259–65.
27. Egan JR, Festa M, Cole AD, Nunn GR, et al. Clinical assessment of cardiac performance in infants and children following cardiac surgery. Intensive Care Med. 2005;31:568–73.
28. Gan H, Cannesson M, Chandler JR, Ansermino JM. Predicting fluid responsiveness in children: a systematic review. Anesth Analg. 2013;117(6):1380–92.
29. Renner J, Broch O, Duetschke P, et al. Prediction of fluid responsiveness in infants and neonates undergoing congenital heart surgery. Br J Anaesth. 2012;108(1):108–15.
30. Lee JY, Kim JY, Choi CH, et al. The ability of stroke volume variation measured by a noninvasive cardiac output monitor to predict fluid responsiveness in mechanically ventilated children. Pediatr Cardiol. 2014;35:289–94.

31. Kleinman ME, Chameides L, Schexnayder SM. 2010 American Heart Association guidelines for cardiopulmonary resuscitation and emergency cardiovascular care. Circulation. 2010;122:S876–908.
32. Rumball CJ, MacDonald D. The PTL, combitube, laryngeal mask, and oral airway: a randomized prehospital comparative study of ventilatory device effectiveness and cost-effectiveness in 470 cases of cardiorespiratory arrest. Prehosp Emerg Care. 1997;1:1.
33. Kattwinkel J, Perlman JM, Aziz K, et al. Neonatal resuscitation 2010 American Heart Association guidelines for cardiopulmonary resuscitation and emergency cardiovascular care. Pediatrics. 2010;126(5):e1400–13.
34. Bhende MS, Thompson AE. Evaluation of an end-tidal CO_2 detector during pediatric cardiopulmonary resuscitation. Pediatrics. 1995;95:395.
35. Langer JC. Abdominal wall defects. World J Surg. 2003;27(1):117–24.

Part III
Cases Resulting in Perioperative Serious Complications

Chapter 12
Postoperative Respiratory Distress in the PACU: A Unique Differential Diagnosis

Brittany Grovey and Jonathan L. Benumof

Case Summary

This is a case of a patient with likely obstructive sleep apnea (OSA), perioperative anxiety, and questionable residual neuromuscular blockade, who experienced vocal cord dysfunction in the postanesthetic care unit (PACU) leading to respiratory distress. In order to understand the patient's postoperative respiratory distress, it is necessary to have a good understanding of the preoperative and intraoperative risk factors present in this patient.

Case Specifics

The patient is a 54-year-old male who is 5′11″ and 129 kg with a BMI of 39.7 kg/m^2 scheduled for laparoscopic umbilical hernia repair under general anesthesia.

His cardiopulmonary history was significant for well-controlled hypertension with >4 metabolic equivalents (METS) exercise tolerance without cardiac symptoms. Although the patient had not been formally diagnosed with OSA, he had an elevated STOP-Bang questionnaire score of 7 and was therefore considered at high risk for having OSA (see **Lesson 1, [L-1]**). He was HIV positive with a history of Kaposi sarcoma of the foot treated with chemotherapy and radiation. He also had anxiety with attacks usually manifesting as palpitations, but had occasionally experienced attacks with palpitations and stridorous breathing (see **[L-2]**). He had taken

B. Grovey (✉)
Department of Anesthesiology, University of California, San Diego, CA, USA

J. L. Benumof
Department of Anesthesiology, University of California, UCSD Medical Center, UCSD School of Medicine, San Diego, CA, USA

J. L. Benumof, G. R. Manecke (eds.), *Clinical Anesthesiology II*,
https://doi.org/10.1007/978-3-030-12365-9_12

all prescribed medications on the morning of surgery, including metoprolol, atazanavir, ritonavir and lorazepam.

On physical exam, the patient was an anxious, obese male lying on a gurney with a room air oxygen saturation of 97%. He had a class III Mallampati airway score, but an otherwise favorable airway exam. The cardiac and pulmonary exams were unremarkable.

His preoperative laboratory results, vital signs, and electrocardiogram were within normal limits.

The patient was pre-medicated with midazolam 2 mg IV and taken to the operating room. Upon arrival to the operating room, the patient self-transferred to the operating table, and standard ASA monitors were placed. Vital signs were noted to be within the patient's baseline values. A two-lead peripheral nerve stimulator was placed to stimulate the left orbicularis oculi muscle (see **[L-3]**), and the patient was positioned on an intubating ramp in order to optimally align the oral, pharyngeal, and laryngeal axes. He was preoxygenated with 100% FiO_2 for >5 min prior to induction, and a time-out verifying the patient, procedure, and intraoperative plan was performed.

The patient underwent an uneventful intravenous induction with fentanyl, hydromorphone, lidocaine, and propofol via a peripheral IV. The patient was hand ventilated via mask with an oral airway in place. A train-of-four (TOF) stimulus was administered via the peripheral nerve stimulator and noted to produce moderate contractions of the orbicularis oculi muscle, which served as a control prior to administration of rocuronium 80 mg IV. Once complete loss of single twitches was achieved (see **[L-4]**), direct laryngoscopy was performed, yielding a Grade 2 view with atraumatic placement of an 8.0 mm internal diameter, cuffed endotracheal tube. Partial pressure end tidal CO_2 ($PetCO_2$) and bilateral breath sounds were verified prior to placing the patient on the ventilator. Anesthesia was maintained with sevoflurane via the anesthesia machine ventilator with volume control settings titrated to maintain a $PetCO_2$ of 33–40 mmHg.

The case proceeded uneventfully. Upon successful completion of the case, the patient's neuromuscular blockade was reversed with a dose of neostigmine (5 mg) plus glycopyrrolate (0.8 mg) after two twitches of the orbicularis oculi muscle were verified with the peripheral nerve stimulator (see **[L-4]**).

Prior to emergence, four twitches plus a sustained 5-s tetanic response at 100 Hz were confirmed (see **[L-4]**). The oropharynx was suctioned. Prior to extubation, the patient was spontaneously ventilating with tidal volumes of 550–600 cc with a $PetCO_2$ of 47 mmHg. During emergence, the patient demonstrated emergence agitation, requiring multiple nurses to keep him from reaching up and self-extubating. Once the patient was following commands appropriately, he was extubated with an oral airway in situ and placed on 6 L/min of oxygen delivered via a simple facemask.

Upon transport to the PACU, the patient became extremely anxious and developed stridorous breath sounds. The oral airway was removed per the patient's request upon arrival to PACU. Standard ASA monitors were placed with SpO_2 > 95% on 6 L O_2 via simple facemask. The patient was very anxious with visibly increased work of breathing. His main mode of communication was with hand gestures – indicating that he felt his throat was closing. Pulmonary exam during this time revealed poor air movement with inspiratory stridor. Given the patient's increased work of breathing and continued stridor, he was placed on 100% FiO_2 via a Mapleson circuit. The patient reported subjective improvement with the gentle, hand-delivered pressure support (PS) and positive end expiratory pressure (PEEP) administered via the Mapleson circuit. Neuromuscular strength testing demonstrated 5/5 strength in the upper extremities, although he demonstrated abnormal movements similar to a "floppy fish" (see **[L-4]**) in the lower extremities. The patient denied subjective feelings of weakness and, although visibly anxious, continued to maintain an appropriate level of consciousness – nodding appropriately in response to questions. Neostigmine 1.5 mg with glycopyrrolate 0.3 mg IV was given for concern of residual neuromuscular paralysis without improvement in respiratory mechanics. Noninvasive positive ventilation (NIPPV) via a ventilator was initiated and titrated to bi-level positive airway pressure (BiPAP) settings of PS/PEEP of 10/5 cmH_2O with resultant tidal volumes of 600–700 cc and FiO_2 of 30%. Midazolam 1 mg IV was given with resolution of stridor and improvement of respiratory mechanics (see **[L-2]** and Table 12.1).

Table 12.1 Differential diagnosis of patient's respiratory distress with supporting and conflicting evidence

Differential diagnoses	Evidence	Proposed mechanism
Paradoxical vocal cord dysfunction (PVCD)	History of anxiety and anxiety-induced stridor[a] Resolution with low-dose sedative/anxiolytic and NIPPV/BiPAP[a] Note: No fiber-optic laryngoscopy performed to verify inspiratory vocal cord adduction	Postoperative anxiety producing paradoxical vocal cord dysfunction
Obstructive sleep apnea (OSA)	High STOP-bang score[a] Improvement with NIPPV/BiPAP[a] Alert mental status[b] Would usually be worsened by administration of sedatives/anxiolytics[b]	(1) Soft tissue obstruction leading to upper airway obstruction and respiratory distress (2) Soft tissue obstruction leading to upper airway obstruction and anxiety, fueling PVCD
Residual neuromuscular blockade	"Floppy fish" movements in PACU[a] Underdosing of neostigmine[a] 5-s sustained tetany demonstrated prior to extubation[b] No improvement with a repeat dose of reversal agent[b]	(1) Residual paralysis producing soft tissue obstruction leading to upper airway obstruction and respiratory distress (2) Residual paralysis producing soft tissue obstruction leading to upper airway obstruction and anxiety, fueling PVCD

NIPPV noninvasive positive pressure ventilation, *BiPAP* bi-level positive airway pressure, *PACU* postanesthetic care unit
[a]Evidence in favor of diagnosis
[b]Evidence against diagnosis

Table 12.2 Timeline of perioperative events

Time	Events
08:15	Arrival to operating room
08:16	Induction (IV)
08:16	Fentanyl 100 mg
08:29	Hydromorphone 1 mg
08:29	Lidocaine 100 mg
08:30	Propofol 300 mg (2.3 mg/kg)
	Rocuronium 80 mg (0.6 mg/kg)
08:25	Intraoperative management
08:50	Cefazolin 2000 mg
09:05	Inhaled sevoflurane
09:10	Two twitches demonstrated
09:18	Ondansetron 4 mg
09:21	Neostigmine 5 mg, glycopyrrolate 0.8 mg
	Four twitches, +5-s sustained tetany (50 Hz)
	Extubation
09:23	Arrival in PACU
09:26	Neostigmine 1.5 mg
09:26	Glycopyrrolate 0.3 mg
09:33	Midazolam 1 mg

Vital signs remained within the patient's baseline ranges throughout this event. After 30 min of BiPAP, the patient's abnormal floppy fish movements had resolved, his emotional status had normalized, and his respiratory function had returned to normal. The NIPPV was discontinued, and the patient was placed on 2 L/min O_2 delivered via nasal cannula. The patient had no further events in the PACU and was discharged home 6 h later without complications (see **[L-5]**) after meeting PACU discharge criteria. Please see Table 12.2 for a timeline of preoperative, intraoperative, and postoperative events.

Lesson 1: What Tools Are Available for Obstructive Sleep Apnea (OSA) Risk Stratification?

Obstructive sleep apnea is the most common type of sleep-disordered breathing and is associated with a variety of conditions that increase perioperative morbidity. The incidence of OSA is estimated to be between 9% and 25% in the general American population [1]. Many studies demonstrate an independent association between OSA and increased incidence of adverse perioperative events including, but not limited to, postoperative hypoxemia, re-intubation, pneumonia, arrhythmias, ischemia, cardiac arrest, hypotension, hypertension, and unintended intensive care unit (ICU) admission [2, 3]. Given these risks, it is important to identify patients with OSA for appropriate perioperative management and postoperative discharge (see **[L-5]**).

The gold standard for measuring the severity of OSA is the polysomnography-determined Apnea-Hypopnea Index (AHI). Apneas are typically defined as an 80–100% cessation of airflow lasting ≥10 s with associated arousal and/or 3% decrease in arterial oxygen saturation. Hypopneas are typically defined as a 25–79% reduction of flow or volume from baseline breathing for ≥10 s with associated arousal and/or 3% decrease in arterial oxygen saturation. The AHI represents the number of apnea and hypopnea events per hour of sleep. Although polysomnography labs may differ in their measurement definitions, generally speaking, an AHI ≥5 and <15 is considered mild OSA, AHI ≥15 and <30 is considered moderate OSA, while an AHI ≥30 is considered severe OSA.

Many screening questionnaires have been developed in an attempt to best identify patients at risk for sleep-disordered breathing, the most popular of which are the Epworth Sleepiness Scale (ESS) (Fig. 12.1), the STOP and STOP-Bang questionnaires (Fig. 12.2), the Berlin Questionnaire (Fig. 12.3), the American

The Epworth Sleepiness Scale

Use the following scale to choose the most appropriate number for each situation

0: would never doze
1: slight chance of dozing
2: moderate chance of dozing
3: high chance of dozing

Score:
0–10: normal
11–12: borderline
12–24: abnormal

Situations	Chance of dozing
Sitting and reading	
Watching TV	
Sitting, inactive in a public place	
As a passenger in a car for an hour without a break	
Lying down to rest in the afternoon when circumstances permit	
Sitting and talking to someone	
Sitting quietly after a lunch without alcohol	
In a car, while stopped for a few minutes in traffic	
Total	

Fig. 12.1 Epworth Sleepiness Scale questionnaire – used to evaluate daytime sleepiness as a screening for sleep-disordered breathing

STOP-Bang questionnaire

	Yes / No
S (Snoring): Do you snore loudly (louder than talker or loud enough to be heard through closed doors)?	
T (Tired): Do you often feel tired (tired, fatigued or sleepy during the daytime)?	
O (Observed): Has anyone observed you stop breathing during your sleep?	
P (Pressure): Do you have or are you being treated for high blood pressure?	
B (BMI): Is your BMI > 35 kg/m^2?	
A (Age): Age over 50 years old?	
N (Neck Circumference): Neck circumference > 40 cm?	
G (Gender): Gender male?	

High risk of OSA: answering yes to three or more questions
Low risk of OSA: answerign yes to less than three questions

Fig. 12.2 STOP-Bang questionnaire example – used as a screening tool for sleep-disordered breathing

Berlin Questionnaire

Category 1

Do you snore?
- ❑ Yes
- ❑ No
- ❑ I don't know

If you snore...
Your snoring is?
- ❑ Slightly louder than breathing
- ❑ As loud as talking
- ❑ Louder than talking
- ❑ Very loud, can be heard in adjacent rooms

How often do you snore?
- ❑ Nearly every day
- ❑ 3–4 times per week
- ❑ 1–2 times per week
- ❑ 1–2 times per month
- ❑ Never or nearly never

Has your snoring ever bothered other people?
- ❑ Yes
- ❑ No

Has anyone ever noticed that you quit breathing in your sleep?
- ❑ Nearly every day
- ❑ 3–4 times per week
- ❑ 1–2 times per week
- ❑ 1–2 times per month
- ❑ Never or nearly never

Category 2

How often do you feel tired or fatigued after your sleep?
- ❑ Nearly every day
- ❑ 3–4 times per week
- ❑ 1–2 times per week
- ❑ 1–2 times per month
- ❑ Never or nearly never

During your wakefulness do you feel tired, fatigued or not up to par?
- ❑ Nearly every day
- ❑ 3–4 times per week
- ❑ 1–2 times per week
- ❑ 1–2 times per month
- ❑ Never or nearly never

Have you ever nodded off or fallen asleep while driving a vehicle?
- ❑ Yes
- ❑ No

If yes, how often does it occur?
- ❑ Nearly every day
- ❑ 3–4 times per week
- ❑ 1–2 times per week
- ❑ 1–2 times per month
- ❑ Never or nearly never

Category 3

Do you have high blood pressure
- ❑ Yes
- ❑ No
- ❑ I don't know

BMI: ______

Scoring:
Scoring Questions: Any answer in the highlighted text is considered a positive answer

Category 1 is positive with ≥ 2 positive responses
Category 2 is positive with ≥ 2 positive responses

Category 3 is positive with a positive response and a BMI ≥ 30 kg/m^2

Final Result: a positive result in ≥ 2 categories indicates a high likelihood of sleep disordered breathing

Fig. 12.3 Berlin Questionnaire example – used as a screening tool for sleep-disordered breathing

Society of Anesthesiologists (ASA) checklist (Fig. 12.4), and the Sleep Disorders Questionnaire (SDQ), which is a complex, 175-item scale adapted from the Sleep Questionnaire and the Assessment of Wakefulness tool. Head-to-head comparisons of the various questionnaires demonstrated the superiority of the Berlin Questionnaire and the SDQ in identifying patients who are at higher risk for moderate-severe and severe OSA [4]. The ASA checklist and STOP-Bang questionnaire have higher sensitivities in these analyses than the ESS and STOP questionnaire [4, 5]. The STOP-Bang questionnaire is more user-friendly than the other checklists and maintains comparable or improved sensitivity, so it is more commonly used as an OSA screening tool in practice.

In this case, we utilized the STOP-Bang questionnaire as the preoperative screening modality for OSA. The results for the patient presented above are shown (Fig. 12.5). Based on the results of his STOP-Bang score of 7, he is at high risk for undiagnosed moderate-severe and severe OSA with estimated odds ratios (ORs) of 6.9 and 14.9 compared to a STOB-Bang score of 0–2 [6]. Although this patient's respiratory distress was multifactorial, soft tissue upper airway obstruction was likely a contributing factor (see Table 12.1). After application of BiPAP, the patient reported a subjective improvement in respiratory mechanics, and this was the first intervention that began to alleviate the patient's respiratory distress.

a ASA checklist for OSA screening

Table 1. Identification and assessment of OSA:

A. Clinical signs and symptoms suggesting the possibility of OSA
   1. Predisposing physical characteristics
      a. BMI 35 kg/m^2 (95th percentile for age and gender)
      b. Neck circumference 17 inches (men) or 16 inches (women)
      c. Craniofacial abnormalities affecting the airway
      d. Anatomical nasal obstruction
      e. Tonsils nearly touching or touching in the midline
   2. History of apparent airway obstruction during sleep (two or more of the following are present, if patient lives alone or sleep is not observed by another person, then only one of the following needs to be present)
      a. Snoring (loud enough to be heard through closed door)
      b. Frequent snoring
      c. Observed pauses in breathing during sleep
      d. Awakens from sleep with choking sensation
      e. Frequent arousals from sleep
      f. [Intermittent vocalization during sleep]
      g. [Parental report of restless sleep, difficulty breathing, or struggling respiratory efforts during sleep]
   3. Somnolence (one or more of the following is present)
      a. Frequent somnolence or fatigue despite adequate "sleep"
      b. Falls asleep easily in a non-stimulating environment
      c. [Parent or teacher comments that child appears sleepy during the day, is easily distracted, is overly aggressive, or has difficulty concentrating]
      d. [Child often difficult to arouse at usual awakening time]

Scoring:

If a patient has signs or symptoms in two or more of the adjacent categories, there is a significant probability that he or she has OSA. The severity of OSA may be determined by sleep study (see below). If a sleep study is not available, such patients should be treated as though they have moderate sleep apnea unless one or more of the signs or symptoms above is severely abnormal (e.g. markedly increased BMI or neck circumference, respiratory pauses that are frightening to the observer, patient regularly falls asleep within minutes after being left unstimulated) in which case they should be treated as though they have severe sleep apnea.

B. If a sleep study has been done, the results should be used to determine the perioperative anesthetic management of a patient. However, because sleep laboratories differ in their criteria for detecting episodes of apnea and hypopnea, the ASA Task Force believes that the sleep laboratory's measurement (none, mild, moderate or severe) should take precedence over the actual AHI. If the overall severity is not indicated, it may be determined by utilizing the table below:

* Items in brackets refer to pediatric patients

Severity of OSA	Adult AHI	Pediatric AHI
None	0–5	0
Mild OSA	6–20	1–5
Moderate OSA	21–40	6–10
Severe OSA	> 40	> 10

Fig. 12.4 (**a**): ASA checklist for OSA screening example. (**b**) ASA checklist for OSA screening example continued

b ASA checklist for OSA screening cont.

Table 2. OSA scoring system

A. Severity of OSA based on sleep study (or clinical indicators if sleep study not available).

Point score ____ (0–3)*T

Severity of OSA (Table 1)	
None	0
Mild	1
Moderate	2
Severe	3

B. Invasiveness of surgery and anesthesia.

Point score ____ (0–3)

Type of surgery and anesthesia	
Superficial surgery under local or peripheral nerve block anesthesia without sedation	0
Superficial surgery with moderate sedation or general anesthesia	1
Peripheral surgery with spinal or epidural anesthesia (with no more than moderate sedation)	2
Peripheral surgery with general anesthesia	2
Airway surgery with moderate sedation	2
Major surgery, general anesthesia	3
Airway surgery, general anesthesia	3

C. Requirement for postoperative opioids.

Point score ____ (0–3)

Opioid requirement	
None	0
Low-dose oral opioids	1
High-dose oral opioids, parenteral or neuraxial opioids	2

Scoring:

D. Estimation of perioperative risk.

Overall score = the score for A plus the greater of the score for either B or C.

Point score ____ (0–6) Ŧ

A scoring system similar to this table may be used to estimate whether a patient is at increased risk of complications from OSA. This example, which has not been clinically validated, is meant only as a guide, and clinical judgment should be used to assess the risk of an individual patient.

* One point may be subtracted in a patient has been on continuous positive airway pressure (CPAP) or noninvasive positive-pressure ventilation (NIPPV) before surgery and will be using his or her appliance consistently during the postoperative period.

T One point should be added if a patient with mild or moderate OSA also has a resting arterial carbon dioxide tension ($PaCO_2$) greater than 50mmHg.

Ŧ Patients with score of 4 may be at increased perioperative risk from OSA: patients with a score of 5 or 6 may be at significantly increased perioperative risk from OSA.

Fig. 12.4 (continued)

STOP-Bang questionnaire

	Yes / No
S (Snoring): Do you snore loudly (louder than talker or loud enough to be heard through closed doors)?	Yes
T (Tired): Do you often feel tired (tired, fatigued or sleepy during the daytime)?	Yes
O (Observed): Has anyone observed you stop breathing during your sleep?	Yes
P (Pressure): Do you have or are you being treated for high blood pressure?	Yes
B (BMI): Is your BMI > 35 kg/m^2?	Yes
A (Age): Age over 50 years old?	Yes
N (Neck Circumference): Neck circumference > 40 cm?	No
G (Gender): Gender male?	Yes

High risk of OSA: answering yes to three or more questions
Low risk of OSA: answering yes to less than three questions

Score: 7

Fig. 12.5 Patient's results in STOP-Bang questionnaire

Lesson 2: What Is Paradoxical Vocal Cord Dysfunction (PVCD)?

Paradoxical vocal cord dysfunction is known by a multitude of names including paradoxical vocal cord motion, laryngeal dyskinesia, inspiratory adduction, periodic occurrence of laryngeal obstruction, Munchausen's stridor, episodic paroxysmal laryngospasm, psychogenic stridor, functional stridor, hysterical croup, emotional laryngeal wheezing, factitious asthma, pseudo-asthma, and irritable larynx syndrome, just to name a few. It is a clinical phenomenon of abnormal movement of the true vocal cords leading to partial or complete airway obstruction [7]. The abnormal vocal cord movement usually manifests as adduction during inspiration, presenting as inspiratory stridor, but may occur during expiration, producing expiratory or biphasic stridorous breathing. Paradoxical vocal cord dysfunction differs from laryngospasm in that in PVCD, the vocal cord adduction has respiratory variation, as opposed to the sustained adduction throughout all phases of the respiratory cycle seen in laryngospasm. Although a patient with paradoxical vocal cord dysfunction may appear anxious and in severe respiratory distress, hypoxemia is rarely seen in PVCD, and arterial blood gases are either normal or demonstrate a mild respiratory alkalosis.

Although the mechanism of PVCD is incompletely understood, the leading hypothesis is that increased laryngeal hypersensitivity, induced by external irritants, or abnormal autonomic regulation may promote abnormal true vocal cord closure and glottis narrowing, leading to the dysfunctional movement seen in PVCD [8]. In addition to obstruction at the level of the vocal cords, patients experiencing PVCD are at an increased risk of soft tissue airway obstruction. During inspiration, extrathoracic intraluminal pressure decreases relative to atmospheric pressure, resulting in some degree of narrowing of the upper airway and pharyngeal structures. In patients without PVCD, this narrowing is normally offset with the coordinated contraction of the posterior cricoarytenoid muscles, which serves to enlarge the glottis opening [9]. The dynamic airway constriction seen in PVCD may be worse in patients with OSA or residual neuromuscular blockade due to concomitant soft tissue obstruction, which further narrows the upper airway. Agitation and anxiety cause increased respiratory effort and inspiratory flow, which worsens the obstruction, forming the basis of an agitation – stridor loop (Fig. 12.6)

Paradoxical vocal cord dysfunction is associated with a variety of conditions. Although the vocal cord dysfunction is an organic, involuntary disorder, it has a high association with psychological disorders such as acute anxiety, generalized anxiety disorder, depression, personality disorders, and post-traumatic stress disorder [10]. The irritant-induced laryngeal hypersensitivity theory is supported in the association of PVCD with laryngopharyngeal reflux and inhalational irritant exposure (smoke, ammonia, fumes, dust, etc.) [11]. Also supporting a hypersensitivity etiology is its association with asthma, and in some cases, the ability of PVCD to be induced with exercise [12]. There are also case reports of postoperative PVCD associated with thyroid surgery, suggesting that irritation of the recurrent laryngeal

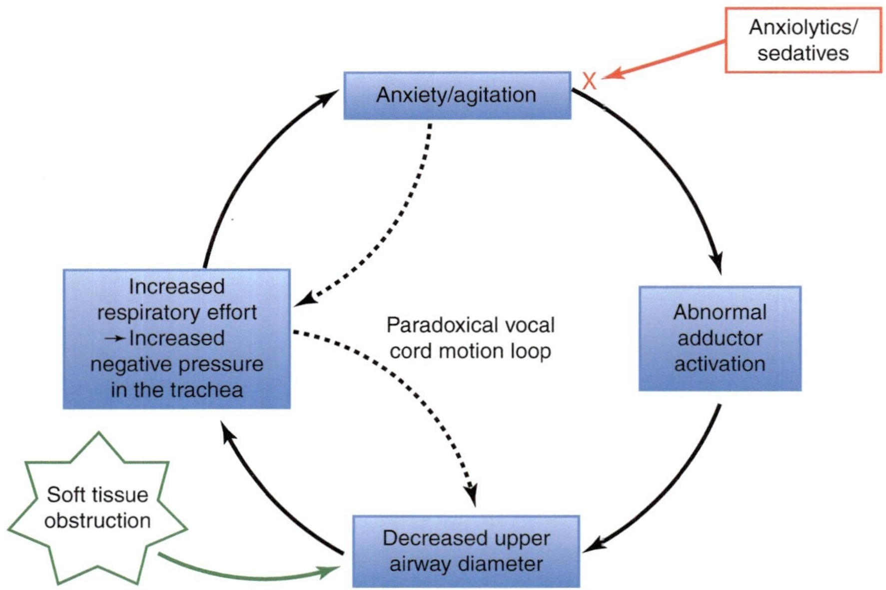

Fig. 12.6 Factors contributing to the self-propagating anxiety-induced paradoxical vocal cord motion loop. (1) Anxiety and agitation trigger abnormal adductor activation, most commonly manifesting as inspiratory vocal cord adduction. Anxiolytic and sedative interventions can reduce anxiety, returning adductor activation to normal function, thus relieving the vocal cord obstruction. (2) Abnormal adductor activation during inspiration decreases upper airway diameter causing airway obstruction, resulting in inspiratory stridor and respiratory distress. (3) Narrowed upper airway diameter and respiratory distress result in increased respiratory effort and elevated negative pressure in the trachea which can cause further airway narrowing and contribute to anxiety. Soft tissue obstruction, as seen in OSA or residual neuromuscular blockade feed into the loop by decreasing the upper airway diameter and producing increased respiratory effort and potentially worsening anxiety. (4) The increased work of breathing can worsen anxiety, which, in turn, results in stronger respiratory effort and worsens upper airway narrowing as described above

nerve may play a role in some cases [13]. Although the exact mechanism of PVCD is unknown, it is clear that it is a complex clinical phenomenon resulting from combinations of psychological and organic etiologies that vary depending on the particular situation.

The clinical presentation and patient history may suggest the diagnosis, but a definitive diagnosis is made with direct visualization of inspiratory vocal cord adduction with nasal fiber-optic laryngoscopy. Spirometry is neither sensitive nor specific, but may show a variable extra-thoracic obstruction on inspiration [8].

The treatment of acute and chronic paradoxical vocal cord motion differ, and only acute treatment will be discussed here. As with any case of respiratory distress, the primary treatment of acute PVCD focuses on ensuring adequate oxygenation and ventilation with proper patient positioning and supplementing with oxygen therapy or NIPPV as needed. The application of NIPPV during an episode of paradoxical vocal cord dysfunction has been shown to decrease the glottis narrowing, as less inspiratory effort is required to achieve satisfactory tidal volumes [14]. NIPPV with continuous positive airway pressure (CPAP) or BiPAP may also be beneficial if the patient has an element of glottis narrowing secondary to soft tissue upper airway obstruction, as in patients with OSA. Given the association of PVCD and psychological disorders, it is not surprising that a reduction in anxiety via psychological measures, such as reassurance and breathing techniques, or pharmacologic measures, such as benzodiazepines, is usually beneficial. Indeed, many patients with postoperative PVCD saw dramatic improvement in respiratory status after administration of small doses of benzodiazepines and/or opioids [15–17]. Of note, it is prudent to identify the cause of respiratory distress prior to careful titration of sedating medications to avoid worsening of respiratory status. If the diagnosis is confirmed, and these interventions fail to work, the patient may require more invasive measures to ensure adequate respiratory function, including paralysis and re-intubation.

The differential diagnosis for stridor in the PACU is extensive and includes more common etiologies such as soft tissue obstruction, bronchospasm, laryngospasm, and aspiration, in addition to the immediately life-threatening etiologies such as anaphylaxis and angioedema. Given the presentation of stridor and respiratory distress, PVCD is often misdiagnosed as reactive airway disease.

Although etiologies such as hypocalcemic tetany and paradoxical vocal cord dysfunction are less common causes of postoperative stridor, prompt recognition is important to avoid unnecessary interventions (intubation, tracheostomy) and hospitalizations in these patients.

In this case, strong suspicion of PVCD based on the patient's exam and history of anxiety-induced stridor led to appropriate treatment with NIPPV/BiPAP and carefully titrated doses of midazolam (Table 12.1). The resolution of stridor with low doses of a sedative/anxiolytic supports the diagnosis. Soft tissue airway obstruction from OSA +/− mild residual neuromuscular blockade may have exacerbated the inspiratory obstruction, contributing to further anxiety and obstruction at the level of the vocal cords via the PVCD obstruction loop described in Fig. 12.6.

Lesson 3: What Is the Proper Use of a Peripheral Nerve Stimulator?

Muscle contraction is a complex series of events that first begins with initiation and propagation of a presynaptic action potential. The resting membrane potential of a nerve cell is approximately –70 mV, meaning that the intracellular space is relatively negatively charged when compared to the extracellular space. This negative membrane potential difference serves as the driving force for ion movement during depolarization and action potential initiation. The negative potential difference is established by the sodium (Na^+) and potassium (K^+) ion exchanger, which moves three Na^+ ions into the extracellular space for every two K^+ ions moved into the intracellular space. This unequal ion exchange results in a net negative intracellular space or membrane potential. When this negative potential is reduced (less voltage difference between the intracellular and extracellular spaces), as during a depolarization, voltage-gated Na^+ channels allow for an influx of Na^+ ions down their electrical and chemical concentration gradients. This further reduces the negative potential, allowing the inside of the cell to become positive relative to the outside of the cell, which in turn results in depolarization of the next segment of the membrane. These currents are responsible for the propagation of an action potential down an axon, ultimately resulting in release of acetylcholine (ACh) from the nerve terminal and initiating the postsynaptic events that culminate in muscle contraction. In summary, reduction of the negative potential of a nerve cell to a threshold level can initiate an action potential and result in a muscle contraction.

A reduction in the negative membrane potential of a nerve cell can be accomplished via the intrinsic, centrally mediated mechanism described above or through a peripherally mediated mechanism via the addition of extracellular negative ions with a peripheral nerve stimulator (via the negative electrode/cathode) (Fig. 12.7). The negative pole/cathode of a peripheral nerve stimulator donates electrons to the extracellular space, thus reducing the negative potential (decreasing the charge difference between the intracellular and extracellular space by making the extracellular space more negative) of the cell and initiating an action potential that then propagates distally to the axon terminals in the normal fashion. Alternatively, the positive pole/anode donates protons to the extracellular space, thus increasing the negative potential (making the extracellular space more positive relative to the intracellular space, effectively increasing the charge difference), which results in hyperpolarization of the cell and slightly increases the level of stimulus needed to initiate an action potential (Fig. 12.8). For these reasons, it is important to apply the electrodes along the course of the nerve with the negative pole/cathode placed distal to the positive pole/anode for the most efficient action potential propagation.

Neuromuscular-blocking drugs (NMBDs) effectively inhibit postsynaptic depolarization by either blockage of the postsynaptic nicotinic ACh receptor (nondepolarizing NMBDs) or by causing depolarization of the postsynaptic membrane (the depolarizing NMBD/succinylcholine) and thereby inducing "desensitization" of the postsynaptic membrane. Peripheral nerve stimulators measure the respon-

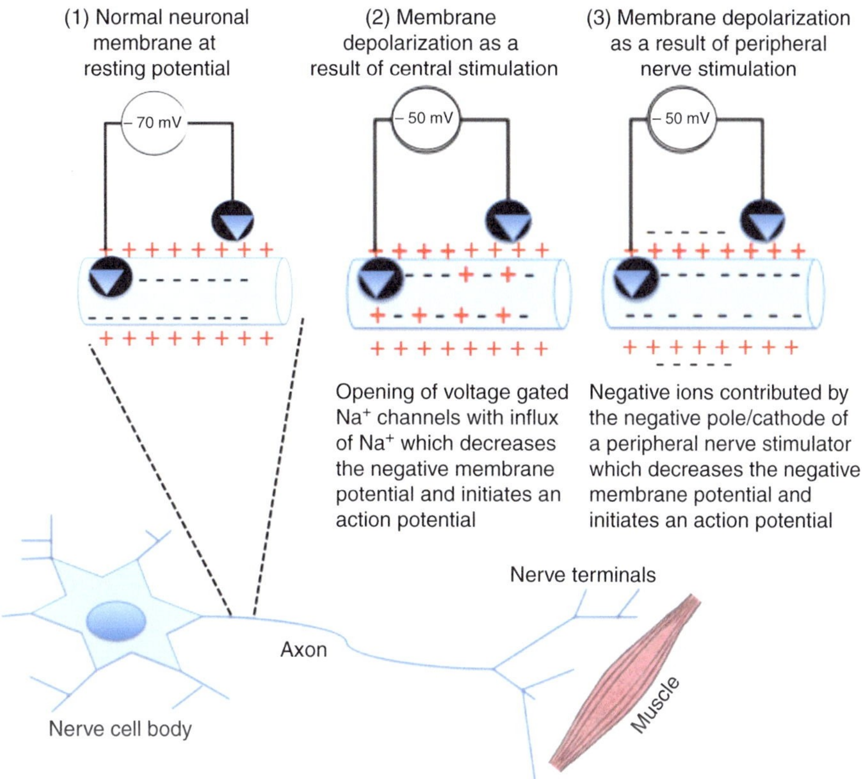

Fig. 12.7 Schematic representation of ion potentials of a neuronal membrane

siveness of a muscle cell to a programmed stimulus and are able to generate multiple levels of stimulation at different frequencies. This results in different patterns of muscle contraction that are used to assess the depth of neuromuscular blockade in a patient (see **[L-4]**).

Peripheral nerve stimulators can be used to stimulate any muscle with a nerve running superficially enough to be affected by its electrical current. Ideally we would monitor those muscles of physiologic importance (i.e., the muscles of the upper airway, muscles of respiration, or abdominal muscles during a laparoscopic surgery), but usually, this isn't feasible. Clinically, there are a few muscles that are widely used for monitoring of neuromuscular blockade: the adductor pollicis muscle located in the mid-forearm (thumb adduction), innervated by the ulnar nerve; the extensor halluces longus muscle located in the leg with extension to the ankle (big toe extension), innervated by the posterior tibial nerve; and the orbicularis oculi (eyelid closure) and corrugator supercilii muscles located in the face (medial eyebrow), both innervated by the facial nerve**.**

Because different muscle groups have different responses to NMBDs, it is important to know which of the muscles above correlates with the paralysis and recovery

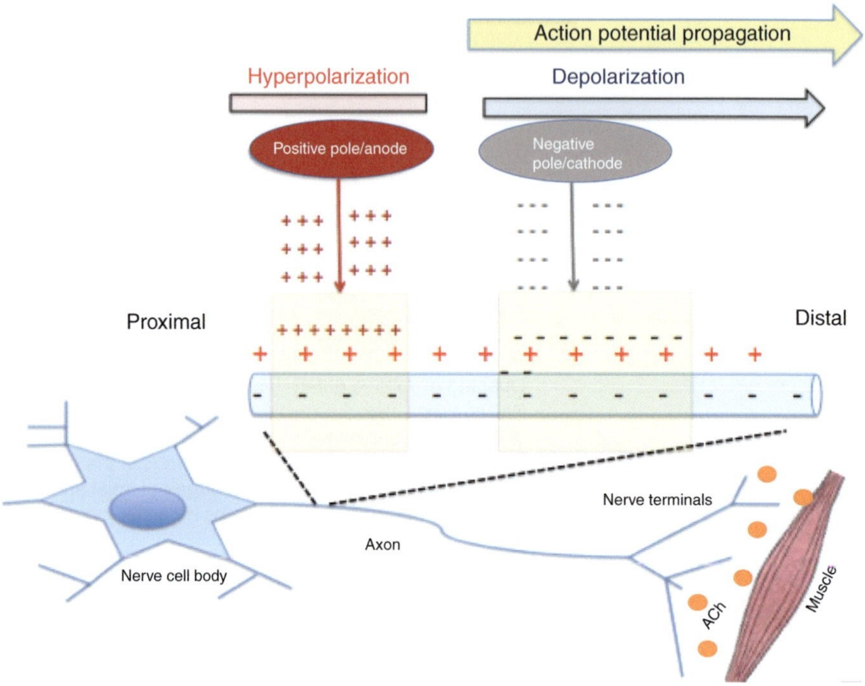

Fig. 12.8 Schematic representation of correct placement of peripheral nerve stimulator leads. The negative pole contributes negative ions which leads to depolarization and action potential propagation which results in ACh release and muscle contraction. The positive pole contributes positive ions and hyperpolarizes the cell membrane. ACh, Acetylcholine in neuromuscular synapse

of the muscles of physiologic interest. The muscles of the larynx and diaphragm correlate well with the corrugator supercilii, making this location ideal for monitoring patient muscle relaxation for intubation. For assessing the recovery of the muscles of the upper airway and diaphragm in preparation for extubation, monitoring the adductor pollicis (AP) gives an added layer of security, because as seen below, it has a long recovery time. Therefore, if AP is fully recovered, there is a high likelihood that the other muscle groups have recovered as well. On the other hand, if during a laparoscopic procedure, measurements made at the AP demonstrate complete neuromuscular relaxation, there may be recovery of the abdominal muscles, preventing optimal surgical conditions.

The location of neuromuscular monitoring may also be influenced by patient factors (i.e., acute bilateral upper extremity burns preventing access to the ulnar nerves), surgical procedure, or positioning (i.e., prone positioning may prevent monitoring of the facial nerve muscles or tucking of bilateral arms may prevent monitoring of the adductor pollicis).

In drawing conclusions of level of neuromuscular blockade of muscles of physiologic interest, it is important to consider factors that may have regional influence on neuromuscular blockade. A patient with significant upper extremity edema may demonstrate falsely elevated levels of neuromuscular paralysis with ulnar nerve stimulation secondary to poor nerve stimulation rather than actual neuromuscular blockade. The same may occur with poor electrode pad contact or inappropriate placement of the leads as discussed above. Resistance to non-depolarizing NMBDs occurs in peripheral and central nerve damage so that monitoring neuromuscular function in regions supplied by these nerves may lead to NMBD overdose.

Finally, it is of utmost importance to assess a baseline response to stimulation prior to administration of NMBDs for future reference. For example, if the pre-paralysis control response to train-of-four (TOF) stimulation (see **[L-4]**) is four strong twitches, and your post-neuromuscular blockade reversal response is four weak twitches, there is a high probability of residual neuromuscular blockade even though the patient has regained a four twitch response. Without assessing a control response, you sacrifice valuable information that may assist your decision-making when determining if post-reversal neuromuscular function is adequate.

In this case, the orbicularis oculi muscle was used throughout the case for monitoring of neuromuscular blockade, which may have given us false reassurance of the full recovery of the muscles of the upper airway. Even mild residual neuromuscular paralysis may have contributed to the patient's unanticipated airway obstruction in the PACU (see **[L-4]**).

Lesson 4: How Do you Diagnose Residual Neuromuscular Blockade?

Neuromuscular-blocking drugs (NMBDs) were first introduced into clinical practice in 1942 and are an important component of current anesthetic practice. NMBDs improve surgical conditions by creating immobility and improving surgical exposure, which is beneficial to our surgical colleagues. Of particular benefit to the anesthesiologist is the improvement in intubating conditions that occurs with NMBD administration [18]. While neuromuscular paralysis may be desired intraoperatively, even mild residual postoperative weakness can have deleterious effects. Even mild residual neuromuscular blockade can cause (1) upper airway obstruction, (2) vocal cord dysfunction, (3) decreased ability to cough which results in retention of secretions, (4) decreased ability to prevent aspiration, and (5) decreased hypoxic response which all contribute to the increased morbidity associated with incomplete reversal of neuromuscular blockade [19]. A vital role of the anesthesiologist is to develop the knowledge and skills to titrate NMBDs to desired effect and accurately verify return of neuromuscular function.

Physical exam findings can help assess the degree of neuromuscular paralysis at high levels of blockade, but are not as informative at lower depths of blockade (Table 12.3). The peripheral nerve stimulator (PNS) is the primary means by which we monitor the depth of neuromuscular blockade (see **[L-3]**). Peripheral nerve stimulators are usually programmed to deliver a maximum current between 60 and 80 mA at various frequencies to produce different patterns of muscle contraction including a single twitch, a train of four (TOF) which is a series of four twitches, and a sustained muscle contraction called tetanus. Numerous modalities

Table 12.3 Clinical tests of neuromuscular transmission and correlation with receptor occupancy

Clinical tests of neuromuscular transmission		
Test	Normal function	% of receptor occupied[a]
Tidal volume	5 mL/kg	80
Train of four	No fade	70
Vital capacity	≥20 mL/kg	70
Sustained tetanus (50 Hz)	No fade	60
Head lift	180° for 5 s	50
Handgrips	Sustained for 5 s	50

[a]Approximate percentage of receptors occupied when the response returns to its normal value

are available to quantify the muscle response to stimulation including mechanomyography (MMG) which directly measures force, electromyography (EMG) which measures the electrical response of the target muscle, and accelerometry which measures acceleration (as acceleration is proportional to force if the mass remains constant per Newton's law). Although the quantitative modalities discussed above are more accurate at detecting residual neuromuscular blockade, visual and tactile evaluation is the most clinically used modality due to the low cost and ease of use. Because intraoperative neuromuscular blockade monitoring is primarily performed when non-depolarizing NMBDs are utilized, the following discussion will focus on monitoring muscle response in the presence of non-depolarizing neuromuscular blockade. It is important to note that full recovery of neuromuscular function should always be verified after any class of NMBDs is used.

Single Twitch Stimulation

A single twitch muscle response is produced from a single current of stimulation provided by the PNS. A baseline single twitch muscle response is recorded prior to administration of NMBDs and is used for comparison against single twitches performed after NMBD administration. It is important to note that in order to accurately evaluate a single twitch response after administration of a non-depolarizing NMBD, measurements should be performed at least >10 s (<0.1 Hz frequency) apart to allow for full recovery of the neuromuscular junction. Visual and/or tactile assessment of the differences between single twitch responses is crude, and in the authors' experiences, difference in twitch height <70% can be difficult to detect with visual or tactile endpoints [20].

Train-of-Four Stimulation

For a train-of-four (TOF) response, a series of four stimulations is applied at a frequency of 2 Hz, which results in four sequential twitches of the muscle of interest. The number of twitches and the ratio between the first and last twitches (TOF ratio)

Table 12.4 Correlation between TOFR, depression of single twitch, and response to 5-s tetanus stimulation

Correlation of response between single twitch, tetanic stimulation, and train-of-four stimulation					
	1 twitch	2 twitches	3 twitches	4 twitches	TOFR ≥ 0.7
Single twitch height depression (% block)	90–100%	80–90%	70–80%	60–70%	0%
Response to tetanus	Fade	Fade	Fade	Fade	Sustained

TOFR train-of-four ratio

provide information on the depth of neuromuscular blockade (Table 12.4). In the absence of neuromuscular blockade, no fade will be present between the first and fourth twitches, and the TOF ratio will be 1. However, when non-depolarizing NMBDs are present at the neuromuscular junction, the amount of acetylcholine (ACh) present in the synapse during the TOF stimulation is not enough to outcompete the NMBD for receptor binding sites. In this case, fade will be observed, resulting in a TOF ratio <1. A TOF ratio >0.9 is accepted as full return of neuromuscular function. Determining the exact TOF ratio with visual or tactile measurements is difficult, and studies demonstrate that ratios as low as 0.3 can be misinterpreted as sustained [20].

Tetanic Stimulation

A stimulus delivered at ≥30 Hz does not allow enough time for complete muscle relaxation between stimuli and thus results in a sustained contraction called tetanus. If no neuromuscular blockade is present, the force of the tetanic contraction is sustained for the duration of the stimulus. In clinical practice, a 5-s tetanic stimulation at 50–100 Hz is generally used. Tetanic contractions are painful and should only be performed at an appropriate anesthetic depth. A 100 Hz stimulus is more effective in diagnosing residual neuromuscular blockade than a 50 Hz stimulus, but because of the high frequency of stimulation, fade may be seen even in the absence of neuromuscular blockade. A tetanic stimulation floods the neuromuscular junction with ACh, which produces a phenomenon called post-tetanic facilitation. Any nerve stimulus occurring after a tetanic stimulation will be markedly exaggerated – with the level of response enhancement dependent on the strength and frequency of the tetanic stimulation. Clinically, this comes into play when monitoring recovery from neuromuscular blockade. Take, for instance, an anesthetized patient who has received non-depolarizing NMBDs. Fade is noted when a tetanic stimulus is delivered to assess depth of neuromuscular blockade. A TOF stimulus performed directly after the tetanic stimulus results in four twitches due to post-tetanic facilitation. Because of this, the TOF result may give you an underestimation of neuromuscular blockade depth, resulting in incorrect clinical decision-making (i.e., overdosing NMBDs). A 2–5-min interval between stimuli is generally sufficient to abolish this effect.

Although direct-acting NMBD antagonists are available outside of the United States, at the time of this writing, the actions of the NMBDs are reversed by administration of acetylcholinesterase inhibitors in the United States. By decreasing metabolism of ACh, acetylcholinesterase inhibitors allow ACh to outcompete NMBDs for binding sites on the postsynaptic membrane, thus restoring neuromuscular function. The ability of the excess ACh to outcompete the NMBDs is affected by the concentration of the NMBD at the synaptic cleft, and indeed, longer recovery times are seen when intermediate-acting (neostigmine) acetylcholinesterase inhibitors are given at deeper depths of neuromuscular blockade. Acetylcholinesterase inhibitors are not site specific and will produce effects of cholinergic stimulation (bradycardia, salivation, increased GI motility, etc.) and so must always be concomitantly administered with an anticholinergic (atropine, glycopyrrolate).

The residual paralysis secondary to incomplete neuromuscular blockade reversal is often first detected in the PACU. These patients may complain of subjective weakness or may demonstrate what is described as a "floppy fish" appearance. With residual neuromuscular blockade, a patient is able to generate an initial movement but lacks the strength to sustain or complete the movement leading to extremity motions that have a similar appearance to a fish flopping out of water. Even mild residual neuromuscular blockade can cause (1) upper airway obstruction, (2) vocal cord dysfunction, (3) decreased ability to cough which results in retention of secretions, (4) decreased ability to prevent aspiration, and (5) decreased hypoxic response which all contribute to the increased morbidity associated with incomplete reversal of neuromuscular blockade [19].

Although the patient in this case denied subjective feelings of weakness, his "floppy fish" movements suggested that undiagnosed residual neuromuscular blockade played a role in his PACU respiratory distress (Table 12.1). Studies in obese patients demonstrate prolonged recovery after dosing of NMDs at total body weight. In this case, the incorrect use of the patient's ideal body weight for dosing of the acetylcholinesterase inhibitor may have led to insufficient reversal of neuromuscular blockade [21]. As discussed earlier, sustained tetanic contraction as measured by tactile sensation does not guarantee complete return to normal neuromuscular function. Post-extubation soft tissue obstruction and vocal cord dysfunction due to residual paralysis may have contributed to the patient's upper airway narrowing and anxiety, feeding into the vocal cord dysfunction loop demonstrated in Fig. 12.7.

Lesson 5: What Are the Postanesthetic Care Unit (PACU) Guidelines for Discharge After an Episode of Respiratory Distress?

Postoperative respiratory events are usually quickly recognized in the PACU owing to the low patient-to-nursing ratios, continuous pulse oximetry monitoring, and the proximity of the nurses and physicians to the patients. However, a potentially very dangerous time period begins once the patient is discharged from the highly monitored area of the PACU to a less monitored area such as a step-down unit, a surgical ward, or home. In these environments, unrecognized abnormalities of oxygenation and ventilation can have catastrophic consequences. Ultimately, it is the role of the anesthesiologist to apply sound clinical judgment when deciding the appropriate disposition location for a patient who has experienced, or is at increased risk for experiencing, perioperative respiratory distress.

There are many causes of postoperative respiratory distress, and the management of the various etiologies differs. However, once resolved, there are a few common steps that must be taken to decide the appropriate discharge location for the patient. It is imperative to ensure resolution of respiratory distress and also assess the risk for recurrence prior to discharging a patient to a less monitored environment. For example, the patient who experienced respiratory distress secondary to residual neuromuscular blockade, which has since resolved, may not need to be discharged to a monitored environment. However, the patient with OSA who experienced respiratory distress secondary to upper airway obstruction in the postoperative period is at risk for recurrence and may need to be discharged to a more monitored environment with low patient-to-nursing ratios. The PACU discharge should always be tailored to the clinical scenario, but extending the PACU stay for patients who have experienced or who are at risk for experiencing respiratory distress (i.e., patients with OSA), an extra amount of time after meeting the standard modified Aldrete criteria is a safe practice. Indeed, the American Society of Anesthesiology (ASA) guidelines recommend keeping an OSA patient 3 h longer than an otherwise completely matched control who does not have OSA.

Obstructive sleep apnea deserves special mention due to both the prevalence of the disorder and the lethal consequences of mismanagement. Patient with diagnosed or suspected OSA is especially vulnerable in the perioperative period due to effects of anesthesia and the use of sedating medications such as opioids that increase the risk for soft tissue upper airway obstruction. If unrecognized, this hypoventilation can have deleterious consequences like hypoxemia, hypercarbia, cardiovascular collapse, and even death. In addition to continuous monitoring of oxygenation and ventilation with continuous pulse oximetry and potentially capnography, patient-to-nursing ratios play an important role in preventing perioperative death. Oftentimes, desaturation as noted by continuous pulse oximetry is a later sign of airway obstruction and may not be noticed if a patient is not under close, direct observation by a medical professional. In 2014, the American Society of Anesthesiologists published practice guidelines for the perioperative management of patients with OSA and concluded that patients should not be discharged to unmonitored settings until they are no longer at risk for postoperative respiratory depression; expert opinion deemed this to be 3 h longer than otherwise matched controls [22]. Risk can also be assessed in terms of the severity of OSA, respiratory behavior in the PACU, type of surgery, and opioid requirement (see Fig. 12.9).

In this case, the patient had an episode of respiratory distress related to a combination of factors including paradoxical vocal cord dysfunction, residual neuromuscular blockade, and likely obstructive sleep apnea (STOP-Bang score of 7). After weaning from initial NIPPV/BiPAP, he did not experience any further adverse respiratory events, including desaturations ($SpO_2 < 90\%$), bradypnea (<8 breaths/

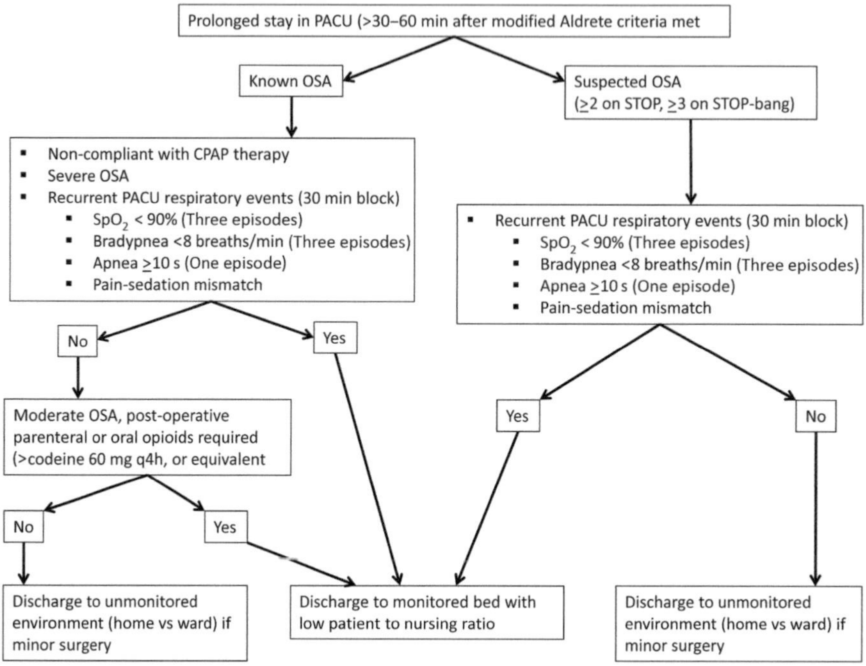

Fig. 12.9 Clinical decision pathway for discharge of patients with OSA

min), or apnea >10 s. He had adequate pain control from his laparoscopic procedure on low-dose oral opioid medications (<60 mg codeine equivalents every 4 h) and displayed no evidence of sedation with these medications. He remained in the PACU an additional 60 min after meeting modified Aldrete criteria, for a total of 6 h without additional documented perioperative complications.

References

1. Peppard PE, Young T, Barnett JH, et al. Increased prevalence of sleep disordered breathing in adults. Am J Epidemiol. 2013;177:1006–14.
2. Chung F, Mokhlesi B. Postoperative complications associated with obstructive sleep apnea: time to wake up! Anesth Analg. 2014;118:251–3.
3. Benumof JL. Mismanagement of obstructive sleep apnea results in finding these patients dead in bed. Can J Anesth. 2016;63:3–7.
4. Ramachandran SK, Josephs LA. A meta-analysis of clinical screening tests for obstructive sleep apnea. Anesthesiology. 2009;110:928–39.
5. Silva GE, Vana KD, Goodwin JL, et al. Identification of patients with sleep disordered breathing: comparing the four-variable screening tool, STOP, STOP-bang, and Epworth Sleepiness Scales. J Clin Sleep Med. 2011;7(5):467–72.
6. Chung F, Subramanyam R, Liao P, et al. High STOP-bang score indicates a high probability of obstructive sleep apnoea. Br J Anaesth. 2012;108(5):768–75.

7. Rogers JH, Stell PM. Paradoxical movement of the vocal cords as a cause of stridor. J Laryngol Otol. 1978;92:157–8.
8. Truong A, Truong DT. Vocal cord dysfunction: an updated review. Otolaryngology. 2011;S1:002. https://doi.org/10.4172/2161-119x.S1-002.
9. Murkami Y, Kirchner JA. Mechanical and physiological properties of reflex laryngeal closure. Ann Otol Rhinol Laryngol. 1972;81:59–72.
10. Husein OF, Hussein TN, Gardner R, et al. Formal psychological testing in patients with paradoxical vocal fold dysfunction. Laryngoscope. 2008;118:740.
11. Perkner JJ, Fennely KP, Balkissoon R, et al. Irritant-associated vocal cord dysfunction. J Occup Environ Med. 1998;40:136.
12. Chiang T, Marcinow AM, deSilva BW, et al. Exercise-induced paradoxical vocal fold motion disorder: diagnosis and management. Laryngoscope. 2013;123:727.
13. Harbison J, Dodd J, McNichols WT. Paradoxical vocal cord motion causing stridor after thyroidectomy. Thorax. 2000;55:533–4.
14. Collett PW, Brancatisano T, Engel LA. Spasmodic croup in the adult. Am Rev Respir Dis. 1983;127:500–4.
15. Baldwin M, Benumof JL. Paradoxical vocal cord motion: a unique case of occurrence in treatment. Anesth Analg. 2015;120(2):451.
16. Larsen B, Carus LJ, Villariet DB. Paradoxical vocal cord motion: an often misdiagnosed cause of postoperative stridor. J Clin Anesth. 2004;16:230–4.
17. Neustein SM, Taitt-Wynter LM, Rosenblatt MA. Treating stridor with opioids: a challenging case of paradoxical vocal cord movement. J Clin Anesth. 2010;22:130–1.
18. Barash PG. Clinical anesthesia. 7th ed. Philadelphia: Lippincott Williams & Wilkins. Chapter 20; 2013. p. 524–5.
19. Hagberg CA. Benumof and Hagberg's airway management. 3rd ed: Philadelphia: Elsevier. Chapter 47; 2013. p. 1147–8.
20. Capron F, Fortier LP, Racine S, et al. Tactile fade detection with hand or wrist stimulation using train-of-four, double-burst stimulation, 50-hertz tetanus, 100-hertz tetanus, and acceleromyography. Anesth Analg. 2006;102:1578–84.
21. De Baerdemaeker LEC, Mortier EP, Struys M. Pharmacokinetics in obese patients. Br J Anaesth. 2004;4(5):152–5.
22. American Society of Anesthesiologists Task Force on Perioperative Management of patients with obstructive sleep apnea. Practice guidelines for the perioperative management of patients with obstructive sleep apnea: an updated report by the American Society of Anesthesiologists Task Force on Perioperative Management of patients with obstructive sleep apnea. Anesthesiology. 2014;120:268–86.

Chapter 13
An Undiagnosed Intraoperative Pheochromocytoma

Bjorn Benjamin Jensen and Seth Herway

Case Presentation

A 35-year-old Caucasian female (height 157.5 cm, weight 58.5 kg, BMI 23.6 kg/m^2) with a past medical history significant for asthma and beta thalassemia presented to the operating room for a left adrenalectomy. She initially presented to the emergency room with abdominal and left-sided shoulder pain. A CT scan was done which demonstrated a very large 18.0 × 17.3 × 21.1 cm solid/cystic complex multicomponent heterogeneously enhancing mass in the left upper quadrant centered at the left adrenal gland which displaced the spleen, left kidney, stomach, and pancreas due to mass effect (see Fig. 13.1). It was believed to be a primary left adrenal gland neoplasm of adrenal origin [**L-1**]. Her vital signs when seen by the consulting surgical team were blood pressure (BP) 146/90 mmHg, heart rate (HR) 105 beat per minute (bpm), RR 18 breaths/min, and SpO_2 98% on room air. She denied syncope, headache, chest pain, weight loss, or diaphoresis [**L-2**]. She was otherwise feeling in good health. Based on the patient's presentation, the size of the tumor, and the CT images, the surgical team determined that further evaluation of the mass was unnecessary and the only labs indicated prior to surgery were a complete blood count (CBC) and basic metabolic panel (BMP) [**L-3**] .

She denied anesthetic issues with her previous knee arthroscopy 6 years prior. She had a good exercise tolerance (>4 METS) which included running and biking without any shortness of breath or chest pain. She characterized her asthma as mild and intermittent, never requiring emergency department visits with very rare inhaler use. She was not taking any iron supplements for her beta thalassemia and denied any coagulation issues. She was otherwise healthy, with a negative cardiac, neurologic, renal, endocrine, and GI history. Current medications included loratadine for seasonal allergies and jolessa for contraception [**L-4**].

B. B. Jensen (✉) · S. Herway
Department of Anesthesiology, University of California, San Diego, CA, USA

J. L. Benumof, G. R. Manecke (eds.), *Clinical Anesthesiology II*,
https://doi.org/10.1007/978-3-030-12365-9_13

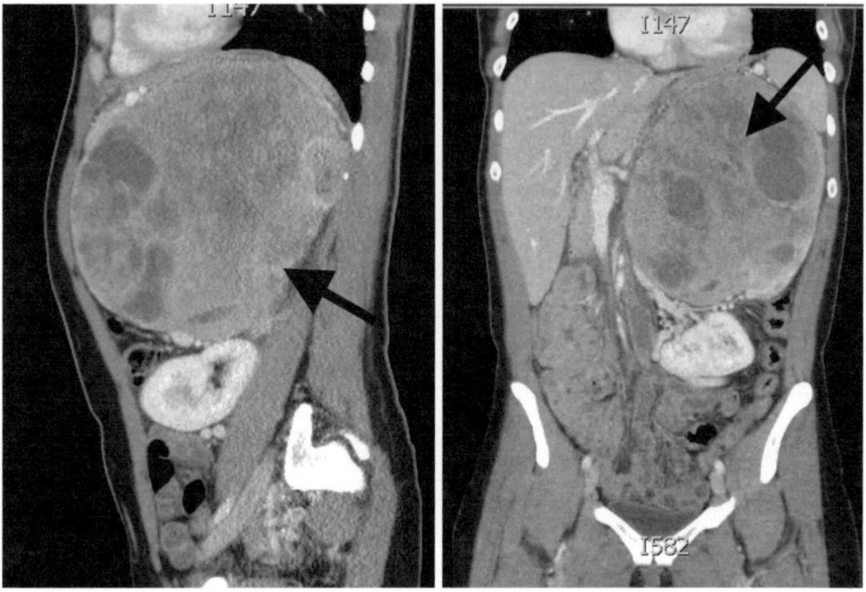

Fig. 13.1 CT scan prior to surgery. Left image: midline sagittal view. Right image: midline frontal view. Arrows: demonstrates a 18.0×17.3×21.1 cm adrenal mass

Her physical exam was unremarkable including clear breath sounds bilaterally on auscultation and normal cardiac and airway examinations. Her CBC and BMP results were unremarkable including a hemoglobin of 9.8 mg/dL and hematocrit of 31.1. The anesthesia team contacted the surgical team prior to surgery to confirm that their assessment was that the mass was nonsecretory and that no further labs or evaluation were indicated. The attending surgeon confirmed that this was the case.

On the day of surgery, the patient's vital signs were BP 135/90 mmHg, HR 82 bpm, RR 18 breaths/min, and SpO_2 100% on room air. In the preoperative holding area, a thoracic epidural was placed at the T6–T7 interspace with the catheter left at 14 cm with a plan to bolus with 0.125% Marcaine near the end of the procedure for pain control. The patient received 2 mg of midazolam and 50 mcg of fentanyl for sedation during placement of the thoracic epidural. In addition, the patient was typed and crossed for two units of packed red blood cells and two units of fresh frozen plasma.

General anesthesia was induced using a mask induction with 8% sevoflurane and 50% nitrous with a goal of facilitating a more hemodynamically stable induction. An arterial line was placed by one provider while the other simultaneously performed the mask induction. A grade 1 view was obtained using a MAC 3 blade, the vocal cords were sprayed with 4 cc of 2% lidocaine, and a 7.0 mm internal diameter endotracheal tube was inserted without difficulty. Vital signs remained stable throughout induction and intubation. Two additional 18-gauge peripheral IVs were placed after intubation. A Vigileo monitor (Edwards Lifesciences, Irvine, California,

USA) was attached to the arterial line to monitor cardiac output and stroke volume variation, with the initial readings being 7.6 L/min and 3%, respectively. A Foley catheter was placed, weight-based cefazolin and Flagyl were given for antibiotic prophylaxis, and subcutaneous heparin was administered prior to incision **[L-5].**

Incision was uneventful with patient's systolic blood pressures averaging 110–120 mmHg, mean arterial pressures (MAPs) averaging 70–80 mmHg, and HR averaging 70–80 bpm (see Fig. 13.2). Approximately 20 min after incision, systolic blood pressures began to rise to 150–160 mmHg with the MAPs increasing to approximately 110 mmHg. Additional boluses of fentanyl (100 mcg) and propofol (100 mg) were administered with only a mild reduction in blood pressures. Systolic pressures continued to increase to 180 mmHg, and heart rate increased to 100 bpm. Additional boluses of propofol (200 mg) and fentanyl (250 mcg) were administered, and the volatile anesthetic depth was increased as well from 2.3% to 3.2%. Nicardipine boluses of 250 mcg at a time were also administered for a total of 1000 mcg. The acute changes in hemodynamics were discussed with the surgeon who reported that they were dissecting around the mass at this time. The surgery team stopped dissecting, and the blood pressures remained elevated but stabilized. However, upon resuming surgical dissection around the mass, blood pressures began to rise again to as high as 200 mmHg systolic despite anesthetic and antihypertensive dosing as described. The patient continued to become more tachycardic, with a HR up to 120 bpm. The hemodynamic instability was communicated to the surgeon, and the likelihood that the mass was secretory and could be a pheochromocytoma was discussed. Two nitroprusside boluses of 10 mcg (20 mcg total) were administered, and a nitroprusside drip (0.3 mcg/kg/min) was started. In addition, a phentolamine drip was ordered from pharmacy **[L-6].** At this time, the Vigileo monitor showed a cardiac output of 10.0 L/min and a stroke volume variation of 3%. About 10 min after the drip was started, the surgeons were able to ligate the primary blood supply to the mass, and soon thereafter the blood pressures began to decrease to as low as 80 mmHg systolic, necessitating the discontinuation of the nitroprusside drip and the administration of a phenylephrine drip. The heart rate also normalized to 70–80 bpm. After mass removal (see Figs. 13.1 and 13.3), the Vigileo monitor showed a cardiac output of 6.9 L/min and a stroke volume variation of 7%.

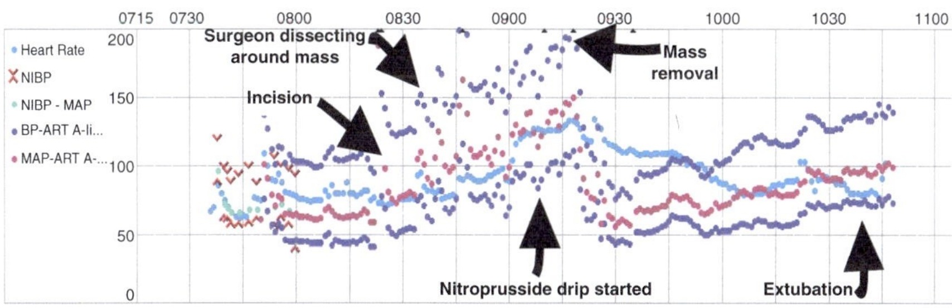

Fig. 13.2 Anesthetic record

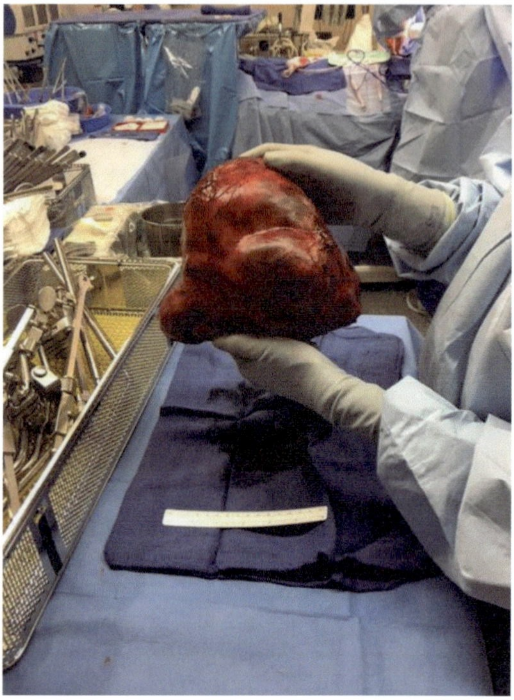

Fig. 13.3 Image of pheochromocytoma after removal

The patient was weaned off of the phenylephrine drip prior to extubation and emerged from anesthesia without administration of any further vasoactive agents. The thoracic epidural was bolused for pain control, and she was successfully extubated and taken to the ICU.

Other than replacement of her thoracic epidural for improved pain control, the patient's postoperative course was uneventful. The pathology report on the mass stated that the tumor cells were diffusively positive for synaptophysin, chromogranin, CD56, and sustentacular cells, and it was confirmed to be a pheochromocytoma with biologically aggressive behavior with a potential for recurrence. The patient was discharged on POD#5 and is currently doing well. Initial genetic testing did not show an obvious phenotype for neurofibromatosis or Von Hippel-Lindau. However, the patient is scheduled to receive a more extensive genetic evaluation.

Lesson 1: Types of Adrenal Masses

Adrenal masses can be thought of in the categories of nonfunctioning masses, functioning masses, and masses of that are not adrenal in origin (see Table 13.1). Of the three categories, it is often the functioning masses that can have the greatest

Table 13.1 Three types of adrenal masses

Types of adrenal masses		
Nonfunctioning mass	Functioning mass	Nonadrenal mass
Abscess	Nonclassical congenital adrenal hyperplasia	Renal
Granuloma	Pheochromocytoma	Pancreatic
Cyst	Other endocrine tumor	Gastric
Hemorrhage	Carcinoma	
Lipoma	Cortisol-secreting adenoma	
Myelolipoma	Aldosterone-secreting adenoma	
Primary malignancy	Sex hormone-secreting adenoma	
Metastatic malignancy		

Based on data from Ref. [1]

effect on anesthetic management. Three major products often secreted by functioning adrenal masses include excess glucocorticoids, mineralocorticoids, and catecholamines.

Glucocorticoid excess, also known as Cushing syndrome, may demonstrate characteristics such as truncal obesity, hypertension, hyperglycemia, increased intravascular fluid volume, hypokalemia, fatigability, abdominal striae, osteoporosis, and muscle weakness. It is often either due to the overproduction of cortisol or exogenous glucocorticoid therapy. Most cases that occur spontaneously are due to excess ACTH produced by an anterior pituitary microadenoma or nonendocrine tumor (e.g., lung, pancreas, kidney), which leads to bilateral adrenal hyperplasia. An adrenal neoplasm is the cause of excess cortisol secretion in 20–25% of Cushing syndrome patients. Approximately half of these adrenal tumors are malignant, and they are usually unilateral. Anesthetic management considerations include treating diabetes, hypertension, and electrolyte abnormalities (e.g., hypokalemia) preoperatively. Normalizing volume status through diuresis and evaluation of the patient's cardiac reserve may also be required prior to surgery. Glucocorticoid replacement therapy should be initiated at a dose equal to full replacement of adrenal output during periods of high stress when either bilateral or unilateral adrenalectomy is planned.

In patients with mineralocorticoid excess, it is primarily the hypersecretion of aldosterone that leads to the peripheral effects. Aldosterone works through the exchange of sodium for potassium and hydrogen ions in the renal tubule. Its increased secretion leads to hypertension, hypokalemic alkalosis, fatigue, and skeletal muscle weakness. As many as 1% hypertensive patients have primary hyperaldosteronism. The increase in sodium reabsorption and extracellular volume expansion is a contributor to the high incidence of diastolic hypertension in these patients. Anesthetic considerations involve restoring the patient's intravascular volume and electrolyte concentrations (e.g., hypokalemia) to normal, as well as treating hypertension. Aldosterone antagonists (spironolactone) may be used along with restricting sodium intake to control hypertension and hypokalemia preoperatively.

The overproduction of the catecholamines, epinephrine and norepinephrine, are what lead to the characteristics of pheochromocytomas. Pheochromocytomas occur in <0.2% of hypertensive patients, but their diagnosis is essential as surgical removal is curative in >90% of patients. Complications are often lethal in undiagnosed cases. The majority (85–90%) of pheochromocytomas are localized to a single adrenal gland (primarily the right). Approximately 25% of children and 10% of adults possess bilateral tumors. These tumors are extremely vascular, and malignant spread occurs in approximately 10% of cases. In approximately 5% of cases, the tumor may inherited as a part of a syndrome known as multiple endocrine neoplasia (MEN) IIA or IIB. The pheochromocytoma in type IIA is associated with medullary carcinoma of the thyroid and parathyroid hyperplasia. Meanwhile, the pheochromocytoma in type IIB is associated with neuromas of the oral mucosa and medullary carcinoma of the thyroid. In addition, pheochromocytomas may arise in association with von Hippel-Lindau disease (retinal and cerebellar angiomatosis) or von Recklinghausen neurofibromatosis [2]. The anesthetic management of a pheochromocytoma will be covered in the following lessons.

Lesson 2: Symptom-Based Diagnosis of Pheochromocytoma

A pheochromocytoma is a rare endocrine tumor originating from chromaffin tissue, with a published incidence of two to eight diagnoses per million people per year [3]. Chromaffin cells are postganglionic sympathetic neurons which produce catecholamines [4]. It is the secretion of catecholamines such as epinephrine and norepinephrine (and their subsequent interaction with α_1, α_2, β_1, and β_2 receptors) that lead to the systemic effects associated with a pheochromocytoma (see Fig. 13.4). It is important to pay attention to these symptoms, because a pheochromocytoma presenting to the operating room undiagnosed can result in sudden hypertensive crises which may be life-threatening. The published mortality for an undiagnosed pheochromocytoma presenting intraoperatively is 80% [3]. This highlights the seriousness of the problem encountered in the above case.

Patients may present with a variety of symptoms, including hypertension, headache, palpitations, diaphoresis, anxiety, dyspnea, chest/abdominal/flank pain, tremor, flushing, blurred vision, orthostatic hypotension, diarrhea, weakness, paresthesias, and vomiting. The most prevalent symptoms include hypertension, headache, palpitations, and diaphoresis, with the latter three symptoms being described as a classic triad in these patients. However, recent literature suggests there is no group of symptoms that guarantees the diagnosis of a pheochromocytoma. Instead, it is a combination of these symptoms, signs, and para-clinical exams that is most valuable in making the diagnosis [6].

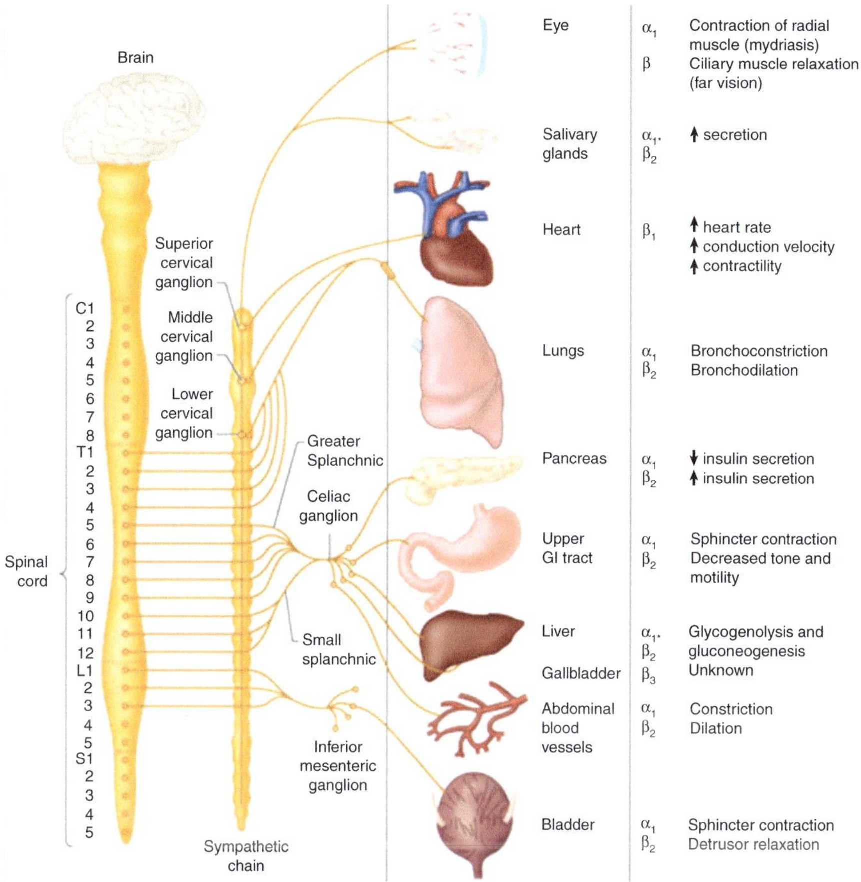

Fig. 13.4 Systemic effects of catecholamines through their interactions α_1, α_2, β_1, and β_2 receptors. (Reprinted from Butterworth et al. [5]. With permission from McGraw-Hill Education)

Lesson 3: Diagnosis of Pheochromocytoma Using Laboratory Values

Laboratory tests for a pheochromocytoma are taken from the urine or plasma and are based on the excess of catecholamines and their metabolites released by the tumor. Vanillylmandelic acid [VMA] is the final common product of the catecholamine metabolic pathways (see Fig. 13.5) and would be a reliable laboratory test in theory [8]. However, the most common practice is to perform initial screening using plasma-free metanephrines or urine-fractionated metanephrines. Although studies have shown that plasma-free metanephrines are a more sensitive test than the urine

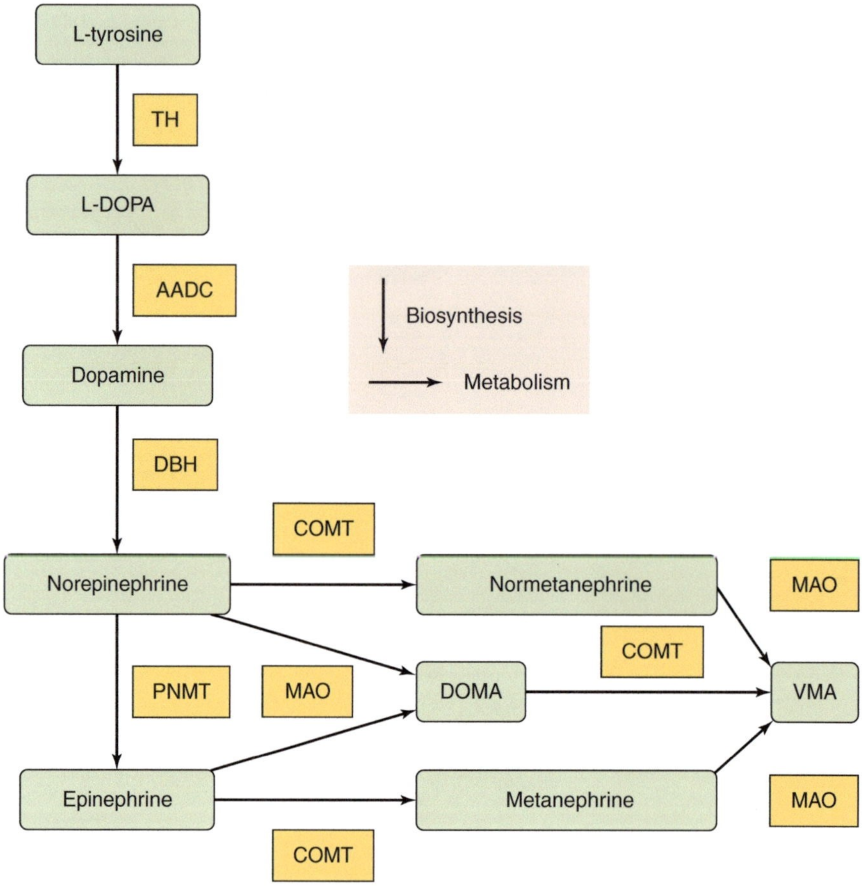

Fig. 13.5 Catecholamine biosynthetic and metabolism pathways. Precursors, catecholamines, and metabolites are shown in square boxes. Enzymes are shown in stippled boxes. Enzyme gene symbol designations are as follows: *TH* tyrosine hydroxylase, *AADC* aromatic-L-amino acid decarboxylase, *DBH* dopamine β hydroxylase, *PNMT* phenylethanolamine-N-methyltransferase, *COMT* catechol-O-methyltransferase, *MAO* monoamine oxidase, *VMA* 3-methoxy-4-hydroxy-mandelic acid. (Adapted with permission from Wolters Kluwer Health: Mulholland [7])

test, the differences were small and did not reach significance. It continues to be debated whether one test is superior to the other or under what conditions one is more preferable [8, 9].

Lesson 4: Preoperative Management

Preoperative alpha blockade is the mainstay of preparation for a pheochromocytoma resection. Beta blockade should never be used in isolation and only after adequate alpha blockade has been established. A potentially catastrophic hypertensive crisis could ensue with unopposed alpha stimulation, which may result in heart failure and other end-organ damage. In preparation for an elective adrenalectomy for a pheochromocytoma, phenoxybenzamine is the drug most commonly used in the United States for alpha blockade, and it is commonly started 10–14 days prior to surgery [3].

Roizen et al. in 1982 put forward criteria to objectively gauge the adequacy of alpha blockade prior to surgery. The criteria include:

1. No in-hospital blood pressure >160/90 mmHg for 24 h prior to surgery.
2. No orthostatic hypotension with blood pressure <80/45 mmHg.
3. No ST or T wave changes for 1 week prior to surgery.
4. No more than five premature ventricular contractions per minute.

His group reported that mortality from pheochromocytoma resection decreased to 0–3% from 13% to 45% once alpha blockade was instituted prior. These criteria have remained reliable over the years, and most centers use some (if not all) of the criteria during the preoperative evaluation process [3].

Once adequate alpha blockade has been established, β-blocker therapy may be initiated, and calcium channel blockade has also been used successfully. A preoperative echocardiogram may be useful to evaluate global systolic, diastolic, and valvular function. If the patient's cardiac function is acceptable, liberal fluid and salt intake is encouraged in order to facilitate volume replacement and minimize postural hypotension [3, 8].

Lesson 5: Intraoperative Management

Pheochromocytoma resection is among the most challenging procedures in anesthetic practice, with the primary goal of delivering a hemodynamically stable anesthetic both prior to and after tumor removal. Key areas to focus on include induction, incision, tumor handling, and tumor removal (see Table 13.2).

Relief from anxiety and hemodynamic stress during laryngoscopy are the goals to key in on during induction. A long-acting benzodiazepine (lorazepam/diazepam) the night before and/or midazolam prior to induction can help relieve preoperative anxiety. A pre-induction arterial line is indicated to aid in monitoring any large swings in blood pressure during induction and throughout the rest of the procedure. Hemodynamic stress during laryngoscopy may be limited with adequate amounts of intravenous anesthetics and opiates. Adjuncts including lidocaine and/or esmolol may also be considered. Airway instrumentation should only be attempted after adequate anesthetic depth is achieved [3].

Anesthesia may be maintained using volatile agents with sevoflurane and isoflurane being the most common. Desflurane is often avoided due to irritation and sympathetic stimulation. Anesthetics, vasoactives, and paralytics to be avoided include ketamine (sympathomimetic effects), histamine-releasing agents (e.g., morphine, curare, atracurium), succinylcholine (stimulation of autonomic ganglia and possible

Table 13.2 Anesthetic considerations in removal of a pheochromocytoma

Induction	
Anxiolytics	Pre-induction long benzodiazepine (e.g., midazolam/diazepam)
Arterial line	Placed pre-induction to closely monitor hemodynamic changes
Additional lines	Large-bore IV access (peripheral and/or central)
Induction agents	Propofol and/or etomidate along with opioids
Adjuvants	Consider lidocaine or esmolol (airway reflexes/tachycardia)
Laryngoscopy	Only after adequate depth of anesthesia
Incision/tumor manipulation	
Anesthetic maintenance	Volatiles (sevoflurane/isoflurane), adequate opioids (consider remifentanil drip), propofol
Antihypertensives (see Table 13.4 as well)	Calcium channel blockers (nicardipine), sodium nitrates (nitroprusside), β-blockers (labetalol), magnesium, alpha-antagonists (phentolamine)
Hydration	To prepare for tumor removal and possible hypotension
Tumor removal	
Consider steroid replacement	Especially in bilateral adrenalectomies
Vasopressors available	E.g., phenylephrine, vasopressin, epinephrine
Pain control post-op	Opioids, adjuvants (NSAIDS, a_2 agonists), and/or consider neuraxial

Based on data from Ref. [3]

Table 13.3 Medications to avoid in patients with a pheochromocytoma

Medication	Effect
Ketamine	Sympathomimetic effects – catecholamine release
Morphine	Histamine release
Curare	Histamine release
Atracurium	Histamine release
Ephedrine/epinephrine	Sympathomimetic effects – Catecholamine release
Pancuronium	Vagolytic effect
Halothane	Arrhythmogenic – Sensitizing the heart to catecholamines
Desflurane	Sympathetic stimulation due to irritation

Based on data from Refs. [3, 8]

mechanical compression of the tumor with fasciculations), halothane (arrhythmogenic), ephedrine (increase in catecholamines), and pancuronium (vagolytic effect) (see Table 13.3) [3, 8].

Hypertension may occur during any period including intubation, patient positioning, and incision, but tumor manipulation usually generates the most dramatic pressor response. Treating the resulting hypertensive crisis involves increasing anesthetic depth and the use of antihypertensives with direct arterial vasodilators being the most common (see Tables 13.3 and 13.4). However, following tumor removal and the loss of the catecholamine stimulation, sudden hypotension may occur. Contracted plasma volume, surgical bleeding, and anesthetic-induced vaso-

Table 13.4 Intravenous drugs to control intraoperative hypertension

Medication	Dosages	Half-life IV
Nicardipine	Infusion 5–15 mg/h. Increase 2.5 mg/h. Q15 min to effect [8, 10]	2.7 min
Phentolamine	1 mg IV boluses Q5–10 min. Infusion 0.1–2 mg/min and titrate [8, 11]	19 min
Nitroglycerin	20–40 mcg boluses Q5–10 min to effect. Infusion 5–20 mcg/min initially with max dose 400 mcg/min [8, 12]	2.3 ± 0.6 min
Nitroprusside	Infuse initially 0.5–1.5 mcg/kg/min to maximum 8 mcg/kg/min over 1–3 h [8, 13]	2 min
Propranolol	1 mg boluses to total of 10 mg [8, 14]	2–3 h
Esmolol	Load with 5–10 mg boluses and infuse 0.25–0.5 mcg/kg/min [8, 15]	2 min
Labetalol	5–10 mg boluses Q20–30 min up to max dose 150 mg [8, 16]	5.5 h

dilation may confound the issue as well. Post-removal hypotension may be counteracted using fluid boluses prior to tumor ligation, vasoactive agents, and steroid replacement especially following bilateral adrenalectomies [3].

Lesson 6: Commonly Used Antihypertensives Intraoperatively

The typical hemodynamic crisis during tumor resection is due to epinephrine or norepinephrine (depending on which one is predominately secreted by the tumor) and can manifest as hypertension associated with either tachycardia or bradycardia. In addition to increasing the anesthetic depth, the administration of antihypertensives is important to counteracting the hemodynamic changes. Direct arterial vasodilators have been shown to be very effective intraoperatively. Sodium nitroprusside and nitroglycerin are the most commonly used agents. Both drugs are easily titratable and have a rapid onset of action. Nicardipine and/or fenoldopam have also been used with success. Additional antihypertensive adjuvants include phentolamine and magnesium [3].

Phentolamine is a direct arterial vasodilator that is used in refractory situations and/or hypertensive emergencies where preferential alpha blockade is critical (e.g., cocaine intoxication, pheochromocytoma) [17–19]. Magnesium sulfate is a potent vasodilator and calcium antagonist which helps counteract the catecholamine-stimulated hemodynamic swings. A short-acting beta blocker such as esmolol may be included for heart rate control being careful to avoid unopposed alpha blockade [3]. Although labetalol is a commonly used antihypertensive in practice, one must consider the ratio of beta to alpha antagonism when treating someone with a pheochromocytoma. Labetalol has greater beta than alpha receptor antagonism, with the ratio of beta-alpha antagonism being 3:1 after oral and 7:1 after intravenous administration [20]. Lastly, it is important to recognize the drug half-life when using antihypertensive medications. Upon removal of the catecholamine-secreting tumor, the associated hypotension will be worsened by any long-active antihypertensive medications (see Table 13.4).

Conclusion

The case described above demonstrates the importance of early diagnosis and proper planning for the surgical removal of a pheochromocytoma. As previously stated, the published mortality for an undiagnosed pheochromocytoma presenting intraoperatively is as high as 80% [3]. Nevertheless, remaining adequately prepared for the unexpected intraoperative pheochromocytoma can help turn an imminent disaster into a successful anesthetic.

References

1. Sabatine S, Marc MD. Pocket medicine. 4th ed. Philadelphia: Lippincott Williams & Wilkins; 2011. Print
2. Barash PG. Clinical anesthesia. Philadelphia: Wolters Kluwer Health/Lippincott Williams & Wilkins; 2013. p. 1334–42. Print
3. Ramakrishna H. Pheochromocytoma resection: current concepts in anesthetic management. J Anaesthesiol Clin Pharmacol. 2015;31(3):317–23. PubMed. Web. 20 Oct 2016
4. Ilias I, Pacak K. A clinical overview of pheochromocytomas/paragangliomas and carcinoid tumors. Nucl Med Biol. 2008;35(Suppl 1):S27–34.
5. Butterworth JF, Mackey DC, Wasnick JK, editors. Morgan and Mikhail's clinical anesthesiology. 5th ed. New York: The McGraw-Hill Companies, Inc.; 2013.
6. Pourian M, Mostafazadeh DB, Soltani A. Does this patient have pheochromocytoma? A systematic review of clinical signs and symptoms. J Diabetes Metab Disord. 2015;15:6.
7. Mulholland MW. Greenfield's surgery: scientific principles and practice. In: Lillemoe KD, Doherty GM, Maier RV, editors. Adrenal gland. 5th ed. Philadelphia: Lippincott Williams & Wilkins; 2010.
8. Yao F-SF, Malhotra V, Fontes ML. Endocrine system: pheochromocytoma, Yao & Artusio's Anesthesiology: Problem-Oriented Patient Management. 8th ed. Philadelphia: Wolters Kluwer Health/Lippincott Williams & Wilkins; 2012. p. 501–11. Print
9. Eisenhofer G, Peitzsch M. Laboratory evaluation of pheochromocytoma and paraganglioma. Clin Chem. 2014;60(12):1486–99.
10. Curran MP, Robinson DM, Keating GM. Intravenous nicardipine its use in the short-term treatment of hypertension and various other indications. Drugs. 2006;66(13):1756–82. Web
11. Phentolamine. PubChem. National Center for Biotechnology Information, n.d. Web. 1 Dec 2016. https://pubchem.ncbi.nlm.nih.gov/compound/phentolamine#section=Top.
12. Nitroglycerin. Pubchem. National Center for Biotechnology Information, n.d. Web. 1 Dec 2016. https://pubchem.ncbi.nlm.nih.gov/compound/4510.
13. Nitroprusside. Pubchem. National Center for Biotechnology Information, n.d. Web. 1 Dec 2016. https://pubchem.ncbi.nlm.nih.gov/compound/11963622.
14. Propranolol. PubChem. National Center for Biotechnology Information., n.d. Web. 1 Dec 2016. https://pubchem.ncbi.nlm.nih.gov/compound/4946.
15. Esmolol. PubChem. National Center for Biotechnology Information., n.d. Web. 1 Dec 2016. https://pubchem.ncbi.nlm.nih.gov/compound/59768.
16. LABETALOL HYDROCHLORIDE INJECTION USP. Product Monograph. Sandoz Canada Inc, 23 Aug 2011. Web. 1 Dec 2016. http://www.sandoz.ca/cs/groups/public/@sge_ca/documents/document/n_prod_1301125.pdf.
17. Chan GM, Sharma R, Price D, Hoffman RS, Nelson LS. Phentolamine therapy for cocaine-association acute coronary syndrome (CAACS). J Med Toxicol. 2006;2(3):108–11.

18. Hollander JE, Henry TD. Evaluation and management of the patient who has cocaine-associated chest pain. Cardiol Clin. 2006;24(1):103–14.
19. Tuncel M, Ram VC. Hypertensive emergencies. Etiology and management. Am J Cardiovasc Drugs. 2003;3(1):21–31.
20. Maccarthy EP, Bloomfield SS. Labetalol: a review of its pharmacology, pharmacokinetics, clinical uses and adverse effects. Pharmacother: J Hum Pharmacol Drug Ther. 1983;3(4):193–217.

Chapter 14
LMA Morbidity: A Case of Unilateral Recurrent Laryngeal Nerve Palsy

Ryan Suda and Seth Herway

Case Presentation

A 23-year-old male with no past medical history presented for an elective open reduction and internal fixation of the left ankle for treatment of a left medial malleolus fracture. The patient was 5′9″, 73 kg (BMI = 24) with a favorable airway and a neurovascularly intact left lower extremity.

The patient was premedicated with intravenous (IV) midazolam 2 mg and ketamine 20 mg for severe anxiety prior to transport to the operating room. Standard ASA monitors were placed, and he was preoxygenated for 5 min. He received IV fentanyl 150 mcg and propofol 160 mg for induction of anesthesia. A Cookgas 4.5 laryngeal mask airway (LMA) was placed easily with air leak seen at 20 cm H_2O, and ventilation was maintained via pressure control with driving pressure of 10 cm H_2O and PEEP of 4 cm H_2O (**Lesson 1**). Peak inspiratory pressures were less than 14 cm H_2O. General anesthesia was maintained with sevoflurane and a 50/50 mixture of oxygen and air. Vecuronium 5 mg was given for muscle relaxation, and cefazolin 1 gm was given for antimicrobial prophylaxis at the surgeon's request prior to incision (**Lesson 2**). Surgery proceeded uneventfully, and muscle relaxation was fully reversed prior to LMA removal when the patient was alert, following commands, and adequately spontaneously ventilating. The patient had an unremarkable course in the PACU and was discharged home later that day.

During the patient's orthopedic surgery clinic visit on postoperative day (POD) 22, he reported voice hoarseness and difficulty swallowing that had persisted since the day of his procedure. His voice was hoarse and barely audible. He reported three episodes of difficulty swallowing liquids with subsequent coughing and choking. He was immediately referred to otolaryngology for evaluation of these symptoms. On POD 33, a videostroboscopy exam was performed in the otolaryngology office

R. Suda (✉) · S. Herway
Department of Anesthesiology, University of California, San Diego, CA, USA

J. L. Benumof, G. R. Manecke (eds.), *Clinical Anesthesiology II*,
https://doi.org/10.1007/978-3-030-12365-9_14

which revealed an immobile left vocal fold positioned laterally with incomplete glottic closure during sustained phonatory tasks (**Lesson 3**). He was diagnosed with left vocal cord paralysis, and treatment was to be initiated after a 2-week surveillance period for return of vocal cord function (**Lesson 4**). On POD 40, the patient reported complete spontaneous resolution of voice changes, and no further intervention or management was required.

Lesson 1: Laryngeal Mask Airway Placement and Utilization Is Associated with Morbidity Including Sore Throat, Trauma to the Oropharynx, and Nerve Injury

Sore Throat

The incidence of sore throat following laryngeal mask airway (LMA) use varies from 4% to 50% and is highly dependent on the study methods, which may differ in insertion skills and techniques, lubricants, and cuff pressure [1]. Factors contributing to the incidence of sore throat include the insertion technique, type of lubricant, type of ventilation (spontaneous or controlled), use of dry airway gases, and intracuff pressure [2]. These risk factors will be discussed in detail in Lesson 2. Sore throat usually resolves after 24–36 h and does not have long-term sequelae. Utilizing the fewest number of insertion attempts, minimizing the intracuff pressure, and inserting the LMA fully inflated or with a special insertion aid to prevent the tip of the LMA from folding back can help decrease the incidence of sore throat [2–4].

Oropharyngolaryngeal Injury

Any foreign body that comes into contact with the airway structures can potentially cause trauma. The LMA passes through and occupies anatomic areas from the oral cavity to the hypopharynx (Fig. 14.1a, b). The mucous membranes, soft tissues of the pharynx, and larynx are structures at high risk for injury [2]. However, trauma to the uvula, tonsils, posterior pharyngeal wall, epiglottis, and larynx has been reported after LMA use [2, 5]. Good insertion technique is crucial in minimizing trauma to the sensitive pharyngeal structures. Similarly, choosing an appropriately sized LMA can minimize pharyngeal trauma as one too large may create insertion difficulties and one too small may require an increased intracuff volume thus increasing pressure and thereby increasing the chance of LMA morbidity [6]. Preventing the tip of the LMA from folding back by using an insertion aid reduced the incidence of trauma, defined by the presence of blood on the LMA after removal, from 22% to 4% [4]. Similarly, the fully inflated technique decreased the presence of blood after removal to 0% compared with 15.3% using the standard

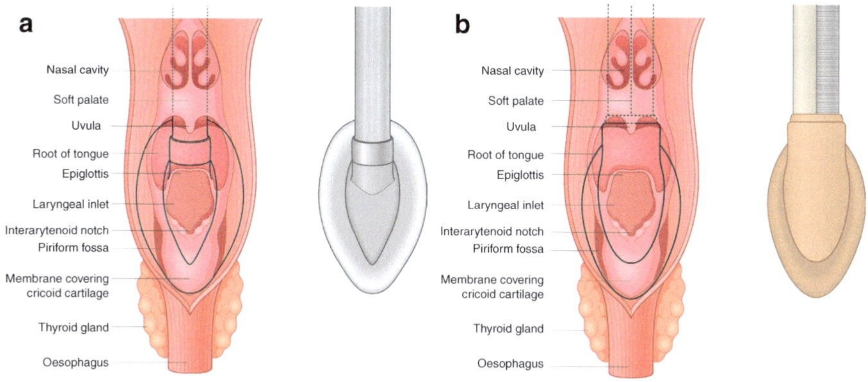

Fig. 14.1 (**a**) Pharyngeal structures adjacent to LMA® Unique™, a first-generation device. LMA® Unique™ is a trademark or registered trademark of Teleflex Incorporated or its affiliates. Image generated by, and used with permission from, Teleflex®. Author note: the author's intent is to show the LMA can exert pressure on a large surface area of delicate pharyngeal structures. (**b**) Pharyngeal structures adjacent to LMA® Proseal™, a second-generation device. Author note: the author's intent is to show the LMA can exert pressure on a large surface area of delicate pharyngeal structures. (LMA® Proseal™ is a trademark or registered trademark of Teleflex Incorporated or its affiliates. Image generated by, and used with permission from, Teleflex®)

technique [3]. When placing an LMA, good insertion technique utilizing one of above methods with appropriate lubrication and a gentle hand can minimize trauma to the airway.

Nerve Injury

Some of the more serious complications from LMA use are nerve palsies. The injuries usually manifest from emergence to 48 h after surgery. The majority of nerve palsies resolve in 1 h to 18 months. Pressure neuropraxia from the tube or cuff is the most common cause [1]. Injuries can occur with appropriate LMA use, despite previous thoughts that nerve injuries were related to suboptimal use. Other etiologies are chemical neuritis by use of the wrong lubricant or cleaning fluid, local inflammation due to insertion trauma, and stretch neuropraxia from head, neck, or body positional changes [7]. Injuries to the lingual, recurrent laryngeal, and hypoglossal nerves have been reported with the Classic (Teleflex Medical, Research Triangle Park, NC, USA), ProSeal (Teleflex Medical, Research Triangle Park, NC, USA), and Supreme (Teleflex Medical, Research Triangle Park, NC, USA) LMAs [8–10]. Both unilateral and bilateral injuries have been reported. Unilateral inferior alveolar and infraorbital nerve injuries have been described with the Classic and Supreme LMAs, respectively [10].

The lingual nerve is at risk of compression as it enters the mouth below the inferior border of the superior pharyngeal constrictor muscle and continues against the periosteum of the mandible posterior to the third molar (Table 14.1, Fig. 14.2).

Table 14.1 Anatomical site and clinical manifestation of reported nerve injuries from LMA use

Nerve at risk	Anatomical site	Clinical manifestation
Lingual	Entering the mouth below the inferior border of the superior pharyngeal constrictor muscle	Loss of taste and sensation over the anterior tongue
Inferior alveolar	Superficially between the last molar tooth and the ramus of the mandible or direct compression over the lower lip	Lower lip numbness
Hypoglossal	Crossing over the hyoid bone	Difficulty swallowing
Recurrent laryngeal	Entering the larynx deep to the lower border of the inferior pharyngeal constrictor muscle	Hoarseness, aphonia, stridor, dyspnea, or aspiration

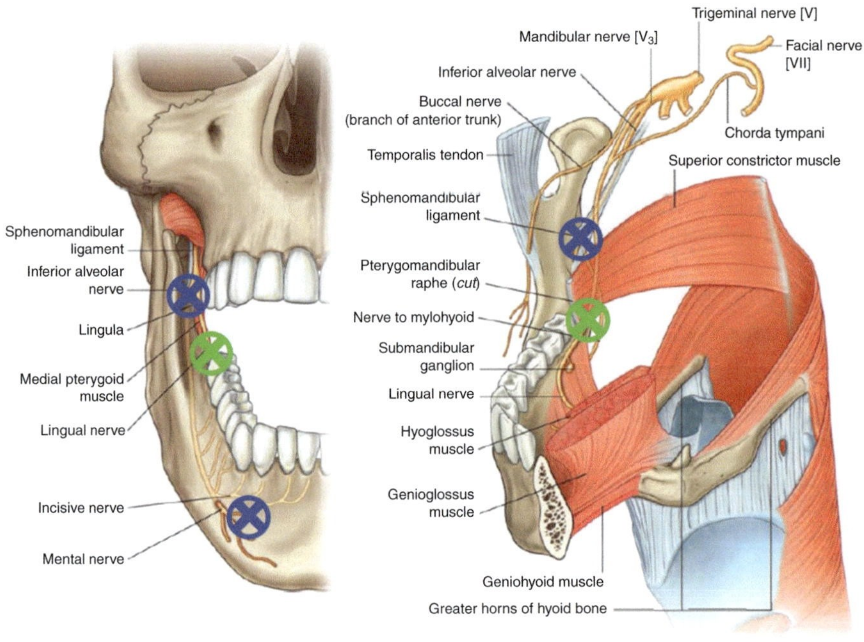

Fig. 14.2 LMA pressure neuropraxia site of lingual (X) and inferior alveolar (X) nerve injury. (Adapted from Drake et al. [33]. With permission from Elsevier)

Lingual nerve injury usually presents as loss of taste, and sensation over the anterior tongue. The inferior alveolar nerve is at risk of compression where it lies superficially between the last molar tooth and the ramus of the mandible or direct compression of the LMA over lower lip (Fig. 14.2). Inferior alveolar nerve injury usually presents as numbness to the lower lip [9]. The hypoglossal nerve is at risk of compression as it crosses the hyoid bone (Fig. 14.3). Hypoglossal nerve injury usually presents as difficulty in swallowing. The recurrent laryngeal nerve is at risk of compression as it enters the larynx, where it passes deep to the lower border of the inferior pharyngeal constrictor muscle (Fig. 14.4) [8]. Recurrent laryngeal nerve injury can manifest as hoarseness, aphonia, stridor, dyspnea, or postoperative aspiration, but presentation is dependent on presence of unilateral or bilateral injury

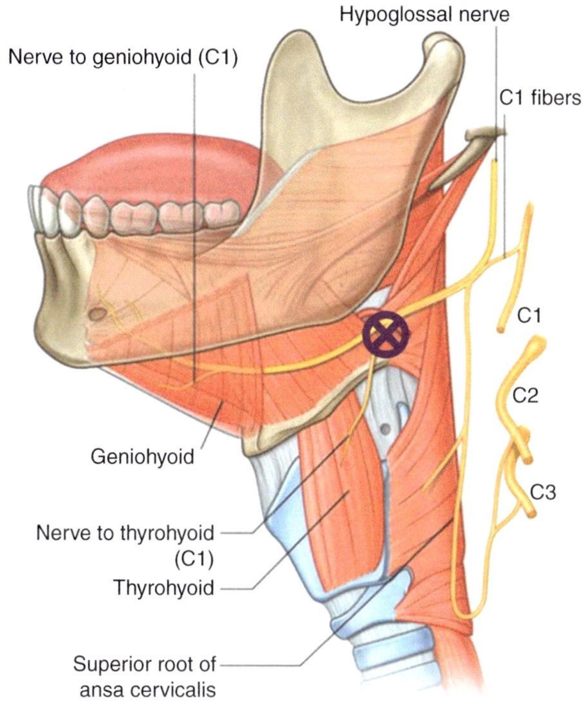

Fig. 14.3 LMA pressure neuropraxia site of hypoglossal nerve (X) injury. (Adapted from Drake et al. [33]. With permission from Elsevier)

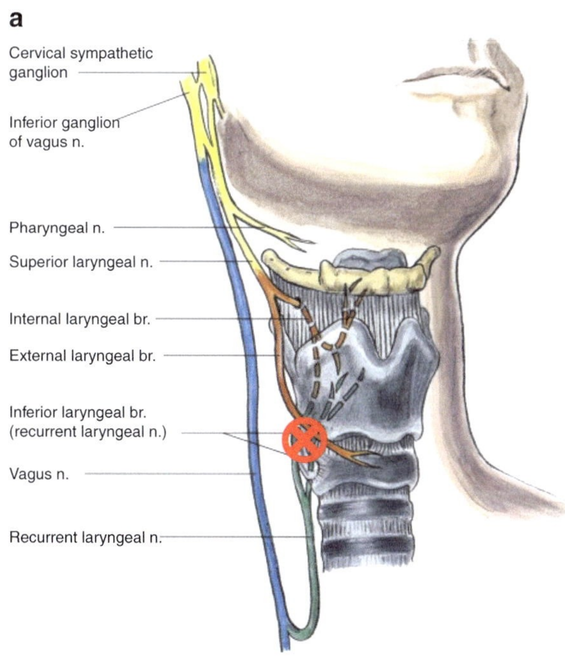

Fig. 14.4 (**a**, **b**) Schematic illustration of the anatomy of laryngeal innervation. (Adapted from Brown [34]. With permission from Elsevier)

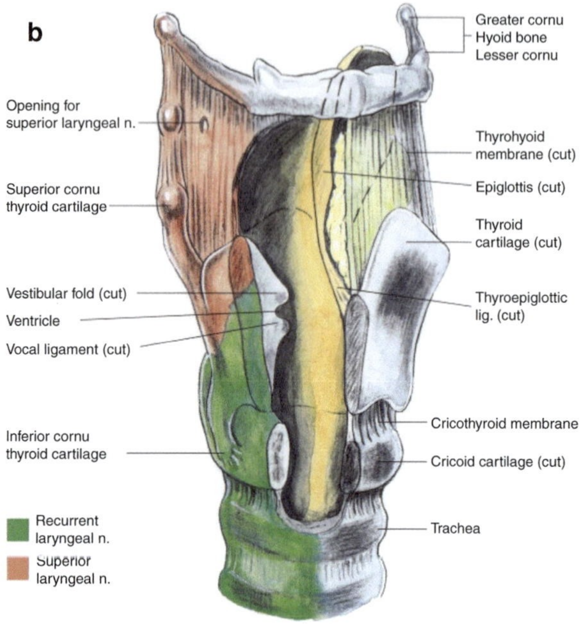

Fig. 14.4 (continued)

(see Lesson 4). Permanent nerve injury is rare, and minimizing LMA morbidity risk factors will provide the optimal environment for LMA use.

Lesson 2: Certain Risk Factors Increase the Prevalence of LMA Morbidity

High Intracuff Pressures

Pressure exerted by the LMA can be transferred onto the pharyngeal mucosa causing a decrease in pharyngeal perfusion [11]. Pharyngeal capillary perfusion pressures have not been measured, but they are assumed to be similar to those in the trachea at 30 mmHg (41 cm H_2O). The extent of pharyngeal mucosal injury is likely determined by the level of pressure and its duration of application [12]. When LMAs are positioned correctly, and using minimal intracuff pressures, capillary perfusion pressure is rarely exceeded. The highest mucosal pressures are in the distal oropharynx, where the curved tube is pressed firmly into the vertebral body by the expanding cuff and its own elastic recoil [12]. Efficacy of the LMA seal depends on the degree of conformity with pharyngeal tissues. Using an appropriately sized and positioned LMA with the minimal cuff volume required to create a seal is ideal for minimizing LMA morbidity.

The ProSeal LMA may decrease the risk of injury as the pressure against the mucosa (i.e., mucosal pressure) is lower than with the classic LMA for a given seal pressure [8]. In both paralyzed and non-paralyzed patients, the ProSeal LMA may be a more effective ventilation device than the LMA Supreme since it delivers greater positive pressure before an oropharyngeal leak, albeit with increased intracuff pressure [13, 14]. While increased intracuff pressure of LMAs may improve oropharyngeal leak pressure, they may result in more postoperative pharyngolaryngeal adverse events. The intubating LMA Fastrach (Teleflex Medical, Research Triangle Park, NC, USA) can provide a more effective seal than the classic LMA, but pressures on the pharyngeal mucosal are higher and always exceed capillary perfusion pressure [12]. Therefore, it is recommended that the LMA Fastrach be removed after successful endotracheal intubation. Pharyngeal mucosal pressures have not been measured directly in the newer LMAs capable of facilitating endotracheal intubation, such as the Cookgas air-Q (Cookgas, Lucas Ave, St. Louis, MO, USA). Mucosal pressure increases with increasing intracuff volume, but there is no correlation between mucosal pressures and leak pressures [15]. Intracuff pressures <60 cm H_2O are unlikely to cause pharyngeal damage from excessive mucosal pressure. Postoperative pharyngolaryngeal complications (sore throat, dysphagia, dysphonia) from LMA use can be reduced, up to 70%, when cuff pressure is frequently monitored and maintained with the lowest intracuff pressure feasible [11, 16, 17].

LMA Size

If the LMA is too small, there is increased frequency of malposition and a tendency for the user to overinflate the cuff in an attempt to create a better seal, which can predispose the patient to oropharyngolaryngeal morbidity and nerve damage [8]. However, larger LMA sizes may be associated with more frequent incidence of sore throat due to difficult insertion [6]. A deeper plane of anesthesia or use of muscle relaxation may facilitate easier insertion of larger LMAs due to decreased pharyngeal muscle tone. When choosing an LMA size, the user must also consider if the patient will be spontaneously ventilating or if positive pressure ventilation is necessary. If positive pressure ventilation is necessary, a larger LMA can be beneficial as it creates a better seal at a lower intracuff volume and pressure [18]. If spontaneous ventilation is planned, a smaller LMA can be beneficial as insertion is easier and airway sealing pressure is less critical to effective LMA function, assuming optimal positioning [6]. Choosing the appropriate LMA size can be challenging, and multiple factors must be taken into consideration to minimize LMA morbidity.

Non-supine Positioning

The LMA was originally intended to be inserted and used in the supine position [19]. As LMA familiarity increased, it began being used in various patient positions. LMAs have been used in a variety of patient positions, ranging from supine, to lateral, to prone. However, lateral positioning and extreme head-side rotation are risk factors for oropharyngolaryngeal morbidity and nerve injury [8]. Multiple types of nerve injuries have been reported when using an LMA in a lateral position, and many of the hypothesized mechanisms focus on localized nerve compression. Similar nerve injuries have been reported with extreme head-side rotation with the proposed mechanism being localized nerve compression or stretch neuropraxia [8, 9, 20]. Anytime a patient's position is changed, there is an opportunity for the airway device to alter position. The LMA can become slightly malpositioned when turning lateral, creating an unbalanced increased in pressure on certain pharyngeal structures. Additionally, external forces may alter internal interaction between the LMA and pharyngeal structures such as a pillow, neck roll, or extreme head positions. The appropriateness of using an LMA should be carefully considered if there are additional LMA morbidity risk factors present when the lateral position is surgically necessary. If there are no other risk factors, extra vigilance should be taken to prevent extreme head-side rotation and minimize any intra- or extra-oropharyngeal pressure points.

Nitrous Oxide

Nitrous oxide is routinely used as part of a balanced anesthetic for procedures. If nitrous oxide is used, it rapidly diffuses into the cuff of reusable LMA devices, causing an increase in intracuff pressure [8]. The intracuff pressure, if not monitored, can rise to levels where pharyngeal mucosal perfusion may be impaired, causing morbidity. There is a significant increase in intracuff pressure during the first 60 min from the diffusion of nitrous oxide [11]. The increase in intracuff pressure seems to plateau over a period of 1–2 h [21]. Interestingly, disposable (polyvinyl chloride) LMAs have more stable intracuff pressures than reusable (silicone) LMAs during nitrous oxide administration [22]. Given the morbidity potential, monitoring LMA intracuff pressures with manometry is recommended when administering nitrous oxide [17]. Vigilant removal of cuff air may be necessary throughout a procedure utilizing nitrous oxide to keep intracuff pressures to a minimum. Postoperative morbidity from LMA use can be reduced, up to 70%, when cuff pressure is frequently monitored and maintained with the lowest intracuff pressure feasible [11, 16, 17].

Lidocaine Lubricants

Adequate lubrication of LMAs assists in gentle and successful insertion. There are various types of lubricants such as normal saline, water based, silicone based, and local anesthetic based. These lubricants serve a similar function as saliva, which aids in swallowing and helps prevent sticking to the oropharynx. Water-soluble and normal saline lubricants are recommended for use in LMA insertion. Lubricants composed of local anesthetic gel can cause paresthesia and damage the integrity of protective airway reflexes in some patients [23]. Similarly, transient nerve injury has been reported with the use of local anesthetic lubricants [24]. Avoiding local anesthetic lubricants can decrease LMA morbidity by preserving the integrity of the protective airway reflex and minimizing the possibility of transient nerve injury.

Difficult or Alternate Insertion Techniques

The standard technique of inserting the LMA by the manufacturer and inventor includes complete LMA deflation with lubrication of the back of the mask, placement of the LMA using the palate as a guide, and then inflation of the LMA with enough air to obtain an adequate seal. The standard technique is most successful in obtaining appropriate position (assessed with fiber-optic bronchoscopy) and function when compared to semi-inflated, fully inflated, or back-to-front (deflated with 180° rotation) LMA insertion [19]. Multiple insertion attempts increase the chance of traumatizing oropharyngeal structures, which may lead to sore throat. However, fully inflating the LMA with recommended volume of air prior to insertion decreased sore throat from 21.4% to 4.1%, which may be due to the presentation of a softer leading edge to the posterior pharyngeal wall [3]. A similar effect was observed when a special insertion aid was used to prevent the tip of the LMA from folding back, reducing the incidence of trauma (blood on the LMA after removal) from 22% to 4% [4]. Therefore, optimizing insertion technique to minimize insertion attempts, and trauma to the posterior pharyngeal wall, should be employed to reduce the chance of sore throat.

The ProSeal LMA may carry greater risk of injury, in principle, than the classic LMA, as it is more difficult to insert and the larger cuff will be in contact with a greater portion of the oral and pharyngeal cavities [8]. However, malposition is less likely with the ProSeal LMA as it can be easily detected.

Cervical Bone or Joint Disease

Cervical bone or joint disease decreases the flexibility of the neck and can cause inhibition in its range of motion. The sniffing position facilitates LMA insertion and is recommended according to its manufacturer and inventor [19]. LMA insertion may be challenging if conditions are not optimized, such as with impaired neck extension. Similar to cervical joint or bone disease, a cervical collar intended to maintain cervical spine stability can create challenging conditions for LMA placement. As previously discussed, difficult insertion is a risk factor for LMA morbidity. Traumatic LMA placement can cause oropharyngolaryngeal trauma or nerve injury [25]. Optimal, atraumatic insertion can be accomplished with the previously described techniques. In patients with cervical bone or joint disease, the practitioner should balance the risks of LMA morbidity when determining the best method to secure the airway.

Lesson 3: Airway Innervation

Five nerves innervate the airway. The lingual nerve and chorda tympani provide sensation to the anterior two thirds of the tongue. The glossopharyngeal nerve supplies sensation to the posterior one third of the tongue and upper pharynx. The internal branch of the superior laryngeal nerve receives sensory input from the epiglottis, aryepiglottic folds, and larynx as inferior as the vocal cords. The recurrent laryngeal nerve provides sensation to the larynx below the vocal cords to the trachea. Knowledge of airway anatomy and innervation is critical to the anesthesia provider not only for airway management but also in preventing nerve palsies due to pressure neuropraxia. The following text highlighted in red indicates anatomic locations prone to pressure neuropraxia in the course of the various nerves. Complete knowledge of airway innervation can distinguish between pressure neuropraxia from LMA use and other sources (i.e., surgical).

Trigeminal/Lingual Nerve

The trigeminal nerve is composed of three branches, the ophthalmic, maxillary, and mandibular nerves. The mandibular nerve is a mixed nerve carrying motor and sensory fibers. The lingual nerve is a branch of the mandibular nerve and supplies somatic sensory afferent innervation from the mucous membrane of the anterior two thirds of the tongue, the lingual mucosa on the floor of the oral cavity, and the lingual gingiva associated with the lower teeth. After it courses through the infratemporal fossa, the nerve continues between the mandibular ramus and the medial pterygoid before joining with the chorda tympani branch of the facial nerve. The nerve proceeds along the surface of the medial pterygoid until it reaches the bone located a few millimeters below and behind the junction of the vertical and horizontal rami of the mandible. The lingual nerve then passes below the mandibular attachment of the superior pharyngeal constrictor and pterygomandibular raphe until it lies opposite to the posterior root of the third molar where it is covered only by the gingival mucoperiosteum (Fig. 14.2, see green X). The nerve continues along the superior surface of the mylohyoid muscle until it divides into numerous terminal branches entering the hyoglossus, genioglossus, and lingual mucosa [26].

Facial Nerve/Chorda Tympani

The facial nerve is composed of intracranial and extracranial branches that perform a variety of functions. The chorda tympani is an intracranial branch that provides special sensory fibers providing taste sensation from the anterior two thirds of the tongue. The nerve arises anterolaterally below the facial nerve to the stapedius, passing anterosuperiorly in the posterior canaliculus to the middle ear. It exits the tympanum via the anterior canaliculus before exiting the skull by a minute foramen behind the base of the spine of the sphenoid. The chorda tympani descends medial to the spine of the sphenoid and angles forward to join the lingual nerve a few centimeters below the base of the skull, just above the lower border of the lateral pterygoid. It continues to join the fibers of the lingual nerve [27].

Glossopharyngeal Nerve

The glossopharyngeal nerve is a mixed nerve consisting of both sensory and motor nerve fibers. The general sensory component carries afferent pain, temperature, and touch from the walls of the upper pharynx and posterior one third of the tongue. The glossopharyngeal nerve exits the skull through the jugular foramen and runs superficial to the internal carotid artery but deep to the jugular vein, external carotid artery, and styloid process to cross the deep surface of the stylopharyngeus muscle, which it innervates. It gives off a branch to the pharyngeal plexus and then continues around the lateral border of the stylopharyngeus muscle traveling toward the tongue base where, deep to the hyoglossus muscle, it divides into its terminal lingual and tonsillar branches [28].

Superior Laryngeal Nerve

The superior laryngeal nerve is a branch of the vagus nerve and itself branches into an external and internal laryngeal nerve. The external branch supplies innervation to the cricothyroid muscle, which functions to tense the vocal cords, increasing pitch. The internal branch carries sensory afferent fibers from the epiglottis, mucous membranes in the aryepiglottic fold, and mucous membranes lining the larynx as inferior as the vocal cords. The superior laryngeal nerves arise from the inferior ganglion of the vagus nerve, descend alongside the pharynx posterior to and then medial to the internal carotid artery, and then divide into a larger internal branch and a smaller external branch. The external branch descends posterior to the sternothyroid muscle and the superior thyroid artery, passing superficially to the inferior constrictor and then piercing it to supply the cricothyroid muscle as well as the inferior constrictor. The internal branch pierces the thyroid-hyoid membrane and subsequently divides into the upper and lower branches, which provide terminal fibers to the mucous membrane of the larynx from the epiglottis to the focal folds [29].

Recurrent Laryngeal Nerve

The recurrent laryngeal nerve is a branch of the vagus nerve. The recurrent laryngeal nerve supplies innervation to all the intrinsic muscles of the larynx, with the exception of the cricothyroid muscles. It also carries sensory afferent fibers from the larynx below the vocal cords to the trachea, (Fig. 14.2). The recurrent laryngeal nerves emerge from the vagus nerve at the level of the aortic arch, and the right and left nerves are not symmetrical (Fig. 14.3). The left nerve loops posterior and medially under the aortic arch and then ascends within the tracheoesophageal groove before coursing between the thyroid gland and trachea before entering the larynx (Fig. 14.4; see red X). The right nerve loops posterior and medially under the right subclavian artery, then ascends along the superior lobe of the pleura, and approaches the tracheoesophageal groove behind the common carotid artery where it continues superiorly between the trachea and thyroid gland before entering the larynx [30].

Lesson 4: How Do You Diagnose a Recurrent Laryngeal Nerve Injury?

Lesson 4-A: How Does a Unilateral Recurrent Laryngeal Nerve Injury Present?

To diagnose a recurrent laryngeal nerve (RLN) injury, an objective clear undisturbed view of the vocal cords during spontaneous ventilation must be obtained. The view can be obtained via flexible fiber-optic laryngoscopy with the patient awake or under general anesthesia. If done awake, the airway should be adequately anesthetized to tolerate the passage of the flexible fiber-optic bronchoscope. The nasal route is usually more comfortable for patients. Once there is a good view of the vocal cords with the fiber-optic bronchoscope, watch the vocal cords abduct with inspiration and passively adduct with expiration or, if possible, actively adduct by having the patient say "eeee."

If done under general anesthesia, either at the end of a case to see if there is an RLN injury or for other reasons, ensure the patient is under an adequate depth of anesthesia prior to changing the endotracheal tube to a LMA. Through the LMA, confirm a good view of the vocal cords with a fiber-optic bronchoscope. While the patient is still under general anesthesia, reverse the muscle relaxant completely and allow the $PETCO_2$ to increase so the patient begins to breathe spontaneously. Lighten the general anesthesia until spontaneous ventilation is well established; then vocal cords will abduct with inspiration and will passively adduct with expiration (Fig. 14.5) [31].

A unilateral recurrent laryngeal nerve injury presents with dysphonia such as hoarseness or breathiness and may be associated with dysphagia and aspiration [32]. A partial injury of a unilateral recurrent laryngeal nerve will result in the injured side remaining fixed in adduction toward the midline, and it does not abduct

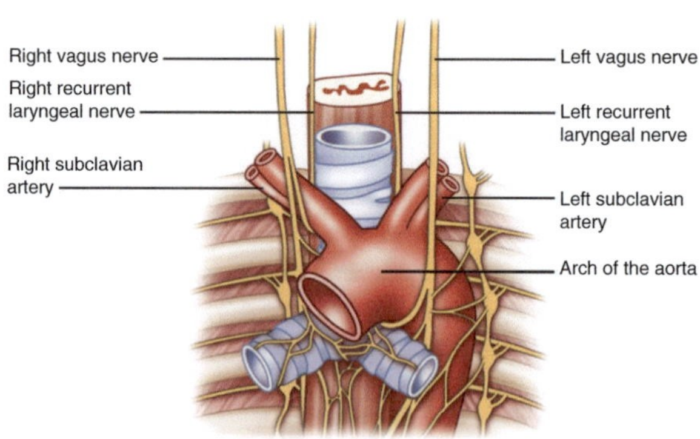

Fig. 14.5 Schematic illustration of the course of the recurrent laryngeal nerve. (Adapted from Daly [31]. With permission from Springer-Verlag)

(Fig. 14.6c). The uninjured side abducts and adducts normally. A total transection of a unilateral recurrent laryngeal nerve will result in no vocal cord movement on the injured side, and the injured vocal cord is fixed in the cadaveric 45° position (Fig. 14.6b) [31].

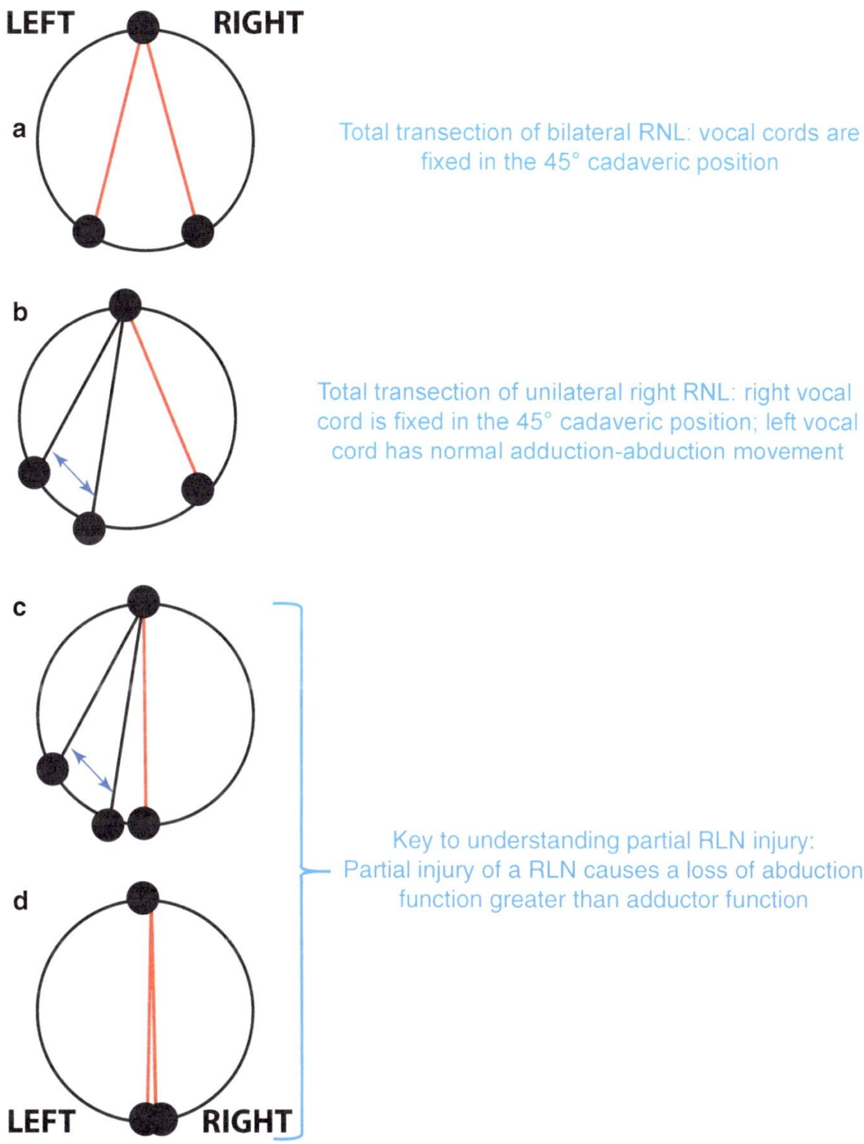

Fig. 14.6 Various types of recurrent laryngeal nerve injury. (**a**) Total transection of bilateral recurrent laryngeal nerves. (**b**) Total transection of unilateral recurrent laryngeal nerve. (**c**) Partial injury of unilateral recurrent laryngeal nerve. (**d**) Partial injury of bilateral recurrent laryngeal nerves. Red line indicates vocal cord with nerve injury. Black line indicates vocal cord without nerve injury. The blue arrows show movement of uninjured vocal cord. (Adapted from Daly [31]. With permission from Springer-Verlag)

Lesson 4-B: How Does a Bilateral Recurrent Laryngeal Nerve Injury Present?

A partial injury of bilateral recurrent laryngeal nerves will result in no movement of both vocal cords, and both sides are in adduction toward the midline (Fig. 14.6d). A bilateral recurrent laryngeal nerve injury presents immediately after extubation as biphasic stridor, respiratory distress, or both [24]. A complete transection of bilateral recurrent laryngeal nerves will result in no vocal cord movement; both vocal cords are fixed in the cadaveric 45° position (Fig. 14.6a) [31]. The diagnostic procedures for bilateral injury are identical to the ones described in Lesson 4-A.

References

1. Rosenblatt WH, Sukupragarn W. Airway management. In: Barash PG, editor. Clinical anesthesia. 7th ed. Philadelphia: Wolters Kluwer Health/Lippincott Williams & Wilkins; 2013. p. 762–99.
2. Ferson DZ, Brain AIJ. Chapter 21: Laryngeal mask airway. In: Hagberg CA, editor. Benumof's airway management. 2nd ed. Philadelphia: Mosby; 2007. p. 476–501.
3. Wakeling HG, Butler PJ, Baxter PJ. The laryngeal mask airway: a comparison between two insertion techniques. Anesth Analg. 1997;85:687–90.
4. Dingley J, Whitehead MJ, Wareham K. A comparative study of the incidence of sore throat with the laryngeal mask airway. Anaesthesia. 2007;49:251–4.
5. Emmett SR, Lloyd SD, Johnston MN. Uvular trauma from a laryngeal mask. Br J Anaesth. 2012;109:468–9.
6. Grady Deirdre M, McHardy F, Wong J, Jin F, Tong D, Chung F. Pharyngolaryngeal morbidity with the laryngeal mask airway in spontaneously breathing patients: does size matter? Anesthesiology. 2001;94:760–6.
7. Brimacombe JR. Problems laryngeal mask anesthesia: principles and practice. 2nd ed. London: Saunders; 2005. p. 552–76.
8. Brimacombe J, Clarke G, Keller C. Lingual nerve injury associated with the ProSeal laryngeal mask airway: a case report and review of the literature. Br J Anaesth. 2005;95:420–3.
9. Hanumanthaiah D, Masud S, Ranganath A. Inferior alveolar nerve injury with laryngeal mask airway: a case report. J Med Case Rep. 2011;5:122.
10. Thiruvenkatarajan V, Van Wijk RM, Rajbhoj A. Cranial nerve injuries with supraglottic airway devices: a systematic review of published case reports and series. Anaesthesia. 2015;70:344–59.
11. Burgard G, Möllhoff T, Prien T. The effect of laryngeal mask cuff pressure on postoperative sore throat incidence. J Clin Anesth. 1996;8:198–201.
12. Keller C, Brimacombe J. Pharyngeal mucosal pressures, airway sealing pressures, and fiberoptic position with the intubating versus the standard laryngeal mask airway. Anesthesiology. 1999;90:1001–6.
13. Eschertzhuber S, Brimacombe J, Hohlrieder M, Keller C. The laryngeal mask airway Supreme – a single use laryngeal mask airway with an oesophageal vent. A randomised, cross-over study with the laryngeal mask airway ProSeal in paralysed, anaesthetised patients. Anaesthesia. 2009;64:79–83.
14. Zhang L, Seet E, Mehta V, Subramanyam R, Ankichetty S, Wong D, Chung F. Oropharyngeal leak pressure with the laryngeal mask airway Supreme™ at different intracuff pressures: a randomized controlled trial. Can J Anesth. 2011;58:624–9.

15. Brimacombe J, Keller C. A comparison of pharyngeal mucosal pressure and airway sealing pressure with the laryngeal mask airway in anesthetized adult patients. Anesth Analg. 1998;87:1379–82.
16. Reed I, Walker E, Oliver Rose B. An implementation program targeted at non-physician, anaesthesia assistants improves the quality of laryngeal mask anaesthesia. BMJ Qual Improv Rep. 2014;2:1–4.
17. Seet E, Yousaf F, Gupta S, Subramanyam R, Wong DT, Chung F. Use of manometry for laryngeal mask airway reduces postoperative pharyngolaryngeal adverse events: a prospective, randomized trial. Anesthesiology. 2010;112:652–7.
18. Asai T, Howell TK, Koga K, Morris S. Appropriate size and inflation of the laryngeal mask airway. Br J Anaesth. 1998;80:470–4.
19. Brain AJ. The intavent laryngeal mask instruction manual. Henley-on-Thames: Intavent International; 1991. p. 7–16.
20. Takahoko K, Iwasaki H, Sasakawa T, Suzuki A, Matsumoto H, Iwasaki H. Unilateral hypoglossal nerve palsy after use of the laryngeal mask airway supreme. Case Rep Anesthesiol. 2014;2014:4.
21. Brimacombe J, Berry A. Laryngeal mask airway cuff pressure and position during anaesthesia lasting 1 to 2 hours. Can J Anaesth. 1994;41:589–93.
22. Brimacombe J, Keller C, Morris R, Mecklem D. A comparison of the disposable versus the reusable laryngeal mask airway in paralyzed adult patients. Anesth Analg. 1998;87:921–4.
23. Edwards ND. Lignocaine gel and the laryngeal mask airway. Anaesthesia. 1995;50:746–7.
24. Inomata S, Nishikawa T, Suga A, Yamashita S. Transient bilateral vocal cord paralysis after insertion of a laryngeal mask airway. Anesthesiology. 1995;82:787–8.
25. King C, Street MK. Twelfth cranial nerve paralysis following use of a laryngeal mask airway. Anaesthesia. 1994;49:786–7.
26. Piagkou M, Demesticha T, Piagkos G, Georgios A, Panagiotis S. Lingual nerve entrapment in muscular and osseous structures. Int J Oral Sci. 2010;2:181–9.
27. McManus LJ, Dawes PJ, Stringer MD. Clinical anatomy of the chorda tympani: a systematic review. J Laryngol Otol. 2011;125:1101–8.
28. Goodwin WJ Jr, Arnold D, Wachholz J. Surgical anatomy of the glossopharyngeal nerve. Laryngoscope. 1993;103:1302–4.
29. Sakorafas GH, Kokoropoulos P, Lappas C, Sampanis D, Smyrniotis V. External branch of the superior laryngeal nerve: applied surgical anatomy and implications in thyroid surgery. Am Surg. 2012;78:986–91.
30. Haller JM, Iwanik M, Shen FH. Clinically relevant anatomy of recurrent laryngeal nerve. Spine. 2012;37:97–100.
31. Daly SC. Possible recurrent laryngeal nerve injury. In: Benumof JL, editor. Clinical anesthesiology. 1st ed. New York: Springer; 2014. p. 81–3.
32. Chan TV, Grillone G. Vocal cord paralysis after laryngeal mask airway ventilation. Laryngoscope. 2005;115:1436–9.
33. Drake R, Vogl AW, AWM M, editors. Gray's anatomy for student's. 3rd ed. Philadelphia: Churchill Livingstone; 2014.
34. Brown DL. Airway block anatomy. In: Brown DL, editor. Atlas of regional anesthesia. 4th ed. Philadelphia: Saunders; 2010. p. 191–6.

Chapter 15
Management of Local Anesthetic Systemic Toxicity (LAST)

Preetham J. Suresh

A 70 kg otherwise healthy 32-year-old G4P0 at 22 weeks of gestation who is status post a motor vehicle accident with multiple rib fractures, L2 and L3 burst fractures, and an open right distal tibia and fibular fracture is scheduled for an open reduction and internal fixation of her right leg. The patient is very worried about general anesthesia given her prior miscarriages. Because of her strong preference for regional anesthesia and concern with performing a neuraxial anesthetic immediately after spinal trauma, peripheral nerve blocks were chosen as the anesthetic plan. Ultrasound-guided femoral and sciatic nerve blocks were performed using 25 cc of 2% lidocaine with epinephrine for the femoral and 20 cc of 2% lidocaine with epinephrine for the sciatic done in the popliteal fossa.

Approximately 10 min after the second block is completed, the patient becomes very anxious, and she complains that her tongue and lips are tingling (L1–22).

L-1. What Are the Symptoms of LAST, and How Do They Correlate with Plasma Concentrations?

Older studies suggest a biphasic sequence of symptoms for both central nervous system (CNS) and cardiovascular system (CVS) toxicity. Typically, there is CNS stimulation followed by depression and CVS stimulation followed by collapse (Fig. 15.1).

This relationship is based on data from volunteers who were given infusions of local anesthetics and monitored for symptoms [1, 2]. Five volunteers got infusions of intravenous bupivacaine at 10 mg/min until 125 mg was given or symptoms were severe enough to stop the infusion. One week later, they received lidocaine at 20 mg/min until 250 mg was given. This was compared to symptoms using etidocaine.

P. J. Suresh (✉)
Department of Anesthesiology, University of California, San Diego, CA, USA
e-mail: pjsuresh@ucsd.edu

J. L. Benumof, G. R. Manecke (eds.), *Clinical Anesthesiology II*,
https://doi.org/10.1007/978-3-030-12365-9_15

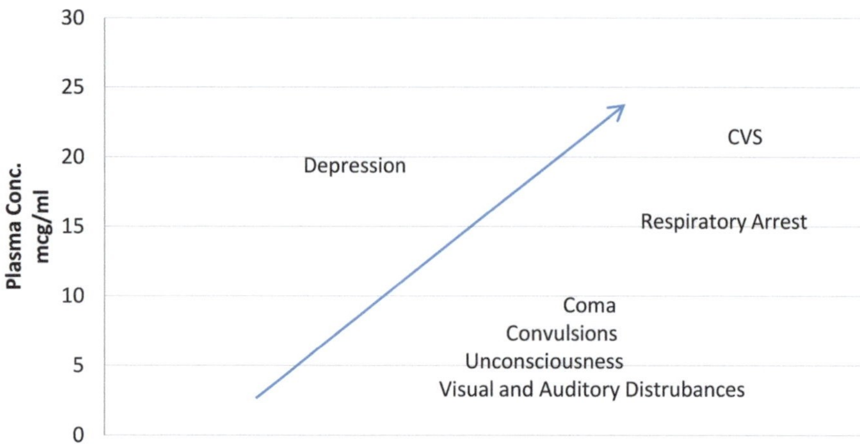

Fig. 15.1 Relationship of signs and symptoms of local anesthetic toxicity to plasma concentrations of lidocaine. (Based on data from Refs. [1, 2])

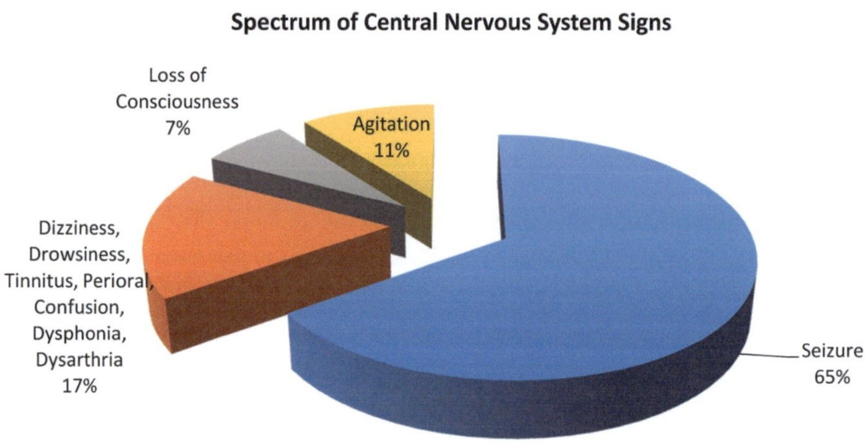

Fig. 15.2 The range of presenting CNS symptoms in confirmed cases of LAST. (Adapted from Di Gregorio et al. [3]. With permission from Wolters Kluwer Health, Inc.) [5]

The first finding is the local effect on the tongue and mouth from the local anesthetic (LA) leaving the vascular space and anesthetizing the nerve endings causing tongue or perioral numbness. Following this, neuroexcitatory symptoms were seen due to blocking inhibitory pathways followed by neurodepression due to blockage of inhibitory and facilitatory pathway. CVS effects have a similar excitatory effect with hypertension and tachycardia, followed by myocardial depression and decreased cardiac output.

In situations where large doses or rapid injections are given, this gradual progression of symptoms is less likely as evidenced by more recent data describing the presenting symptoms in known LAST cases (see Figs. 15.2 and 15.3) [3]. Rather than seeing the gradual onset of symptoms described in the controlled setting, patients may present with symptoms such as seizure loss of consciousness [4].

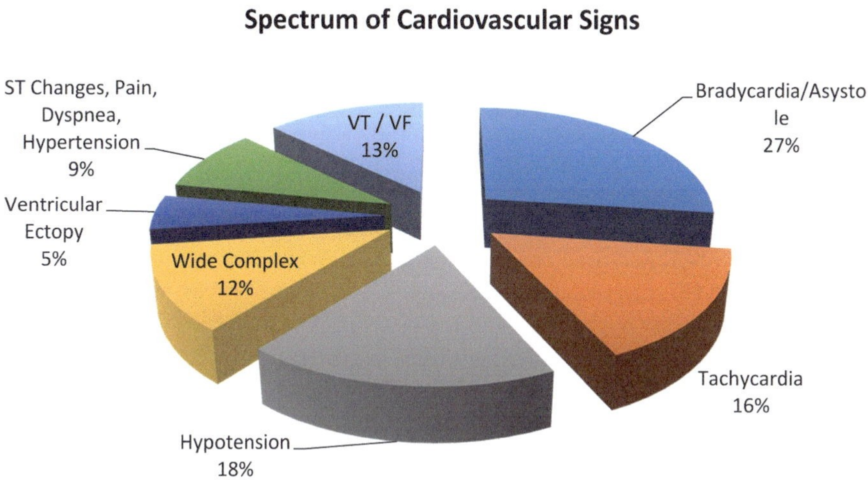

Fig. 15.3 Spectrum of presenting cardiovascular symptoms in confirmed cases of LAST. (Adapted from Di Gregorio et al. [3]. With permission from Wolters Kluwer Health, Inc.) [5]

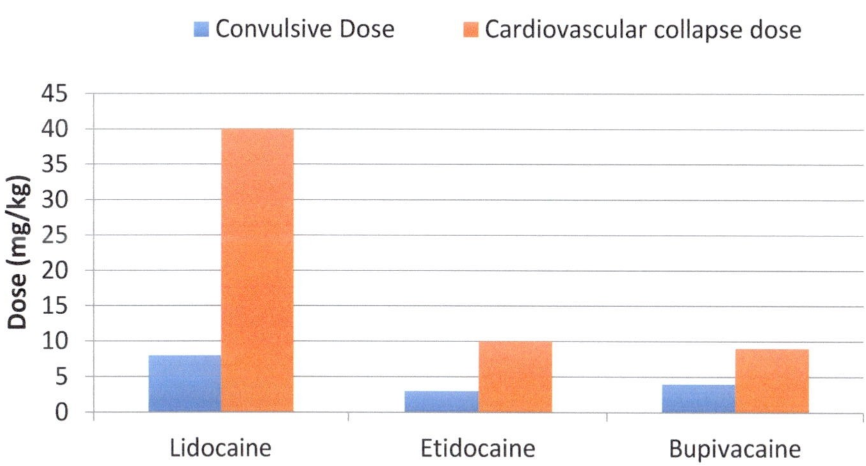

Fig. 15.4 Relative toxic doses to cause convulsions versus cardiovascular collapse of three different local anesthetics. (Reprinted from Rogers et al. [7]. With permission from Elsevier)

L-2. In the Presence of CNS Symptoms with Lidocaine, What Is the Likelihood of Impending Cardiac Instability?

The likelihood of CVS instability from LAST depends on the local anesthetic used. With lidocaine, the dose at which CVS symptoms are seen is approximately four times the dose required to generate CNS symptoms. For the more potent lipophilic local anesthetics like bupivacaine, the dose to generate CVS collapse is much closer to the one required for CNS toxicity and convulsions (see Fig. 15.4) [6].

L-3. If There Is CV Instability with Lidocaine, What Is the Likelihood of a Successful Resuscitation?

The rate of successful resuscitation in dogs after cardiovascular collapse from intravenous infusions of lidocaine, bupivacaine, levobupivacaine, and ropivacaine was evaluated [8, 9]. Success rates (see Fig. 15.5) were greater for resuscitations from lidocaine (100%), than ropivacaine (90%), than levobupivacaine (70%), and than bupivacaine (50%). Required doses to induce cardiovascular collapse were greater for lidocaine (127 mg/kg), than ropivacaine (42 mg/kg), than levobupivacaine (27 mg/kg), and than bupivacaine (22 mg/kg). From this data we can see that the dose required to generate CVS toxicity from lidocaine is extremely high, and if it were to occur, the likelihood of a successful resuscitation is also high.

L-4. Your Colleague Suggests Giving Lipid Emulsion, How Does Lipid Emulsion Work?

The understanding of the mechanism for how a lipid emulsion works for LAST has evolved from a static lipid sink and metabolic substrate hypothesis [10] to one that involves dynamic shuttling, hemodynamic, and postconditioning effects [11]. The lipid shuttle allows for local anesthetics to be transferred from highly vascular organs like the brain and heart that are sensitive to local anesthetics to the muscle and liver for storage and metabolism. The metabolic mechanism suggests that the lipid emulsion provides the fatty acid substrate required from ATP generation by the mitochondria. The theory is based on the fact that local anesthetics inhibit carnitine-acylcarnitine translocase (CAT). CAT is the intracellular enzyme responsible for the transfer of long-chain fatty acids into mitochondria for ATP production (see Fig. 15.6). The theory is that the enzymatic inhibition by local anesthetics is overwhelmed by the massive amounts of fatty acids allowing ATP production to resume. This is supported by evidence from a patient with carnitine deficiency who was particularly sensitive to developing arrhythmias with low-dose bupivacaine. Additionally, lipid emulsion improves contractility in a rat model of LAST and a canine model of myocardial stunning. Additionally, lipid has been shown

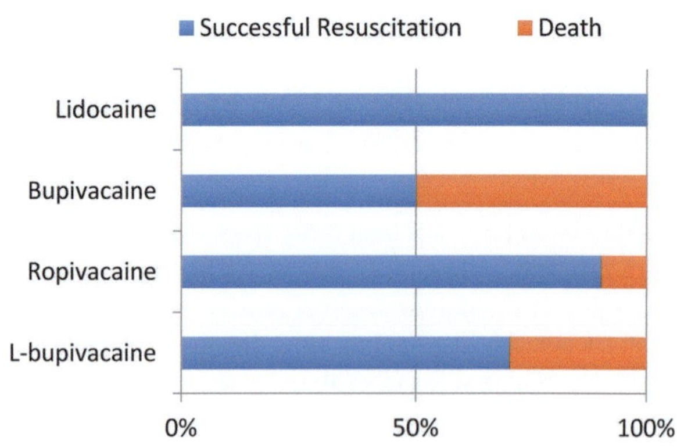

Fig. 15.5 Likelihood of death vs. successful resuscitation after various local anesthetics in dogs. (Based on data from Refs. [9, 10])

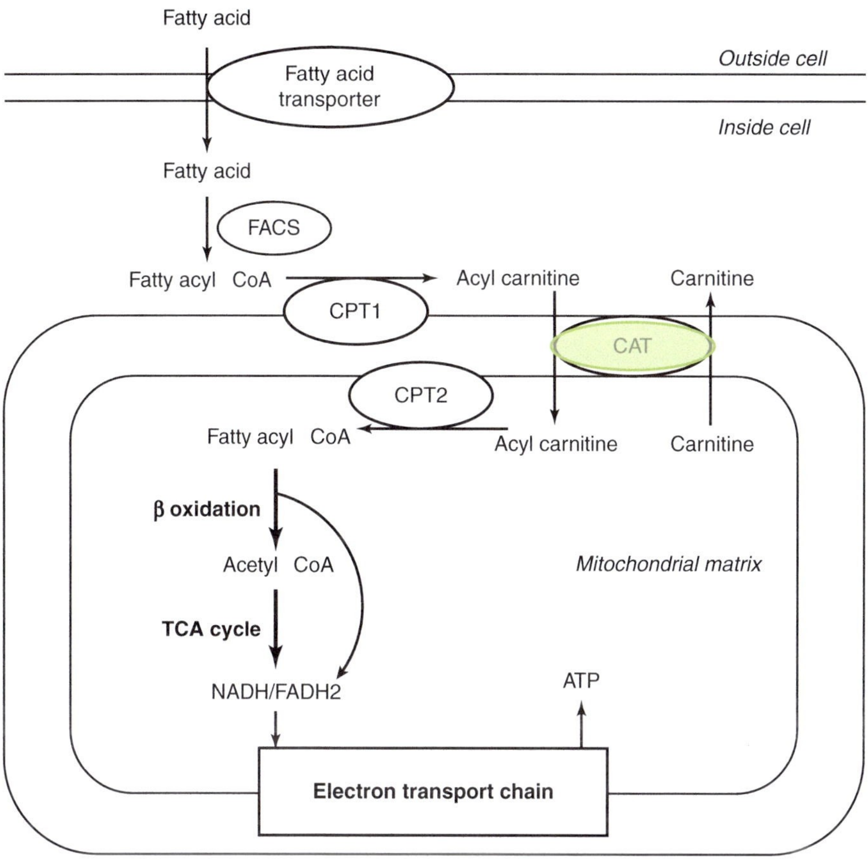

Fig. 15.6 The steps required for a fatty acid to get into the mitochondria and be utilized to generate ATP via the electron transport chain. *FACS* fatty acyl CoA synthetase, *CPT1* carnitine palmitoyltransferase 1, *CPT 2* carnitine palmitoyltransferase 2, *CAT* carnitine acyltransferase, *TCA* the citric acid cycle

to reduce myocardial ischemia-reperfusion injury and may also be acting in this way during treatment of LAST. Using mathematical computer modeling, the need for the additional factors impacting recorvery were identified. The beneficial effects of lipid infusion via volume expansion and improved cardiac performance help satisfy the model [11].

L-5. What Physiochemical Property of the Local Anesthetic Will Predict the Utility of Lipid Emulsion in LAST?

Lipid solubility is the primary determinant of a local anesthetic getting absorbed by an infusion of lipid emulsion. Lipid solubility is secondary to the carbon groups on the benzene ring (see Fig. 15.7). The more lipid soluble a local anesthetic is, the

Fig. 15.7 Comparison of amide and ester local anesthetics. The chemical structure of the local anesthetics determines its class (amide or ester) and its physiochemical properties like lipophilicity and pKa. The lipophilicity comes from the benzene ring at one end, and the pKa is related to the amine group at the other

Amide		Ester
Dibucaine Lidocaine Mepivicaine Prilocaine Bupivicaine Ropivicaine		Benzocaine Cocaine Procaine (Novocain) Tetracaine Chloroprocaine
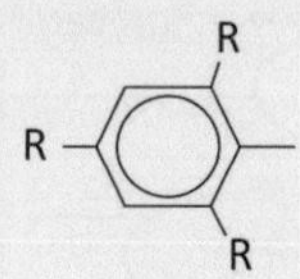	Ester: -C(=O)-O-C- Amide: -NH-C(=O)-C-	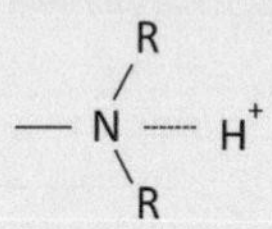
Lipophilicity	Intermediate linkage	pKa

Table 15.1 Table of chemical properties of various local anesthetics

	pKa	% unionized @ pH 7.4	Onset (fast or slow)	Typical conc (%)	Lipid solubility	Protein binding (%)
Mepivacaine	7.7	33	Fast	1.5	130	77
Lidocaine	7.8	28	Fast	1	366	64
Ropivacaine	8.1	17	Slow	0.5	775	94
Bupivacaine	8.1	17	Slow	0.25	3420	95
Tetracaine	8.4	9	Slow	0.2	5822	93

As lipid solubility increases reflecting an increase in potency, the concentrations needed in clinical use decrease

more easily it can cross through a neural membrane allowing it to be more potent. This is reflected by more lipid-soluble local anesthetics being used at lower concentrations than the less potent ones. See Table 15.1 for relative lipid solubilities measured in octanol/water binding coefficients.

L-6. What Is the Likelihood That Lipid Emulsion Will Work on Less Lipid-Soluble Local Anesthetics?

In vitro studies have revealed that local anesthetics will inhibit the flow of a current across a membrane by inhibiting a voltage-gated proton pumps. When exposed to lipid emulsion, this effect is blocked for bupivacaine but not significantly for lidocaine [12]. Similarly, when rat hearts were pretreated with lipid emulsion (0.25 ml/kg/min × 10 min) prior to the administration of bupivacaine, the onset of asystole was delayed. No such beneficial effects were seen in preventing mepivacaine-induced cardiotoxicity, and the recovery period was prolonged in the rats that got lipid emulsion [13]. This would suggest that lipid emulsion was actually detrimental to the resuscitative efforts from mepivacaine.

Furthermore an earlier study from the same group showed that lipid emulsion hastens the electrical and hemodynamic recovery of isolated rat hearts from bupivacaine but not for ropivacaine or mepivacaine [14]. Despite the lack of experimental evidence supporting the use of lipid emulsion for the resuscitation from less lipophilic local anesthetics and animal data to suggest potential for harm, there are several case reports and anecdotes on the lipidrescue.org supporting its success and encouraging its use.

L-7. Despite the Lack of Evidence Supporting Lipid Emulsion Therapy in the Context of Lidocaine Toxicity, Are There Any Risks of Giving Lipid Emulsion to the Mother?

There have been no reported adverse effects from giving lipid emulsion for clinical treatment of LAST. Most risks associated with lipid emulsion are from long-term use except anaphylaxis, which can occur acutely [15, 16]. In rats, the LD50 for lipid emulsion was 68 ml/kg which was approximately three times the therapeutic dose [17]. The plasma triglycerides were noted to be elevated for less than 48 h, and there was a subsequent increase in amylase 1816–2804 U/L (40–140 U/L) and AST 45–284 U/L (8–35 U/L). The histologic appearance of the brain, heart, pancreas, and kidneys was all normal. The lung had thickening of the alveolar septae and a few intra-alveolar foamy histiocytes at 60 ml/kg and hemorrhagic vascular congestion at 80 ml/kg. There was also a dose-related finding of hepatic microvascular steatosis with extensive necrosis at the highest dose.

It has been suggested that other possible consequences of high-dose lipid emulsion may be extrapolated from findings associated with the use of lipid infusion for nutrition [16]. Of note, the typical duration of exposure is much longer when used for nutritional purposes than for toxicity treatment, but the peak dosing is less. For example, the dosing for infants who had received TPN and had histopathologic evidence of pulmonary fat embolism is shown in Table 15.2 [19].

Table 15.2 Patient data for cases of pulmonary fat embolism after infusion of lipid emulsion [18]

	Case 1	Case 2	Case 3	Case 4
Body weight (kg)	1.65	1.48	2.76	3.13
Mean rate (ml/kg/h)	0.7	0.75	0.4	0.6
Max rate (ml/kg/h)	0.9	1.05	2.55	3.5
Total duration (days)	11	14	12	18

Adapted from Barson et al. [19]. With permission from BMJ Publishing Group Ltd

The max hourly rate given to the infants is less than the max dose recommended for the first 30 min in LAST of 10 ml/kg, but the cumulative dose given over the course of several days far exceeds the LAST doses

Another consideration when giving a large dose of lipid emulsion is allergic reaction. Lipid emulsion contains soybean oil 20% = 200 mg/ml (long-chain triglycerides), egg yolk-derived phosphatides 12 mg/ml, and glycerin 22 mg/ml. Phosphatides serve the purpose of emulsification or mixing of two immiscible materials. The phosphatide in lipid emulsion comes from egg lecithin. Typically, allergic individuals are sensitive to the glycoproteins in soy or egg white albumin and not to the lecithin. Regardless, there is a theoretical risk of protein contamination in the lipid and subsequent allergic reaction in a sensitive individual.

L-8. What Factors Affect Whether Local Anesthetics Will Cross the Placenta?

Local anesthetics cross the placenta by simple diffusion, not active transport or pinocytosis. The factors that affect how much crosses are protein binding, lipid solubility, maternal plasma concentration, maternal pH, and fetal pH [18]. At equilibrium the fetal/maternal ratio is approximately 0.3 for bupivacaine and 0.6 for lidocaine. However, the lower fetal concentrations of plasma proteins like $\alpha 1$ acid glycoprotein cause a higher fetal free fraction of drug and a similar concentration of drug capable of causing toxicity [20]. In the context of fetal acidosis, ion trapping can take place through protonation of the local anesthetic making it unable to diffuse back to the maternal circulation and eventual accumulation on the fetal side [21].

L-9. Are There Any Risks to the Fetus in Utero by Giving the Mother Lipid Emulsion?

Triglycerides are too large to cross the placenta and are broken down by the placenta into fatty acids, which do cross. There is currently only one report in the literature of giving lipid emulsion for LAST in pregnancy, and it worked effectively without any known negative effects [22]. That case was an 18-year-old G1P0, 86 kg at 38 weeks of gestation for induction of labor. The patient's blood pressure (BP) was 160/81 mmHg, and she had mild proteinuria with occasional fetal heart rate (FHR) decelerations. An epidural was placed, and negative test dose of 4 cc 2% lidocaine was administered. Six milliliters of 0.25% bupivacaine was given with good pain relief. Over the next 15 min, the BP increased to 172/114 mmHg and HR 86 bpm with pronounced FHR decelerations. After negative aspiration, 100 mcg fentanyl +10 cc of 0.5% bupivacaine is given via epidural in preparation for cesarean section (CS). Following injection the patient became restless and agitated and then began twitching and became unresponsive. Aspiration of catheter at that time was clearly positive for blood. At that time, two 50 cc boluses of 20% lipid emulsion were given, and the patient regained full consciousness, but there was ongoing fetal bradycardia. An emergency CS was performed under general anesthesia resulting in a delivery of a 6 lbs infant with APGAR scores of 0^1, 7^5, and 10^{10}. Both mother and baby were discharged home on POD#4 without complication.

With only one case report of its use in pregnancy, the potential fetal risks could be extrapolated from data on the use of total parenteral nutrition (TPN) in pregnancy [23]. TPN also contains 10–20% lipid solutions and has been evaluated in malnourished pregnant women who required TPN for a range of 14–220 days. In the study group of 26 women all with conditions significant enough to require TPN, 7 were delivered preterm without congenital malformations, and 1 psychiatric patient with diabetes who developed a hyperglycemic coma resulted in an intrauterine fetal demise (IUFD). In all patients there was ultrasound evidence of improved fetal growth after starting TPN [24].

In another study looking at the effect of TPN on the placenta in 20 women, all but one had a normal placenta. That patient received TPN for 8 weeks and had placental fat deposits noted prior to a 22 week IUFD [25].

There is data from the pediatric literature that administration of lipid emulsion to a newborn can result in pulmonary lipid emboli [26] and potentially an increase in pulmonary vascular resistance [27].

L-10. To Prevent the Progression of the CNS Symptoms to a Seizure, What Are the Options for Treatment?

The best option for treatment of LAST-induced seizure is midazolam. In the absence of immediate access to midazolam, propofol could be used while carefully considering its potential impact on the blood pressure. Please note, propofol can**not** be used as a lipid sink in place of a lipid emulsion. It contains 10% lipid so to give the equivalent amount of lipid as is recommended for the initial bolus to treat LAST (1.5 ml/kg of 20% lipid emulsion), one would be giving 200 ml of propofol at once (ten 20 ml syringes).

L-11. Why Is Prevention of a Seizure Important?

There can be rapid development of hypoxia and respiratory and metabolic acidosis during immediately after a seizure [28]. A clinical report of two cases of seizures from LAST where rapid blood gas values were obtained was published by Moore et al. [29]. In the first patient, 3 min after the first seizure, the blood gas was 7.09/59/33/17 (pH/pCO_2(mmHg)/PO_2(mmHg)/HCO_3(mEq/L). In the other patient, 1 min after the onset of the seizure, the blood gas was 6.99/76/87/17 (pH/pCO_2(mmHg)/PO_2(mmHg)/HCO_3(mEq/L). Between convulsions, attempts at ventilating both patients with 100% O_2 were being made.

These rapid rises in CO_2 are significantly faster than what had been reported in apneic awake or anesthetized patients where the expected rate of rise in the CO_2 is 13 mmHg in the first min and 6 mmHg/min after that [30].

L-12. What Effect Does Acidosis Have on Local Anesthetics?

Local anesthetics are weak bases and cross the lipid bilayer in the uncharged form (see Fig. 15.8). Once intracellular, they can become protonated depending on their pKa relative to the surrounding pH. Once protonated, they bind the intracellular portion of the Na channel to prevent depolarization and signal conduction along the nerve.

In the context of acidosis, the local anesthetics may be less likely to cross the membrane, but the ones that have will stay protonated and bound to the sodium channel.

L-13. Resuscitation Guidelines for LAST Emphasize the Primacy of Oxygenation and Ventilation. Is There Evidence to Support that Hypoxia and Acidosis Is Especially Harmful in the Recovery from LAST?

A study that sheds light on this took ewes, performed a tracheostomy, and invasively monitored electrocardiograms, encephaloelectrogram, and arterial pressure [31].

They then received either lidocaine at low (5.7 mg/kg) or high doses (11.4 mg/kg) or bupivacaine at low (2.1 mg/kg) or high doses (4.2 mg/kg).

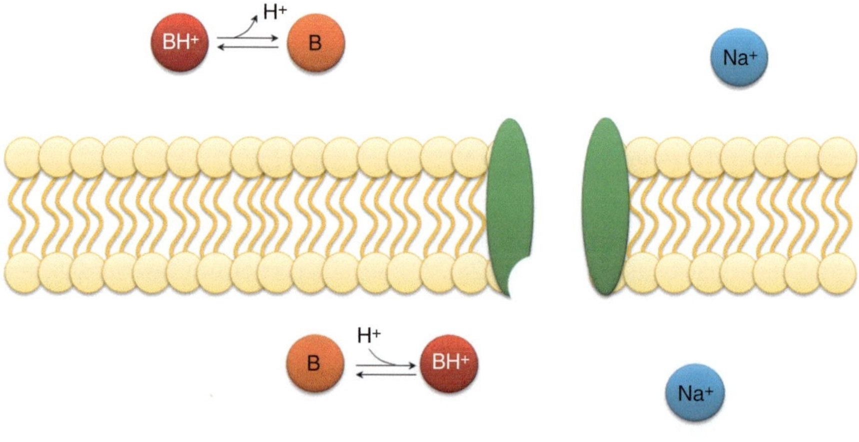

Fig. 15.8 Steps required for a local anesthetic (B) to give up a proton (H+) and cross the lipid bilayer to get the site of action at the intracellular portion of the sodium channel

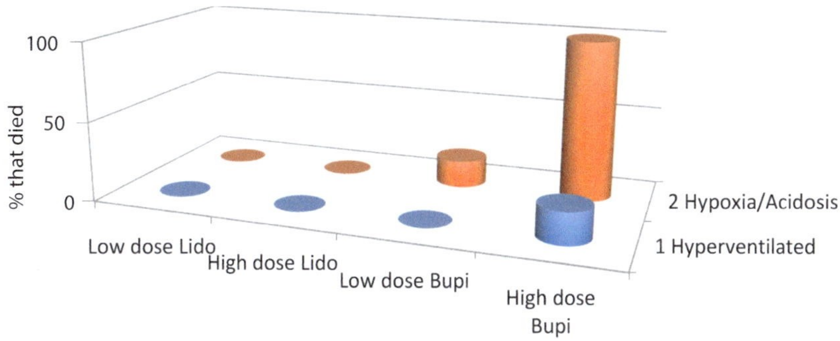

Fig. 15.9 Survival rates of sheep after LAST in the context of the sheep that spontaneously hyperventilated vs. the ones with induced hypoxia (PO_2 50 mmHg) and acidosis (pH 7.15 and CO_2 85 mmHg). (Based on data from Refs. [31, 32])

Their findings showed that the ewes spontaneously hyperventilated during a LAST-induced seizure and maintained pH > 7.35 and all survived. In a subsequent study, the investigators induced hypoxia and a respiratory acidosis by ventilating with CO_2 until the pH was 7.15, the PO_2 was 50 mmHg, and the CO_2 was 85 mmHg. They then administered one of the four local anesthetic regimens listed above [32].

In contrast to the hyperventilating sheep, they found that all of the acidotic and hypoxic ones in high-dose bupivacaine group died (see Fig. 15.9).

L-14. For This Patient, Who Got Lidocaine Alone and Showed Early Signs of CNS Toxicity, Would You Give Any Medications to Treat Her?

The priorities in management are first to ensure oxygenation and ventilation and second to prevent the seizure. Given the potential for cardiac depression from propofol, midazolam would be a preferable option for treating seizures from LAST. If midazolam was not immediately available, judicious use of propofol would also be a reasonable option.

L-15. Take the Same Scenario, and Let's Assume She Got Her Peripheral Nerve Injections with 0.5% Bupivacaine (Instead of Lidocaine) and She Developed the Same CNS Symptoms. Would You Treat? With What?

In the presence of neurological symptoms from a lipid-soluble local anesthetic that causes cardiotoxicity and CNS toxicity at similar doses, it would be appropriate to move rapidly to lipid emulsion to prevent the progression of symptoms.

L-16. What Is the Evidence that Lipid Emulsion Works?

The initial report by Dr. Guy Weinberg in 1998 described an incidental discovery that a lipid infusion significantly increased the LD50 of bupivacaine in rats [33]. Subsequently, the findings have been confirmed in other animal models and supported by multiple clinical reports of its use during resuscitation from LAST and other lipid-soluble drug overdoses. As a result, it has been adopted into the resuscitation guidelines by multiple professional societies including the American Society for Regional Anesthesia guidelines published in 2010 with revisions in 2012 and 2018. This widespread acceptance has preceded full understanding of the mechanism of action(s) or its specific indications. The rapid expansion of its use has been hastened from additional research from Dr. Weinberg's group and others cautioning against the use of what would otherwise be the drugs of choice during resuscitation like epinephrine and vasopressin.

L-17. What Is the Dose of Lipid Emulsion?

The dose of 20% lipid emulsion is as follows for a patient below 70 kg: First, bolus 1.5 ml/kg over 2–3 min, and then repeat after 5 min. Second, infuse 0.25 mg/kg/min or 15 ml/kg/h. Third, stop infusion after CVS stability has been present for more than 10 min. Fourth, keep dose less than 10 ml/kg in the first 30 min. For a patient above 70 kg: First, bolus 100 mL over 2–3 min. Second, infuse 200–250 mL over 15–20 min.

L-18. This Patient Was Supposed to Go Home After Their Procedure, Would You Still Send Them Home? Would You Still Do the Procedure?

The recommendation from the Checklist for Treatment of LAST [34] is to monitor for at least 4–6 h after a cardiovascular event or at least 2 hours after an isolated neurological event. The decision to proceed with the case should be based on the severity of the reaction and the magnitude of treatment that was required. If there was accompanying hemodynamic instability, it seems prudent to avoid further complicating the situation by proceeding with surgery.

L-19. Is Using a Checklist Effective?

Trainees who used the ASRA checklist for management of LAST were twice as likely to complete medical management steps correctly [35]. Of note, of the trainees using the checklist, 40% only partially used it. It is recommended to have a copy of a LAST treatment along with lipid emulsion immediately available in any area where local anesthetics are given in significant doses.

L-20. Can We Follow Standard ACLS Protocols? What Aspects Are the Same/Different?

As with ACLS, the LAST management algorithm starts with airway management with the goal of avoiding hypoxia and acidosis. There are subsequent steps and considerations that deviate from standard ACLS and are unique to the management of LAST (Table 15.3).

Table 15.3 Recommendations for treatment of LAST

If signs and symptoms of LAST occur, prompt and effective airway management is crucial to preventing hypoxia, hypercapnia, and acidosis, which are known to potentiate LAST. (I; B)
Lipid emulsion therapy *(I; B)*:
Administer at the first signs of LAST, after airway management
Timeliness of lipid emulsion is more important than the order of administration modality (bolus vs. *infusion)*
20% lipid emulsion BOLUS
100 mL over 2–3 min if patient is over 70 kg
1.5 mL/kg over 2–3 min if patient is less than 70 kg
20% lipid emulsion INFUSION
200–250 mL over 15–20 min if patient is over 70 kg
0.25 mL/kg/min if patient is less than 70 kg (ideal body weight)
If circulatory stability is not attained, consider rebolus or increasing infusion to 0.5 mL/kg/min
Continue infusion for at least 10 min after circulatory stability is attained
Approximately, *12 mL/kg* lipid emulsion is recommended as the upper limit for initial dosing *(IIb; B)*
Propofol is not a substitute for lipid emulsion (*III. B*)
Seizure control:
If seizures occur, they should be rapidly halted with benzodiazepines. If benzodiazepines are not readily available, *lipid emulsion* or small doses of propofol are acceptable (I; B)
Although propofol can stop seizures, large doses further depress cardiac function; propofol should be avoided when there are signs of cardiovascular compromise (III; B)
If seizures persist despite benzodiazepines, small doses of succinylcholine or similar neuromuscular blocker should be considered to minimize acidosis and hypoxemia (I; C)
If cardiac arrest occurs:
If epinephrine is used, small initial doses (≤1 μg/kg) are preferred (*IIa: B*)
Vasopressin is not recommended (III; B)
Avoid calcium channel blockers and β-adrenergic receptor blockers (III; C)
If ventricular arrhythmias develop, amiodarone is preferred (IIa: B): treatment with local anesthetics (lidocaine or procainamide) is not recommended (III: *B*)
Failure to respond to lipid emulsion and vasopressor therapy should prompt institution of CPB (*I*; *B*). Because there can be considerable lag in beginning CPB, it is reasonable to notify the closest facility capable of providing it when cardiovascular compromise is first identified during an episode of LAST

(continued)

Table 15.3 (continued)

Patients with a significant CV event should be monitored for at least 4–6 h. If the event is limited to CNS symptoms that resolve quickly, they should be monitored for at least 2 h (IIa; B)
Use written or electronic checklists as cognitive aids during the management of LAST. A dedicated reader improves adherence to the checklist (I; A)

These recommendations are intended to encourage optimal patient care but cannot ensure the avoidance of adverse outcomes. As with any practice advisory recommendation, these are subject to revision as knowledge advances regarding specific complications
The class of recommendation and level of evidence for each intervention are given in parenthesis (see Table 1)
Changes from the 2010 LAST practice advisory [42] are italicized
CPB indicates cardiopulmonary bypass

L-21. Why Is the Dose of Epinephrine Reduced?

This is based primarily on animal studies that revealed that lower doses of epinephrine (1–2 mcg/kg) were associated with better metabolic and hemodynamic profiles after resuscitation from LAST than higher doses (10–25 mcg/kg) [36].

Lower doses of epinephrine resulted in a return of spontaneous circulation (ROSC) faster than with saline and allowed for maintenance of hemodynamics stability without the decompensation that was seen with higher doses of epinephrine.

It should be noted the studies that showed higher doses of epinephrine to be detrimental, gave a single high dose, and did not give subsequent vasopressors to support the hemodynamics. Also of note, there is animal data to show that in the context of hypoxia or compromised coronary perfusion and LAST, epinephrine is superior to lipid for resuscitation [38, 39].

L-22. Why Is Vasopressin Discouraged in Context of LAST?

In animal studies evaluating the use of vasopressors in resuscitation from LAST (20 mg/kg of bupivacaine), rats that got vasopressin (0.4 U/kg) or vasopressin and epinephrine (30 mcg/kg) developed "red-tinged" pulmonary edema and had a measurable increase in their wet/dry lung weight ratios [40]. Also of note, the resuscitations were less successful from a metabolic and hemodynamic perspective when compared to lipid emulsion alone. As a result, the resuscitation guidelines caution against its use because of these worse outcomes and the association with "pulmonary hemorrhage." In the paper that is referenced, however, the diagnosis of pulmonary hemorrhage is never used, but rather, the mice that received vasopressin were noted to have red-tinged pulmonary edema fluid in the expiratory limb of the breathing circuit.

Regardless, the worse outcomes with vasopressin are indirect contrast to a study done in pigs where resuscitation from LAST was more successful with vasopressin and epinephrine compared to lipid emulsion. These conflicting findings may be related to differences in experimental protocols. In the experiments with rats by Di Gregorio and Weinberg et al. [40], asystole occurred immediately with injection of 20 mg/kg of bupivacaine and CPR initiated without delay. In the study by Mayr et al. [41], a lower dose of 5 mg/kg was used and CPR was not initiated until approximately 3 min later during which time the pigs were apneic for all of that time and pulseless for 1 min. This study design was intended to more accurately reflect what would happen clinically in the context of seizure and a more realistic subsequent treatment time course.

References

1. Neal JM, Bernards CM, Butterworth JF, et al. ASRA practice advisory on local anesthetic systemic toxicity. Reg Anesth Pain Med. 2010;35:152–61.
2. Cousins MJ. Cousins & Bridenbaugh's neural blockade in clinical anesthesia and pain medicine. 4th ed. Philadelphia: Wolters Kluwer/Lippincott Williams & Wilkins; 2009.
3. Di Gregorio G, et al. Clinical presentation of local anesthetic systemic toxicity: a review of published cases, 1979 to 2009. Reg Anesth Pain Med. 2010;35(2):181–7.
4. Gitman M, Barrington MJ. Local anesthetic systemic toxicity. Reg Anesth Pain Med:1.
5. Neal JM, Barrington MJ, Fettiplace MR, Gitman M, Memtsoudis SG, Mörwald EE, Rubin DS, Weinberg G. The Third American Society of Regional Anesthesia and pain medicine practice advisory on local anesthetic systemic toxicity. Reg Anesth Pain Med. 43(2):113–23.
6. Finucane BT. Complications of regional anesthesia. 2nd ed. New York: Springer; 2007.
7. Rogers MC, Tinker IH, Covino BG, et al. Principles and practice of anesthesiology. Philadelphia: Mosby; 1993.
8. Groban L, et al. Cardiac resuscitation after incremental overdosage with lidocaine, bupivacaine, levobupivacaine, and ropivacaine in anesthetized dogs. Anesth Analg. 2001;92(1):37–43.
9. Barash PG. Clinical anesthesia. 6th ed. Philadelphia: Wolters Kluwer/Lippincott Williams & Wilkins; 2009.
10. Garrett R, Kaura V, Kathawaroo S. Intravenous lipid emulsion therapy–the fat of the land. Trends Anaesthesia Crit Care. 2013;3(6):336–41.
11. Fettiplace MR, Weinberg G. The mechanisms underlying lipid resuscitation therapy. Reg Anesth Pain Med. 43(2):138–49.
12. Hori K, et al. The effect of lipid emulsion on intracellular bupivacaine as a mechanism of lipid resuscitation: an electrophysiological study using voltage-gated proton channels. Anesth Analg. 2013;117(6):1293–301.
13. Aumeier C, Kasdorf B, Gruber M, Busse H, Wiese CH, Zink W, et al. Lipid emulsion pretreatment has different effects on mepivacaine and bupivacaine cardiac toxicity in an isolated rat heart model. Br J Anaesth. 2014;112(4):735–41.
14. Zausig YA, Zink W, Keil M, Sinner B, Barwing J, Wiese CH, et al. Lipid emulsion improves recovery from bupivacaine-induced cardiac arrest, but not from ropivacaine- or mepivacaine-induced cardiac arrest. Anesth Analg. 2009;109(4):1323–6.
15. Brull SJ. Lipid emulsion for the treatment of local anesthetic toxicity: patient safety implications. Anesth Analg. 2008;106(5):1337–9.
16. Mirtallo JM, et al. State of the art review: intravenous fat emulsions: current applications, safety profile, and clinical implications. Ann Pharmacother. 2010;44(4):688–700.
17. Hiller DB, Di Gregorio G, Kelly K, Ripper R, Edelman L, Boumendjel R, et al. Safety of high volume lipid emulsion infusion: a first approximation of LD50 in rats. Reg Anesth Pain Med. 2010;35(2):140–4.
18. Hamshaw-Thomas A, Rogerson N, Reynolds F. Placental transfer of bupivacaine, pethidine and lignocaine in the rabbit. Effect of umbilical flow rate and protein content. BJOG Int J Obstet Gynaecol. 1985;92(7):706–13.

19. Barson AJ, Chistwick ML, Doig CM. Fat embolism in infancy after intravenous fat infusions. Arch Dis Child. 1978;53(3):218–23.
20. Kearns GL, Abdel-Rahman SM, Alander SW, et al. Developmental pharmacology: drug disposition, action, and therapy in infants and children. N Engl J Med. 2003;349(12):1157–67.
21. Miller RD. Miller's anesthesia. 7th ed. Philadelphia: Churchill Livingstone/Elsevier; 2010.
22. Spence AG. Lipid reversal of central nervous system symptoms of bupivacaine toxicity. Anesthesiology. 2007;1079(3):516–7.
23. Bern S, Weinberg G. Local anesthetic toxicity and lipid resuscitation in pregnancy. Curr Opin Anesthesiol. 2011;24(3):262–7.
24. Caruso A, et al. Pregnancy outcome and total parenteral nutrition in malnourished pregnant women. Fetal Diagn Ther. 1998;13(3):136–40.
25. Jasnosz KM, Pickeral JJ, Graner S. Fat deposits in the placenta following maternal total parenteral nutrition with intravenous lipid emulsion. Arch Pathol Lab Med. 1995;119(6):555–7.
26. Puntis JW, Rushton DI. Pulmonary intravascular lipid in neonatal necropsy specimens. Arch Dis Child. 1991;66(1):26–8.
27. Lloyd TR, Boucek MM. Effect of intralipid on the neonatal pulmonary bed: an echographic study. J Pediatr. 1986;108(1):130–3.
28. Weinberg GL. Treatment of local anesthetic systemic toxicity (LAST). Reg Anesth Pain Med. 2010;35(2):188–93.
29. Moore DC, Crawford RD, Scurlock JE. Severe hypoxia and acidosis following local anesthetic-induced convulsions. Anesthesiology. 1980;53(3):259–60.
30. Stock MC, Downs JB, McDonald JS, Silver MJ, McSweeney TD, Fairley DS. The carbon dioxide rate of rise in awake apneic humans. J Clin Anesth. 1988;1(2):96–103.
31. Kotelko DM, et al. Bupivacaine-induced cardiac arrhythmias in sheep. Anesthesiology. 1984;60:10–8.
32. Rosen MA, Thigpen JW, Shnider SM, Foutz SE, Levinson G, Koike M. Bupivacaine-induced cardiotoxicity in hypoxic and acidotic sheep. Anesth Analg. 1985;64(11):1089–96.
33. Weinberg GL, et al. Pretreatment or resuscitation with a lipid infusion shifts the dose-response to bupivacaine-induced asystole in rats. Anesthesiology. 1998;88(4):1071–5.
34. https://www.asra.com/advisory-guidelines/article/3/checklist-for-treatment-of-local-anesthetic-systemictoxicity
35. Neal JM, Hsiung RL, Mulroy MF, Halpern BB, Dragnich AD, Slee AE. ASRA checklist improves trainee performance during a simulated episode of local anesthetic systemic toxicity. Reg Anesth Pain Med. 2012;37(1):8–15.
36. Feinstein DL, et al. Resuscitation with lipid versus epinephrine in a rat model of bupivacaine overdose. Anesthesiology. 2008;108(5):907–13.
37. Neal JM, Mulroy MF, Weinberg GL. American Society of Regional Anesthesia and Pain Medicine checklist for managing local anesthetic systemic toxicity: 2012 version. Reg Anesth Pain Med. 2012;37(1):16–8.
38. Hicks SD, et al. Lipid emulsion combined with epinephrine and vasopressin does not improve survival in a swine model of bupivacaine-induced cardiac arrest. Anesthesiology. 2009;111(1):138–46.
39. Mayr VD, et al. A comparison of the combination of epinephrine and vasopressin with lipid emulsion in a porcine model of asphyxial cardiac arrest after intravenous injection of bupivacaine. Anesth Analg. 2008;106(5):1566–71.
40. Di Gregorio G, Schwartz D, Ripper R, Kelly K, Feinstein DL, Minshall RD, et al. Lipid emulsion is superior to vasopressin in a rodent model of resuscitation from toxin-induced cardiac arrest*. Crit Care Med. 2009;37(3):993–9.
41. Mayr VD, Mitterschiffthaler L, Neurauter A, Gritsch C, Wenzel V, Müller T, et al. A comparison of the combination of epinephrine and vasopressin with lipid emulsion in a porcine model of asphyxial cardiac arrest after intravenous injection of bupivacaine. Anesth Analg. 2008;106(5):1566–71.
42. Neal JM, et al. The third American Society of Regional Anesthesia and Pain Medicine practice advisory on local anesthetic systemic toxicity: executive summary 2017. Reg Anesth Pain Med. 2018;43(2):113–23.

Chapter 16
Pseudocholinesterase Deficiency in a Patient with Subglottic Stenosis

Lawrence Weinstein

Case Description

The patient is a 64-year-old, 68-kg woman with a past medical history significant for hypertension, hypothyroidism, and subglottic stenosis secondary to remote neck trauma 10 years prior to admission **(L-1, L-2)**. She underwent multiple procedures to treat the tracheal narrowing and at one time had a Montgomery T-tube **(L-3)**. The T-tube was removed about 5 years ago, and the patient last had a tracheal dilation 4 years ago. She presented to the pulmonology service with shortness of breath and increasing fatigue over the preceding 2 weeks **(L-4, L-5)**. A bronchoscopy demonstrated subglottic narrowing, and she was scheduled for a rigid bronchoscopy with dilation under general anesthesia **(L-6, L-7)**.

On the day of surgery, the patient's history and medications were reviewed. In addition to the above, her surgical history was notable for a hysteroscopy 2 years prior. The patient denied personal and family history of complications related to general anesthesia. Current medications included low-dose aspirin, levothyroxine, hydrochlorothiazide, and a multivitamin. Physical exam demonstrated normal, regular, heart sounds and clear lungs. Notably, there was stridor of the upper airway when the neck was auscultated. Airway assessment showed a Mallampati II score, full neck range of motion, 4–5 cm thyro-mental distance, and a good mouth opening. The patient's dentition was intact and solid. Preoperative EKG demonstrated normal sinus rhythm with no acute ST nor T wave changes, and laboratory values (complete blood count, basic chemistry, and liver function tests) were all within normal limits. The benefits and risks of general anesthesia were reviewed with the patient in the holding area. A plan for general anesthesia was discussed with the interventional pulmonologist, who estimated that the case duration would be 30–45 min.

L. Weinstein (✉)
Department of Anesthesiology, University of California, San Diego, CA, USA
e-mail: lsweinstein@ucsd.edu

J. L. Benumof, G. R. Manecke (eds.), *Clinical Anesthesiology II*,
https://doi.org/10.1007/978-3-030-12365-9_16

As premedication, the patient received midazolam 2 mg for anxiolysis. Upon arrival in the operating room, standard ASA monitors were placed. Baseline vital signs showed a normal sinus rhythm at 80 bpm, blood pressure of 115/64 mmHg, and oxygen saturation of 98% on room air. She was then preoxygenated for 3 min, and anesthesia was induced with fentanyl 100 mcg, lidocaine 80 mg, and propofol 200 mg. After demonstration of easy mask ventilation and four strong twitches with train-of-four stimulation of the right ulnar nerve, the patient was paralyzed with succinylcholine 100 mg (**L-8, L-9, L-10**). She was ventilated via mask until complete muscle relaxation was achieved, at which point the pulmonologist inserted a rigid bronchoscope into the trachea, and we hooked up the anesthesia circuit to the scope's side port to deliver positive pressure ventilation. Maintenance anesthesia was provided via infusion of propofol at 160 mcg/kg/min.

The surgery and anesthetic proceeded smoothly over the next 40 min. At the conclusion of the procedure, the rigid bronchoscope was removed, and the anesthesia team stopped the propofol infusion and resumed mask ventilation with an oral airway in place. At this point, the patient had four barely perceptible twitches with train-of-four stimulation of the ulnar nerve. After 15 more minutes, train-of-four stimulation showed four equal but significantly diminished twitches when compared with baseline twitch strength (**L-11**). The patient would open her eyes to command but had significantly reduced grip strength and could not lift her head off the bed (**L-12, L-13, L-14**). She was re-sedated with propofol 50 mg IV push, and a #3.5 laryngeal mask airway (LMA) was placed to provide pressure support ventilation. A propofol infusion was restarted at a rate of 75 mcg/kg/min, and the patient was transported to the postanesthesia care unit (PACU) with the LMA in place and hand ventilation via a Mapleson circuit connected to an oxygen tank with flows set to 8 l/min. Upon arrival in the PACU, the anesthesia team were met by a respiratory therapist with a ventilator, and the patient was placed on pressure support ventilation of 10 cm H_2O with PEEP of 5 cm H_2O on 50% oxygen. Vital signs were stable throughout transport and drop off in recovery. At the time of PACU report, blood pressure was 94/50, pulse 66, respiratory rate 18, and oxygen saturation 98%. The patient was still on pressure support ventilation with a propofol infusion for sedation and amnesia at this time.

Roughly 1 h later, the patient had recovered four full twitches with train-of-four stimulation and no fade on tetanus. Pressure support was weaned, and the patient breathed spontaneously. The propofol sedation was weaned, and the patient woke up, expressing desire to have the LMA removed by nodding when questioned. She was taking tidal volumes of 200–250 cc at a rate of 18 breaths/min and still exhibited reduced grip strength and an inability to sustain head lift for more than 2 s. The anesthesiologist administered midazolam 2 mg IV to prevent recall, and the propofol sedation and pressure support were restarted. From this point on, sedation was weaned every 20 min to assess grip strength. Ultimately, 150 min after arrival in the PACU, the patient demonstrated good grip strength and sustained head lift and was able to generate tidal volumes of 330–370 cc without support. The LMA was removed, and the patient was able to breathe well without evidence of weakness or airway obstruction. She remained in the recovery area for one more hour. Prior to discharge, the patient was counseled about the events of the anesthetic and the prolonged recovery following neuromuscular blockade with succinylcholine **(L-15, L-16)**. She was instructed to inform future anesthesia providers about the prolonged weakness after anesthesia and to obtain a test for pseudocholinesterase deficiency if possible **(L-17)**.

Several weeks later the anesthesia team received an email from the patient's primary care provider with the results of a pseudocholinesterase study. The total pseudocholinesterase level came back low at 1245 U/L (reference range 2900–7100 U/L). The finding provides evidence that she indeed has an enzyme deficiency that most likely contributed to the prolonged muscular weakness following a single dose of succinylcholine. The lab results were reported back to the patient so she can inform future providers of the enzyme activity deficiency **(L-18)**.

Learning Points

L-1. Where Is the Subglottic Space and What Are the Clinical Manifestations of Subglottic Stenosis?

The subglottic space, extending from the inferior border of the vocal cords to the lower border of the cricoid cartilage, is the narrowest part of the airway above the carina [1]. The space is normally circular in shape and bound posteriorly by the cricoid cartilage. Normal diameter of the subglottic space in adults is about 13–16 mm in males and roughly 12 mm in females.

Subglottic stenosis is a congenital or acquired narrowing of this area below the true vocal folds [2]. Patients with subglottic stenosis will often present with a complaint of dyspnea. Sometimes this may be accompanied by hoarseness or cough as well. Dyspnea with exertion typically occurs at airway diameters of 8 mm or less, while patients with dyspnea at rest will usually have diameters of 5 mm or less at the narrowest point of the subglottic region [2].

Subglottic stenosis represents a fixed airway obstruction that will affect both parts of the normal respiratory cycle. On inspiration, audible stridor may be evident. Stridor is caused by turbulent, non-laminar, airflow through the stenotic region and is loudest at times of maximal airflow, such as with deep breaths and exercise [3]. During exhalation, flow is limited by the stenotic region, such that, with very small tracheal diameters, exhalation time will be prolonged and air trapping may occur. This carries clinical significance for the anesthesia provider providing ventilation to a patient with severe tracheal stenosis. Without allowing for adequate exhalation time, a provider could cause air trapping with eventual volume trauma to the overinflated lungs. At tracheal diameters less than 5 mm, the time needed for complete exhalation increases dramatically (Fig. 16.1) [4].

To diagnose subglottic stenosis, both noninvasive and invasive studies can be useful. Narrowing of the airway can sometimes be seen on X-rays of the neck

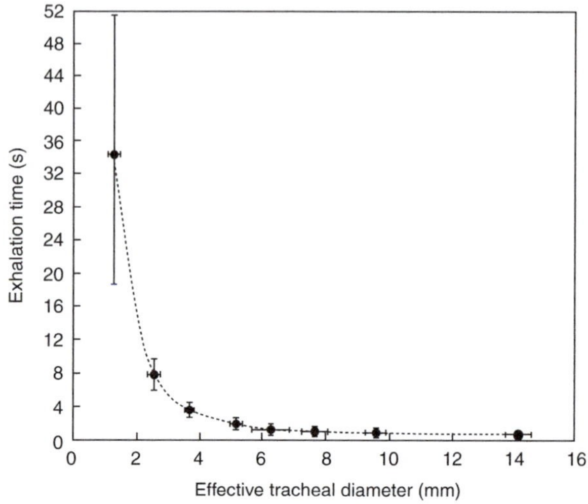

Fig. 16.1 Exhalation time as a function of effective tracheal diameter. (Reprinted from Dworkin et al. [4]. With permission from Elsevier)

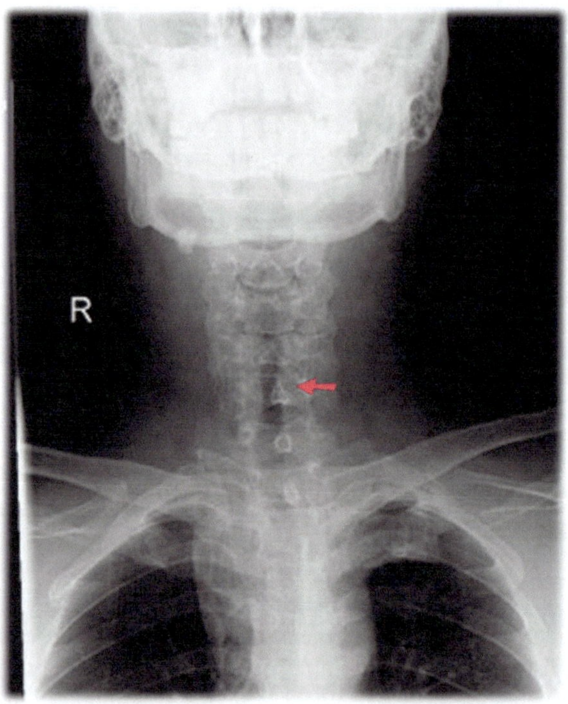

Fig. 16.2 X-ray demonstrating airway narrowing secondary to subglottic stenosis – note arrow pointing to arrowed airway. (Reprinted from https://en.wikipedia.org/wiki/File:Subglottic_stenosis_(X-ray).jpg. with permission from Creative Commons License 3.0: https://creativecommons.org/licenses/by-sa/3.0/)

(Fig. 16.2) [5]. More precise imaging studies like CT and MRI can be useful to view cross-sectional images of the narrowed subglottic space, in addition to being able to elucidate the soft tissue structures surrounding the trachea to assess for evidence of external compression of the airway (Figs. 16.3 and 16.4). The *gold standard* for diagnosis, evaluation, and severity classification of subglottic stenosis is direct

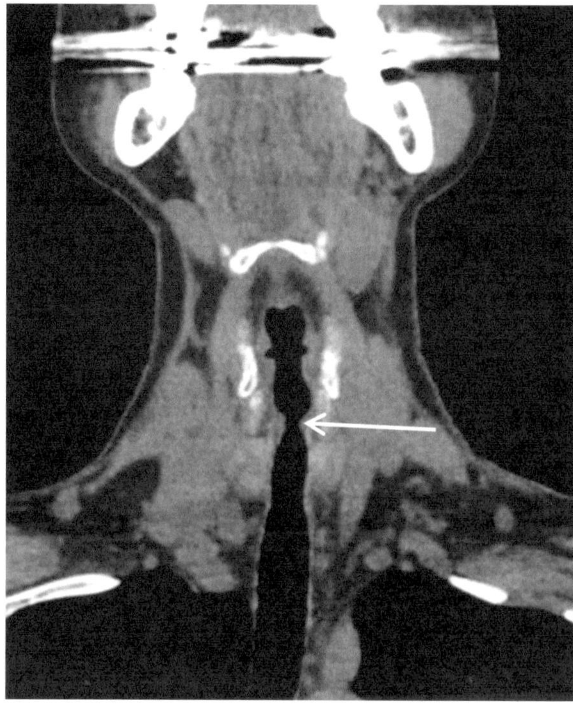

Fig. 16.3 Coronal neck CT of the case patient demonstrating subglottic narrowing

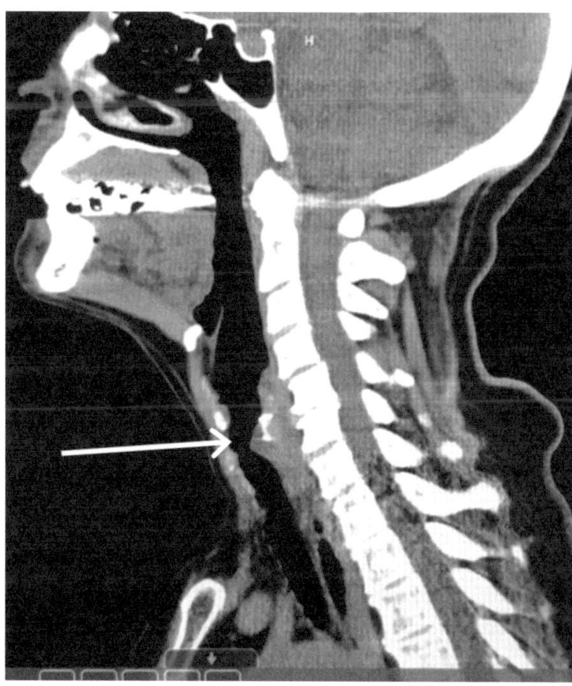

Fig. 16.4 Sagittal neck CT of the case patient demonstrating subglottic narrowing

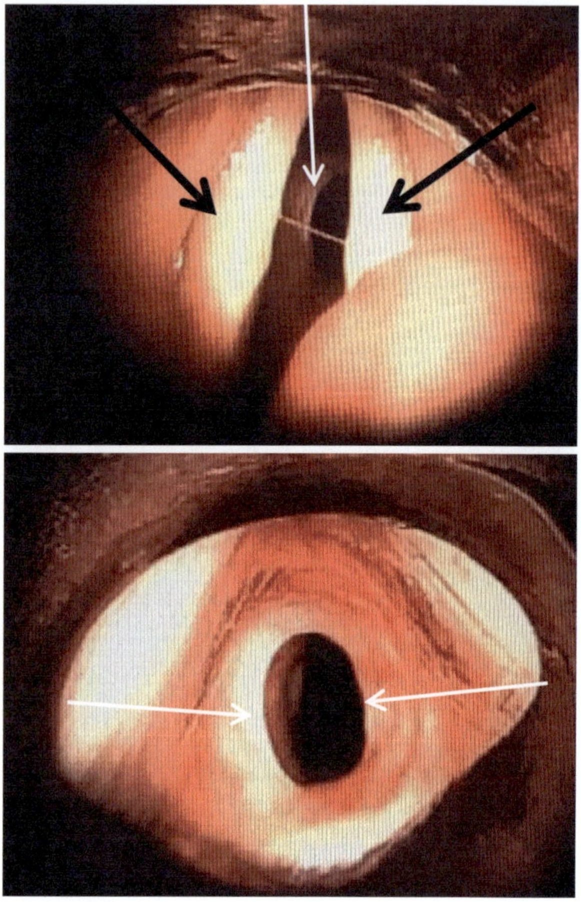

Fig. 16.5 Fiberoptic image of subglottic stenosis secondary to tissue web in the case patient. Black arrows, vocal folds; white arrows, subglottic stenosis area

laryngoscopy and bronchoscopy under general anesthesia [2] (Fig. 16.5). Utilizing this invasive technique, the pulmonologist or thoracic surgeon can assess the location and degree of airway stenosis. Measurements should be taken to determine the largest bronchoscope or endotracheal tube that can easily pass through the stenotic segment; such information is vital going forward should the patient need additional procedures under general anesthesia.

L-2. What Are the Potential Causes of Adult-Onset, Acquired Subglottic Stenosis?

The most common cause (90%), by far, of acquired subglottic stenosis is *endotracheal intubation*. Following intubation, the subglottic mucosal tissue may be damaged and undergo an inflammatory healing process resulting in eventual proliferation of granulation tissue and scarring with consequent narrowing of the subglottic region. The most important risk factor for development of airway narrowing is *duration* of intubation. Endotracheal tube size, cuff pressure, number of intubations, traumatic intubation, and concurrent infection also contribute to the likelihood of post-intubation stenosis formation [2].

Other causes of acquired subglottic stenosis include laryngeal trauma, prior airway surgery (particularly a high tracheotomy or cricothyroidotomy), airway infection, gastroesophageal reflux disease (GERD), inflammatory diseases, radiation therapy, and idiopathic stenosis [2].

L-3 What Is a Montgomery T-Tube?

A Montgomery T-tube is a device used as an airway and stent after laryngeal trauma or surgery. It is "T" shaped and has laryngeal arm, a tracheal projection, and an extra-tracheal portion that extends anteriorly out through a tracheostomy stoma (Fig. 16.6). It allows a patient to move air via either the upper "natural" airway through the laryngeal piece or via the stoma (as is necessary in the case of upper airway obstruction) [6]. The laryngeal projection also serves to stent the stenotic region of the subglottis, maintaining airway patency.

Very symptomatic patients with subglottic stenosis may require a temporary Montgomery T-tube or tracheostomy as a bridge to more definitive treatment. While minimally invasive, these options have the disadvantage of potentially increasing the extent of the tracheal narrowing and can predispose to bacterial colonization and infection. They are typically utilized as a short-term palliative treatment prior to an intervention or when surgical treatment is not a viable option [6].

L-4. How Is Subglottic Stenosis Classified in Terms of Disease Severity?

The *Myer-Cotton* staging is the most useful and widely used classification system for stenosis confined to the subglottis. It categorizes stenosis based on the percent reduction in cross-sectional area of the subglottic space. Four grades are recognized ranging in severity from *grade I lesions (<50% occlusion)* to *grade IV*, in which there is no detectable lumen with complete stenosis [2] (Table 16.1, Fig. 16.7).

Table 16.1 Myer-Cotton grades for subglottic stenosis

Myer-Cotton grade	Subglottic occlusion
Grade I	Less than 50%
Grade II	51–70%
Grade III	71–99%
Grade IV	Complete

Based on data from Ref. [2]

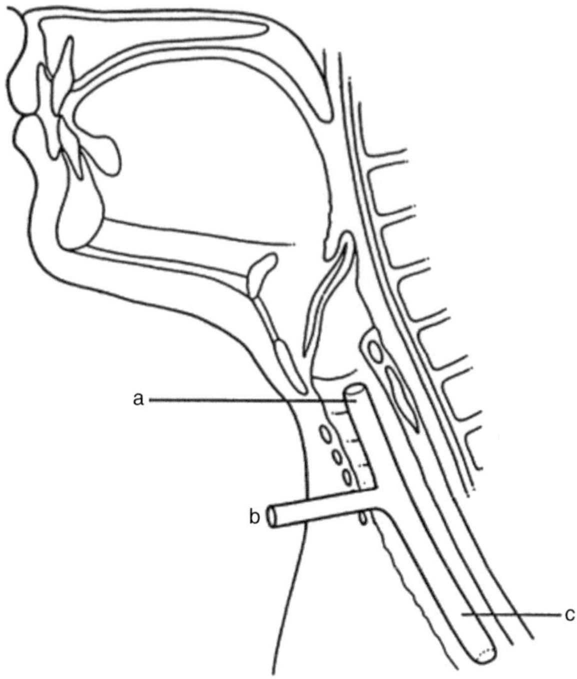

Fig. 16.6 Montgomery T-tube 1: (a) short laryngeal arm, (b) extra-tracheal part through stoma, (c) long tracheal projection. (Reprinted from Guha et al. [6]. With permission from Elsevier)

L-5. How Is Resistance *Defined and What Is the Effect of Subglottic Stenosis on Airway Resistance and Flow?*

Resistance can be defined by the relationship of a pressure change or gradient divided by a flow rate:

$$\mathbf{R} = \frac{\Delta \mathbf{P}}{\dot{\mathbf{V}}}$$

R = resistance, **ΔP** = driving pressure, $\dot{\mathbf{V}}$ = flow rate
ΔP is expressed in cm H_2O and $\dot{\mathbf{V}}$ in L/min, so **R = ($\mathbf{cmH_2O}$)/(L/min)**

Rearranging, $\dot{\mathbf{V}}$ = **ΔP/R**; it can be seen that with a constant ΔP, increases in resistance lead to a decrease in flow. Such is the case in the stenotic airway, with significant stenosis greatly increasing airway resistance leading to reduced flow necessitating an increased work of breathing to generate a larger **ΔP** [3].

In order to better understand this, it is important to understand the relationship between airway diameter and resistance to flow in a cylindrical pipe. The *Poiseuille equation* gives the pressure drop in a fluid flowing in a laminar fashion through a cylindrical pipe. This can be applied to respiratory physiology at low velocity flow rates through the roughly cylindrical trachea and upper airways. The equation follows:

$$\mathbf{\Delta P} = \frac{8\eta\iota\dot{\mathbf{V}}}{\pi\mathbf{r}^4}$$

ΔP, pressure difference; **ι**, pipe length; **η**, viscosity; $\dot{\mathbf{V}}$, flow rate; **r**, radius

Dividing both sides by FLOW gives us an expression of resistance, since $\mathbf{R = \Delta P/}\ \dot{\mathbf{V}}$:

$$\mathbf{R} = \frac{8\eta\iota}{\pi\mathbf{r}^4}$$

The important take-home point of the equation is that airway resistance in the trachea and subglottic space is inversely related to radius by a power of four [7]. Therefore small reductions in subglottic cross-sectional area can have a profound impact on increasing the resistance to airflow and consequently the work of breathing and symptoms of dyspnea. Additionally, the narrowed airway often causes more turbulent flow, which in turn produces the auditory stridor heard on auscultation of the stenotic airway.

L-6. What Are the Treatment Options for Subglottic Stenosis?

There are both medical and surgical management options for subglottic stenosis. For patients with non-severe symptoms and a decent level of activity, medical therapy is aimed at preventing disease progression [2]. These therapies include controlling underlying processes contributing to the stenosis (inflammatory disease, infection, etc.) and anti-esophageal reflux management (proton pump inhibitors, dietary modification).

Once subglottic stenosis has progressed to a consistently symptomatic problem, medical intervention is not usually sufficient to provide resolution of symptoms. In an acute exacerbation, heliox may be useful in decreasing the work of respirations until a temporizing or more permanent surgical treatment can be performed. Heliox is a mixture of helium and oxygen at varying ratios, which has a much lower density than air or oxygen alone. Heliox utility stems from its much lower density than air or oxygen (Table 16.2). While laminar flow resistance is dependent on viscosity (lower viscosity = lower resistance = better flow),

Table 16.2 Carrier gas properties for air, oxygen, and various heliox mixtures

Carrier gas	Density (g/L)	Viscosity (μP)
Room air	1.20	183
Oxygen 100%	1.429	203
Heliox 70/30	0.52	199
Heliox 80/20	0.40	198

Based on data from Ref. [8]

turbulent flow is related to the density of a fluid or gas. Since subglottic stenosis causes a turbulent, non-laminar, flow pattern, the less dense heliox mixture will result in improved flow with decreased work of breathing. The other potential benefit of the less dense heliox is that, at a given flow velocity and airway diameter, it has a lower Reynolds number, which will produce a tendency toward more laminar flow [9].

Interventional management options can be subcategorized into endoscopic and open procedures. Endoscopic treatment, such as was used in this case, typically involves flexible or, more often, rigid bronchoscopy under general anesthesia. Palliative and corrective options via this approach include balloon dilation, laser resection of granulomatous tissue, and stenting of stenotic regions [2]. These non-open surgical approaches tend to be more effective when the stenotic lesion is limited in scope (Myer-Cotton grades I–II) and distribution. Also, they may not be permanent solutions; with balloon dilation and laser treatment, there is a possibility of recurrence necessitating future procedures.

When endoscopic techniques cannot be utilized, then patients may be candidates for more invasive open surgical procedures. These surgeries involve *expansion* of the stenotic area with or without a cartilage graft or *resection* of the stenotic region with tracheal reconstruction [2]. The details of these procedures are beyond the scope of this chapter.

Regardless of what operative approach is taken, very symptomatic patients may require a temporary Montgomery T-tube or tracheostomy as a bridge to more definitive treatment. While minimally invasive, these options have the disadvantage of potentially increasing the extent of the tracheal narrowing and can predispose to bacterial colonization and infection. However, they are useful as a short-term treatment prior to an intervention or for palliative purposes [6].

L-7. What Are the Anesthetic Considerations for Rigid Bronchoscopy?

A rigid bronchoscope is a straight, hollow metal tube that can be inserted through the vocal cords in order to visualize the upper and central airway structures. It consists of a cylindrical or oval tube through which a rigid or flexible optic device can pass, allowing direct observation of the airway. Many rigid scopes also have an oblique lateral entrance to allow for passage of instruments such as stents, dilation balloons, clips, and lasers. Therefore, rigid bronchoscopy is utilized for both diagnosis and treatment of airway masses and obstructions [10].

Rigid bronchoscopy is a very stimulating procedure and is most often performed under general anesthesia. The base of the bronchoscope contains a lateral side port,

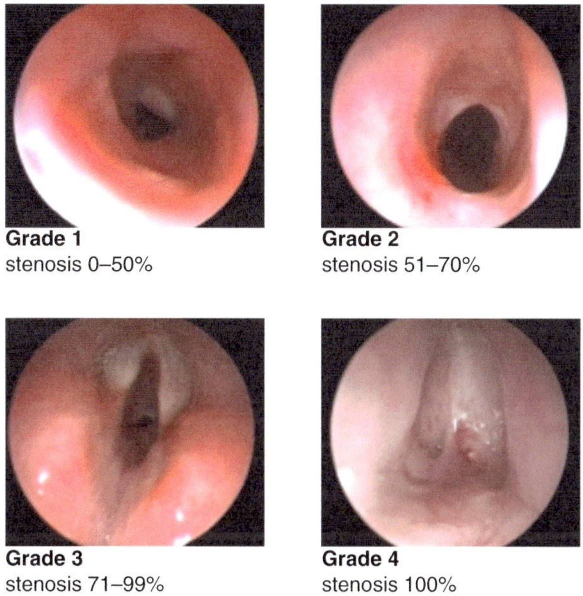

Fig. 16.7 Bronchoscopy images of Myer-Cotton grades. (Reprinted from Subglottic Stenosis [11]. Retrieved from http://www.chop.edu/conditions-diseases/subglottic-stenosis. 17 Dec 2017. ©2018 The Children's Hospital of Philadelphia)

which can be accessed to ventilate the patient during the procedure. This lateral arm is compatible with the breathing circuit of the anesthesia machine, an Ambu bag, or most portable Mapleson circuits [10] (Fig. 16.8). Constant communication between the bronchoscopist and anesthesia provider is essential to maintain consistent and safe ventilation throughout the procedure.

With rigid bronchoscopy under general anesthesia, a deep plane of anesthesia is necessary, and neuromuscular blockade makes for optimal operating conditions [12]. Most often, total intravenous (TIVA) techniques are employed because the airway is shared between the surgeon and anesthesia provider [12]. This can create a number of issues with the reliable delivery of inhaled anesthetic drugs. Further, there can be difficulty providing adequate ventilation and oxygenation during rigid bronchoscopy (Table 16.3) [10, 12].

For the reasons listed in Table 16.3, TIVA with propofol and a short-acting narcotic is frequently utilized as the anesthetic of choice since it provides a reliable way to establish and maintain consistent anesthetic depth and analgesia [12]. Muscle relaxation is generally achieved with succinylcholine for very short procedures or with a moderate duration non-depolarizing muscle relaxant for longer cases (Fig. 16.8).

Table 16.3 Ventilation and oxygenation concerns during rigid bronchoscopy

Problem	Solution
Airway disconnects or interruptions in ability to ventilate (e.g., during balloon dilation)	Thorough preoxygenation prior to scope placement Use 100% oxygen when able to ensure adequate reserve Constant communication with surgeon to maximize ventilation while connected
Gas leaks around bronchoscope → inability to provide positive pressure ventilation	Ensure that the scope's cap is securely in place High fresh gas flows to keep anesthesia bag well inflated Use oxygen flush button to rapidly achieve airway pressure Saline-soaked gauze throat pack to close off airway from above, creating a closed system for positive pressure ventilation Use jet ventilation if necessary
Suctioning during procedure decreases ability to maintain positive pressure for ventilation	High fresh gas flows to maintain circuit gas volume Use oxygen flush button to rapidly achieve airway pressure Close pop-off valve to maximize circuit pressures Communicate with surgeon to stop suctioning if unable to ventilate for a prolonged time or if there is oxygen desaturation
End-tidal carbon dioxide tracings frequently interrupted by suctioning and airway disconnects	Pay attention to other signs of ventilation such as chest rise and fogging on the bronchoscope image Auscultate lungs to ensure adequate air movement
Interruptions in ventilation and frequent use of oxygen flush make delivery of inhalational anesthetics unreliable and difficult to monitor	Total intravenous anesthetic technique
Use of cautery or lasers via bronchoscope poses a risk for airway fire	Communicate preoperatively with surgeon about fire risk Use FiO_2 of 30% or lower to minimize fire risk If using jet ventilation, hook a second jet ventilator to the AIR outlet to maintain $FiO_2 < 30\%$

L-8. Describe the Neuromuscular Junction and the Role of Acetylcholine at the Nicotinic Junction

A neuromuscular junction is a synapse formed between a motor neuron and a skeletal muscle cell. As the presynaptic motor neuron approaches the synapse, it divides into terminal buttons that contain many small vesicles housing the neurotransmitter acetylcholine. The terminal endings align with the motor end plate of the muscle cell. Within the end plate are junctional folds, which serve to provide an abundance of surface area for densely packed nicotinic acetylcholine receptors and their associated voltage-gated sodium channels [13] (Fig. 16.9).

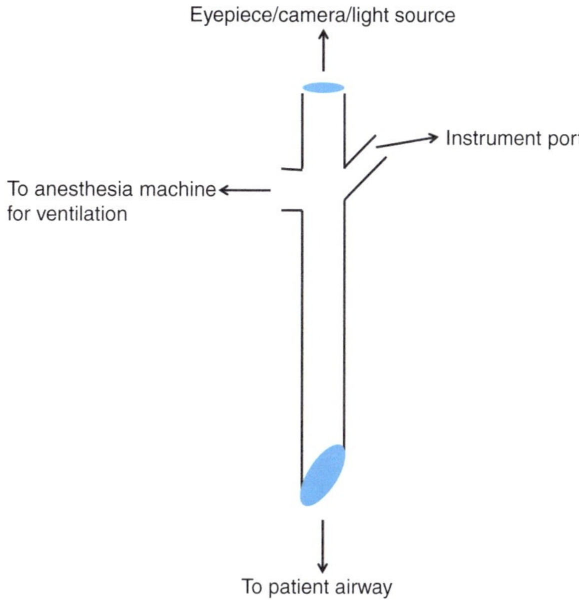

Fig. 16.8 Rigid bronchoscope

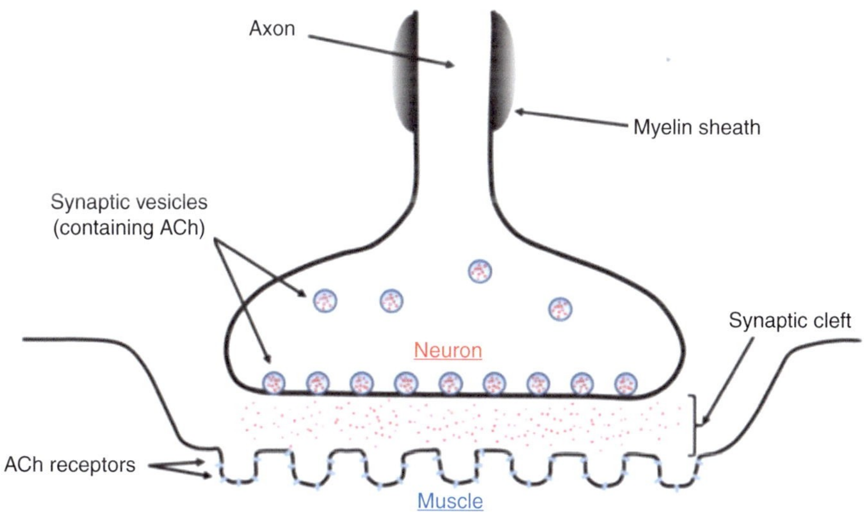

Fig. 16.9 Neuromuscular junction. (Reprinted from https://openi.nlm.nih.gov/detailedresult.php?img=PMC3093673_2046-1682-4-5-1&req=4. with permission from Creative Commons License 2.0: https://creativecommons.org/licenses/by/2.0/)

When an action potential impulse arrives at the terminal end of a presynaptic motor neuron, the permeability to Ca^{2+} increases, resulting in an influx of calcium, which in turn triggers the release of acetylcholine from the vesicles within the terminal buttons. Acetylcholine diffuses across the synaptic neuromuscular junction and binds to receptors on the junctional folds of the motor end plate of the muscle cell. This binding of acetylcholine produces a conformational change in a membrane ion channel that causes a net influx of positively charged Na^+ ions, resulting in *depolarization* of the postsynaptic muscle cell membrane. The depolarization, called the *end-plate potential*, subsequently generates action potentials on either side of the motor end plate which are conducted across the muscle fiber in both directions. The muscle action potential then initiates muscle contraction [13].

Under normal conditions, acetylcholine is rapidly metabolized by the enzyme acetylcholinesterase, which is abundant in the folds of the motor end plate, in close proximity to the site of neurotransmitter action [14]. The rapid hydrolytic breakdown of acetylcholine limits the duration of increased membrane sodium permeability and results in repolarization of the muscle fiber to its baseline transmembrane potential. This in turn limits the duration of muscle contraction.

L-9. What Is the Mechanism of Action of Succinylcholine?

Succinylcholine is the only clinically available *depolarizing* muscle relaxant. The drug is structurally similar to acetylcholine and binds to the nicotinic receptors on the motor end plate (Fig. 16.10).

Binding causes the opening of ion channels and widespread depolarization of muscle fibers with resultant action potentials and disorganized muscle contraction seen clinically as fasciculations. After this initial depolarization and muscle contraction, succinylcholine remains at the nicotinic receptor, preventing repolarization of the muscle cell membrane. The depolarized muscle fiber is unresponsive to subsequent acetylcholine agonism, and a flaccid paralysis ensues until the succinylcholine diffuses away from the end plate into extracellular fluid [15] (Fig. 16.11).

For most patients, succinylcholine has a short duration of action. The majority of administered drug is rapidly broken down by pseudocholinesterase in the plasma before ever reaching the active site at the neuromuscular junction. As only a small

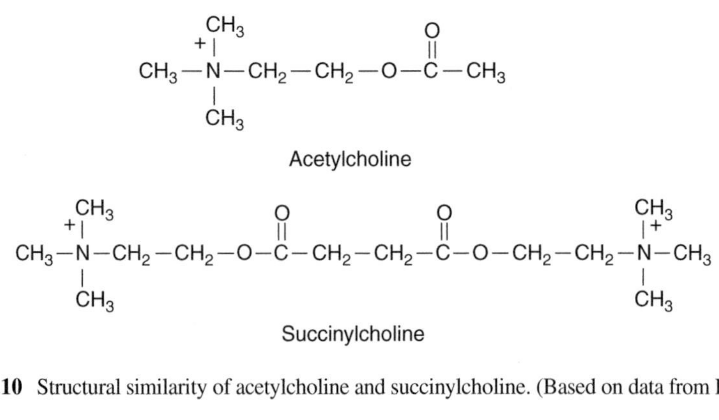

Fig. 16.10 Structural similarity of acetylcholine and succinylcholine. (Based on data from Ref. [14])

fraction of succinylcholine reaches the acetylcholine receptors, the limited (about 8.5 min) duration of succinylcholine-induced muscle relaxation is due to a paucity of drug reaching the active sites [16]. Once succinylcholine has bound to an acetylcholine receptor and caused depolarization, its termination of action is dependent on diffusion away from the active site, as pseudocholinesterase is not present at the neuromuscular junction. Conditions that decrease the initial hydrolytic breakdown of succinylcholine result in an increased amount of drug reaching the neuromuscular junctions and a consequently prolonged duration of flaccid paralysis following initial depolarization and fasciculation. Another cause of prolonged muscle weakness following succinylcholine

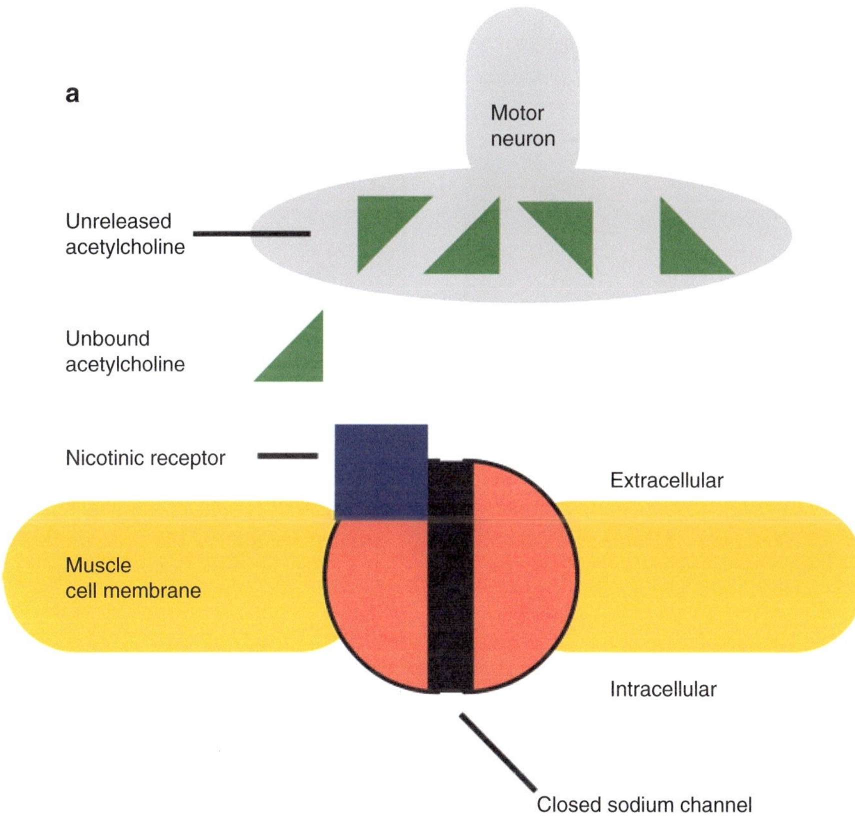

Fig. 16.11 Mechanism of action of acetylcholine and succinylcholine at the neuromuscular junction. (**a**) The neuromuscular junction prior to the binding of acetylcholine to the nicotinic receptor. Note that the sodium ion channel is closed. The muscle cell is in its native, polarized resting state. (**b**) When acetylcholine from the motor neuron binds the nicotinic receptor on the muscle cell, the sodium channel opens, and the muscle cell is depolarized, leading to contraction. Under normal conditions the acetylcholine is rapidly metabolized by acetylcholinesterase, permitting repolarization. (**c**) When bound by succinylcholine, the sodium channel opens, and the muscle cell is depolarized. However, the succinylcholine molecule stays bound, preventing repolarization until the drug diffuses away. It is during this "bound and blocked" period that succinylcholine causes flaccid muscle paralysis

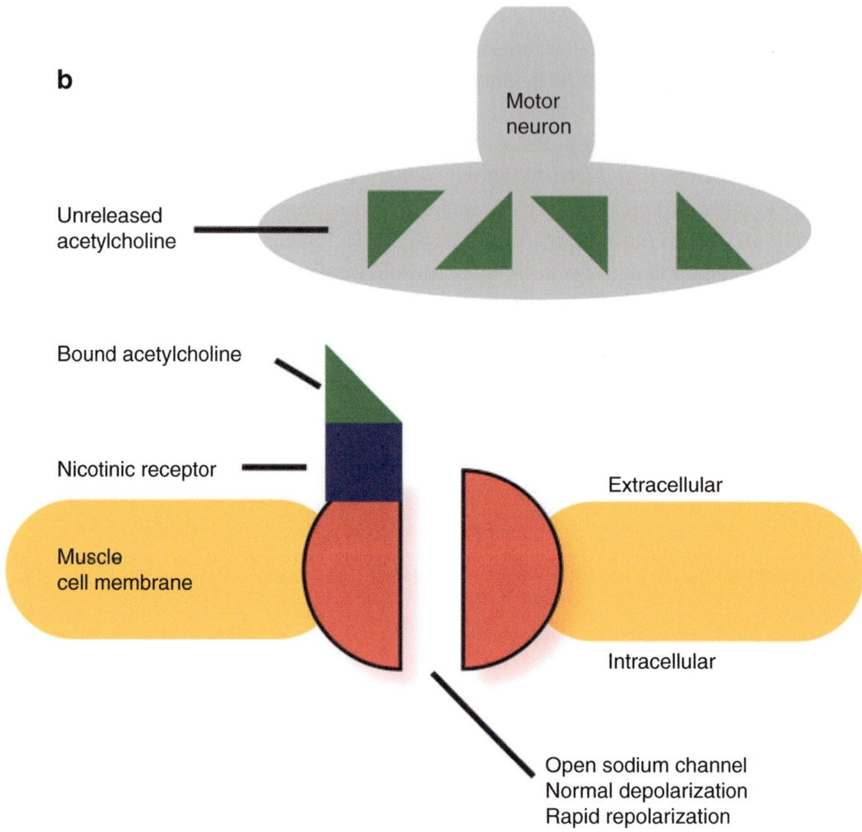

Fig. 16.11 (continued)

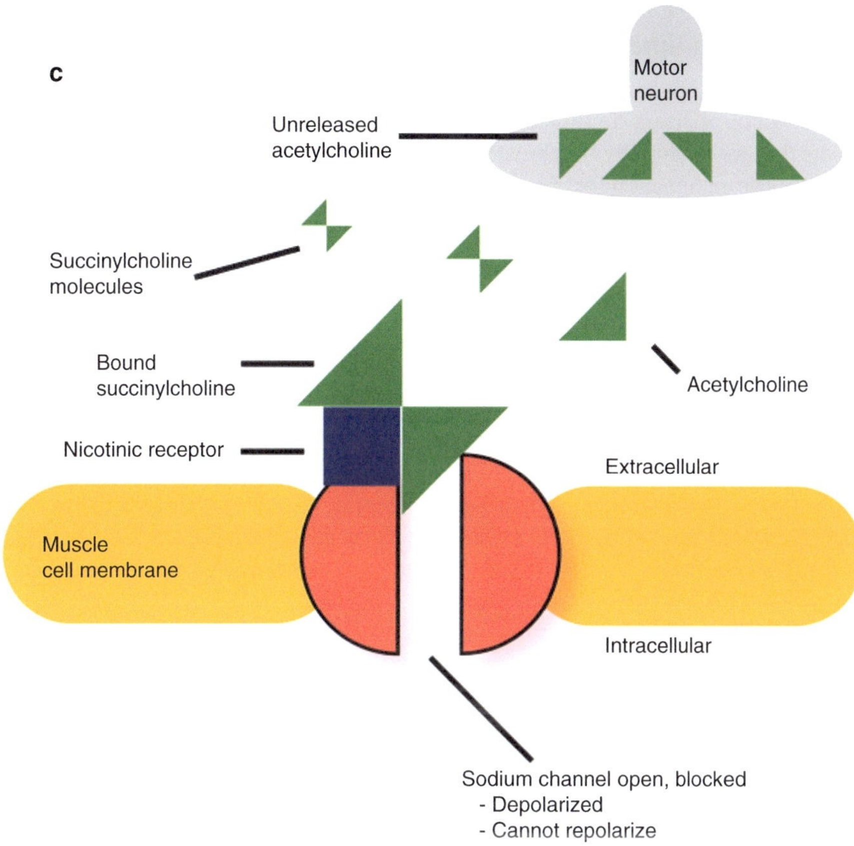

Fig. 16.11 (continued)

is the development of a phase II block, which typically follows administration of excessively large (3–5 mg/kg) or repeated doses of the drug [15].

Note that the *depolarizing blocker* is representative of the action of succinylcholine. The ion channel is *open* but *blocked* until the drug diffuses away, preventing repolarization of the membrane for the duration of flaccid paralysis.

With the *non-depolarizing blocker* (e.g., rocuronium, vecuronium, cisatracurium), the drug binds and blocks the nicotinic acetylcholine receptor, but the channel does not open. Thus there is no depolarization.

L-10. Are There Any Side Effects or Contraindications to Succinylcholine?

Succinylcholine has a multitude of side effects, some of which are common and others that are potentially life threatening. It is also the only intravenous drug that is a trigger for malignant hyperthermia [8].

Cardiac Side Effects

Succinylcholine is notorious for its ability to cause bradycardia. Given its structural similarity to acetylcholine, succinylcholine can act at postganglionic cardiac muscarinic receptors mimicking the effects of vagus nerve stimulation with resultant bradycardia, junctional rhythm, or even sinus arrest [15]. This is more likely with repeated dosing and can be prevented by pretreatment with an anticholinergic agent such as glycopyrrolate or atropine. Succinylcholine-associated bradycardia is particularly worrisome for pediatric patients, as cardiac output in neonates is heart rate dependent since they do not have the ability to increase stroke volume to sufficiently compensate for low pulse rates.

Conversely, succinylcholine can also act at autonomic nervous system sympathetic ganglia, resulting in an increase in sympathetic outflow with resulting tachycardia. This potential side effect can be troublesome in the patient with coronary artery disease or other heart conditions making tachycardia undesirable (e.g., aortic stenosis, diastolic heart failure).

Hyperkalemia

Under normal conditions, neuromuscular acetylcholine receptors are concentrated at the motor end plates. When acetylcholine or succinylcholine binds the receptor, ion channels open, and there is a large influx of sodium Na^+ into the muscle fiber causing depolarization. Concurrently, there is an efflux of potassium K^+ out of the cell, transiently increasing plasma K^+ concentration. In a healthy individual administered a standard intubating dose of succinylcholine, the plasma potassium concentration increases by about 0.5–1.0 mEq/l. The temporary elevation in plasma K^+ concentration is non-problematic for the vast majority of healthy individuals, though practitioners should exercise caution in patients with pre-existing elevated potassium [15].

Clinically significant hyperkalemia following succinylcholine administration is a greater risk in patient populations that demonstrate exaggerated potassium release in response to drug administration. Medical conditions that result in *denervation* or *prolonged loss of muscle excitation* and contraction lead to a spread of *extrajunctional* acetylcholine receptors along the entire muscle membrane (rather than just confined to the neuromuscular junctions). Despite a lack of clustered density of the extrajunctional acetylcholine receptors, the surface area of the muscle is so large that there is a dramatic net increase in the total number of receptors, such that when succinylcholine is administered, many more acetylcholine receptors are bound with a resulting dramatic increase in extracellular (plasma) potassium levels.

Conditions associated with extrajunctional acetylcholine receptors and the potential for exaggerated potassium release with succinylcholine include upper motor neuron injury (spinal cord trauma, stroke), severe burns, prolonged immobilization, muscular dystrophies, severe infection, direct muscle trauma, and disuse atrophy [15]. Due to the potential for clinically significant hyperkalemia in these patients, a careful history and physical is crucial to avoid administration of succinylcholine to anyone at risk for exaggerated potassium elevation.

Myalgia

Postoperative muscle soreness is among the most common side effects of succinylcholine administration. It is thought to be a result of the unsynchronized skeletal muscle contractions that occur following succinylcholine receptor occupation before the onset of flaccid muscle paralysis. These fasciculations may cause muscle damage that manifests postoperatively as myalgia. Young, muscular patients seem to be at particular risk for postoperative muscle soreness following succinylcholine use [15].

Malignant Hyperthermia

Succinylcholine is the only intravenous drug known to trigger malignant hyperthermia in genetically susceptible patients. A careful personal and family history regarding anesthetic complications can help to identify patients potentially at risk for developing malignant hyperthermia upon exposure to succinylcholine or volatile anesthetic agents [17].

Increased Intraocular Pressure

Succinylcholine causes an elevation in intraocular pressure. This is of theoretical concern for patients with an open globe injury, as an elevated ocular pressure could potentially extrude globe contents. However, there has been little to no clinical correlation to support this potential complication [17].

Increased Intracranial Pressure

Studies are conflicted as to the effects of succinylcholine on intracranial pressure in the setting of a brain tumor or emergent craniotomy for bleeding. Clinically, many practitioners still consider succinylcholine an acceptable neuromuscular blocker when rapid airway establishment is prioritized, such as in the setting of acute head trauma or a full stomach.

L–11. What Is the Difference Between a Phase I and Phase II Succinylcholine Block?

The typical block following administration of succinylcholine is called a phase I block. As mentioned above, succinylcholine binding to the acetylcholine receptors at the neuromuscular junction produces a depolarization event followed by a period of flaccid paralysis until the drug diffuses away from the active site [14]. With very high or repeated doses of succinylcholine, a patient may develop a phase II block. Prolonged exposure of the end plate to succinylcholine will result in desensitization to the depolarizing action of succinylcholine, as well as to the chemical transmitter acetylcholine. Therefore, the block will change from a depolarizing (phase I) block into a desensitized (phase II) block [14]. Phase II blocks tend to be much longer in duration and demonstrate different responses to neuromuscular twitch monitors.

Phase I blocks can be differentiated from a phase II block by using a twitch monitor. After administration of succinylcholine and initial fasciculation, there is a brief period of profound block density during which there may be no twitches upon train-of-four stimulation of the ulnar nerve. As succinylcholine molecules diffuse away from the neuromuscular junction, acetylcholine receptors begin to repolarize and regain sensitivity to native acetylcholine. This is the mechanism by which the flaccid paralytic block resolves. As the block resolves, patients will regain twitches upon train-of-four nerve stimulation.

A phase I *depolarizing* block with succinylcholine will demonstrate four EQUAL twitches with diminished twitch height compared with baseline twitch height [17]. This is in contrast to the train-of-four recovery pattern seen with non-depolarizing muscle relaxants and a succinylcholine-produced phase II block. In these situations, train-of-four stimulation will demonstrate fade from the first through fourth twitches, producing a TOF ratio less than 1 (the fourth twitch has a smaller amplitude than the first) [17] (Fig. 16.12).

Phase I and phase II blocks also differ in the response to tetanic stimulation with a twitch monitor. When a patient has a depolarizing phase I block, tetanic nerve stimulation will produce a diminished but constant muscle response, *without* fade. Additionally, there is no post-tetanic potentiation of twitch height with a phase I depolarizing block. Phase II desensitizing blockades demonstrate fade with sustained tetany as well as post-tetanic potentiation of twitch height [17]. In this respect, a phase II succinylcholine block demonstrates the same response to train of four as a non-depolarizing muscle relaxant.

Finally, phase I and II blocks differ in the response to reversal with neostigmine or other acetylcholinesterase inhibitors. Phase I blockade is noncompetitive and does not show resolution with neostigmine, whereas a phase II block will demonstrate improved twitch amplitude and TOF ratio when the local concentration of acetylcholine is increased [17]. Despite the presence of a response to neostigmine, the pharmacologic reversal of a phase II succinylcholine block should be carried out with great caution as it may potentiate any residual phase I block.

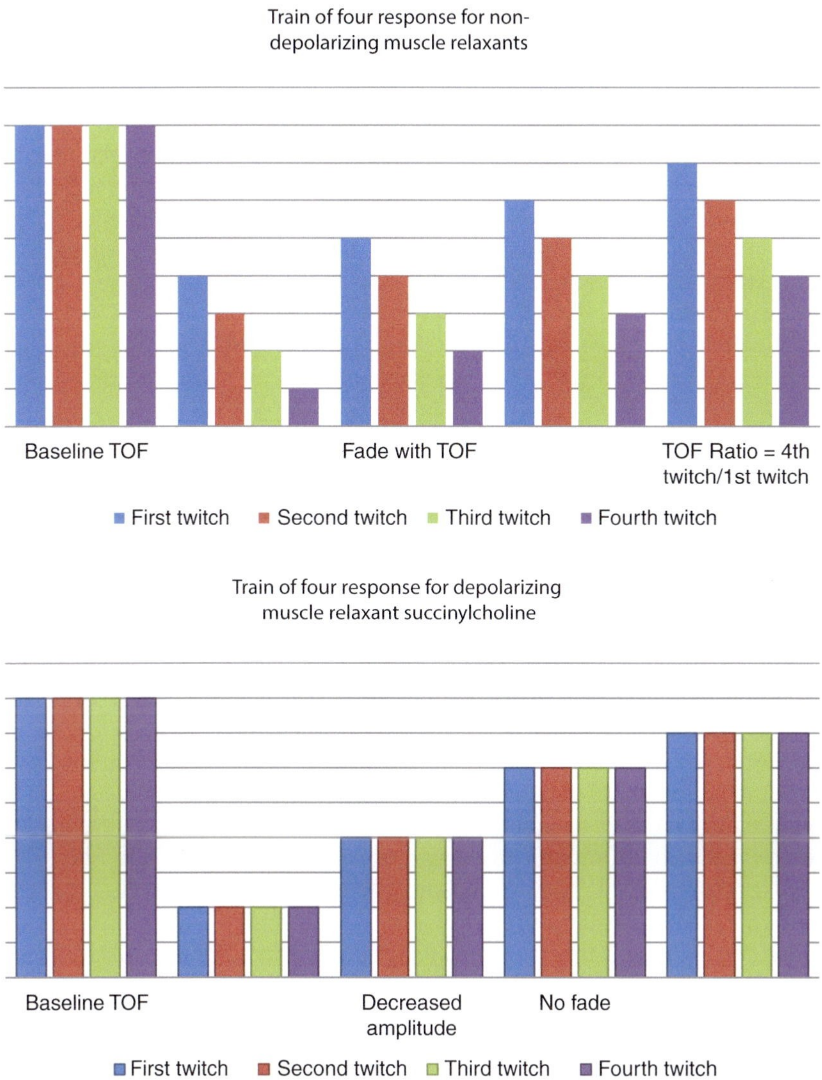

Fig. 16.12 Train-of-four (TOF) response patterns of non-depolarizing muscle relaxants and succinylcholine. (Based on data from Ref. [17])

L-12. What Are the Characteristics of a Patient That Is Not Fully Recovered from Neuromuscular Blockade?

Patients not fully recovered from neuromuscular blockade will manifest objective findings with nerve stimulation (train-of-four and tetany with the twitch monitor). For patients with a succinylcholine-associated depolarizing block, TOF will demonstrate four equal twitches whose amplitude is diminished from baseline [17]. In other words, they will have four equal, but weaker, twitches. In response to 5-s tetanic stimulation, there will be contraction with diminished amplitude from baseline, but *no* fade.

The twitch monitor findings in depolarizing blockade differ from those in patients who are weak secondary to a non-depolarizing block or succinylcholine-induced phase II block. The latter group will demonstrate *fade* on TOF testing, where there is diminishing twitch amplitude from the first through fourth twitches. A TOF ratio (amplitude of fourth twitch/amplitude of first twitch) less than 0.9 is consistent with incomplete recovery from non-depolarizing neuromuscular blockade [18]. In response to tetanic stimulation, there will be amplitude fade within 5 s during nerve stimulation. A lack of fade with full 5-s tetanic stimulation is consistent with complete recovery from blockade.

Both train-of-four and tetanic nerve monitoring can be problematic in that they are difficult to objectively measure and practitioners are often not very accurate in their ability to detect fade or small differences in twitch/contraction amplitudes. Nerve monitor findings should be correlated with other clinical criteria for adequate muscle strength. Unfortunately, most of these require patient cooperation and so are difficult to perform until the patient is fully awake. Clinical findings *consistent with adequate* recovery from neuromuscular blockade include eye opening to command, sustained 5-s head lift, strong grip strength, effective cough, vital capacity of at least 15 ml/kg, generation of negative inspiratory force of at least 30 cm H_2O, and coordinated purposeful movement [19].

Patient inability to perform or demonstrate the above may be secondary to muscular weakness in the setting of residual neuromuscular blockade. The weakened patient will often have “floppy,” uncoordinated extremity movements resembling a “fish out of water.” Extubated patients will report feeling weak and short of breath and may have diminished voice volume. If a patient is not fully recovered from neuromuscular blockade, it is important to intervene.

L-13. What Is the Management of the Patient with Prolonged Neuromuscular Blockade?

The treatment of patients with residual weakness following muscle relaxants will vary based on the degree of weakness and patient comorbidities. The common goals of treatment across all situations are summarized in Table 16.4 [20].

Table 16.4 Treatment goals for the patient with residual muscle weakness

Treatment goal	Intervention
Adequate minute ventilation Prevents hypercarbia and respiratory acidosis Enhances oxygenation	Ventilatory support Intubated/LMA → volume control, pressure control, or pressure support Non-intubated → BIPAP
Adequate oxygenation	Ventilatory support Supplemental oxygen PEEP to decrease atelectasis
Prevention of airway obstruction	Intubation/LMA Oral of nasal airway if not intubated
Minimize aspiration in patients at risk Bowel obstruction Full stomach GERD	Endotracheal intubation
Provide sedation Avoid recall Decrease stress response	Intravenous sedation Propofol Benzodiazepines Dexmedetomidine Narcotics

As one can see, much of the management for the patient with residual neuromuscular blockade will be support of the airway and respiratory effort. For patients at elevated risk for aspiration (bowel surgery, GERD, full stomach pre-op, etc.), protecting the airway with an endotracheal tube is likely the best option, as reduced pharyngeal muscle strength and coordination is associated with a weakened gag reflex. If possible, such patients should be re-intubated without the administration of additional neuromuscular blocking drugs, as that would potentially prolong the time to complete recovery of baseline strength. Under these conditions it is important to provide adequate sedation to prevent awareness and recall of the intubation and weakness. Patients should remain intubated and sedated in the operating room, PACU, or ICU until full resolution of neuromuscular blockade is evident.

When the patient with prolonged weakness does not have risk factors for aspiration, endotracheal intubation may not be necessary to provide airway and ventilatory support. As long as airway obstruction is prevented and adequate minute ventilation is maintained, supraglottic airway support such as a laryngeal mask airway or BiPAP may be considered. In either case, ventilatory support should be set to achieve adequate tidal volumes (about 8 cc/kg ideal body weight) and minute ventilation (use end-tidal CO_2, if available as a guide). As in the intubated patient, sedation should be used for prevention of recall and anxiolysis.

No matter how one chooses to manage the airway and provide respiratory support, patience is an important virtue when caring for the patient with residual neuromuscular blockade. It is crucial to wait for evidence of complete block resolution prior to removing support, as post-extubation weakness is associated with upper airway obstruction, reduced pharyngeal muscle coordination, hypoxemia, and hypercarbia [18].

L-14. Would a Reversal Agent Be Beneficial in This Case?

The case presented above is consistent with a prolonged phase I blockade secondary to a single dose of succinylcholine. Phase I blockade does not improve with administration of acetylcholinesterase (e.g., neostigmine, physostigmine). In fact, neostigmine can potentially prolong the effect of succinylcholine by exerting an inhibitory action on pseudocholinesterase [21].

L-15. What Causes a Prolonged Neuromuscular Blockade to Succinylcholine? What Are Quantitative and Qualitative Pseudocholinesterase Deficiencies?

A prolonged effect of succinylcholine can be due to a defect in either the quantity or quality of the enzyme pseudocholinesterase [21]. Causes of decreased *quantity* of pseudocholinesterase are myriad, as illustrated by the accompanying chart (Table 16.3). Despite the many possible factors that can lower serum pseudocholinesterase levels, most of these patients will not demonstrate prolonged paralysis following succinylcholine. ***Quantitative*** enzyme deficits must be extreme (<20% normal level) before clinically significant block prolongation occurs with succinylcholine. Keep in mind, however, that an acquired quantitative deficiency in combination with a mildly abnormal *qualitative* deficiency may result in a prolonged response to succinylcholine (Table 16.5).

Qualitative defects of pseudocholinesterase refer not to the amount of enzyme in the plasma but to the ability of the enzyme to effectively metabolize succinylcholine and other drugs. In other words, there is sufficient amount of enzyme, but it is abnormal or *atypical*. Qualitative pseudocholinesterase deficiencies are inherited via mutations of the butyrylcholinesterase (*BChE*) gene located on the long arm of chromosome 3 [22]. In addition to the normal, or wild-type, gene, there are over 60 named variants of the gene that vary in their effects on prolongation of succinylcholine block. Of these, four are most frequently encountered and discussed. These are *atypical or dibucaine-resistant*, *fluoride-resistant*, *silent*, and *K* varieties [22]. See the accompanying chart for more information about these alleles (Table 16.8). Importantly, combinations of all the various alleles are possible, yielding differing clinical consequences (Table 16.6).

L-16. Aside from Pseudocholinesterase Deficiency, Are There Any Drugs That Can Predispose to Prolonged Weakness Succinylcholine Administration?

Pharmacologic inhibition of normal pseudocholinesterase will result in more succinylcholine molecules reaching neuromuscular junction active sites and consequently prolonged duration of paralysis. There are both noncompetitive and

Table 16.5 Causes of acquired quantitative pseudocholinesterase deficiency

Liver failure	Synthesized by liver. 30–50% decrease with acute hepatitis, 50% decrease with cirrhosis. Little clinical relevance until end stage
Pregnancy	Roughly 25% decrease during pregnancy, not usually clinically significant
HELLP syndrome	≈60% HELLP syndrome patients demonstrate below normal pseudocholinesterase activity, possibly due to liver damage from preeclampsia
Malnutrition	Secondary to decreased hepatic production, usually concurrent with low albumin
Renal disease	≈60% renal failure patients have decreased pseudocholinesterase activity up to two standard deviations below normal. Values improve with transplantation
Malignancy	Decreased activity related to site of primary lesion and degree of spread. Hepatic tumors have greatest reduction, followed by lung, GI, and genitourinary
Burns	Reduction correlates with severity of burn, with up to 80% reduction 5–6 days postburn. Little clinical significance since succinylcholine contraindicated in major burn injury patients due to hyperkalemia risk
Cardiopulmonary bypass	Reductions in enzyme activity of up to 37% with initiation of bypass. May be of limited significance due to length of cases
Oral contraceptives	Activity decreased about 20%
Monoamine oxidase inhibitor	Case reports of prolonged paralysis after electroconvulsive therapy in patients treated with the MAO inhibitor phenelzine. Rarely used currently

Based on data from Refs. [22, 23]

Table 16.6 Pseudocholinesterase phenotype interpretation

Phenotype	Frequency	Prolonged succinylcholine block	Comments
U	96%	No	Normal, wild-type phenotype
UA	3%	Variable, moderate prolongation	More susceptible with large dose + short surgery
A	1/3000	Yes, always	
US	0.7%	Variable, moderate prolongation	More susceptible with large dose + short surgery
S	1/40,000	Yes, always	"U" with organophosphate poisoning will look same
AS	1/8000	Yes, always	
FS	Very rare	Yes	More susceptible with large dose + short surgery
AF	Very rare	Yes	More susceptible with large dose + short surgery
UF	Very rare	Variable	More susceptible with large dose + short surgery

Based on data from Ref. [24]

Key: *U* usual (normal), *A* atypical, *S* silent, *F* fluoride sensitive

Table 16.7 Drug and electrolyte effects on neuromuscular blockade characteristics

Drug class/electrolyte/ vital issue	Depolarizing block effect	Non-depolarizing block effect	Comment
Hypothermia	Increased block	Increased block Prolonged duration	Dose in small increments when hypothermia present
Acute hypokalemia	Little effect	Increased sensitivity	Acutely decreased plasma K^+ hyperpolarizes muscle cell membrane, making it resistant to depolarization by Ach
Plasma calcium	Little effect	Little effect	Intracellular, not plasma, Ca^{2+} more important in muscle activation
High magnesium	No effect on single dose duration Diminishes fasciculations	Increased sensitivity Prolonged duration	Causes weakness even in the absence of concurrent NMB administration. Titrate blockade with caution
Antibiotics (aminoglycosides, tetracycline, clindamycin, etc.)	Little effect	Increased sensitivity Prolonged duration	
Beta blockers	Little effect	Prolonged duration	
Calcium channel blockers	Little effect	Increased sensitivity Prolonged duration	
Local anesthetics	Increased sensitivity	Increased sensitivity	Even normal doses of epidural local anesthetic can potentiate non-depolarizing neuromuscular blockers

Based on data from Ref. [25]

competitive *cholinesterase inhibitors* known to prolong the effect of succinylcholine secondary to their inhibitory effect on pseudocholinesterase.

Competitive cholinesterase inhibitors include edrophonium, pyridostigmine, neostigmine, and physostigmine. Pyridostigmine is commonly used in the pharmacologic treatment of patients with myasthenia gravis, so succinylcholine should be used with great caution, if at all, in that population. Neostigmine is very commonly used in modern anesthesia practice as a reversal agent for non-depolarizing competitive muscle relaxants. Administration of succinylcholine following block reversal with neostigmine may result in a prolonged block [25]. *Noncompetitive* cholinesterase inhibitors include organophosphate insecticides and echothiophate eye drops, which had been used to treat glaucoma [25].

There is a long list of drugs and electrolyte abnormalities that potentiate or prolong non-depolarizing neuromuscular blockade. Many have little to no effect on duration of succinylcholine-induced blockade (Table 16.7).

L-17. What Studies Are Available to Evaluate for the Presence of Pseudocholinesterase Deficiency?

When a patient demonstrates prolonged paralysis following a single, appropriate dose of succinylcholine, it is important to find out what factors led to the lengthened drug effect. Succinylcholine is a very commonly used muscle relaxant with anesthesia, so the patient should be aware if they are at risk for an adverse drug effect so that they can advise future providers accordingly.

The patient in this case did not have any of the comorbidities associated with acquired pseudocholinesterase deficiency. Likewise, she did not present with electrolyte abnormalities known to potentiate the action of depolarizing muscle relaxants. That leaves a *qualitative*, inherited pseudocholinesterase deficiency as a probable cause of the markedly prolonged duration of succinylcholine-produced paralysis in this instance.

The first step in the workup for inherent pseudocholinesterase deficiency is to send a biochemical assay testing for the amount of *pseudocholinesterase activity* in the plasma. The value range of normal enzyme activity (roughly 3000–7000 IU/L) will vary based on the lab facility running the test. In the above case, the patient's pseudocholinesterase activity level was definitively low at 1245 IU/L, suggesting a lack of ability to effectively metabolize succinylcholine [23].

The *pseudocholinesterase activity assay* result is sufficient to prove that a patient is at risk for a prolonged weakness following administration of succinylcholine. However, to determine whether the deficiency is secondary to *atypical dibucaine-resistant pseudocholinesterase* or another mutation requires further testing.

The *dibucaine inhibition test* determines the presence or absence of atypical dibucaine-resistant pseudocholinesterase [23]. Dibucaine is an amide local anesthetic that inhibits the enzymatic activity of normal, fully functional pseudocholinesterase. When exposed to dibucaine, normal pseudocholinesterase activity is decreased by 80%. Thus, normal wild-type pseudocholinesterase has a *dibucaine number* of 80. Dibucaine does not inhibit *atypical dibucaine-resistant* pseudocholinesterase to the same extent. A dibucaine number of 20 is found in individuals homozygous for dibucaine-resistant pseudocholinesterase (atypical enzyme is only inhibited 20% by dibucaine). Such patients are at high risk for prolonged paralysis with succinylcholine. Heterozygous patients have dibucaine numbers from 40 to 60 and are at variable risk for prolonged succinylcholine block [17].

In learning point **L-15**, several pseudocholinesterase mutations were mentioned (see Table 16.8). Some of the more common mutations shown in Table 16.8 can be identified using *pseudocholinesterase phenotype interpretation*. The analysis is based on total pseudocholinesterase activity *and* the dibucaine inhibition number [24]. Phenotypes that can be identified using this method are shown in Table 16.6.

Table 16.8 Genetic variants for abnormal pseudocholinesterase

Common genetic variants in pseudocholinesterase deficiency and effects on succinylcholine duration

Variant	Frequency	Activity	Sensitivity to succinylcholine	Estimated block duration
Wild-type NORMAL (U)	≈98% of population	Normal enzyme	Normal response	≈8–10 min
Atypical dibucaine resistant (A)	Homozygote: 1/3000–1/10,000	Homozygote (AA): Decreased 70%	Homozygote (AA): very sensitive	≥2 h
	Heterozygote: Up to 1/25		Heterozygote (UA): Occasional prolonged block	≈20 min
Fluoride resistant (F)	Homozygote: 1/150,000	Decreased 60%	Homozygote (FF): moderately sensitive	1–2 h
	Heterozygous: More common but less clinical significance			
Silent (S)	Homozygous 1/10,000–8/100,000	No enzyme activity	Homozygote (SS): extremely sensitive	3–4 h
	Heterozygous: more common but less clinical significance			
Kalow (K)	Homozygous: 1/65	Decreased 30%	Homozygotes (KK): mildly sensitive	<1 h

Based on data from Ref. [23]

L-18. How Should the Patient in This Case Be Counseled Going Forward?

As mentioned in **L-16**, it is important to communicate significant clinical and laboratory findings to the patients so that they can advise future providers accordingly. In this case, the patient was contacted with the abnormal pseudocholinesterase activity results and advised to make a point of informing all future providers about the condition. With a low pseudocholinesterase activity level and the prolonged response to succinylcholine, it is known that the patient is at high risk for prolonged muscle weakness should she receive succinylcholine again. It was recommended to carry a note with her identification so that medical providers can be aware of the enzyme deficiency in the event of an emergency. However, a medical alert bracelet would be the best way to inform future providers of the condition since it is always readily visible on the patient's body.

At this point the patient could seek further lab work, including a dibucaine number and pseudocholinesterase phenotype interpretation. The studies might help to elucidate the precise nature of an underlying mutation but would be unlikely to change the way anesthesiologists care for her in the future. With the data and history already available, providers should know to avoid succinylcholine.

References

1. Ernst A, FJF H. Principles and practice of interventional pulmonology. New York: Springer Science + Business Media; 2013. https://doi.org/10.1007/978-1-4614-4292-9_9.
2. Quinn F, Ryan M, Pou A, Muller C. Subglottic stenosis: grand rounds presentation, UTMB Dept. of Otolaryngology [pdf]. 2002. Retrieved from http://utmb.edu.
3. Ernst A, FJF H. Principles and practice of interventional pulmonology. New York: Springer Science + Business Media; 2013. https://doi.org/10.1007/978-1-4614-4292-9_7.
4. Dworkin R, Benumof JL, Benumof R, Karagianes TG. The effective tracheal diameter that causes air trapping during jet ventilation. J Cardiothorac Anesth. 1990;4(6):731–6.
5. Subglottic stenosis. 2017. Retrieved 17 Dec 2017, from https://en.wikipedia.org/wiki/Subglottic_stenosis.
6. Guha A, Mostafa SM, Kendall JB. The Montgomery T-tube: anaesthetic problems and solutions. Br J Anaesth. 2001;87:787–90.
7. Ganong W. Dynamics of blood and lymph flow. In: Review of medical physiology. Norwalk: Appleton and Lange; 1995. p. 525–41.
8. Gamard S. US Patent Application No. W02010019467 A1 2010.
9. Mcgarvey JM, Pollack CV. Heliox in airway management. Emerg Med Clin North Am. 2008;26(4):905–20.
10. Themes U. Otolaryngology-head and neck surgery. 2016. Retrieved 15Nov 2017, from https://aneskey.com/otolaryngology-head-and-neck-surgery/.
11. Subglottic stenosis. Philadelphia; 2014. Retrieved 17 Dec 2017, from http://www.chop.edu/conditions-diseases/subglottic-stenosis.
12. Pathak V, Welsby I, Mahmood K, Wahidi M, MacIntyre N, Shofer S. Ventilation and anesthetic approaches for rigid bronchoscopy. Ann Am Thorac Soc. 2014;11:628–34.
13. Ganong W. Synaptic and junctional transmission. In: Review of medical physiology. Norwalk: Appleton and Lange; 1995. p. 75–104.
14. Themes U. Skeletal muscle relaxants. 2016. Retrieved 15 Nov 2017, from https://basicmedicalkey.com/skeletal-muscle-relaxants/.
15. Appiah-Ankam J, Hunter J. Pharmacology of neuromuscular blocking drugs. Contin Educ Anesth Crit Care Pain. 2004;4(1):2–7. https://doi.org/10.1093/bjaceaccp/mkh002.
16. Benumof JL, Dagg R, Benumof R. Critical hemoglobin desaturation will occur before return to an unparalyzed state following 1 mg/kg intravenous succinylcholine. Anesthesiology. 1997;87(4):979–82.
17. Stoelting R, Miller R, editors. Neuromuscular blocking drugs. In: Basics of anesthesia. 4th ed. New York: Churchill Livingstone; 2000. p. 89–106.
18. Murphy G, Szokol J, Marymount J, Greenberg S, Avram M, Vender J. Residual neuromuscular blockade and critical respiratory events in the post anesthesia care unit. Anesth Analg. 2008;107:130–7.
19. Leonard P, Whittier T, Sokoll M. Monitoring neuromuscular blockade. In: Longnecker D, Tinker J, Morgan G, editors. Principles and practice of anesthesiology. 2nd ed. Philadelphia: Mosby; 1998. p. 907–22.
20. Moi. 290 residual neuromuscular blockade. Anaesthesia, UK: FRCA. n.d. Retrieved 15 Nov 2017, from http://www.frca.co.uk/Documents/290%20Residual%20Neuromuscular%20Blockade.pdf.
21. Binkley C. Unknown pseudocholinesterase deficiency in a patient undergoing TIVA with planned motor evoked potential monitoring: a case report. AANA J. 2016;84:198–200.
22. Soliday F, Conley Y, Henker R. Pseudocholinesterase deficiency: a comprehensive review of genetic, acquired, and drug influences. AANA J. 2010;78:313–20.
23. Hackett P, Sakai T. Pseudocholinesterase deficiency: a case report and literature review. Open J Anesthesiol. 2012;2:188–94.
24. ARUP Laboratories. Lab test directory. Pseudocholinesterase, dibucaine inhibition. ltd.aruplab.com/tests/pub/print/0020159.
25. Zwer F. Factors affect neuromuscular transmission and block. J Anesth Crit Care Open Access. 6(1):00216. https://doi.org/10.15406/jaccoa.2016.06.00216.

Part IV
Cases Requiring Difficult and/or Unusual Anesthetic Management

Chapter 17
Cesarean Section in a Heart Failure Patient with Previous Lumbosacral Spine Surgery

John J. Finneran IV, Thomas Archer, and Alyssa Brzenski

The patient is a 29-year-old, 69-kg female with a history significant for nonischemic cardiomyopathy (NICM) and surgical resection of a lumbosacral teratoma with subsequent chemotherapy at age 18 months who presented for elective Cesarean section.

At age 28, the patient was diagnosed with NICM after undergoing an uncomplicated laparoscopic cholecystectomy. Approximately 2 weeks after the procedure, the patient presented to the emergency department complaining of a 20-pound weight gain and severe dyspnea. She was found to have an ejection fraction (EF) of 10% on transthoracic echocardiogram (TTE). After treatment with spironolactone, carvedilol, and digoxin, the patient's symptoms improved, and a repeat TTE showed improved EF to 45%.

Approximately 1 year later, the patient became pregnant. Two months into the pregnancy, she presented to the cardiology clinic for regular monitoring through delivery **(L1, L2)**. The cardiologist recommended she continue carvedilol and restrict sodium intake to avoid fluid overload **(L3, 4)**. The patient's subsequent antenatal course was uncomplicated until she presented to her obstetrician at 35 weeks complaining of 3 days of progressively worsening dyspnea; at this time she was admitted to the hospital for further evaluation.

Significant findings from transthoracic echocardiogram performed on admission (see Fig. 17.1):

- Ejection fraction of 35%
- Severe pulmonary hypertension (pulmonary artery systolic pressure 61 mmHg)
- Severe mitral regurgitation
- Moderate tricuspid regurgitation

J. J. Finneran IV (✉) · T. Archer · A. Brzenski
Department of Anesthesiology, University of California, San Diego, CA, USA
e-mail: jfinneran@ucsd.edu

J. L. Benumof, G. R. Manecke (eds.), *Clinical Anesthesiology II*,
https://doi.org/10.1007/978-3-030-12365-9_17

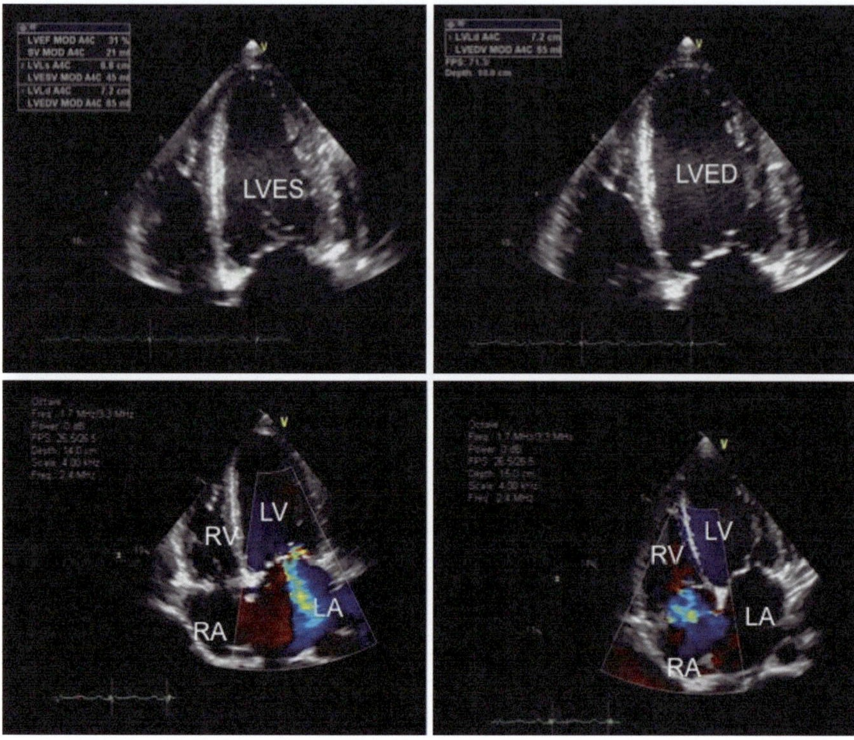

Fig. 17.1 Transthoracic echocardiographic images on admission showing left ventricular end-systolic volume (left upper), left ventricular end-diastolic volume (right upper), mitral regurgitation as Doppler flow from left ventricle to left atrium (left lower), and tricuspid regurgitation as Doppler flow from right ventricle to right atrium (right lower)

Right heart catheterization showed (normal values [1]):

- Right atrial mean pressure: 15 mmHg (1–10 mmHg)
- Right ventricular pressure: 57/24 mmHg (15–30/0–8 mmHg)
- Pulmonary artery (PA) pressure: 59/35 mmHg (15–30/5–15 mmHg)
- Mean PA pressure: 46 mmHg (10–20 mmHg)
- Pulmonary capillary wedge pressure: 23 mmHg (5–15 mmHg)
- Thermodilution cardiac index: 1.5 L per min/m^2 (2.8–4.2 L per min/m^2)
- Pulmonary vascular resistance: 736 dyne*s/cm^5 (150–250 dyne*s/cm^5)

A central line and pulmonary artery catheter were left in place after the right heart catheterization. The patient was started on a nitroglycerine infusion by the cardiology consultant and diuresed several liters with furosemide three times daily. The cardiologist's recommendation was to proceed with vaginal delivery and epidural analgesia if possible **(L5)**. However, the obstetrician felt the patient was not a candidate for vaginal delivery and would require a scheduled Cesarean section due to small maternal habitus (height 1.499 meters (m), weight 69 kilograms (kg), body

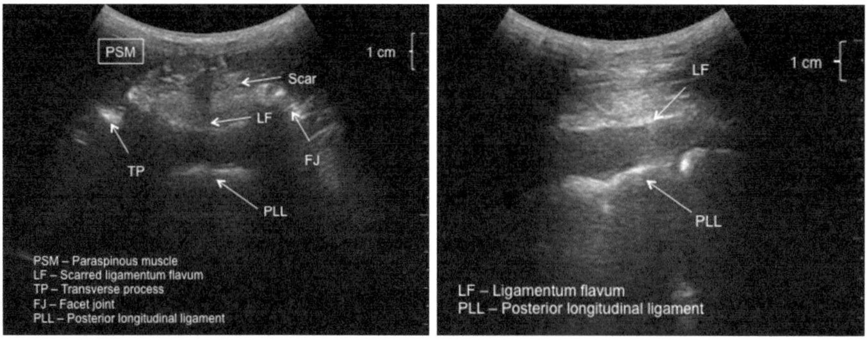

Fig. 17.2 Ultrasonic transverse (left) and parasagittal (right) images of a 29-year-old patient who underwent lumbar laminectomies as infant

mass index 30.71 kg/m^2), large fetal size, unfavorable cervix, and intermittent late decelerations of the fetal heart rate even in the absence of labor **(L6)**.

On the morning of surgery, the patient was brought to the operating room with a nitroglycerine infusion running at 15 micrograms (mcg)/min **(L7)**. A combined spinal/epidural (CSE) anesthetic was planned as the primary anesthetic using a narcotic-only spinal **(L8)** combined with a continuous epidural slowly titrated with local anesthetic drug, using slow dosing to allow the sympathectomy to develop gradually. Ultrasound guidance was employed to facilitate epidural placement **(L9)** due to the fact that the patient had a midline surgical scar extending from the sacrum to the high lumbar region. Ultrasound examination revealed that the patient had undergone laminectomies from L2 to L5 as part of the sacral tumor resection she underwent at 18 months of age (Fig. 17.2). Given the possibility of poor spread of local anesthetic in the epidural space due to scarring from previous laminectomies **(L10)**, it was decided to proceed with epidural placement but to very carefully test the patient's block prior to surgery. If the block was found to be incomplete, the plan was to remove the epidural and proceed with a slowly dosed continuous spinal anesthetic. A continuous spinal was avoided as the initial plan in an attempt to reduce the risk of post-dural puncture headache, while a single injection spinal with local anesthetic was avoided to minimize hemodynamic changes.

A 20-gauge radial artery catheter was placed for tight blood pressure control during the procedure; the patient positioned herself in sitting position for CSE placement. A 17-gauge Tuohy needle was inserted at the level of the iliac crests to a depth of 2 cm based on ultrasound imaging (Fig. 17.3), which estimated the depth of the ligamentum flavum at 3 cm. Ultrasound guidance was particularly helpful in this instance as the patient had no spinal processes to use as landmarks for palpation of the midline and the underlying anatomy of the lumbar spine was unclear. Loss of resistance technique was utilized to locate the epidural space, which was found at a depth of 2.5 cm. A 25-gauge spinal needle was inserted through the Tuohy needle, and 25 mcg of fentanyl and 0.1 milligram (mg) morphine were injected into the intrathecal space. After removal of the spinal needle, an epidural catheter was easily threaded into the epidural space.

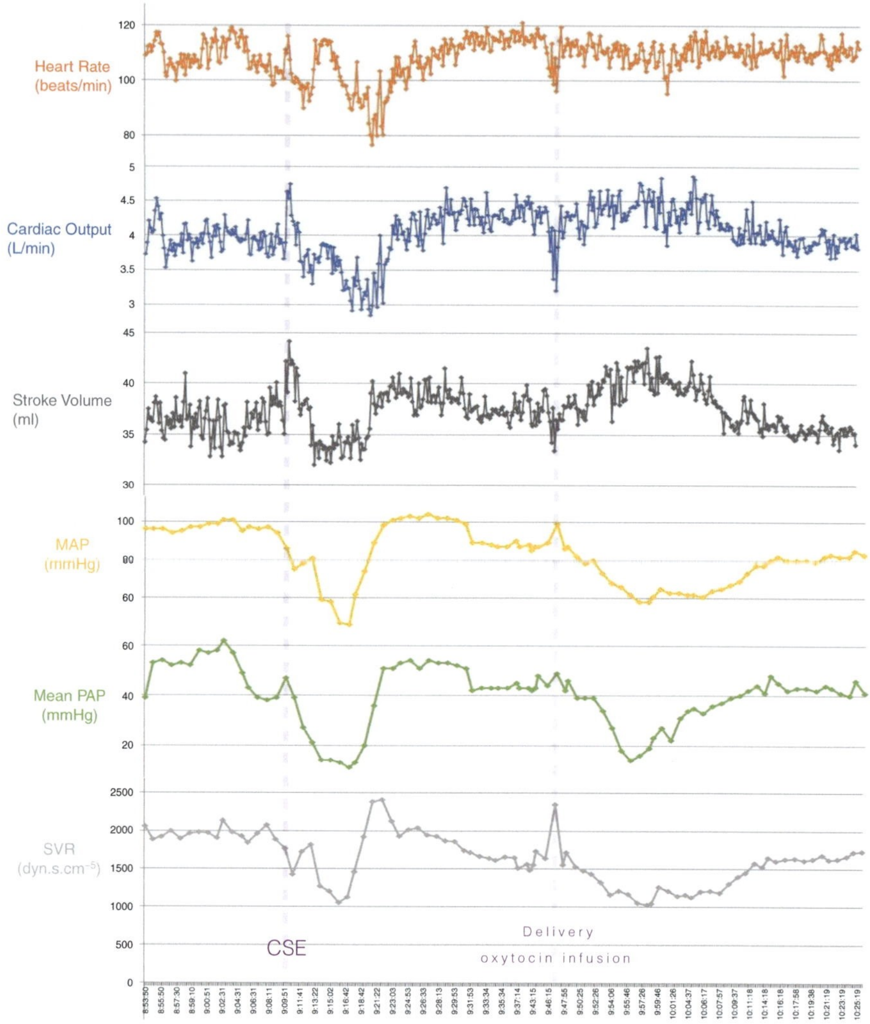

Fig. 17.3 Heart rate recorded from EKG, mean arterial pressure (MAP) from radial arterial line, mean pulmonary arterial pressure (PAP) from PA catheter, cardiac output and systemic vascular resistance (SVR) based on electrical cardiometry (**L11, L12**). Times of combined spinal/epidural (CSE) block administration and delivery with oxytocin infusion denoted by vertical lines

After a negative test dose of 1.5% lidocaine with 1:200,000 epinephrine, the catheter was dosed with 5 milliliters (mL) 2% lidocaine. The patient was found to have a dense block with this dose at approximately a T10 level. The block was therefore supplemented with an additional 7 mL of 2% lidocaine in divided doses. This resulted in a dense T4 block; however the patient's mean arterial pressure (MAP) decreased from approximately 90 mmHg prior to the block to 55 mmHg after the block (Fig. 17.4). Ephedrine was chosen for blood pressure support given

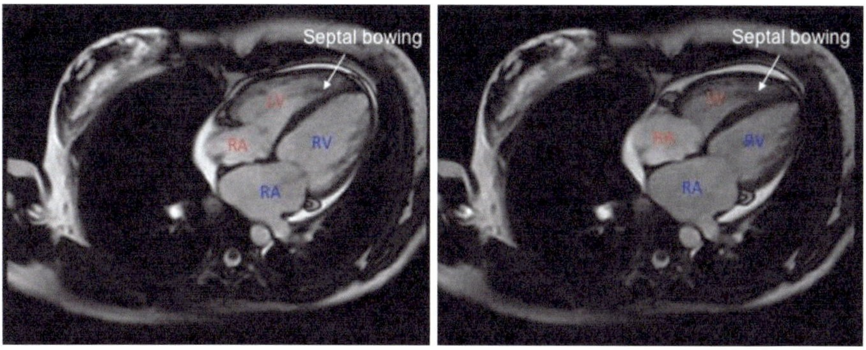

Fig. 17.4 Cardiac MRI during systole (right) and diastole (left) obtained 8 days postoperatively. Demonstrates right atrial (RA) enlargement, right ventricular (RV) enlargement, and hypertrophy and interventricular septal bowing indicating chronic pulmonary hypertension. A mild to moderate pericardial effusion is also noted

its sympathomimetic effects. The patient's MAP subsequently recovered and incision was made with the patient experiencing no discomfort.

The patient remained comfortable through delivery, which occurred 11 min after incision. After delivery, oxytocin infusion was started to support uterine tone, and nitroglycerine infusion was discontinued to facilitate hemostasis and prevent excessive vasodilation in combination with oxytocin infusion **(L13)**.

Over the first 2 postoperative days, the patient's pulmonary capillary wedge pressure (PCWP) progressively increased. She responded well to diuresis and augmentation of cardiac function with milrinone. With diuresis and initiation of an ACE inhibitor, the patient was successfully weaned from milrinone and discharged on the fifth postoperative day. After discharge, the patient underwent cardiac MRI to further evaluate cardiac function (Fig. 17.4). On follow-up 6 months later, both the patient and her baby were doing well. The patient had resumed her previous cardiac medication regimen and had no heart failure symptoms.

- **Lesson 1:** What are the cardiac changes that occur during normal pregnancy?

Cardiac changes begin soon after conception. These alterations are generally well tolerated in normal women; [2] however, they may have great significance in patients with pre-existing cardiac lesions (see Lesson 2) (Table 17.1).

- **Lesson 2:** Which cardiac conditions are most likely to causes problems during pregnancy? Which cardiac lesions are relatively well tolerated in pregnancy?

Regurgitant lesions and those lesions with left to right shunts tend to be well tolerated; while poorly tolerated lesions involve forward flow obstruction or right to left shunting [2] (Table 17.2).

- **Lesson 3:** What factors predict that a pregnant patient with a history of heart failure will decompensate during labor?

Table 17.1 Hemodynamic changes during normal pregnancy

Hemodynamic variable	↑ or ↓	Physiologic explanation
Blood volume	↑	Increases beginning in the 6th week
		Maximum volume, approximately 50% above prepregnancy values, is reached by 30–34 weeks of gestation
		Plasma volume expansion is hormonally mediated, via the renin-angiotensin-aldosterone system
Hematocrit	↓	Red blood cell (RBC) mass increases by 20–40%
		Plasma volume increases to a greater degree, resulting in a decrease in hematocrit
		Normal hematocrit values during the first, second, and third trimesters are 31–41, 30–39, and 28–40, respectively [3]
Cardiac output	↑	Increase begins by 10th week of gestation
		By the third trimester, has increased 40% above prepregnancy levels [4]
		Increases to meet metabolic demands of pregnancy and labor and the increased uterine and placental blood flow associated with pregnancy and labor
Blood pressure	↓	Diastolic pressure decreases more than systolic pressure
		This is related to the effect of progesterone on vascular tone

Table 17.2 Well-tolerated and poorly tolerated cardiac lesions during pregnancy

Well tolerated (Regurgitant lesions/left to right shunts)	Poorly tolerated (Obstructive lesions/right to left shunts)
Mitral and aortic insufficiency	Mitral stenosis
Atrial and ventricular septal defects	Aortic stenosis
Patent ductus arteriosus	Coarctation of the aorta
Mitral prolapse	Unrepaired tetralogy of Fallot
Hypertrophic obstructive cardiomyopathy	Primary pulmonary hypertension

Table 17.3 CARdiac disease in PREGnancy (CARPREG) risk scoring system

Clinical factor	Points
History of prior cardiac event (heart failure, transient ischemic attack, or stroke before pregnancy) or arrhythmia	1
Baseline NYHA class II or greater, or cyanosis	1
Left heart obstruction (mitral valve area <2 cm^2, aortic valve area <1.5 cm^2, or peak left ventricular outflow tract gradient >30 mm Hg by echocardiography)	1
Reduced systemic ventricular systolic function (ejection fraction <40%)	1

The CARdiac disease in PREGnancy (CARPREG) risk score was published in 2001 and can be used to predict severe adverse cardiac events during pregnancy (pulmonary edema, sustained symptomatic tachy- or bradyarrhythmia requiring treatment, stroke, cardiac arrest, or cardiac death). It is based on the presence or absence of four clinical factors (Table 17.3). Using this risk stratification score, each of the risk factors is assigned one point. Severe cardiac event rates associated with 0, 1, and more than 1 point were 5%, 25%, and 75%, respectively [5].

The recommendation from the CARPREG investigators is that any parturient with a risk score of 1 or greater be referred to receive her obstetric care at a regional medical center while parturients without these risk factors are safe to deliver at a community hospital. The patient in this scenario had a history of decompensated heart failure, was NYHA class I prior to pregnancy, had no history of outflow tract obstruction, and did have a reduced ejection fraction on echocardiography, giving her a CARPREG score of 2 and therefore a 75% risk of adverse cardiac event during pregnancy.

- **Lesson 4:** What commonly used cardiac drugs are contraindicated during pregnancy?

Most commonly used anesthetic agents and cardiac drugs are safe for use during pregnancy. Knowledge of which drugs are contraindicated in pregnancy is critical for providers caring for parturients with cardiac disease.

Angiotensin-converting enzyme (ACE) inhibitors such as captopril, enalapril, and lisinopril are commonly used agents in heart failure patients and have been shown to reduce mortality in patients with heart failure. However, very importantly, ACE inhibitors are absolutely contraindicated in pregnancy during the first, second, and third trimesters due to risk of ACE-inhibitor fetopathy, a constellation of congenital malformations that includes oligohydramnios, intrauterine growth retardation, hypocalvaria, renal dysplasia, anuria, renal failure, and death [6].

Warfarin is contraindicated in pregnancy due to concern for fetal warfarin syndrome, a collection of birth defects including nasal hypoplasia, narrowed nasal bridge, and scoliosis. Risk is highest in the first trimester, especially during organogenesis between the 3rd and 9th weeks.

- **Lesson 5:** What are the anesthetic options for delivery in patients with severe pulmonary hypertension? Which anesthetic options should be avoided?

The optimal mode of delivery and anesthetic choice for these patients remains controversial. If a vaginal delivery is attempted, some form of continuous neuraxial anesthesia is important. Alternatively, if the patient undergoes a Caesarian section, both neuraxial techniques and general anesthesia have been advocated. Table 17.4 summarizes these options.

- **Lesson 6:** What are the implications of late fetal heart rate decelerations in the absence of labor?

Uterine contractions decrease perfusion of the placenta. Late decelerations of the fetal heart rate are an indication of inadequate placental perfusion. If the fetus is showing signs of inadequate oxygenation even in the absence of labor, the obstetricians may judge that the fetus may not "tolerate labor"—that is, that the fetus might not tolerate the additional oxygen deprivation caused by uterine contractions.

- **Lesson 7:** What are the hemodynamic effects of nitroglycerine? Describe its mechanism of action.

Table 17.4 Anesthetic options for vaginal delivery or Cesarean section (C-section) in patients with severe pulmonary hypertension

Anesthetic/ delivery option	Acceptable/ unacceptable	Comments
Vaginal delivery with epidural	Acceptable	Contraindicated if patient is a poor candidate for labor due to obstetric issues (i.e., small maternal habitus, large fetus, unfavorable cervix, intermittent late decelerations)
Delivery without neuraxial anesthesia	Unacceptable	Painful labor is contraindicated due to the dramatic increases in blood pressure and cardiac output associated with labor pain
C-section with continuous lumbar epidural	Acceptable	Block should be induced gradually to prevent excessive decrease in systemic vascular resistance (SVR)
		Block must be carefully assessed for patchiness, as block failure with significant pain will result in catecholamine surge
C-section with continuous spinal	Acceptable	Similar to continuous epidural, continuous spinal must be carefully titrated to prevent drop in SVR
		May be advantageous compared to epidural due to denser and more reliable block
C-section under general anesthesia	Acceptable	Some argue that any parturient with severe pulmonary hypertension requires general anesthesia with a cardiac-style induction [7]
		However, concerns of general anesthesia include sympathetic stimulation during laryngoscopy and intubation, inferior postoperative pain control leading to catecholamine increase, aspiration risk, neonatal respiratory depression, and lack of mother/baby interaction in the immediate postpartum period [7]
Single injection spinal for C-section	Unacceptable	Dramatic and poorly controllable reduction in SVR makes this a poor choice for Caesarean anesthesia

Nitroglycerine (NG) and other nitrates (isosorbide dinitrate and isosorbide mononitrate) are potent vasodilators acting on both the capacitance and resistance vessels via nitric oxide (NO). NO is produced by the vascular endothelium by metabolism of nitroglycerin and is a potent activator of the enzyme guanylyl cyclase, which produces cyclic GMP (cGMP). cGMP in turn activates the cGMP-dependent protein kinase, which phosphorylates and activates myosin light chain phosphatase in vascular smooth muscle cells. Activation of myosin light chain phosphatase results in relaxation of the vascular smooth muscle cells producing vasodilation.

The exact mechanism by which NG-mediated vasodilation improves cardiac symptoms has been debated [8]. The antianginal effects of NG are likely multifactorial. Peripheral venous vasodilation reduces preload, LV chamber diameter, and LV wall tension and therefore cardiac work and myocardial oxygen consumption. Vasodilation in the systemic arterioles reduces systolic blood pressure and afterload, also improving left ventricular wall tension and myocardial oxygen consumption. NG also dilates the coronary arteries, improving oxygen delivery to the myocardium.

In patients with heart failure, the beneficial effects of NG likely result from reduced preload, which improves pulmonary capillary wedge pressure, right ventricular and right atrial pressures, and reduced afterload, which may improve forward flow from the heart [8]. This obviously must be balanced against the potential decrease in myocardial perfusion pressure due to decreased diastolic pressure resulting from systemic arterial vasodilation.

- **Lesson 8:** How are the effects of spinal narcotics mediated? Why was intrathecal fentanyl dose chosen to augment the epidural block?

Neuraxially administered opioids redistribute to the spinal cord, epidural fat, CSF, and systemic circulation based on their site of placement (epidural or intrathecal) and relative lipophilicity.

First, in the spinal cord, the analgesic effect of opioids is mediated directly by binding to opioid receptors in the substantia gelatinosa of the dorsal horn in the gray matter.

Second, drug that redistributes to the systemic circulation via venous uptake from epidural fat exerts systemic effects similar to intravenous dosing.

Third, some drug (particularly with more hydrophilic opioids) may reach the medulla and brain via rostral spread within the CSF, where a different subset of opioid receptors produces analgesia [9]. This rostral spread may cause delayed respiratory depression which in the case of morphine can persist up to 18–24 h after administration.

The combination of intrathecal or epidural narcotic with epidural local anesthetics has been demonstrated to provide better analgesia to laboring women than either medication alone [10]. Additionally, it has been observed that subanalgesic concentrations of epidural local anesthetics may be rendered efficacious by the additional of intrathecal opiates [10]. Unlike epidural and intrathecal administration of local anesthetics, intrathecal administration of narcotics generally does not produce significant hemodynamic perturbations [11].

- **Lesson 9:** Use of ultrasound guidance in neuraxial anesthesia.

The first reported use of ultrasound guidance to facilitate epidural catheter placement was by Cork et al. in 1980 [12]. Ultrasound localization during placement of epidural catheters has been demonstrated to reduce both the number of puncture attempts and number of level attempts, reduce the incidence of side effects, and improve patient satisfaction [13].

Our method of ultrasound imaging utilizes transverse views of the spine using the same large curvilinear probe which the obstetricians use for their examinations. Transverse views are usually sufficient for block placement, but the parasagittal view can be used to confirm some of the information from the transverse view (exact interspace level and depth to ligamentum flavum) and is useful in its own right for performing paramedian blocks.

In the transverse view (Fig. 17.5, left), we slowly slide the probe cephalad and caudad while watching the ultrasound screen, in order to visualize the deeper structures, which appear when the probe is located above or below the spinous process and is oriented at the proper angle. These structures are the ligamentum flavum

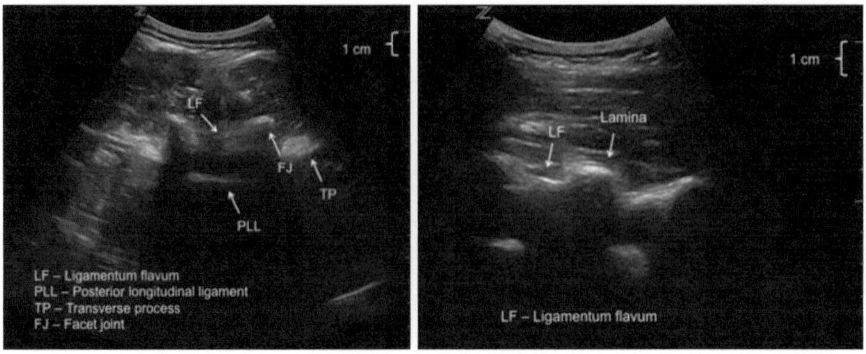

Fig. 17.5 Ultrasonic transverse (left) and parasagittal (right) images of a normal lumbar spine in a 28-year-old healthy volunteer

(LF), posterior longitudinal ligament (PLL), transverse processes (TP), and facet joints (FJ). Optimally visualizing these structures yields a fairly accurate and useful estimation of the depth at which loss of resistance will be found (the depth of the LF) and the ideal angle of needle entry (the angle of the probe that produces the best image). Optimizing the brightness of the PLL demonstrates the best angle of entry for the needle since the angle at which the best view (greatest sound reflection) is obtained will likely be the best trajectory for the needle. It should be emphasized, however, that the final placement of the Tuohy needle in the epidural space is still achieved by the loss of resistance technique and that the measurements taken from the use of ultrasound should serve only as a guide.

In the parasagittal view (Fig. 17.5, right), the lamina and the gaps between adjacent lamina (representing our target interspace) can be confirmed. The parasagittal view is useful for confirming the cephalad-caudad level of needle insertion as well as providing an insertion point and insertion angle if a paramedian approach is desired.

- **Lesson 10:** What are the considerations regarding neuraxial anesthetic options in patients with previous lumbar spine surgery?

The primary concern for performing neuraxial anesthesia in patients with previous spinal surgery is scar tissue in the epidural space limiting spread of local anesthetic. There is evidence that attempting epidural anesthesia in these patients results in increased difficulty in placing the block and increased incidence of a "patchy block" [14]. Spinal anesthesia may be less problematic in these patients.

- **Lesson 11:** Electrical cardiometry to measure cardiac output (CO) and systemic vascular resistance (SVR).

Electrical cardiometry (EC) is a noninvasive mechanism for monitoring hemodynamic variables. It is a more recent version of impedance cardiomyography that works by transmitting insensible, fixed amplitude, high-frequency alternating current through two outer electrodes located on opposite sides of the thorax and then measuring the voltage change that occurs between two inner electrodes. Measurement of the voltage change allows calculation of impedance change across the thorax in different stages of the cardiac cycle. The EC device interprets the thoracic impedance changes in systolic blood acceleration and can use this data to calculate stroke volume, CO, and SVR [15].

- **Lesson 12:** Explain the hemodynamic changes that occur during the course of this anesthetic and surgery. Specifically, what are the effects of neuraxial block and delivery with oxytocin infusion on mean arterial pressure (MAP), systemic vascular resistance (SVR), pulmonary artery pressure (PAP), and cardiac output (CO)?

Both neuraxial block and delivery with oxytocin administration are accompanied by reductions in MAP, PAP and SVR. This is to be expected from the dilation of both capacitance veins and resistance arterioles that results from each of these interventions. Neuraxial block is associated with a decrease in CO (secondary to reduction in preload), whereas delivery and oxytocin administration are associated with an increase in CO (due to autotransfusion of blood from the vasoconstricted uterus and relief of aortocaval compression).

- **Lesson 13:** How should postpartum hemorrhage be treated in a patient with pulmonary hypertension? What common cardiac drugs effect uterine tone?

The first-line medication for postpartum hemorrhage is oxytocin, and an intravenous oxytocin infusion is routinely started immediately on delivery during Cesarean section. In parturients with heart disease, the cardiovascular effect of uterotonic agents must be considered. Simultaneously, one must consider the effects of cardiac drugs on the uterus.

In Fig. 17.3, we demonstrate that there is a dramatic reduction in systemic vascular resistance (SVR) with administration of oxytocin. However, unlike the reduction in SVR seen with induction of the epidural block, there was no decrease in cardiac output after delivery. In fact, the CO increased. We suggest that this is related to augmentation of cardiac output by autotransfusion and the relief of aortocaval compression leading to an increased circulating volume, as well as the afterload reducing effects of oxytocin.

At delivery, nitroglycerin was discontinued due to concern for uterine atony resulting in postpartum hemorrhage. NG has been used in obstetrics for uterine relaxation during obstetric emergencies. There is some evidence from laboratory animals that placental tissue is required for NG-induced uterine relaxation [16], which would suggest decreased concern for postpartum hemorrhage resulting from NG use for cardiac problems in the postpartum period after removal of the placenta. However, given that the effects of nitroglycerin on the postpartum uterus have not been studied in humans, we felt it was prudent to discontinue nitroglycerin after delivery. Table 17.5 summarizes drugs with effects on both uterine and vascular tone.

Table 17.5 Effects of oxytocin, methylergonovine, and nitroglycerine on uterine and vascular tone

Drug	Uterine effect	Effect on vascular tone
Oxytocin	Contraction	Reduced SVR
Methylergonovine	Contraction	Increased SVR
Nitroglycerin	Relaxation	Reduced SVR

References

1. Reich DL, Mittnacht AJC, Manecke GR Jr, Kaplan JA. Monitoring of the heart and vascular system. In: Kaplan JA, Reich DL, Savino JS, editors. Kaplan's cardiac anesthesia. 6th ed. St. Louis: Saunders, Elsevier; 2011.
2. Raymond R, Underwood DA, Moodie DS. Cardiovascular problems in pregnancy. Cleve Clin J Med. 1987;54(2):95–104.
3. Longo D, Fauci A, Kasper D, Hauser S, Jameson J, Loscalzo J. Harrison's principles of internal medicine. 18th ed. New York: McGraw-Hill Professions; 2011.
4. Tenholder MF, South-Paul JE. Dyspnea in pregnancy. Chest. 1989;96:381–8.
5. Siu SC, Sermer M, Colman JM, Alvarez AN, Mercier LA, Morton BC, Kells CM, Bergin ML, Kiess MC, Marcotte F, Taylor DA, Gordon EP, Spears JC, Tam JW, Amankwah KS, Smallhorn JF, Farine D, Sorensen S. Prospective multicenter study of pregnancy outcomes in women with heart disease. Circulation. 2001;104:515–21.
6. Cooper WO, Hernandez-Diaz S, Arbogast P, Dudley J, Dyer S, Gideon PS, Hall K, Ray WA. Major congenital malformations after first-trimester exposure to ACE inhibitors. N Engl J Med. 2006;354:2443–51.
7. Weeks SK, Smith JB. Obstetric anesthesia in patients with primary pulmonary hypertension. Can J Anesth. 1991;38:814–6.
8. Abrams J. Hemodynamic effects of nitroglycerine and long-acting nitrates. Am Heart J. 1985;110(1):217–24.
9. Rathmell JP, Lair T, Nauman B. The role of intrathecal drugs in the treatment of acute pain. Anesth Analg. 2005;101(5S):30–43.
10. Tejwani G, Rattan A, McDonald J. Role of spinal opioid receptors in the antinociceptive interactions between intrathecal morphine and bupivacaine. Anesth Analg. 1992;74:726–34.
11. Grant G, Susser L, Cascio M, Moses M, Zakowski M. Hemodynamic effects of intrathecal fentanyl in nonlaboring parturients. J Clin Anesth. 1996;8(2):99–103.
12. Cork RC, Kryc JJ, Vaughan RW. Ultrasonic localization of the lumbar epidural space. Anesthesiology. 1980;52:513–6.
13. Grau T, Leipold RW, Conradi R, Martin E, Motsch J. Efficacy of ultrasound imaging in obstetric epidural anesthesia. J Clin Anesth. 2002;14(3):169–75.
14. Daley MD, Morningstar BA, Rolbin SH, Stewart JA. Epidural anesthesia for obstetrics after spinal surgery. Reg Anesth Pain Med. 1990;15(6):280–4.
15. Martin A, Anyikam A, Ballas J, Buono K, Mantell K, Covey TH, Archer T. A validation study of electrical cardiometry in pregnant patient using transthoracic echocardiography as the reference standard. J Clin Monit Comput. 2016;30:679.
16. Scott S, Csavoy A, Datta S. Placental tissue enhanced uterine relaxation by nitroglycerin. Anesth Analg. 1998;86(2):304–9.

Chapter 18
Organization Promotes Safety: A Step Forward

Kimberly A. Pollock and Jonathan L. Benumof

Case Description

This is a case of a 31-year-old gravida 1 para 0 female, 5′9″, 67 kg with a body mass index (BMI) of 22 with a gestational age of 39 weeks and 2 days who was admitted for a scheduled primary cesarean section (C-section) for breech presentation of a singleton pregnancy. The plan was to perform a spinal anesthetic block with light sedation for the C-section. The spinal dose was prepared with 1.6 cc of 0.75% bupivacaine, 25 mcg of fentanyl, and 0.1 mg of morphine for a total volume of 2.2 cc. The spinal dose was injected into the tray reservoir and drawn up into a 3 cc syringe and capped with the pink-hubbed 18-gauge needle supplied in the kit. 3 cc of 1% lidocaine was drawn up into a second 3 cc syringe and capped with the blue-hubbed 25-gauge needle also supplied in the kit. Neither syringe was labeled. The patient was seated on the operating room table and positioned appropriately.

The back was prepped with DuraPrep solution and draped with a sterile drape. Landmarks were identified by palpation. The blue-hubbed needle cap to the 1% lidocaine syringe was removed and 1 cc of the 1% lidocaine was then used to anesthetize the skin over the intended insertion site, leaving approximately 2 cc of 1% lidocaine left in the syringe. Both the removed blue-hubbed needle cap and the 1% lidocaine syringe were placed back on the tray separately and not connected. The intrathecal space was accessed (with the aid of an introducer needle) with a 25-gauge spinal needle with return of clear cerebrospinal fluid (CSF). The uncapped, unlabeled 3 cc syringe containing 2 cc of clear solution (1% lidocaine) was then mistakenly administered into the intrathecal space. As the needle was removed from

K. A. Pollock (✉)
Department of Anesthesiology, University of California, San Diego, CA, USA

J. L. Benumof
Department of Anesthesiology, University of California, UCSD Medical Center, UCSD School of Medicine, San Diego, CA, USA

J. L. Benumof, G. R. Manecke (eds.), *Clinical Anesthesiology II*,
https://doi.org/10.1007/978-3-030-12365-9_18

the patient's back, the error was realized (**L1-L5**). The entire spinal anesthetic procedure was repeated, and the intended spinal dose of 2.2 cc of bupivacaine/fentanyl/morphine was administered into the intrathecal space. The patient was placed in the supine position. Heart rate decreased from 70 beats per minute to 50 beats per minute. Blood pressure remained 115–120 mmHg/65–70 mmHg. Fetal heart rate was reassuring. There were no other signs that the intrathecal lidocaine solution, in addition to the bupivacaine solution, had spread to the high thoracic or cervical region, thereby compromising diaphragm function or respirations. The level of the spinal was tested with ice and found to be at approximately the T6 level. The surgical team was notified that the patient was ready to be prepped and draped. When the surgical site was tested using an Allis clamp, the patient indicated that she could feel mild, sharp pain. The patient was then placed in the Trendelenburg position, and after 5 min, a surgical block was achieved. The intraoperative course was uneventful. Following the C-section, the inadvertent administration of intrathecal lidocaine was discussed with the patient. She was reassured that it was unlikely that there would be any long-term neurologic consequences related to this event.

Lessons Learned

L-1: What Is a Drug Error?

In order to address errors involving drug administration, some definitions must be established. According to the Australian Incident Monitoring Study (AIMS), the definition of a drug error is a failure to give the drug or dose of drug that was intended [1]. For the purpose of this chapter, we will focus on incorrect unintentional drug administration instead of incorrect dose administration. There are four categories/types of drug errors (see Table 18.1). First, a syringe swap occurs when the correctly labeled, correct intended drug was drawn up but a correctly labeled, incorrect unintended drug in a different syringe was given to the patient. Second, a drug container swap occurs when an incorrect unintended drug is drawn up from an incorrect unintended drug container and the correct originally intended drug label is used; however and unfortunately use of the correct originally intended drug label

Table 18.1 Four possible combinations of errors leading to incorrect drug administration

Syringe swap	**Labeling error**
Giving a correctly labeled but wrong unintended drug	Placing the wrong unintended label on a drug syringe
Drug container swap	**Colossal error**
Drawing up the wrong unintended drug from the wrong drug container into a syringe and placing the intended drug label on it	Drawing up the wrong unintended drug into a syringe and also placing the wrong label on it

ensures the practitioner will give the incorrect drug (thinking they are giving the correct drug). Third, a labeling error occurs when the correct intended drug is drawn up from the correct intended drug container; however, the incorrect label is placed on the syringe so the practitioner is destined to give the incorrect unintended drug for some given specific future problem/indication. A final possibility of error exists in which the incorrect unintended drug is drawn up into a syringe and the incorrect label is used. If this error occurs, you may want to consider quitting your day job. This would result in a confusing and colossal error.

Studies show that syringe swaps and drug container swaps are the most common cause of medication errors in anesthesia [1] and that syringes of the same size are most frequently involved in giving the wrong drug [2]. Furthermore these studies indicate that many drug errors occur *after* the drug has been correctly drawn up and labeled, indicating a need for workspace organization and a pre-administration check to assure the intended drug is being administered [2]. The main drugs involved in syringe swaps were opioids, neuromuscular blocking agents, reversal agents, benzodiazepines, vasopressors and local anesthetics [1].

L-2: What Is the Incidence of Drug Errors?

According to the Australian Incident Monitoring Study (AIMS), approximately 50% of drug errors were due to syringe and drug preparation errors. Syringe swaps, drug container swaps, and labeling errors were the most common among these errors. Equipment misuse or malfunction, incorrect route of administration and communication error accounted for the remaining incidents of drug error reported [1]. A survey conducted in 2001, showed that one drug administration error was reported for every 133 anesthetics administered [3]. Over 10,000 anesthetics were reviewed and it was found that due to these errors, one patient was aware while under muscle relaxation and two required prolonged ventilation [3]. **Lesson 4a** (Table 18.2) details many other outcome possibilities due to administering the incorrect drug that are known to occur. Although the safety of anesthetic techniques has significantly improved over many decades, techniques for mixing drugs, filling syringes and administration to the patient have not significantly changed [1].

L-3: What Are Major Factors Contributing to Drug Errors?

According to AIMS, the major factors contributing to syringe swaps or drug container swaps are inattention, haste, errors in drug labeling procedure and distraction [1]. The majority of reported events occurred between the hours of 0800 and 1800, which is consistent with the time during which most anesthetics are carried out.

Table 18.2 The most common drugs given in error and effects on patients

Inadvertent drug →	Effect on patient
Opioids →	- Respiratory depression - Bradycardia - Hypotension - Delayed emergence
Neuromuscular blocker →	- Awareness under anesthesia - Respiratory Failure
Reversal agent →	- Inability to re-paralyze - Rigid musculature - Difficulty ventilating - Herniation of tissue
Benzodiazepines →	- Delayed emergence
Vasopressors →	- Vasoconstriction - Hypertension - Tachycardia - Bradycardia
Local anesthetics →	- Delayed emergence - Seizures

What was interesting is that over half of the errors occurred during emergency procedures, which is excessive given the lower relative rate with which these procedures occur. Probable causes for the increased errors during emergency cases include time pressure to proceed with the case, causing the anesthesiologist to potentially "cut corners" and not adhering to their usual routine [1]. Another potential cause of drug error is fatigue, as emergency cases generally proceed after normal hours of operation [1]. In either case, it can be argued that having a standardized way of filling syringes and organizing the location of those syringes within the anesthesia workspace may help reduce these errors.

L-4: Adverse Outcomes Related to a Disorganized Work Station

The Incorrect Drug Is Given

The two most common causes of incorrect drug administration are drug container swap and syringe swap. Unfortunately, drug containers are not standardized. Drug manufacturers are constantly changing the shape, design, size, volume of container, and cap color of the vehicles in which they sell their products and these changes can lead to drug errors if the new design closely resembles the design of a different medication. Drug container shape, volume and color all contribute to selection of the correct medication (in addition to the actual drug label on the container); however, where these drug containers are located within the anesthesia drug tray also determines drug selection. The design and layout of the anesthesia drug tray and how the anesthesia machine tabletop workstation is organized can greatly affect correct drug selection and this consideration, "organization promotes safety," will be discussed in the next section.

Syringe swaps used to be more common than drug container swaps; however in more recent studies, it seems that drug container swaps are now more common (perhaps due to the adoption of a color coded labeling system for syringes). The most common drugs involved in syringe swap are opioids, neuromuscular blocking agents, reversal agents, benzodiazepines, vasopressors, and local anesthetics (see Table 18.2) [1]. Consequences of unknowingly giving opioid include respiratory depression, bradycardia, hypotension, and delayed emergence. Cardiovascular effects of excess opioid are more pronounced in sicker patients (ASA III or IV) due to their lack of physiologic reserve due to depletion of catecholamines. Inadvertent administration of neuromuscular blocking agents could lead to awareness under anesthesia and paralysis of respiratory muscles; both of these complications are unforgivable in the field of anesthesia. Before the introduction of Suggamadex, accidentally administering reversal agent in the middle of a case would lead to potential reversal of the neuromuscular blockade and inability to re-paralyze for some time. If this occurred during an open abdominal case, the anesthesiologist could encounter difficulty ventilating due to rigid abdominal wall musculature and an inability for the surgeons to close the wound adequately, resulting in potential for herniation of tissue through the wound. Administration of benzodiazepines when another agent was intended could lead to delayed emergence, especially in patients undergoing neurologic procedures. Unintentional delivery of vasopressors could lead to vasoconstriction (and perhaps decreased oxygen delivery to vital organs), hypertension, tachycardia, or bradycardia. If these agents were administered to a patient with low intravascular volume or poor cardiac reserve, this could lead to end organ or limb ischemia. Finally, unintended administration of local anesthetics intravenously can cause delayed emergence and seizures (see Table 18.2).

Cross-Contamination Between Patients

Another direct result of picking the wrong syringe is picking up an already used syringe from another patient; this sets up the possibility of cross-contamination and infection. In 1995, a survey of ASA members indicated that 39% of anesthesiologists reported reusing syringes from one patient to another and 36% reported using the same vasopressor syringes for different patients [4]. In the past 15 years, numerous publications have described iatrogenic hepatitis C virus (HCV) transmission unrelated to transfused blood products or transplantation procedures. Nearly all were due to unsafe therapeutic injection practices related to multidose vials (MDVs) and infusion bags contaminated by reinsertion of used needles/syringes, use of a single needle/syringe for intravenous (IV) medication administration to multiple patients, or use of a contaminated finger-stick glucose measurement device on multiple patients [5]. A study was conducted using expired packed red blood cells attached to a basic IV tubing set and connected to a pressure transducer to allow continuous pressure monitoring within the tubing to mimic the backflow exerted by a human vein. At all sample times and at both injection ports on the basic tubing line, fluid in the distal portion of the extension set tested positive for blood by reagent strips as well as spectrophotometric analysis. By cross-contamination with blood, the reuse of syringes from patient to patient increases the risk of transmission of infectious viral particles [6]. It should be noted that syringes and needles are intended for single use only and should be discarded thereafter. Furthermore, attention should be paid to vials marked single dose vs. multidose to avoid cross-contamination between patients. Finally, red caps should be sterilely placed on syringes when not in use since needles contain a hollow bore and therefore have the potential for communication with the environment.

Accidental Needlestick Injury (NSI) Among Anesthesiologists

Here is what we know about NSI in anesthesia personnel. A survey of over 2000 ASA members determined the incidence of accidental NSI. In this study, 88% of respondents reported at least 1 accidental NSI in the past 10 years, 21% of NSI were from a needle used in a high-risk patient, and 4.5% were from a needle used in a known HIV-positive individual [4]. In another study, the most common devices involved in NSI to anesthesia personnel were examined, and it was found that the largest categories of devices causing contaminated percutaneous injuries were needles or syringes, intravenous or arterial catheter needle stylets, suture needles, and standard hollow-bore needles for secondary intravenous infusion. Most of these injuries occurred between steps of a multistep procedure and recapping [7]. Recapping needles is done very commonly and the authors think this is a common cause of NSI. It is likely that there are still other mechanisms of NSIs among anesthesiologists. Practicing routine organization of procedure trays (spinal, epidural/regional, central line kits) and anesthesia machine tabletop workstations to avoid accidental NSI is imperative. One possible approach to standardizing arrangement of these trays will be discussed below.

L-5: Organization Promotes Safety

General Considerations

There are many steps to consider when examining the potential for drug errors to occur (see Fig. 18.1). First, the anesthesiologist must choose the correct drug containers from the anesthesia cart drug drawer (or Pyxis or anesthesia workroom/storage space). These drug drawers are not organized in a way that is standardized from institution to institution or according to a rigorous drug tray wide logic; therefore, errors could occur if the location of the drug container within the anesthesia cart drug drawer has changed or differs from the institution in which the anesthesiologist had trained or was comfortable working in or according to some logic that is in the anesthesiologist's mind. Second, the anesthesiologist must choose syringes to

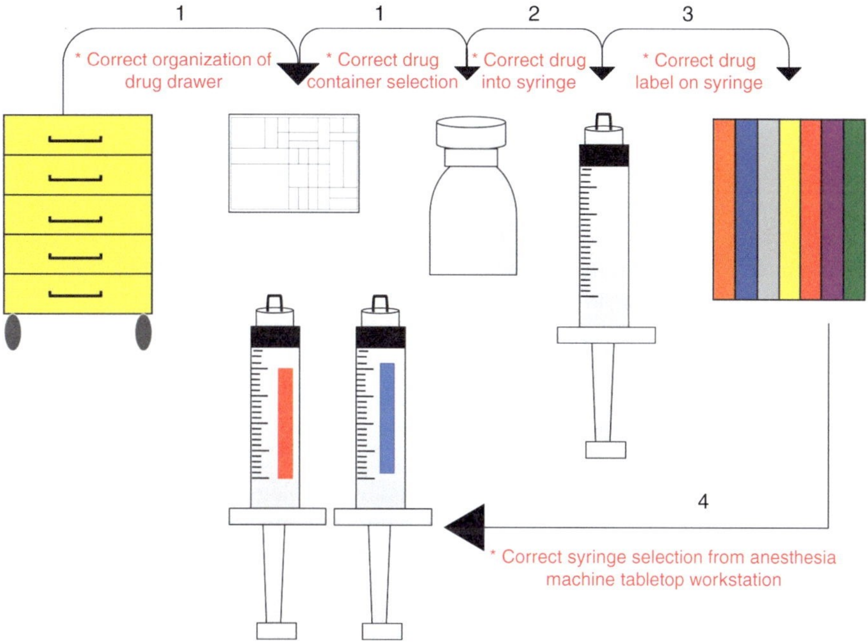

Fig. 18.1 Schematic of potential times of error from cart to patient. Numbers correspond to considerations enumerated in the text

draw up the drugs needed for a particular case. If the drug manufacturing company has recently changed the volume of drug that is distributed to an institution, this could create a possible error. For example, if an anesthesiologist is accustomed to succinylcholine coming in a 5 cc vial and now the manufacturing company is selling succinylcholine in 10 cc vials, the anesthesiologist could mistakenly draw up succinylcholine into a 10 cc syringe labeled with rocuronium leading to a "drug container swap." Third, the anesthesiologist must label the syringe with the appropriate label. This should be done *after* the drug has been drawn up and cross-referenced with the label on the drug container; however, if the anesthesiologist "pre-labels" the syringes prior to drawing up drugs, they could mistakenly draw up the incorrect unintended drug into a syringe with the correct intended drug label of the drug they had intended to draw up leading to a "labeling error." Fourth, even if the anesthesiologist has chosen the correct drug containers, applied the correct labels *after* drawing up their drugs and cross-referenced these labels with the label on the drug container, a "syringe swap" is still very possible and is one of the most common drug errors to occur. The anesthesia machine tabletop workstation is a prime location for a "syringe swap." This last error likely results from lack of organization of drugs atop the anesthesia machine tabletop workstation. In the next few sections, we will address ways to circumvent the aforementioned issues leading to drug error, from the time the drug is removed from the anesthesia drug drawer until the drug is administered to the patient (see Fig. 18.1).

Drug Organization Within the Anesthesia Cart Drug Drawer and Syringe Size Selection

A survey of anesthesiologists and anesthesia assistants has identified incorrectly stocked drugs or drugs arranged in a confusing manner as one of the contributing factors to drug errors [8]. This was supported by a study that showed that one fifth of drug container swaps occurred because the cue to select the correct drug container was a storage location [2] that did not correspond with the expected location in the practitioner's mind; therefore, with the incorrect unintended drug in hand, the likelihood of detecting the incorrect unintended medication before it is administered was relatively low [2].

It would make sense then to develop a standardized way of organizing the anesthesia cart drug drawer in manner that is logical and organizes drugs from left to right in order of category of use as well as places drugs that are potentially dangerous further out of reach. A schematic of the drug drawer currently in use at UCSD is depicted in Fig. 18.2. There are many noticeable problems with the way in which this drug drawer is arranged. First, the left front compartment, which is the easiest and most natural to access, contains a mixture of large propofol bottles, neuromuscular blockers (succinylcholine and rocuronium), as well as syringes of vasopressors (phenylephrine). There is no sequence of use or commonality among drug

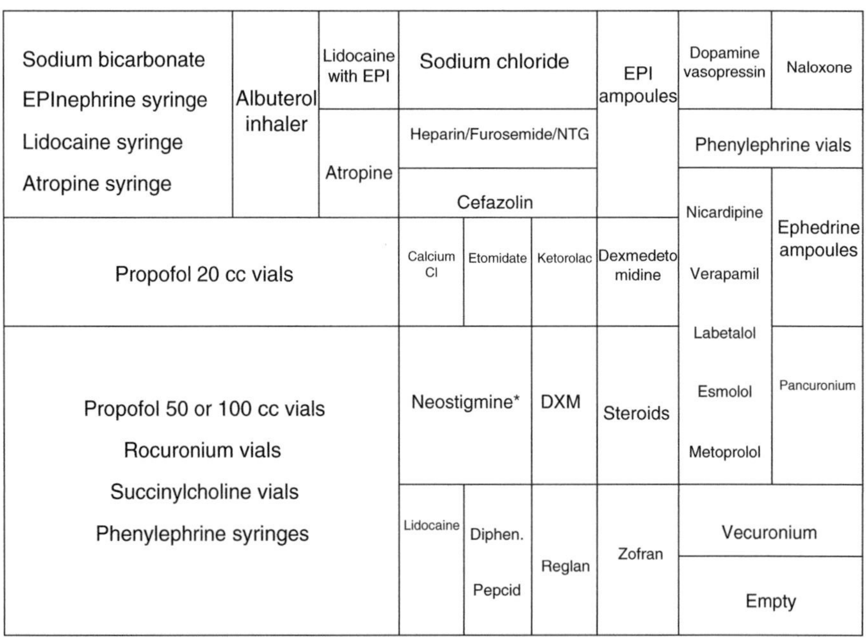

Fig. 18.2 Schematic of the anesthesia cart drug drawer at UCSD. *DXM* dexamethasone, *Diphen* diphenhydramine, *Pepcid* (Famotidine), *Reglan* (Metoclopramide), *Zofran* (Ondansetron), *NTG* nitroglycerine, *EPI* epinephrine. *Note this was before the introduction of Suggamadex

classes in this compartment. Second, moving from left to right, lidocaine is followed by the histamine receptor blockers (H2 blockers) and antiemetics. Although these drugs are fairly benign, it does not seem logical to have H2-blocking agents and antiemetics in the front row when they are generally either effective preoperatively (in the case of the histamine blockers) or toward the end of the case (antiemetics). Timing of the administration of these drugs should place them either in the front far left of the drawer (H2 blockers) or toward the back/right side of the drawer (antiemetics). Furthermore, these vials are all small and resemble each other. Although a drug container swap, syringe swap, or drug labeling error involving these drugs is not necessarily dangerous, it would be considered a drug error nonetheless and the therapeutic effect of the intended drug would be lost. The far right front corner of the drug drawer is empty and therefore is a waste of space, and behind it sits vecuronium, separate from the other neuromuscular blocking agents. Third, cefazolin, a commonly used antibiotic with low potential for adverse reactions (but can still cause anaphylaxis [9]), is located near the back center of the drawer, bordered by atropine, induction agents, heparin/furosemide/NTG, and epinephrine ampoules. There is no reason why this medication should be near the back of the drug drawer given its frequency of use and there is no logic behind its position relative to the surrounding drugs. Fourth, illogical location brings us to the heparin/furosemide/NTG combination compartment. Again, these drugs have no similarity in mechanism of action, and in fact, their vial sizes and shapes are relatively the same, creating increased potential for the occurrence of one of the four drug errors (see **L-1**). Fifth, Fig. 18.2 also contains a section largely dedicated to beta-blockers; however, this compartment also contains verapamil and nicardipine, two potent calcium channel blockers; mixing these two classes of drugs could be potentially harmful depending on the underlying cause of the patient's hypertension. The authors agree with a compartment, located at the left back corner of the drawer, which appears to be designated for some "code drugs."

Although there is no standard, "correct way" to organize a drug drawer, an attempt can be made to do so in a somewhat more logical fashion. We suggest a left-to-right approach, focusing on the order in which drugs are given during a basic general anesthetic and also grouping drugs according to drug class. A schematic of one possible way to organize the anesthesia cart drug drawer to optimize efficiency and limit error is displayed in Fig. 18.3. In this figure, you note that "pre-op" drugs including histamine receptor blockers and albuterol are in the left front corner compartment. Working from left to right, the drawer follows the same layout as the anesthesia machine tabletop workstation (see **L-5e)** with lidocaine in the next drawer, followed by the induction agents and neuromuscular blockers. The next row includes cefazolin followed by (going to the right of the cefazolin compartment) the most commonly used vasopressors, phenylephrine and ephedrine. Neostigmine and glycopyrrolate follow the vasopressors, and the antiemetics, ondansetron, and metoclopramide are on the far right since these are generally given at the end of a case. The next row of drugs includes miscellaneous drugs not necessarily or strictly used for anesthesia purposes. These include steroids, ketorolac, calcium, furosemide, and heparin. The last two rows on the right side of the drug tray are organized in a way that separates the

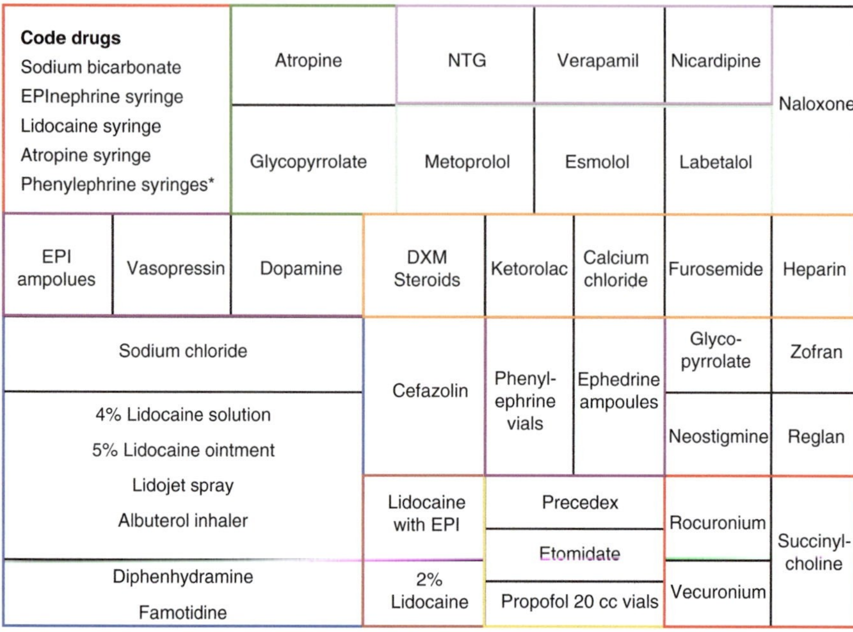

Fig. 18.3 One possible way of organizing an anesthesia cart drug drawer according to order of administration during a general anesthetic as well as grouping drugs according to drug class. *DXM* dexamethasone, *Diphen* diphenhydramine, *Pepcid* (famotidine), *Reglan* (metoclopramide), *Zofran* (ondansetron), *NTG* nitroglycerine, *EPI* epinephrine, *Precedex* (dexmedetomidine). *Note this was before the introduction of Suggamadex

beta-blockers from calcium channel blockers/nitrate vasodilators. Rather than arranging these drugs in line, with one behind the other, these drugs are arranged in a manner that would make it easy to see labels when placed on the drug tray dividers. The authors agreed with the code drugs being in the back left corner; however, the new design places potent vasopressors including epinephrine, vasopressin, and dopamine near these drugs as well as chronotropic agents atropine and glycopyrrolate also in the back, near the other vasoactive drugs. This new layout, arranged in order of use and grouped according to drug class with attention paid to more dangerous drugs being placed further toward the back of the drug drawer, should theoretically decrease the frequency of drug container swaps.

Standardization and careful organization of anesthesia cart drug drawers is one way to combat drug errors at the source (upon selection of the drug container); however, pre-filled syringes provided by drug companies are another approach to drug safety. The problem with pre-filled syringes are that they are expensive and can cost the hospital nearly seven times more money than having the anesthesia providers mix up the drugs themselves. Use of pre-filled syringes does not eliminate the potential for syringe swaps.

Another way to combat incorrect syringe labeling is with a relatively new system, which uses a barcode reader that recognizes a drug vial and prints an appropriate label that complies with the recommendations of regulatory agencies and standards.

This saves time for the anesthesia provider and also ensures that the correct label is paired with the correct drug vial. These labels should be printed individually as each drug is drawn up; however, it is possible to print multiple labels in advance, which theoretically could still result in a labeling error and therefore drug error. Furthermore, this barcode labeling system does not eliminate the issue of syringe swap, which occurs when an incorrect drug is chosen from the anesthesia tabletop workstation. In theory, the syringe itself could be scanned prior to administration to the patient; however, this would be a cumbersome process that is not realistic given the timeliness needed for administration of certain drugs during a given anesthetic. A study of the codonics safe label system (SLS) showed that the drug labeling system resulted in >75% compliant syringe labels. The rate of scanning barcodes was 25% over 13 weeks but increased to 58% over 8 weeks after introduction of a simple (coffee card) incentive [10].

Since syringe swaps frequently occur between syringes of equal size, it is important to have a standardized method for choosing the appropriate syringe size for a given drug so as not to create confusion. One method for syringe selection will be discussed here (see Fig. 18.4a, b), but again, it should be noted that any system would do as long as the anesthesia provider practices it routinely. For a basic case

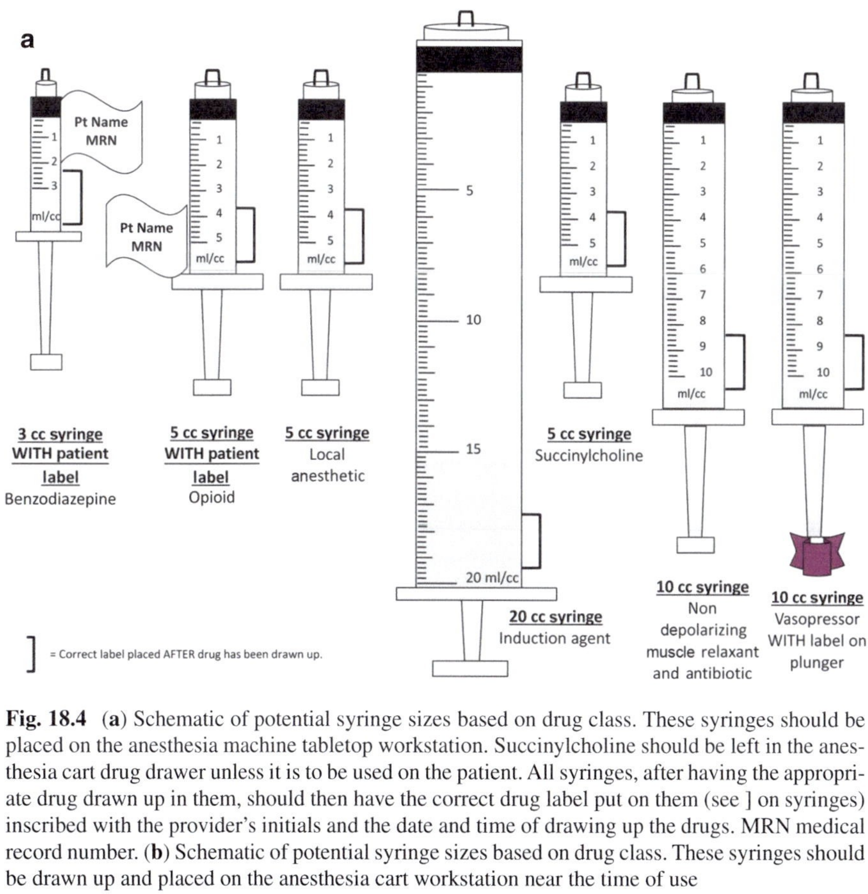

Fig. 18.4 (**a**) Schematic of potential syringe sizes based on drug class. These syringes should be placed on the anesthesia machine tabletop workstation. Succinylcholine should be left in the anesthesia cart drug drawer unless it is to be used on the patient. All syringes, after having the appropriate drug drawn up in them, should then have the correct drug label put on them (see] on syringes) inscribed with the provider's initials and the date and time of drawing up the drugs. MRN medical record number. (**b**) Schematic of potential syringe sizes based on drug class. These syringes should be drawn up and placed on the anesthesia cart workstation near the time of use

Fig. 18.4 (continued)

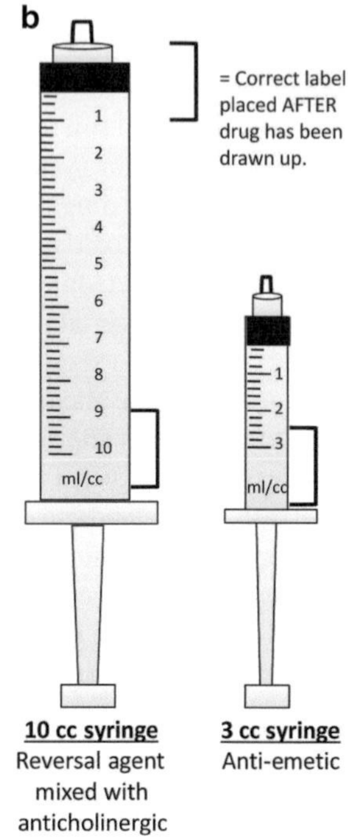

of general anesthesia, benzodiazepines may be drawn up into a 3 cc syringe and opioids may be drawn up into a 5 cc syringe. A patient label should be affixed to the benzodiazepine and opioid syringes so that if not all of the drug is given, the waste will not accidentally be administered to another patient. Two percent lidocaine generally comes in 5 cc vials and therefore can be drawn up into a 5 cc syringe. No patient label should be affixed in order to set it apart from the opioid syringe, which is also 5 cc. Induction agents should be drawn up into a 20 cc syringe. Propofol is very unlikely to be involved in a syringe swap given its white color; however, ketamine and etomidate are clear and thus should be distinguished from other drugs based not only on their label color but also their 20 cc syringe size. Neuromuscular blocking agents are frequently involved in syringe swaps so it is advised that succinylcholine be drawn up into a 5 cc syringe while nondepolarizers be drawn up into 10 cc syringes to set these agents apart. Keeping succinylcholine in the anesthesia cart drug drawer further reduces the risk of accidentally selecting this syringe by accident. Antibiotics may be drawn up into a 10 cc syringe and appropriately labeled. Allergies should be double-checked prior to administration and the syringe discarded after use. Vasopressors (phenylephrine and ephedrine) are typically drawn up into 10 cc syringes; however, their location on the anesthesia machine workspace (to the far right) (see **L-5d**) should reduce the risk of a syringe swap with these drugs and the other 10 cc syringes containing neuromuscular blocking agent and antibiotics. Since it is known that some of the most common drugs involved in “syringe swaps” are vasopressors and neuromuscular blockers, it is reasonable to suggest that the vasopressor syringe have an additional label/cue on the plunger (see **L-5e and** Fig. 18.4a). Finally, reversal agents, anticholinergics, and antiemetics should not be drawn up until near the time of use. Illustrations of these different syringe sizes are displayed in Fig. 18.4a, b.

Drug Labeling and Color-Coding of the Drug Label

Proper labeling technique involves selecting the correct drug container, drawing up the appropriate amount of drug into a given syringe, and labeling the syringe with the appropriate label, while cross-referencing the drug container to assure the drugs match. A drug label should then be inscribed with the anesthesia provider's initials as well as the date and time at which the drug was drawn up. For many years, anesthesia providers have used color-coded labels, which were designed by the American Society for Testing and Materials [11]. These colors are used to differentiate drugs of different drug classes (see Fig. 18.5). For example, orange labels are used to identify benzodiazepines; blue labels are used for opioids; gray for local anesthetics; yellow for induction agents; red for neuromuscular blockers; purple for vasopressors; purple and black for epinephrine; lavender and white stripes for vasodilators (though not available everywhere); red and white stripes for reversal agent; and green for anticholinergics (see Fig. 18.5). While Hirabayashi et al. showed that the use of colored syringes can prevent syringe swaps during anesthesia [12], Fasting et al. showed that syringe swaps occurred most often between syringes of equal size and were not eliminated by color-coding of labels [13]. Although there is mixed evidence regarding whether or not a color-coding system reduces drug errors, it does seem logical that a syringe swap occurring between drugs of the same class (and therefore same colored label) would be less detrimental than a syringe swap occurring between syringes containing drugs from different classes. An easy-to-do obviously/likely effective way to promote safety in drug administration lies in the organization and geography of the location of syringes atop the anesthesia machine tabletop workstation. An example of a standardized order of syringe layout is discussed in the next section.

Label Color-Coding System for Syringes

Drug Class	Color-Code
Benzodiazepines	Orange
Opioids	Blue
Local Anesthetics	Gray
Induction Agents	Yellow
Neuromuscular Blockers	Red
Vasopressors	Purple
Potent Vasopressors (Epi)	**Purple and Black**
Potent Vasodilators	**Lavender/White Stripes**
Reversal Agent	**Red/White Stripes**
Anticholinergics	Green

Fig. 18.5 Figure 18.1 depicts the color-coding labeling system established by the American Society for Testing and Materials. *Epi* epinephrine

The Geography of Location: Syringe Organization Atop the Anesthesia Machine Tabletop Workstation

The geography of location of syringes involves the arrangement of the syringes atop the anesthesia machine tabletop workstation. A proposed mechanism of organization is outlined here; however, it is important to remember that any pattern of organization will work, as long as the anesthesia provider always organizes his/her workplace in the same way. If syringes are physically located and separated based on drug class and/or intended use, it seems likely that the incidence of syringe swaps would decrease. This becomes even more important in high-stress, emergency situations when organization is oftentimes lost.

A left to right organization technique that mirrors the temporal sequence in which anesthetics are administered and also separates syringes based on drug class is a logical way to organize anesthetic drugs (see Fig. 18.6a, b). On the left side of the workstation, the first section or grouping of drugs are those that cause some aspect of intravenous anesthesia. These include the benzodiazepines (if not given in the preoperative area) and opioids. Working left to right, the next medication according to order of administration would be lidocaine to minimize the burning of the induction agent. The induction agent(s) would lie next in the lineup to the right of the local anesthetic. The next section to the right of the intravenous anesthetics contains drugs involved in causing neuromuscular blockade. It should be noted that, due to the few but very serious adverse effects associated with succinylcholine, this drug should be kept in the top drawer of the anesthesia cart drug drawer if not being used for the particular case, so as not to accidentally administer it when contraindicated. To the right of the neuromuscular blocking drug section is the antibiotic syringe which should be given after induction, prior to incision, and the syringe then discarded. To the right of the antibiotics (still in the left to right scheme) are vasoactive drugs (see Fig. 18.6a, b). Vasoactive drugs may be further divided as follows: Vasopressors, vasodilators, and drugs with primarily chronotropic effects. To the far right are miscellaneous drugs commonly used for non-anesthetic reasons (e.g., mannitol, furosemide). Finally, neuromuscular blocking and reversal agents, anticholinergics, and antiemetics should not be drawn up until near the time of use. It is recommended that the reversal agent and the anticholinergic be drawn up into the same syringe because in the rare instance of the patient receiving the reversal agent alone, while the IV simultaneously becomes infiltrated or pulled out, the patient would develop a profound bradycardia or asystole and no IV would be in place. If the anticholinergic agent is mixed with the reversal agent, the risk of profound bradycardia is much lower. Antiemetics work best when administered within 30 min of emergence from anesthesia and therefore should also be drawn up near to the time of use (the end of the case). Once drawn up, these drugs should be placed atop the anesthesia cart (anesthesia cart workstation), separate from the anesthesia machine tabletop workstation, to decrease the possibility of premature intraoperative administration (see Fig. 18.7a, b). Figures 18.6a, b and 18.7a, b constitute the author's general setup for a basic anesthetic case. If your case involves the drawing up of more powerful vasoactive drugs (i.e., vasopressin, epinephrine, dilute nitroprusside

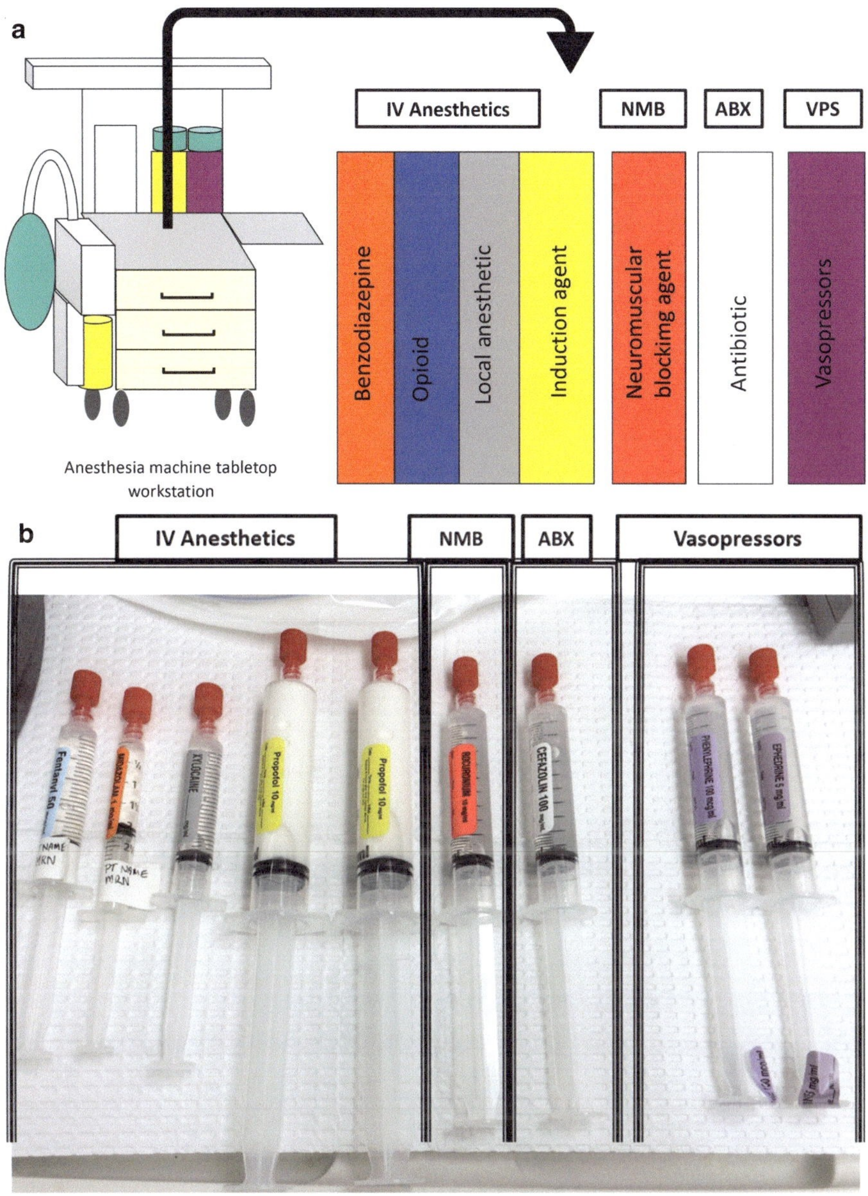

Fig. 18.6 (**a**) Schematic of the anesthesia machine tabletop workstation with drugs organized left to right based on order of use and drug class. NMB neuromuscular blockers, ABX antibiotics, VPS vasopressors. (**b**) Photograph of anesthesia machine tabletop workstation with drugs organized left to right. *NMB* neuromuscular blockers, *ABX* antibiotics

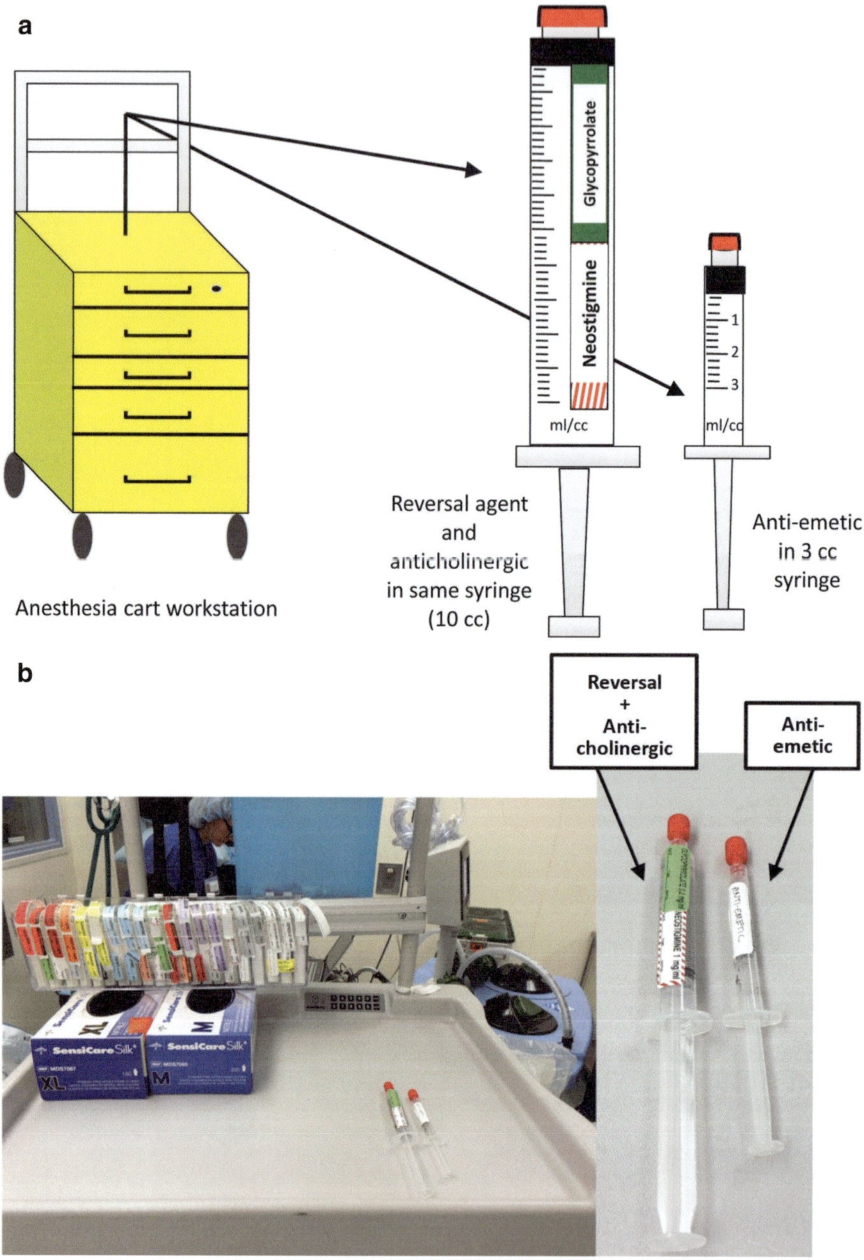

Fig. 18.7 (**a**) Schematic of anesthesia cart workstation with reversal agent and anticholinergic drug (drawn up near the time of use) placed in a separate location from the anesthesia machine tabletop workstation. (**b**) Photographs of the anesthesia cart workstation with reversal agent and anticholinergic drug (drawn up near the time of use) placed in a separate location from the anesthesia machine tabletop workstation. (Note this was before the introduction of Suggamadex)

or nitroglycerine), these drugs should be drawn up, correctly labeled, and placed on the anesthesia machine tabletop workstation above the location of your routine syringes, so not to select them by accident. This more complex setup is displayed in Fig. 18.8a, b.

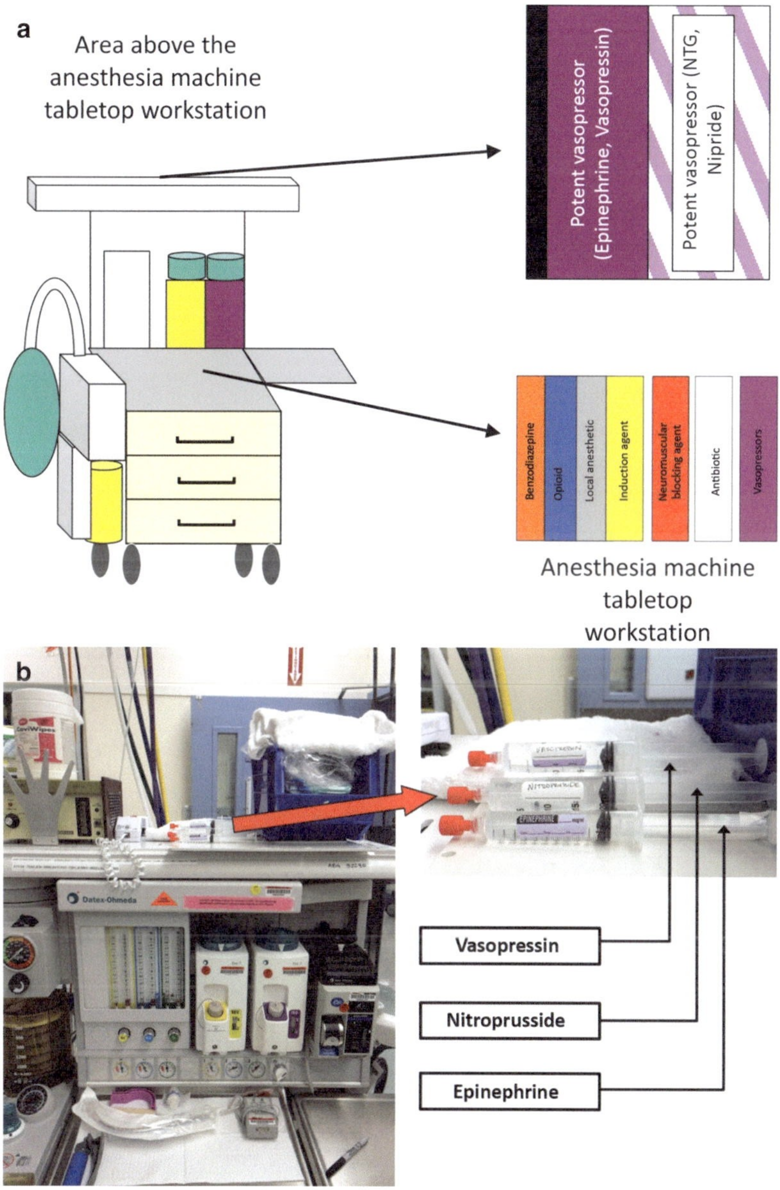

Fig. 18.8 (**a**) Schematic of vasoactive drugs (vasopressors and vasodilators) above the anesthesia machine workstation, separate from the basic setup. NTG nitroglycerine, Nipride nitroprusside. (**b**) Photograph of potent vasoactive drugs (vasopressors and vasodilators) above the anesthesia machine workstation, separate from the basic setup

With an organized anesthesia cart drug drawer, proper labeling technique, and a system for organization of drug syringes atop the anesthesia machine tabletop workstation and anesthesia cart workstation, the rate of administration of incorrect unintentional drugs should be significantly reduced.

How to Prevent Unintentional Drug Delivery to a Patient: One More Step

There is one more step before the drug is actually administered to the patient, and that is depression of the plunger on the syringe. We would recommend one more mechanism for again identifying and confirming that the correct intentional drug is being given by placing the label of vasoactive drugs on the plunger as one more visual cue of what you are administering (see Fig. 18.9).

How to Organize the Central Venous Catheter (CVC) Tray

It is estimated that 90% of catheter-related bloodstream infections (CRBSIs) result from CVC insertion procedures [14]. The Center for Disease Control (CDC) estimates the incidence of these bloodstream infections to be approximately 248,000 per year in US hospitals [14]. Hand hygiene plays an important role in prevention of CRBSIs; therefore, it is important to realize that appropriate setup of the CVC tray prior to catheter insertion is a crucial step in preventing

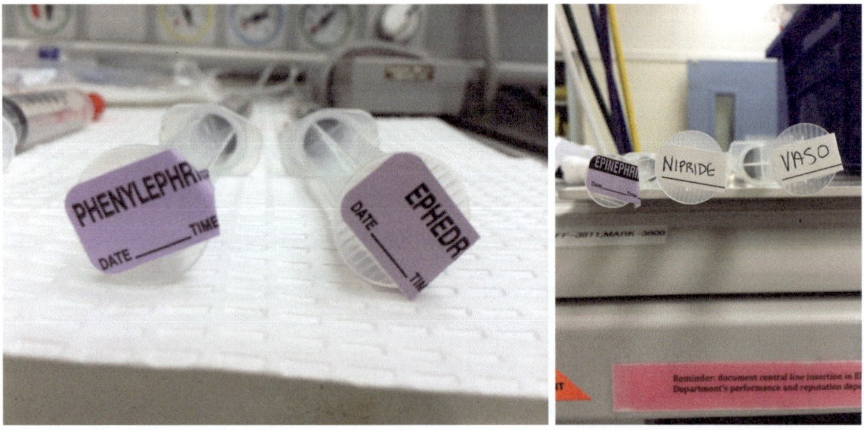

Fig. 18.9 Photograph of vasoactive drug label on plunger end. *Nipride* nitroprusside, *Vaso* vasopressin

breaches in sterility. Furthermore, it can be argued that proper organization of the CVC tray in a way that decreases unnecessary hand movements and manipulation of needles and syringes on the tray will lead to a decrease in incidence of NSI to hospital personnel as well as syringe swaps. A photograph demonstrating the way that the CVC tray comes packaged to the provider is demonstrated in Fig. 18.10a. Once the provider is properly sterilized, gowned, and gloved, they should clean the area of the catheter insertion site in an outward circular manner with chlorhexidine and drape the patient appropriately. Next, the syringes, needles, spring-wire guide, scalpel, and 9 French (Fr.) catheter with tissue dilator placed through it and suture should be removed from the CVC tray and arranged in a left to right manner in order of use, with the needles facing away from the provider but within easy reach on some additionally created sterile field using the sterile drape provided within the CVC tray (see Fig. 18.10b, c). Next, a designated receptacle should be used to receive patient blood, so as to not contaminate the instruments on the tray with slippery or potentially clotted/sticky blood, thus interfering with their ability to safely handle the instruments. Finally, a large receptacle for saline deposition should be designated within the tray that is easily accessible and does not require tilting or tipping of the CVC tray in order to adequately aspirate the fluid into a syringe. The CVC tray should also contain a disposable receptacle that will temporarily hold sharps in a safe manner so that they can be easily kept track of and discarded at the end of the procedure. An example of one way in which the CVC tray can be organized to promote safety is shown in Fig. 18.10a–c.

a

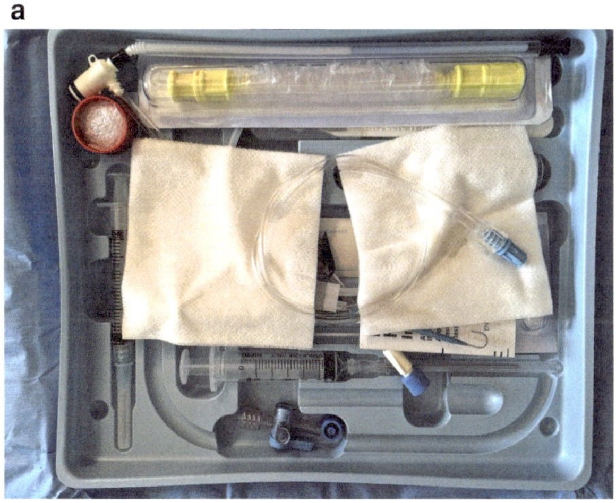

Fig. 18.10 (**a**) Photograph of the central venous catheter tray as it comes packaged to the anesthesiologist. (**b**) Photograph of the central venous catheter tray with equipment removed and organized on a sterile drape. (**c**) Schematic of the central venous catheter tray with syringes removed and organized on a sterile drape

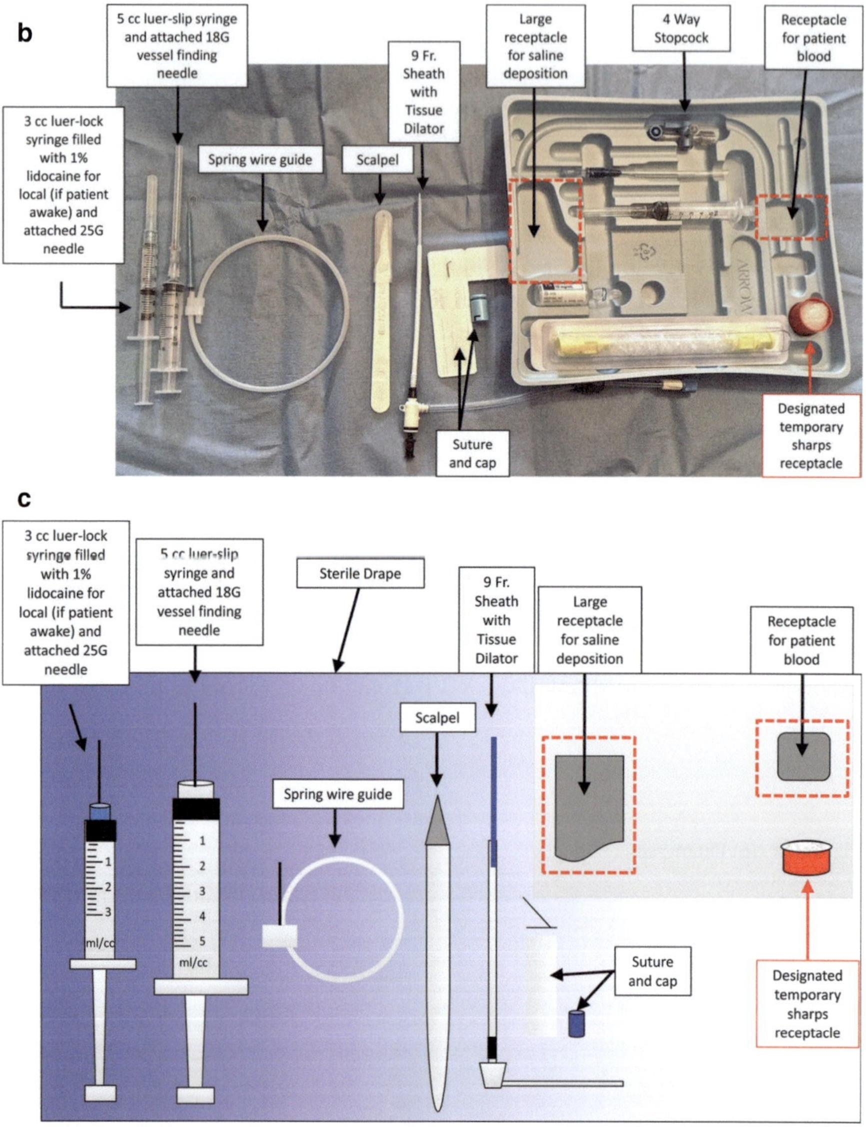

Fig. 18.10 (continued)

How to Organize the Spinal and Epidural Trays

When performing a spinal or epidural, the trays should be arranged in a way that prevents syringe swaps and NSI to anesthesia personnel and also minimizes infection risk to the patient. Figures 18.11a and 18.12a show the spinal kit and epidural kit, respectively, as they come from the manufacturers. Each kit contains syringes

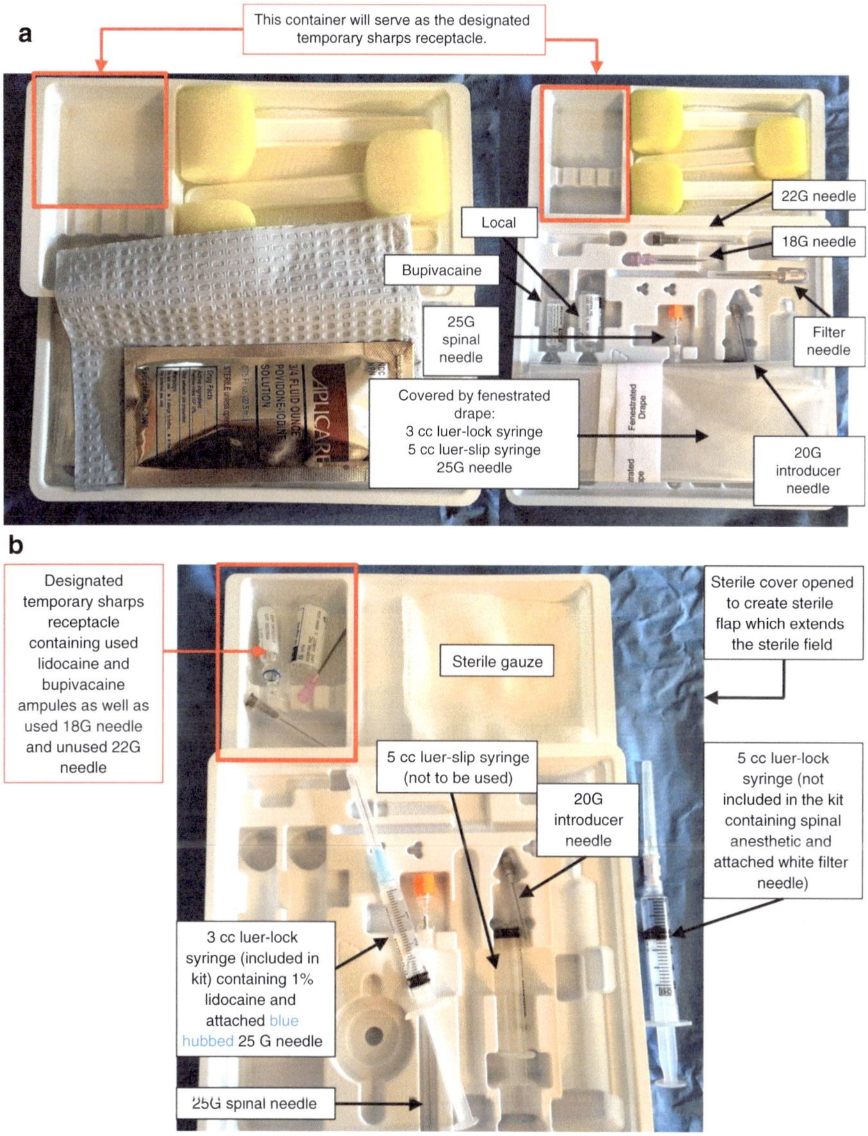

Fig. 18.11 (**a**) Photograph of the spinal tray as it comes packaged to the anesthesiologist. With extra sterile drape and povidone-iodine still present in the kit shown on the left and after removing these items from the kit shown on the right. Bupivacaine, 2 cc of 0.75% bupivacaine with 8.25% dextrose. Local, 5 cc of 1% lidocaine. (**b**) Photograph of the spinal tray with the 3 cc syringe provided in the kit containing the 1% lidocaine to be used for local infiltration. The 5 cc luer lock syringe (not provided in spinal kit) contains the spinal anesthetic and is placed on the sterile drape cover that has been opened up to create flaps to extend the sterile field. Spinal anesthetic, bupivacaine/fentanyl/morphine. (**c**) Schematic of the spinal tray with the 3 cc syringe provided in the kit containing the 1% lidocaine to be used for local infiltration. The 5 cc luer lock syringe (not provided in spinal kit) contains the spinal anesthetic and is placed on the sterile drape cover that has been opened up to create flaps to extend the sterile field. Spinal anesthetic=bupivacaine/fentanyl/morphine

c

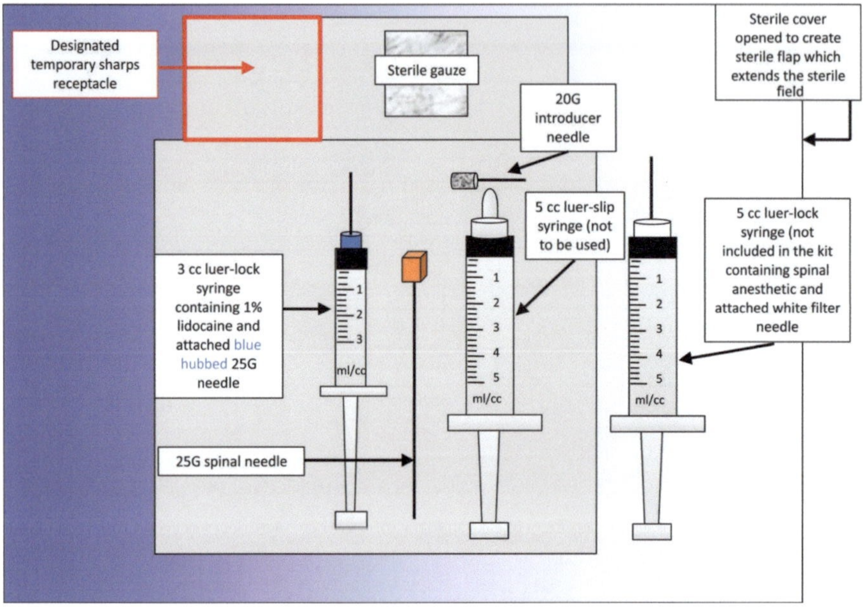

Fig. 18.11 (continued)

of various sizes as well as needles of varying gauges which creates the potential for the provider to pick up the wrong syringe and/or needle; therefore, a method for organization of these items, once removed from the tray, is imperative.

There are three principles to consider when organizing an epidural or spinal tray in order to minimize syringe swaps (see Table 18.1). First, syringes of different sizes should be chosen for each different solution (see Table 18.3, top row) that is to be administered to the patient. For the spinal kit, these two solutions are 1% lidocaine and the actual spinal anesthetic (bupivacaine/fentanyl/morphine) (see Fig. 18.11b, c; Table 18.3). For the epidural kit, the solutions requiring separation based on syringe size include 1% lidocaine, normal saline (NS), and the test dose (1.5% lidocaine with 1:200,000 epinephrine) (see Fig. 18.12b, c; Table 18.3). Figures 18.11b, c and 18.12b, c illustrate the use of different syringe sizes to distinguish the clear solutions mentioned above. When performing a spinal anesthetic, the provider may choose to open a sterile 5 cc luer lock syringe (not provided in the spinal kit) onto the spinal tray at the start of the case. The luer lock provides a more secure connection when administering the spinal anesthetic than does the 5 cc luer-slip syringe provided in the kit and thereby reduces the risk of accidental spilling of spinal anesthetic out of the syringe before it reaches the patient. By using different syringe sizes for each different solution that is to be administered to the patient (whether the syringe is included in the kit or not), the risk of a syringe swap should be diminished (see Table 18.3, top row).

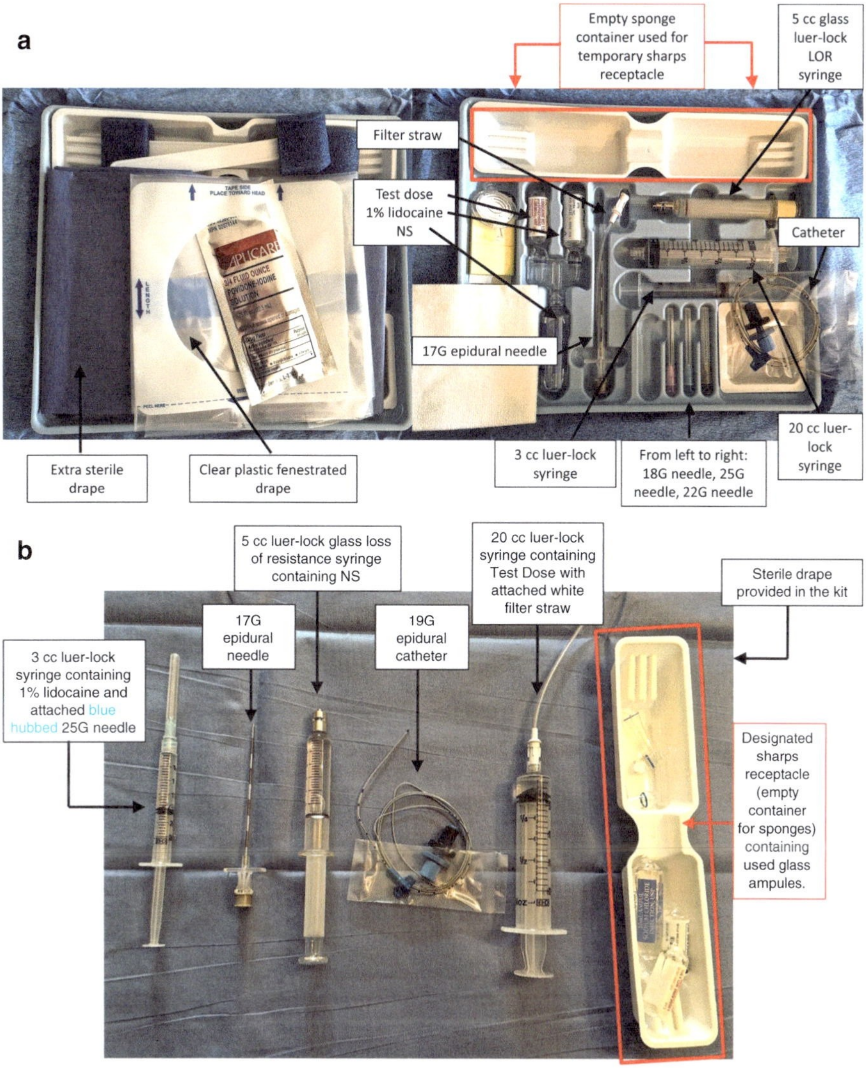

Fig. 18.12 (**a**) Photograph of the epidural tray as it comes packaged to the anesthesiologist. With extra fenestrated patient drape and povidone-iodine still present in the kit shown on the left and after removing these items from the kit shown on the right. LOR loss of resistance; test dose, 5 cc of 1.5% lidocaine with 1:200,000 epinephrine; 1% lidocaine for local infiltration, *NS* 10 cc of normal saline. (**b**) Photograph of the epidural tray with excess materials discarded and syringes organized on the blue sterile drape that is placed on the bed below the clear plastic sheet used to drape the patient. 1% lidocaine for local infiltration; NS normal saline; test dose, 3 cc of 1.5% lidocaine with 1:200,000 epinephrine. (**c**) Schematic of the epidural tray with syringes organized on the blue sterile drape that is placed on the bed below the clear plastic sheet used to drape the patient. 1% lidocaine for local infiltration; NS normal saline; test dose, 3 cc of 1.5% lidocaine with 1:200,000 epinephrine

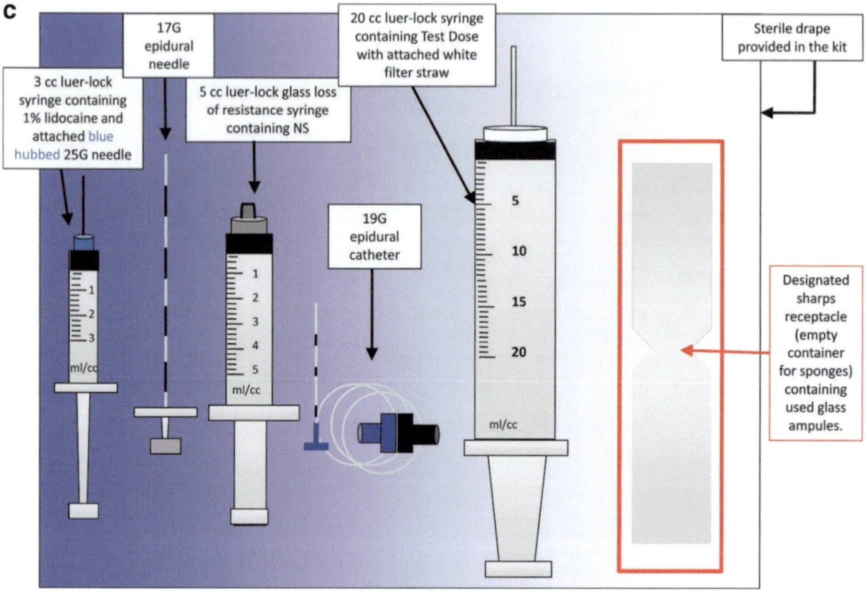

Fig. 18.12 (continued)

Table 18.3 Principles in avoiding syringe swaps

Ways to prevent syringe swaps	Examples: spinal tray	Examples: epidural tray
Differing syringe sizes	3 cc luer lock syringe for 1% lidocaine	3 cc luer lock syringe for 1% lidocaine
	5 cc luer lock syringe for spinal anesthetic	5 cc luer lock glass LOR syringe for normal saline
		20 cc luer lock syringe for test dose
Differing needle gauges and hub color	25G blue needle for 1% lidocaine syringe	25G blue needle for 1% lidocaine syringe
	White filter needle for spinal anesthetic syringe	White filter straw for test dose syringe
Layout on the sterile field	Left to right in order of use	Left to right in order of use

1% lidocaine for local infiltration; spinal anesthetic, bupivacaine/fentanyl/morphine; LOR, loss of resistance; test dose, 1.5% lidocaine with 1:200,000 epinephrine

Second, attaching needles of differing gauges and colored hubs to each syringe will also help distinguish one clear solution from another and should be utilized appropriately (see Table 18.3, middle row) (see also Figs. 18.11b, c and 18.12b, c). For example, syringes containing local anesthetic to be used to anesthetize the skin should contain a blue-hubbed 25 gauge needle, while syringes to be used to inject anesthetic into either the spinal or epidural space should contain a white filter needle or straw. Using different syringe sizes as well as needles with different gauges and hub color should decrease the risk of administering the wrong drug (see Table 18.3).

Third, an effort should be made to arrange syringes with attached needles and other instruments in a way that mirrors their order of use (see Table 18.3, bottom row) (see also Figs. 18.11b, c and 18.12b, c). For a spinal procedure, the 3 cc syringe containing the 1% lidocaine for anesthetizing the skin and subcutaneous tissue should lie to the left of the 5 cc syringe containing the spinal anesthetic (bupivacaine/fentanyl/morphine) (see Fig. 18.11b, c). Similarly, when performing an epidural, syringes and other instruments (epidural needle, epidural catheter) should be arranged on a sterile drape in a similar fashion, from left to right, in order of use (see Fig. 18.12a, b).

In order to prevent accidental needlesticks to anesthesia personnel, a designated area for temporary sharp placement MUST be established (see red outlined areas in Figs. 18.11a and 18.12a). This area should not be easily penetrable by needles or broken glass, should be on an area within the sterile field that is easy to reach, and should serve as a temporary place for all sharps until the procedure is completed, at which time this temporary sharps container should be placed into a large, permanent sharps bin.

Lastly, sterility and patient safety should always be of concern to the anesthesia provider. By extending the flaps of the spinal tray kit cover, the sterile field may be extended to make room for the 5 cc luer lock syringe containing the spinal anesthetic (see Fig. 18.11b). Furthermore, the extra drape provided in the epidural kit may serve as a large sterile field upon which the provider may organize their equipment (see left side of Fig. 18.12a). Having an organized, methodical way of drawing up drugs and arranging them in a way that avoids unnecessary hand movements should, in turn, decrease the likelihood of breaching the sterile field and thus should decrease the potential for infection as well as improve efficiency.

In conclusion, a disorganized workspace introduces the potential for drug errors, accidental needlestick injuries, as well as contamination. These complications place the patient and the provider in danger. In order to establish a well-organized and safe workspace, a systematic approach that addresses the potential for error at all stages is necessary. This chapter proposes a standardized way to organize drugs for a basic general anesthetic case, syringes and instruments for placing a CVC, as well as offers a unique approach for organizing the spinal and epidural trays in a way that should theoretically decrease these potential threats. It is important to note that any method of organization (as long as well thought out and practiced routinely) should achieve the same goals as the methods described in this chapter.

References

1. Abeyekera A, Bergman IJ, Kluger MT, Short TG. Drug error in anaesthetic practice: a review of 896 reports from the Australian incident monitoring study database. Anaesth: J Assoc Anaesthetists Great Brit Ireland. 2005;60(3):220–7.
2. Currie M, Mackay P, Morgan C, Runciman WB, Russell WJ, Sellen A, Webb RK, Williamson JA. The Austrailain incident monitoring study. Anaesth Intensive Care. 1993;21(5):596–601.
3. Webster CS, Merry AF, Larsson L, McGrath KA, Weller J. The frequency and nature of drug administration error during anaesthesia. Anaesth Intensive Care. 2001;29(5):494–500.
4. Rosenberg AD, Bernstein DB, Berntein RL, Skovron ML, Ramanathan S, Turndorf H. Accidental needlesticks: do anesthesiologists practice proper infection control precautions? Am J Anesthesiol. 1995;22(3):125–32.
5. Recommendations for infection control for the practice of anesthesiology (3rd edition) developed by the ASA committee on Occupational Health and Force on Infection Control. 20 Oct 2010. https://asahq.org/~/media/sites/asahq/files/public/resources/asa%20committees/recommendations-for-infection-control-for-the-practice-of-anesthesiology-(1).pdf?la=en. Accessed 12/11/14.
6. Kroll H, Mandell S, Goldman J, Brown M. The use of syringes with a T-port extension set: is it safe? Anesthesiology. 1994;81(3A):A1271.
7. Green ES, Berry AJ, Arnold WP, Jagger J. Percutaneous injuries in anesthesia personnel. Anesth Analg. 1996;83(2):273–8.
8. Shultz J, Davies JM, Caird J, Chrisholm S, Ruggles K, Puls R. Standardizing anesthesia medication drawers using human factors and quality assurance methods. Can J Anesth. 2010;57:490–9.
9. Gibbs M, Kuczkowski K, Benumof J. Complete recovery from prolonged cardiopulmonary resuscitation following anaphylactic reaction to readministered IV cefazolin. Acta Anaesthesiol Scand. 2003;47(2):230–2.
10. Jelacic S, Bowdle A, Nair BG, Kusulos D, Bower L, Togashi K. A system for anesthesia drug administration using barcode technology: the codonics safe label system and smart anesthesia manager. Anesth Analg. 2015;121(2):410–21.
11. Grissinger M. Color-coded syringes for anesthesia drugs–use with care. Pharm Ther. 2012;37(4):199–201.
12. Hirabayashi Y, Kawakami T, Suzuki H, Igarashi T, Saitoh K, Seo N. The effect of coloured syringes and a coloured sheet on the incidence of syringe swaps during anesthetic management. Masui. 2005;54(9):1060–2.
13. Fasting S, Gisvold SE. Adverse drug errors in anesthesia, and the impact of coloured syringe labels. Can J Anaesth. 2000;47(11):1060–7.
14. The road to zero: reducing the incidence of central line associated bloodsream infections and needlestick injuries. http://www.teleflex.com/en/usa/productAreas/vascularAccess/documents/faqs/CVC_2498%20ErgoPack%20Whitepaper%20M1%202011-0283.pdf. Accessed 12/6/2014.

Chapter 19
A Case of Peripartum Cardiomyopathy: Anesthetic Management of Patients on Mechanical Circulatory Support and Status Post Heart Transplantation

Martin Krause and Kimberly S. Robbins

Case Description

A previously healthy 28-year-old woman had an uncomplicated pregnancy and normal spontaneous vaginal delivery of a healthy neonate. The patient noticed new onset of dyspnea and lower extremity edema a week following her delivery. Despite reassurance by her obstetrician, her symptoms progressively worsened to include paroxysmal nocturnal dyspnea, myalgia, fatigue, and rales on auscultation (L1). An urgent care physician diagnosed her with community- acquired pneumonia and treated her with prednisone and azithromycin. Her symptoms continued to worsen and she was admitted to an outside hospital for presumed severe sepsis. A transesophageal echocardiogram (TEE) revealed global hypokinesis, moderate mitral regurgitation, and an ejection fraction of 15%. She was finally diagnosed with peripartum cardiomyopathy (PPCM) (L2, L3). Despite medical therapy, including milrinone and furosemide, her symptoms continued to worsen. Two months after her delivery, the patient was transferred to a cardiac center for advanced heart failure therapy (L4).

The patient arrived awake and lucid. By nightfall, however, her mixed venous saturation (MVO2) had dropped from the 80s to the 30s despite aggressive diuresis and adjustment to her inotropic. A right heart catheterization found the patient in cardiogenic shock with MVO2 at 28%. A percutaneous TandemHeart® left ventricular assist device (LVAD) was placed for temporary mechanical support and a dramatic improvement in her MVO2 was observed. Nevertheless, given her late diagnosis,

M. Krause
Department of Anesthesiology, University of Colorado, Denver, Aurora, CO, USA

K. S. Robbins (✉)
Department of Anesthesiology and Critical Care Medicine, University of California, San Diego, CA, USA
e-mail: krobbins@ucsd.edu

J. L. Benumof, G. R. Manecke (eds.), *Clinical Anesthesiology II*,
https://doi.org/10.1007/978-3-030-12365-9_19

it was believed that her left ventricular (LV) function would not recover without a long-term LVAD. The following day she was taken to the operating room for HeartWare® continuous-flow LVAD implantation and was concurrently listed for a heart transplant (L5). An automatic implantable cardioverter defibrillator (AICD) was implanted to prevent sudden cardiac death and to treat potential dysrhythmias. Upon discharge from the hospital, her medical course was complicated by repeated LVAD driveline infections that required incision and drainage and antibiotic treatment. Five months after her initial presentation, she received a heart transplant and has since done well (L6).

Lesson 1: What Are the Physiologic Changes of the Cardiovascular System During Pregnancy and How Can These Changes Affect Cardiac Disease in Pregnancy?

An increase in blood volume and heart rate and a reduction in systemic vascular resistance bring about the increase in cardiac output necessary to sustain pregnancy [1].

Blood volume begins to increase in week 6 of gestation, and by the end of pregnancy, it will have reached approximately 50% more than in the prepregnant state. During pregnancy, both ventricles dilate allowing for higher end-diastolic ventricular volume. There are also increases in the left atrial and right atrial diastolic dimensions; however cardiac filling pressures remain normal. This eccentric hypertrophy leads to optimization of Frank-Starling dynamics and also to a preload-independent increase in contractility. These changes allow for stroke volume to increase by 25% by the end of the second trimester. By the end of the first trimester, the heart rate has also risen by 25% which results in an overall increase in cardiac output (CO) to 50% by the end of the second trimester until term. Despite elevated CO, the mean arterial blood pressure remains stable due to decreased systemic vascular resistance (SVR). The reduction in SVR is a result of hormonal changes, the low-resistance vascular bed of the placental circuit, and dilutional anemia secondary to increased plasma volume. The resulting increase in blood volume further improves preload and therefore stroke volume [2] (Fig. 19.1).

CO can also dramatically decrease depending on the parturient's position. The supine position results in compression of the inferior vena cava and consequent obstruction of venous return and decreased cardiac output. Not only is the inferior vena cava compressed in the supine position, but the uterus may obstruct the abdominal aorta and the iliac arteries. This compression may be relieved by manual left uterine displacement (Fig. 19.2). Typically, aortocaval compression becomes a concern after 20 weeks of gestation, but may occur as early as 12–13 weeks of gestation [3].

During labor, CO further increases above term levels due to increased sympathetic activity and autotransfusion of 500 mL of blood volume with each contraction. Immediately after delivery, this gain in extra blood volume becomes

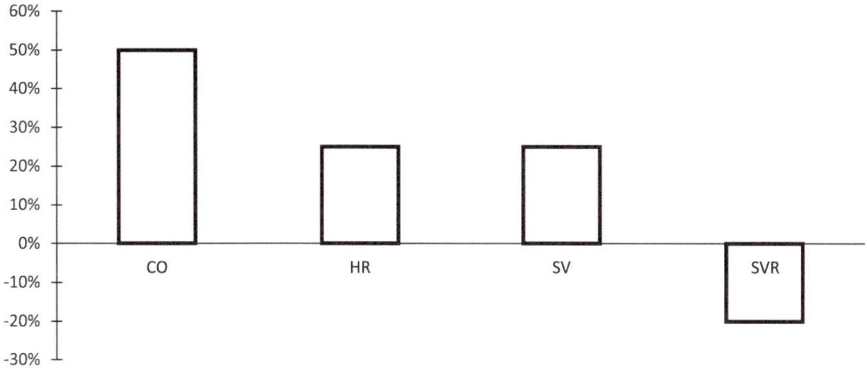

Fig. 19.1 Hemodynamic changes at term compared to nonpregnant values. *CO* cardiac output, *HR* heart rate, *SV* stroke volume, *SVR* systemic vascular resistance. (Based on data from Ref. [2])

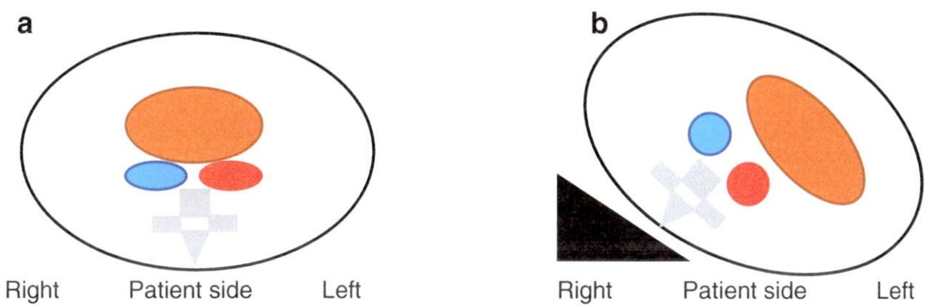

Fig. 19.2 (**a**) Schematic of aortocaval compression; (**b**) schematic of left uterine displacement. In red, aorta; in blue, inferior vena cava; in gray, vertebra; in brown, uterus; in black, ramp

permanent. In addition aortocaval compression is relieved leading to an overall increase in CO of 75% compared to prelabor values. Within the first 24 h, CO returns to its prelabor baseline. However it takes another 24 weeks until CO reaches nonpregnant values [4].

Management of heart failure in pregnant women carries many challenges. Symptoms of progressing heart failure such as dependent edema, dyspnea on exertion, paroxysmal nocturnal dyspnea, and abdominal discomfort mimic symptoms commonly seen during normal pregnancy and may delay the diagnosis [5]. In addition, ACE inhibitors, angiotensin receptor blockers, and beta-blockers, all of which have been shown to improve outcome in heart failure patients, are either contraindicated, or their use is controversial during pregnancy [6, 7]. Parturients with preexisting heart failure are more prone to decompensation secondary to the rise in CO and blood volume. It is also worthwhile to mention that valvular heart lesions have different responses to the physiologic changes of pregnancy. Due to the increase in heart rate and decrease in SVR, stenotic and any other lesions depending on diastolic filling worsen, while regurgitant lesions, which depend on forward flow, improve.

Lesson 2: How Is PPCM Distinct from Other Forms of Heart Failure?

In contrast to other forms of heart failure, PPCM is a form of dilated cardiomyopathy presenting with left ventricular systolic dysfunction toward the end of pregnancy or in the months following delivery, where no other cause for heart failure is found. PPCM is a diagnosis of exclusion and occurs in 1 out of 1149 to 1 out of 4350 live births [8]. There are a myriad of hypotheses attempting to explain the pathophysiology of PPCM. Infection, both bacterial and viral, has been proposed as a mechanism. Additionally, inflammation may play a role in the development of PPCM, as serum markers of inflammation such as IL-6, CRP, IFN-gamma, and sFas/Apo-1 are elevated in patients with PPCM [9]. Autoimmune processes have been implicated as well, as high titers of auto-antibodies against selected cardiac tissue proteins have been found in the majority of women with PPCM [10]. It is not clear, however, whether these findings are causal or secondary to cardiac damage. Some studies have postulated a genetic component to the disease [11, 12].

No clear modifiable risk factors associated with the development of PPCM have been identified. Several associated factors have been noted and may be categorized as general risk factors for cardiovascular disease (hypertension, diabetes, smoking) and pregnancy-related factors (extremes of childbearing age, multiparity, preeclampsia, use of tocolytics, and twin pregnancies) [13]. Certain ethnic groups display a higher incidence of PPCM, suggesting potential genetic or environmental factors. Identifying high-risk patients and understanding the pathophysiology of the disease may one day lead to early diagnoses and improved treatments.

While a little over half of PPCM patients show recovery of LV function, PPCM has a mortality range of 18–54% and can contribute up to 70% of deaths related to cardiomyopathy during pregnancy [14–16] (Fig. 19.3). Decisions about initiating invasive therapies in PPCM such as implantable cardioverter defibrillators and ventricular assist devices can be quite difficult due to the unpredictable time course and incidence of ventricular recovery in this population.

Lesson 3: What Is the Suggested Workup for PPCM?

As stated previously, PPCM is a diagnosis of exclusion and one should take steps to distinguish from other causes of heart failure, as well as noncardiac causes of the patient's symptomatology. Workup parallels that of heart failure from other causes.

Electrocardiogram (ECG) should be performed in all patients with suspected PPCM, as 96% have baseline ECG abnormalities, the most common being T-wave changes (59%), p-wave abnormalities (29%), and QRS axis deviation (25%) [17]. A chest X-ray is not necessary for diagnosis, but if one is obtained during pregnancy, fetal shielding should be used.

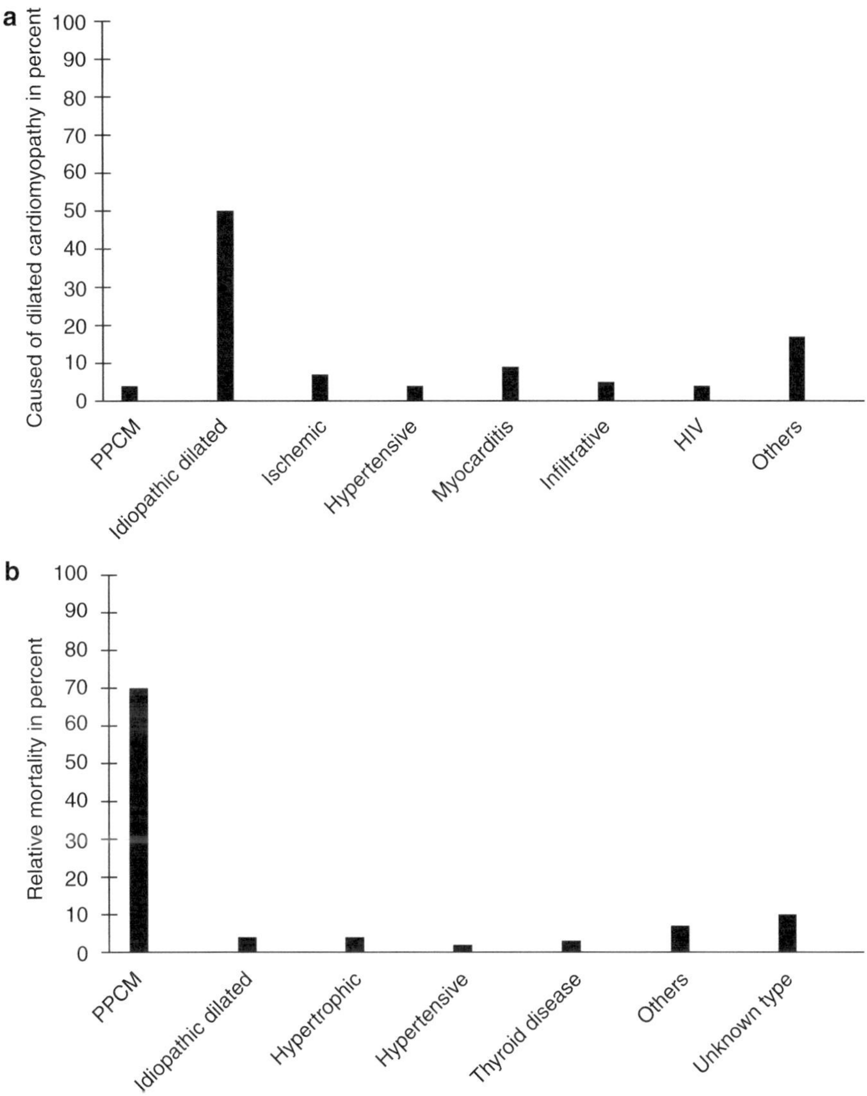

Fig. 19.3 (**a**) Etiology of dilated cardiomyopathy. (**b**) Relative mortality of cardiomyopathy during pregnancy (%) (**a**, Based on data from Ref. [16]). (**b**, Based on data from Ref. [14]). *PPCM* peripartum cardiomyopathy, *HIV* human immunodeficiency virus. Adapted Table with kind permission of Elsevier [24]

B-type natriuretic peptide (BNP) is a neurohormone that is synthesized in ventricular myocardium and released into the circulation in response to ventricular dilatation and pressure overload. BNP is elevated in patients with congestive heart failure and increases in proportion to the degree of left ventricular dysfunction and the severity of symptoms of heart failure. It has been previously demonstrated that a single measure-

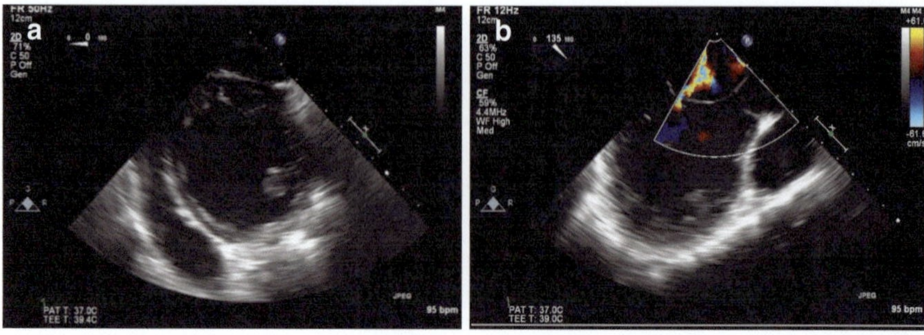

Fig. 19.4 Transesophageal images of a patient with PPCM: (**a**) transgastric midpapillary short axis and (**b**) midesophageal long axis with color flow. Notable are the severely dilated spherical-shaped left ventricle with thin left ventricular wall and functional mitral regurgitation due to dilation of mitral annulus

ment of BNP, obtained in the first few days after the onset of ischemic symptoms, provides predictive information for use in risk stratification across the spectrum of acute coronary syndromes [18]. Patients with PPCM have increased BNP levels, which correlate directly with outcome in PPCM patients [19] (Fig. 19.4).

Cardiac imaging is indicated for women presenting with heart failure symptoms toward the end of pregnancy/in the early postpartum period. This can both help establish a diagnosis and may provide prognostic information. Additionally, imaging is used to screen for LV thrombus, particularly where LV systolic function is severely depressed [20]. A LVEF <30% predicts poor LV recovery as does a LV end-diastolic diameter >60 mm [21]. Echocardiography is the most widely used imaging modality; however cardiac MRI allows for a more accurate measurement of chamber volumes and ventricular function and also has a higher sensitivity for detection of LV thrombus than echocardiography [22, 23]. Follow-up imaging is conducted at regular intervals to assess for recovery of cardiac function. Invasive hemodynamic monitoring with a pulmonary artery (PA) catheter may be necessary to guide therapy in some patients (Fig. 19.5).

Lesson 4: What Is the Management of Acute Decompensated Heart Failure and What Are the Special Considerations for PPCM?

Anesthesiologists may be confronted with patients in acute decompensated heart failure in the intensive care unit or perioperatively. Optimization of medical management is prudent before proceeding with elective cases, but sometimes the benefit of an urgent or emergent procedure outweighs the perioperative risks of acute heart failure. Patients with acute decompensated heart failure may present with signs of poor organ perfusion (“cold”), signs of vascular congestion (“wet”), or both (Table 19.1).

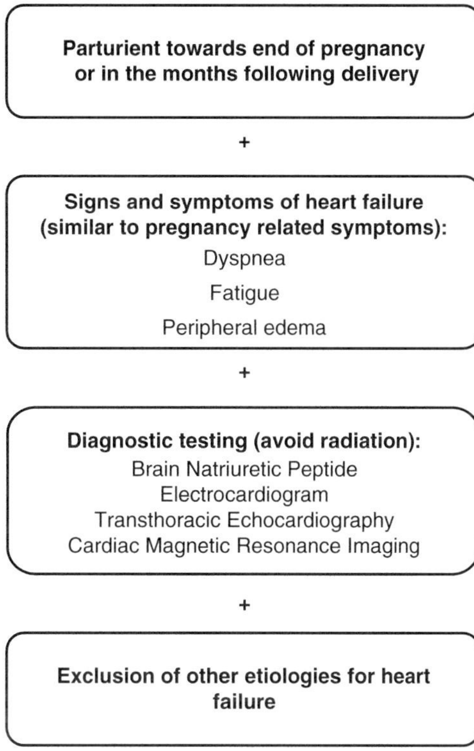

Fig. 19.5 Diagnostic criteria and further workup of peripartum cardiomyopathy. Adapted Table with kind permission of Elsevier [24]

Table 19.1 Treatment options according to volume status and perfusion state

		Congestion at rest	
		Orthopnea, pulmonary rales, S3 gallop, edema	
Low perfusion at rest Cool extremities, hypotension	**No**	**No**	**Yes**
		"Warm and dry"	"Warm and wet"
		Optimized	Diuresis
	Yes	"Cold and dry"	"Cold and wet"
		Inotropes	Inotropes and diuresis

Management of PPCM is similar to that of heart failure due to other causes. Mainstays of therapy include optimizing oxygenation and ventilation, preload reduction with diuretics and nitrates, vasodilator therapy for afterload reduction, and sometimes inotropic support. Long-term treatment includes beta-blockers, angiotensin-converting enzyme (ACE) inhibitors, anticoagulation, aldosterone antagonists, and treatment of other comorbidities such as obesity, hypertension, hyperlipidemia, and diabetes [24, 25].

The following restrictions to these therapies apply during pregnancy: ACE inhibitors and angiotensin II receptor blockers are contraindicated in pregnancy. These medications are associated with teratogenicity, oligohydramnios, renal agenesis, and fetal death. Spironolactone is thought to have antiandrogenic effects on the

Table 19.2 Pharmacologic treatment of heart failure and risk stratification during pregnancy. ACE: angiotensin-converting enzyme. Adapted Table with kind permission of Elsevier [24]

Drug	Risk stratification according to FDA pregnancy categories	Indication in patients with heart failure (55)
ACE inhibitors	D	NYHA I–IV
Angiotensin II blocker	D	If ACE inhibitor not tolerated
Beta-blockers	C	NYHA I–IV
Loop diuretics	C	NYHA II–IV or volume overload
Spironolactone	C	NYHA II–IV or volume overload
Digoxin	C	Atrial fibrillation
Warfarin	X	Atrial fibrillation

fetus and should likewise be avoided. Other diuretics should be used sparingly as they can decrease placental blood flow. Beta-blockers can be used safely, however it is recommended that beta-1 selective agents be used because of the theoretical risk of uterine activity with beta-2 receptor blockade. Both beta-blockers and loop diuretics are risk category C [24].

Anticoagulation should be considered for all patients with PPCM and LVEF <35%. Additionally, women with known LV thrombus and possibly women with atrial fibrillation should be anticoagulated. Warfarin is risk category D and should be avoided during pregnancy. Unfractionated and low-molecular-weight heparins are risk category C and do not cross the placenta and are therefore safe for use during pregnancy [24, 26] (Table 19.2).

In the acute setting, volume overload is suspected with pulmonary capillary wedge pressures (PCWP) >18 mmHg and worsening oxygenation. If oxygenation is critical, positive pressure ventilation is indicated until medical treatment is optimized. Pharmacologic diuresis either with intermittent or continuous intravenous loop diuretics and supplementation with thiazides or aldosterone antagonists should be initiated [27, 28]. If volume overload is resistant to pharmacologic diuresis, hemodialysis might be required. Ultrafiltration is the standard in the treatment of sodium-volume overload especially in the setting of decompensated heart failure. It is superior to loop diuretics in decreasing right atrial pressures and improving pulmonary function [28]. Patients with volume overload and low cardiac index (CI) due to hypertension profit from lowering afterload, which in turn leads to increased CI and reduced pulmonary congestion. Since a decrease in afterload can affect coronary perfusion and oxygen delivery to an already compromised left or right ventricle, vasodilators such as nitroprusside, nitroglycerin, and nesiritide are preferred over afterload-reducing inotropes such as milrinone and dobutamine as inotropy might increase oxygen consumption [29]. Dobutamine and milrinone, however, are synergistic drugs and excellent choices if a patient appears to be in cardiogenic shock suggested by a CI <2.2 l/min/m^2 or MVO2 <75%.

If a patient is dependent on inotropic therapy despite optimal medical therapy, implantation of a mechanical circulatory support device should be considered. Intra-aortic balloon pumps (IABP), venoarterial extracorporeal membrane oxygenation (VA-ECMO), and extracorporeal and low flow percutaneous LVADs have all been proven to be feasible options for temporary cardiac support for cardiogenic shock [30–33] (Figs. 19.6, 19.7, and 19.8)

VA-ECMO is feasible in biventricular failure and requires either central cannulation (similar to cardiopulmonary bypass) or peripheral (usually femoral) cannulation. Independent of the cannulation site, the tip of the venous cannula is positioned close to the right atrium and drains deoxygenated blood into an extracorporeal centrifugal pump. Depending on the pump's settings, a blood flow up to 8 l/min can be produced. Next, blood is pumped through a membrane oxygenator to facilitate gas exchange. From there oxygenated blood returns to the patient's circulation via the arterial cannulation site which is either located at a peripheral artery or the ascending aorta. VA-ECMO decreases myocardial oxygen consumption by decreasing cardiac work. This is achieved by decreasing preload and therefore offloading both ventricles. Special attention has to be paid to patients on VA-ECMO with peripheral cannulation since the retrograde flow from the arterial cannulation site increases afterload and impairs offloading the LV [31].

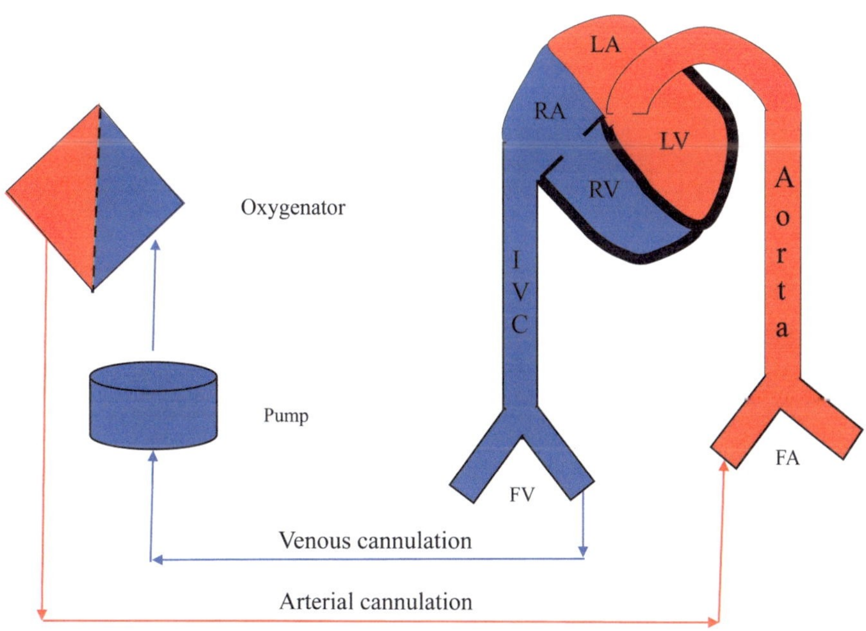

Fig. 19.6 Simplified schematic diagram of peripheral extracorporeal circulatory membrane oxygenation. *RA* right atrium, *RV* right ventricle, *LA* left atrium, *LV* left ventricle, *FA* femoral arteries, *FV* femoral veins

Fig. 19.7 Simplified schematic diagram of an intra-aortic balloon pump during (**a**) systole and (**b**) diastole. *RCA* right coronary artery, *LAD* left anterior descending artery, *CX* circumflex artery. Arrows symbolize blood flow

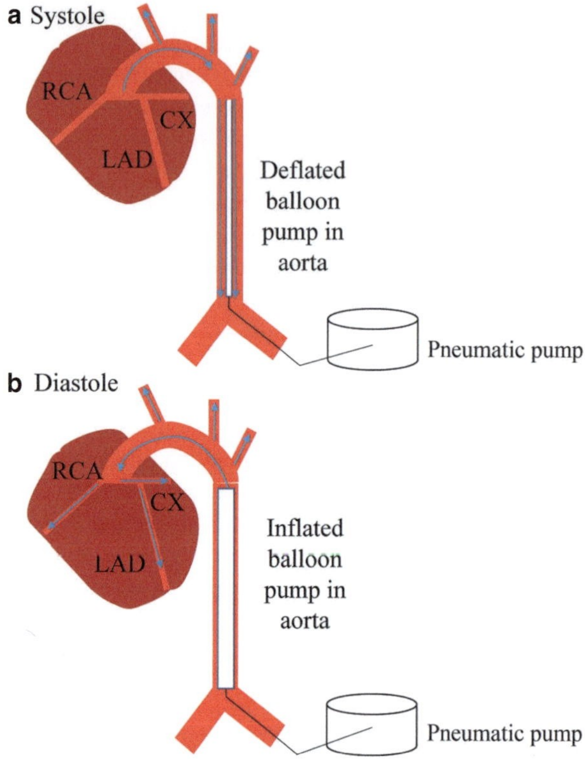

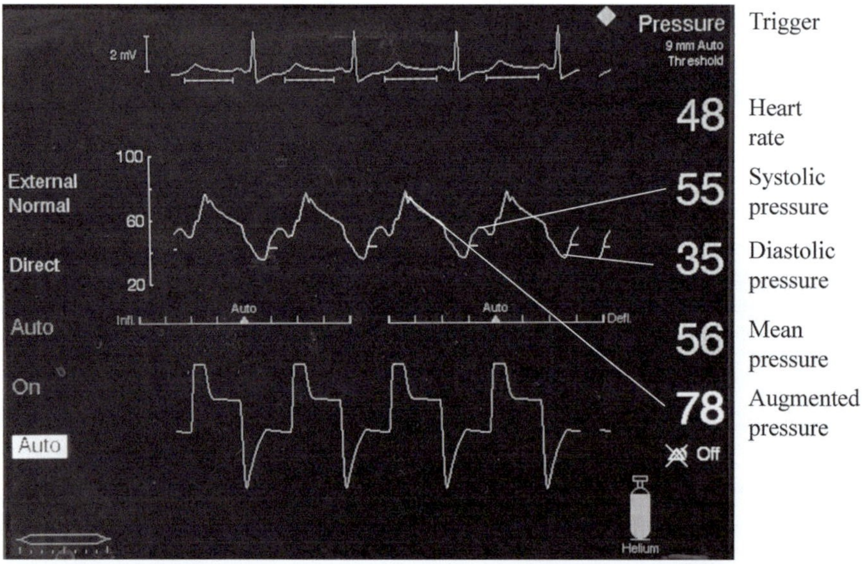

Fig. 19.8 Standard display from a monitor for an intra-aortic balloon pump. Pressures in millimeters of mercury (mmHg)

An IABP is feasible for LV support. It consists of a balloon, which is connected to a helium tank and console. The balloon is placed through the femoral artery and advanced in retrograde direction into the aorta until the tip of the device is positioned just distal to the offcome of the left subclavian artery. Triggered by an EKG or by an arterial pulse pressure wave form, it is filled with helium during diastole and deflated during systole. This leads to decreased afterload and a moreover CO during systole and improved perfusion of the coronary arteries during diastole. Inflation of the balloon can be set for every single, second, or third diastolic period. The augmented diastolic pressures are higher than the systolic pressure [32].

Delivery of the fetus is the ultimate treatment and may be considered regardless of gestation in patients with decompensated heart failure or hemodynamic instability [26]. If symptoms do not resolve after delivery, implantation of a permanent left ventricular assist device (LVAD) either as "destination" therapy or as bridge to heart transplant may be warranted.

Lesson 5: What Are the Anesthetic Implications of Noncardiac Surgery in Patients with Ventricular Assist Device?

Temporary indications for the implantation of a VAD include bridge therapy to either recovery of ventricular function, transplant, or candidacy/decision. In patients with end-stage heart failure who are not candidates for transplantation, implantation of a LVAD has been shown to improve survival and lifestyle compared to medical therapy [34]. This has led to the approval of LVADs for destination therapy and explains why the number of LVAD patients who present for noncardiac surgery is on the rise.

There are a variety of mechanical circulatory support devices, which can grossly be divided into either left, right, or biventricular devices. Depending on the system, it requires either extracorporeal, percutaneous, subdiaphragmatic, or pericardial implantation technique. Placement of extracorporeal or percutaneous devices is less invasive and is usually indicated for temporary circulatory support, whereas intracorporeal devices can provide higher blood flows and have a longer durability [35]. While most devices assist the patient's heart, the total artificial heart requires explantation of the native heart. Last it is important to realize that pumps provide either pulsatile or continuous flow via an axial or centrifugal pump (Table 19.3). Continuous flow has been shown to improve mortality despite other disadvantages including a high prevalence of gastrointestinal bleeds (GIB) [36, 37].

In this short review, we will focus on the most commonly used intracorporeal LVADs, the HeartWare® and Heartmate II/III® devices, as any anesthesiologist might encounter these devices in an outpatient setting. Both have an inflow cannula placed in the left apex of the heart, a pump providing continuous flow, and an outflow cannula placed in the ascending aorta. A driveline connects the pump to the extracorporeal components: batteries as a power source and a controller, which displays pump speed, power, pulsatility of flow or pulsatility index (PI), and flow.

Table 19.3 Most common mechanical ventricular assist devices, implantation site, and pump types. Adapted figure with kind permission of Mabel Chung, MD and Elsevier [24]

Device name	Location	Pump type
CentriMag®	Extracorporeal	Continuous-centrifugal
Impella®	Percutaneous	Continuous-axial
TandemHeart®	Percutaneous	Continuous
HeartMate XVE®	Intracorporeal-subdiaphragmatic	Pulsatile-electric; pusher plate
HeartMate II®	Intracorporeal-subdiaphragmatic	Continuous-axial
HeartMate III®	Intracorporeal-pericardial	Continuous-centrifugal
HeartWare®	Intracorporeal-pericardial	Continuous-centrifugal
SynCardia-total artificial heart®	Intracorporeal-replacing native heart	Pulsatile-pneumatic sac-type

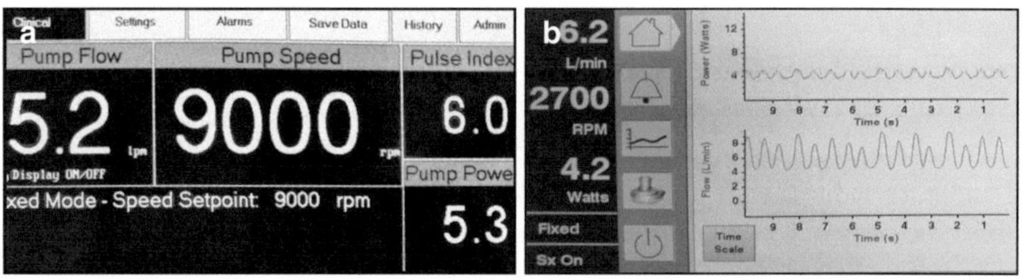

Fig. 19.9 Standard displays from LVAD monitors for (**a**) Heartmate II® and (**b**) HeartWare®. Pump flow in liters per minute, pump speed in rotations per minute, and pump power in watts

In a hospitalized patient, the controller can be connected to a monitor with a larger display (Figs. 19.9 and 19.10).

The LVAD device pumps blood out of the LV and into the ascending aorta. The speed of the pump is the only modifiable variable. It is measured in rotations per minute and can be changed either on the portable controller or a stationary system monitor. The initial pump speed is programmed in the operating room based on septal position and chamber size on TEE.

The motor power required to run the pump depends on the diameter and speed of the pump. It correlates well with blood flow, however there are some exceptions. Flow through the pump is not directly measured but calculated via measured pump power and set pump speed (and in some models blood viscosity/hematocrit). Actual flow through the pump is dependent upon pump speed and also the pressure differential across the pump. For a fixed speed, the difference in mean aortic pressure (afterload) and LV chamber pressure (preload) correlates inversely with flow, with LV intracavitary pressure being the greatest determinant of pump differential pressure. The calculated blood flow may underestimate total cardiac output, as it does not account for blood ejected by the native LV across the aortic valve.

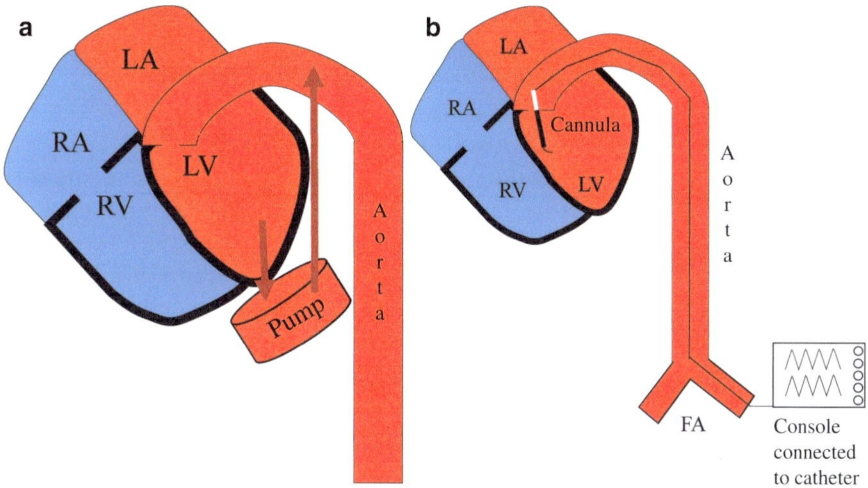

Fig. 19.10 (**a**) Simplified schematic diagram of a pericardial left ventricular assist device (Heartmate III®, Heartware®). *RA* right atrium, *RV* right ventricle, *LA* left atrium, *LV* left ventricle; (**b**) simplified schematic diagram of a percutaneous left ventricular assist device (Heartmate III®, Heartware®). *RA* right atrium, *RV* right ventricle, *LA* left atrium, *LV* left ventricle, *FA* femoral artery. The inflow area of the cannula is positioned in the LV (black part of cannula), and the outlet area, motor, and the pressure sensor are positioned in the aorta (white part of cannula)

The PI is dimensionless and calculated by the flow through the pump:

$$(\text{maximum flow} - \text{minimum flow}) / \text{average flow}$$

The PI is displayed on the monitor of the Heartmate® LVAD (normal values 3–6) (Fig. 19.9a). Pump flow pulsatility is displayed graphically on the monitor of the Heartware® LVAD (Fig. 19.9b). Both provide useful information about LVAD support, LV preload, and contractility: myopathic left ventricles still follow the Frank-Starling principle and increase contractility in response to preload. A higher PI or pulsatility signifies more ventricular filling and thus contractility, less support by the LVAD, or increased afterload. A lower value generally signifies less ventricular filling due to more support from the LVAD, hypovolemia, or decreased right ventricular (RV) function [38].

There are however exceptions, emphasizing that all parameters need to be reviewed in order to troubleshoot the device. An obstruction of the LVAD can lead to more ventricular filling but low PIs. In case of a thrombus located on the rotor, more work would be required to overcome the shear forces of the rotor at a given speed. Since the pump would utilize more power, the calculated flow would be erroneously high compared to the actual flow, which results in a low PI. In another scenario, the inflow or outflow cannulas might be kinked or obstructed. Since the pump would be exposed to less blood, it would utilize less power resulting in lower flows and PIs (Fig. 19.11a, b).

In case of a so-called suction event, the interventricular septum has moved toward the inflow cannula resulting in LV collapse. Suction events usually occur if the blood volume through the pump exceeds LV filling or in other words if speed has been set too high or preload has dropped. Such events present with reduced power and fluctuating speed data as the machine automatically decreases speed until the suction event resolves and then gradually increases speed again.

Pump failure is an acute emergency which requires medical treatment of heart failure until specialized cardiologists, cardiothoracic surgeons, and company representatives are available. Issues which can be resolved right away include checking that the percutaneous lead is connected to the controller and that power supply is warranted either via electrical outlet or battery. It is imperative to exchange one battery at a time as disconnection from both batteries can lead to pump failure itself [35].

Decompression of the LV by the LVAD can lead to problems if LV pressures are too low. Right heart failure is a frequent complication (20–50%) of LVAD implantation [39]. LVAD implantation leads to unloading of the LV, with a resultant change in ventricular septal curvature and RV geometry, thus affecting ventricular interdependence. Additionally, increased venous return from LV unloading increases RV preload. Consequently the RV free wall has to compensate with increased contractility, which carries the risk of RV failure. This is tempered somewhat by the decrease in PCWP and PA pressure seen with LV unloading. Worsening of aortic insufficiency is another common complication seen when LV pressures are too low. This is further exacerbated by increased outflow from the LVAD into the ascending aorta. On the other hand, if the speed of the pump is set too low, the patient might develop LV failure again. In order to determine the appropriate settings of the device, patients are monitored for multiple weeks after implantation before they are discharged home. Even then, frequent interrogation of the pump is mandatory.

All of the commonly used devices in the United States require anticoagulation and antiplatelet therapy to avoid thrombotic occlusion of the pump and to reduce the risk of thromboembolic events. In addition, the sheer force of the pump as well as flow acceleration and interaction of blood with artificial surfaces can lead to acquired von Willebrand deficiency and hemolysis [40]. Therefore GIB and anemia are common complications in patients with a LVAD. This is particularly true of continuous-flow LVADs and is most likely due to decreased arterial pulsatility which causes hypoperfusion of the gastrointestinal mucosa and the formation of arteriovenous malformations. As a consequence, endoscopies are by far the most common noncardiac procedures in these patients [41]. Another common procedure is a device exchange due to infections of drivelines or pump pockets or secondary to thrombosis of the rotor or cannula.

For an elective procedure in a hemodynamically stable patient, routine monitoring may theoretically be sufficient [41]. However, we advocate for arterial line placement for continuous blood pressure and arterial blood gas monitoring. Ultrasound can be helpful in locating the artery in the absence of a palpable pulse. Noninvasive blood pressure monitoring and pulse oximetry are often unreliable because of

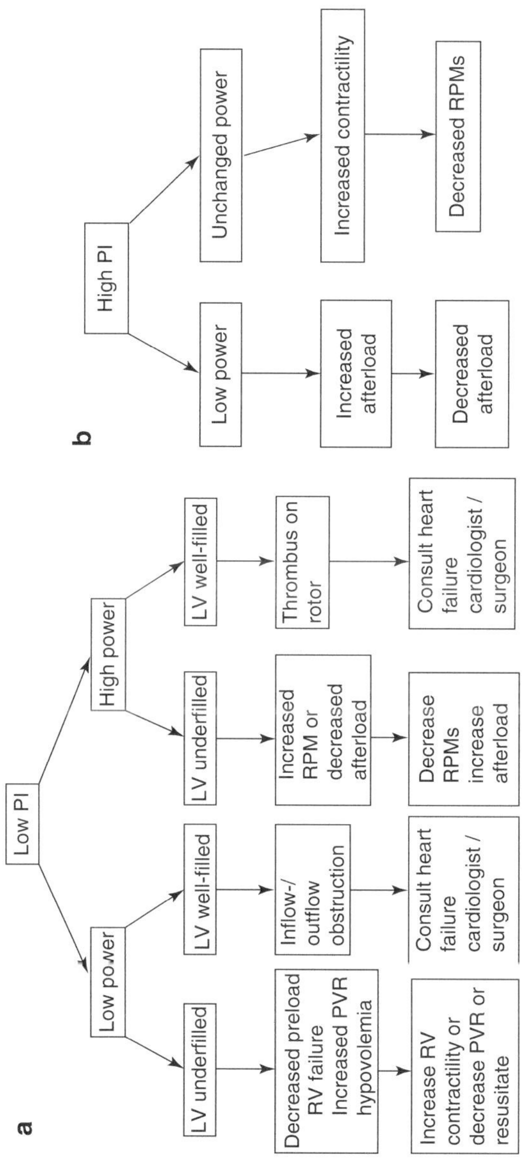

Fig. 19.11 PI pulsatility index. (**a**) Algorithm of decreased PI. (**b**) Algorithm of increased PI. Adapted figure with kind permission by Mabel Chung, MD

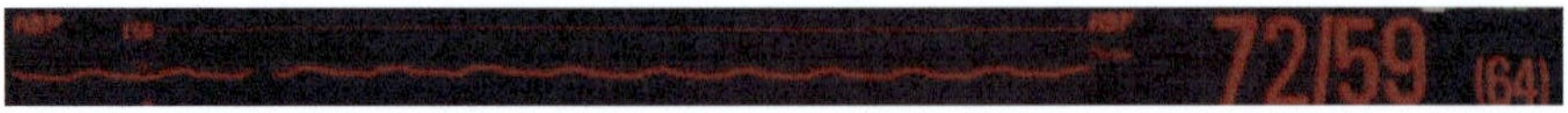

Fig. 19.12 Minimally pulsatile arterial line tracing of a patient after implantation of a ventricular assist device

less pulsatile blood flow, especially with continuous-flow devices (Fig. 19.12). Noninvasive blood pressure measurements may be obtained using a Doppler signal; however it may be impractical in the OR setting to use Doppler for each blood pressure measurement. The anesthesiologist should know the expected battery life of the patient's device and ideally connect the LVAD to a stable power source for the case. The LVAD should be connected to the pump controller console, which will display LVAD flow and may be a rough surrogate for CO. Contact information of the LVAD manufacturer can be useful in case of an emergency. The LVAD coordinator at the nearest heart center is also an invaluable resource. Adequate personnel should be available to assist in the event of an emergency. LVAD patients often have pacemakers/AICDs for cardiac resynchronization therapy and for the treatment of life-threatening arrhythmias, respectively. There are currently no recommendations that are different than those for non-LVAD patients; however it is ideal to maintain biventricular pacing function in order to optimize RV-dependent LVAD filling [42]. Some types of LVADs may impair gastric emptying given their position in the peritoneal space, and a rapid sequence induction should be considered.

Warfarin should be stopped several days in advance and bridged with heparin. Ideally, heparin and antiplatelet therapy would be continued perioperatively; however a multidisciplinary discussion should take place between the surgeon, anesthesiologist, and the patient's cardiologist. Adequate intravenous access and the availability of blood products are crucial in this setting. Postoperatively, anticoagulation and antiplatelet therapy should be reinitiated as early as possible [43].

Intraoperative management of LVAD patients with unstable hemodynamics may require central venous and PA pressure monitoring and/or placement of a TEE probe. Also, central or mixed venous oxygen saturations may be helpful in guiding resuscitation in these patients. Hemodynamic management should include a focus on preload, afterload, and optimization of RV function. Preload should be maintained at high normal values; however caution should be exercised as to not volume overload the vulnerable right ventricle. CVP monitoring and TEE can be used to avoid RV failure but provide adequate preload. A drop in preload may also be detected by hypotension on the arterial line or decreased output or flows on the LVAD. SVR can be calculated as illustrated below. Excessive vasoconstriction will predictably decrease output from a continuous-flow LVAD. A reasonable goal is MAP from 70 to 90, which should assure adequate organ perfusion pressure without excessive afterload. As previously stated, RV failure is a significant cause of morbidity and mortality post-LVAD implantation. The anesthesiologist should work to avoid triggers that would increase pulmonary vascular resistance (PVR). These include hypercarbia, hypoxemia, acidosis, and excessive PEEP. The RV is exquisitely sensitive to perfusion pressure; therefore MAP should be maintained above 70 mmHg. RV contractility can be improved by the addition of an inodilator like dobutamine or milrinone, and PVR/RV afterload may be reduced by the addition of a pulmonary vasodilator like inhaled nitric oxide or epoprostenol. TEE guidance is especially helpful in cases of suspected RV dysfunction [44].

$$\mathrm{SVR} = \left[\left(\mathrm{MAP} - \mathrm{CVP} \right) / \mathrm{LVAD\ output} \right] \times 80\,\mathrm{dynes} / \mathrm{cm}^5$$

In the case of a cardiac arrest, normal ACLS drug dosages and defibrillation energies should be used, and some advocate for placement of defibrillator pads on all LVAD patients undergoing surgery. Manufactures advice that chest compressions must not be performed due to the theoretical risk of dislodgement of VAD cannulae and exsanguination, however evidence is missing [45]. There are case reports of abdominal compressions in the case of cardiac arrest, but this is not yet routinely recommended [46].

Lesson 6: What Are the Anesthetic Implications of Noncardiac Surgery in Patients with Heart Transplant?

Despite the chronic shortage of feasible donors, the quantity of cardiac transplants is expected to increase due to the extension of donor criteria and achievements in preservation solutions and devices [47–49]. As a consequence, the number of heart transplant recipients presenting for noncardiac surgery will continue to rise.

A routine preoperative assessment should be performed ahead of time to allow time for additional testing if needed. There are no specific guidelines for the preoperative evaluation of cardiac transplant recipients. By ACC and ASA guidelines for noncardiac surgery, there is no need for routine testing provided that there is no change in the patient's functional status [50, 51]. Some patients might experience silent ischemia, however, in the setting of sensory denervation of the heart. Given the high incidence of dysrhythmias and the consequences of graft failure, rejection, or ischemia, it is advisable to review or obtain an electrocardiogram within 30 days and functional cardiac testing not older than 3–6 months prior to a planned procedure.

ECGs of heart recipients frequently record two p-waves which are due to the preservation of the native and donor sinoatrial node during the biatrial implantation technique (Fig. 19.13). Other dysrhythmias are also common postoperatively and can be due to implantation approach, surgical trauma, vagolysis, ischemia, rejection, antiarrhythmic drugs, or increased blood levels of catecholamines. Bradyarrhythmias may occur in the early postoperative course. In 10% of biatrial implantations, permanent pacing is required. If a pacemaker (PM) or AICD has been implanted, ASA guidelines for management of cardiac implantable electronic devices advice that the most recent interrogation should be within 6–12 months. Furthermore, the manufacturer should be contacted to clarify PM or AICD settings and how magnet use affects the mode of the device [42]. More recently the need for PM placement has significantly decreased in heart transplanted patients due to

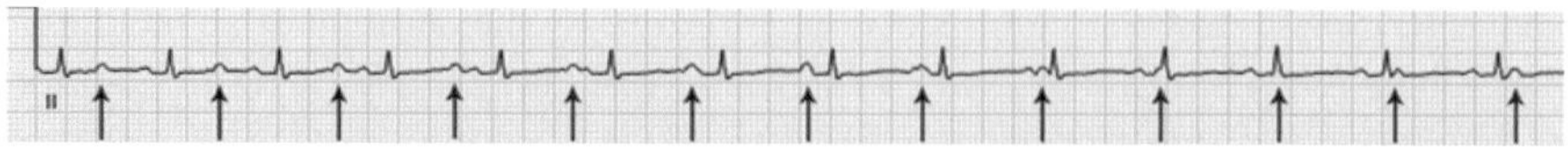

Fig. 19.13 EKG following a heart transplant with biatrial approach: recipient T-waves are marked by arrows. (Courtesy of Jason E. Roediger, CCT, CRAT. Used with permission under the Creative Commons license: https://creativecommons.org/licenses/by-sa/3.0/deed.en) [62]

the bicaval implantation technique [52]. The most common tachyarrhythmias are atrial flutter and fibrillation and require appropriate rate control and anticoagulation. New-onset arrhythmias require further workup before proceeding with surgery [53].

Mortality from rejection is highest for the first 3 months following transplantation. It is common practice to delay the surgery within this time period to avoid additional stress in the perioperative phase [54]. Myocardial biopsies are performed frequently during the first year following transplantation and should carefully be reviewed. After one year, biopsies become less frequent due to lower risk of rejection. Within the first 5 years postoperatively, mortality from cardiac allograft vasculopathy peaks and can potentially lead to intraoperative ischemia. As stated above, preoperative assessment of symptoms might be misleading as cardiac denervation can easily lead to silent episodes of ischemia. Therefore it is prudent to review the most recent stress test and angiography. In general, if there is any suspicion of graft failure, rejection, or ischemia, further workup should precede the scheduled surgery.

In order to avoid the aforementioned complications, immunosuppressive drugs should be continued during the perioperative period. Most immunosuppressive regimens for maintenance are based on a calcineurin inhibitor (CNI), a corticosteroid, and a antiproliferative drug. There are many anesthetic implications for immunosuppressive therapy. Common side effects of antiproliferative drugs are anemia, increased risk of perioperative infection, and increased bleeding risk due to myelosuppression. In addition patients receiving CNIs frequently suffer from hypertension and renal failure. Other nephrotoxic drugs such as gentamycin and ketorolac should therefore be avoided. Common side effects of corticosteroids include hypertension and hyperglycemia. Adrenal suppression occurs with sudden withdrawal of steroids or during physiologic stress such as surgery. Patients on corticosteroids should therefore receive stress dosing in the perioperative period. Hydrocortisone is the preferred option because of its mineralocorticoid activity. Intraoperative etomidate should be used with caution in the light of adrenal suppression [55].

Provided that preoperative findings reveal normal cardiac function with no signs of graft failure or rejection, there is no need for invasive monitoring unless other comorbidities or the procedure justify it. If invasive procedures are indicated, sterile technique should be stressed in the light of immunosuppression. If a dental procedure is planned and preoperative findings include an underlying valvular lesion, infective endocarditis prophylaxis is required [56].

General or regional anesthesia and monitored anesthesia care have been performed successfully in heart transplant patients [57].

Cardiac denervation following a heart transplant has many intraoperative implications [57]. While there has been evidence for reinnervation up to 15 years postoperatively, it appears to be incomplete and regionally heterogeneous with unpredictable clinical relevance [58]. Sympathetic denervation prevents a positive chronotropic response to stress situations such as laryngoscopy, pain, light anesthesia, hypercarbia, or hypoxia. Only a gradual increase of heart rate is noted due to circulating catecholamines secreted from the adrenal glands. For the same reason, compensation for hypotension or hypovolemia mostly occurs by an increase in stroke volume, as the baroreceptor reflex is absent. This makes this patient population highly preload-dependent and vulnerable to induction of anesthesia and bleeding. Volume status should therefore be meticulously evaluated intraoperatively [59]. Temporizing measures to increase inotropy and chronotropy include the administration of direct-acting sympathomimetic drugs such as the beta-agonists epinephrine, isoproterenol, and dobutamine, as well as phosphodiesterase inhibitors such as milrinone. In fact, alpha-1 agonists such as epinephrine and norepinephrine show an exacerbated positive chronotropic and inotropic response via beta-1 receptors because the accompanied increase in blood pressure does not result in a vagal response. Conversely, the effect on blood pressure through alpha-1 receptors is blunted which is most likely due to chronically increased blood levels of catecholamines. In these cases, vasopressin and methylene blue can then be used for refractory hypotension [60]. Vagal denervation leads to a resting heart rate between 90 and 110. The oculocardiac reflex and other vagally mediated reflexes during laryngoscopy, insufflation, and Valsalva maneuvers have no effect.

Early after transplantation indirect-acting drugs show a diminished response. Administration of vagolytic drugs such as atropine might not be accompanied by the positive chronotropic effect seen pretransplant. Ephedrine loses its indirect sympathomimetic and digoxin its indirect vagomimetic effect. Acetylcholinesterase inhibitors and anticholinergic drugs show no effect on chronotropy during reversal of muscle relaxation. However as reinnervation progresses over the years, the autonomic response becomes very unpredictable. The anesthesiologist should therefore be prepared for brady- and tachyarrhythmias [61]. Bradyarrhythmias be can counteracted by the aforementioned beta-agonists. Tachyarrhythmias respond to sotalol and amiodarone and have minimal interaction with immunosuppressive drugs [60]. Intravenous lidocaine should be avoided due to its negative inotropic effect.

During the postoperative course, immunosuppressant drugs need to be continued as soon as possible, and the stress dose of hydrocortisone should be slowly tapered down to baseline requirements [55]. Immunosuppressed patients are particularly vulnerable to postoperative infections and should be monitored prudently for fever and other clinical signs.

References

1. Mabie WC, DiSessa TG, Crocker LG, et al. A longitudinal study of cardiac output in normal human pregnancy. Am J Obstet Gynecol. 1994;170:849e56.
2. Chestnut's Chestnut DH, Polley LS, Tsen LC, Wong CA. Obstetric anesthesia: principles and practice. 4th ed. Philadelphia: Mosby Elsevier; 2009.
3. Bamber JH, Dresner M. Aortocaval compression in pregnancy: the effect of changing the degree and direction of lateral tilt on maternal cardiac output. Anesth Analg. 2003;97(1):256–8.

4. Bucklin BA, Gambling DR, Wlody DJ. A practical approach to obstetric anesthesia. Philadelphia: Lippincott Williams & Wilkins; 2008.
5. Silwa K, Fett J, Elkayam U. Peripartum cardiomyopathy. Lancet. 2006;368:687–93.
6. Petersen KM, Jimenez-Solem E, Andersen JT, et al. β-Blocker treatment during pregnancy and adverse pregnancy outcomes: a nationwide population-based cohort study. BMJ Open. 2012;2:e001185. https://doi.org/10.1136/bmjopen-2012-001185.
7. Karthikeyan VJ, Ferner RE, Baghdadi S, et al. Are angiotensin-converting enzyme inhibitors and angiotensin receptor blockers safe in pregnancy: a report of ninety-one pregnancies. J Hypertens. 2011;29(2):396–9.
8. Elkayam U. Clinical characteristics of peripartum cardiomyopathy in the United States. JACC. 2011;58(7):659–70.
9. Hilfiker-Kleiner D, Kaminski K, Podewski E, et al. A cathepsin D-cleaved 16 kDa form of prolactin mediates postpartum cardiomyopathy. Cell. 2007;128:589–600.
10. Selle T, Renger I, Labidi S, et al. Reviewing peripartum cardiomyopathy: current state of knowledge. Futur Cardiol. 2009;5:175–89.
11. Morales A, Painter T, Li R, et al. Rare variant mutations in pregnancy-associated or peripartum cardiomyopathy. Circulation. 2010;121:2176–82.
12. Van Spaendonck-Zwarts KY, van Tintelen JP, van Veldhuisen DJ, et al. Peripartum cardiomyopathy as a part of familial dilated cardiomyopathy. Circulation. 2010;121:2169–75.
13. Demakis JG, Rahimtoola SH, Sutton GC, et al. Natural course of peripartum cardiomyopathy. Circulation. 1971;44:1053–61.
14. Whitehead SJ, Berg CJ, Chang J. Pregnancy-related mortality due to cardiomyopathy. United States, 1991–1997. Obstet Gynecol. 2003;102(6):1326–31.
15. Leinwand LA. Molecular events underlying pregnancy-induced cardiomyopathy. Cell. 2007;128:436–7.
16. Stergiopoulos K, Shiang E, Bench T, et al. Pregnancy in patients with pre-existing cardiomyopathies. J Am Coll Cardiol. 2011;58(4):337–50.
17. Tibazarwa K, Lee G, Mayosi B, et al. The 12-lead ECG in peripartum cardiomyopathy. Cardiovasc J Afr. 2012;23(6):322–9.
18. DeLemos JA, Morrow DA, Bentley JH, et al. The prognostic value of B-type natriuretic peptide in patients with acute coronary syndromes. N Engl J Med. 2001;345(14):1014–21.
19. Forster O, Hilfiker-Kleiner D, Ansari AA, et al. Reversal of IFN-gamma, oxLDL, and prolactin serum levels correlate with clinical improvement in patients with peripartum cardiomyopathy. Eur J Heart Fail. 2008;10:861–8.
20. Silwa K, Skudicky D, Bergemann A, et al. Peripartum cardiomyopathy: analysis clinical outcome, left ventricular function plasma levels of cytokines, and Fas/APO-1. J Am Coll Cardiol. 2000;35:701–5.
21. Duran N, Gunes H, Duran I, et al. Predictors of prognosis patients with peripartum cardiomyopathy. Int J Gynaecol Obstet. 2008;101:137–40.
22. Mouquet F, Lions C, de Groote P, et al. Characterisation of peripartum cardiomyopathy by cardiac magnetic resonance imaging. Eur Radiol. 2008;18:2765–9.
23. Srichai MB, Junor C, Rodriguez LL, et al. Clinical, imaging, and pathological characteristics of left ventricular thrombus: a comparison of contrast-enhanced magnetic resonance, transthoracic echocardiography, and transesophageal echocardiography with surgical or pathological validation. Am Heart J. 2006;152:75–84.
24. Kimberly S, Robbins MK, Nguyen AP, Almehlisi A, Meier A, Schmidt U. Peripartum cardiomyopathy: current options for treatment and cardiovascular support. J Cardiothorac Vasc Anesth. 2019.
25. Yancy CW, Jessup M, Bozkurt B, et al. ACCF/AHA guideline for management of heart failure. A report of the American College of Cardiology Foundation/American Heart Association Task Force on Practice Guidelines. J Am Coll Cardiol. 2013;62(16):e137–239, 2013
26. Lewey J, Haythe J. Cardiomyopathy in pregnancy. Semin Perinatol. 2014;38:309–17.
27. Clyde WY, Jessup M, Bozkurt B, et al. Report of the American College of Cardiology Foundation/American Heart Association Task Force on Practice Guidelines. J Am Coll Cardiol. 2013;62(16):1495–539.

28. Bart BA. Controversies in heart failure, treatment of congestion in congestive heart failure: ultrafiltration is the only rational initial treatment of volume overload in decompensated heart failure. Circ Heart Fail. 2009;2(5):499–504.
29. Abraham WT, Adams KF, Fonarow GC, et al. In-hospital mortality in patients with acute decompensated heart failure requiring intravenous vasoactive medications: an analysis from the Acute Decompensated Heart Failure National Registry (ADHERE). J Am Coll Cardiol. 2005;46:57–64.
30. Lamarche Y, Cheung A, Ignaszewski A, et al. Comparative outcomes in cardiogenic shock managed with Impella microaxial pump or extracorporeal life support. J Thorac Cardiovasc Surg. 2011;142:60–5.
31. Liden H, Wiklund L, Haraldsson A, et al. Temporary circulatory support with extra corporeal membrane oxygenation in adults with refractory cardiogenic shock. Scand Cardiovasc J. 2009;43:226–32.
32. Yahagi N, Kumon K, Nakatani T, et al. Peripartum cardiomyopathy and tachycardia followed by multiple organ failure. Anesth Analg. 1994;79:581–2.
33. Basra SS, Loyalka P, Kar B. Current status of percutaneous ventricular assist devices for cardiogenic shock. Curr Opin Cardiol. 2011;26:548–54.
34. Rose EA, Gelijns AC, Moskowitz AJ, et al. Long-term use of a left ventricular assist device for end-stage heart failure. N Engl J Med. 2001;345:1435–43.
35. Slaughter MS, Pagani F, Rogers JG, et al. Clinical management of continuous-flow left ventricular assist devices in advanced heart failure. J Heart Lung Transplant. 2010;29(4S): S1–39.
36. Demirozu ZT, Radovancevic R, Hochman LF, et al. Arteriovenous malformation and gastrointestinal bleeding in patients with the HeartMate II left ventricular assist device. J Heart Lung Transplant. 2011;30(8):849–53.
37. Boyle AJ, Russell SD, Teuteberg JJ, et al. Low thromboembolism and pump thrombosis with the HeartMate II left ventricular assist device: analysis of outpatient anti-coagulation. J Heart Lung Transplant. 2009;28:881–7.
38. Pratt AK, Shah NS, Boyce SW. Left ventricular assist device management in the ICU. Crit Care Med. 2014;42(1):158–68.
39. Meineri M, Van Rensburg AE, Vegas A. Right ventricular failure after LVAD implantation: prevention and treatment. Best Pract Res Clin Anaesthesiol. 2012;26(2):217–29.
40. Heilmann C, Geisen U, Benk C, et al. Hemolysis in patients with ventricular assist devices: major differences between systems. Eur J Cardiothorac Surg. 2009;36(3):580–4.
41. Eric W, Nelson DO, Heinke T, et al. Management of LVAD patients for noncardiac surgery: a single institution study. To be printed in Journal of Cardiothoracic and Vascular Anesthesia.
42. Crossley GH, Poole JE, Rozner MA, et al. The heart rhythm society (HRS)/American society of Anesthesiologists (ASA) Expert Consensus Statement on the perioperative management of patients with implantable defibrillators, pacemakers and arrhythmia monitors: facilities and patient management. Heart Rhythm. 2011;8(7):e1–18.
43. Apfelbaum JL, Nuttall GA, Connis RT, et al. American Society of Anesthesiologists Task Force on perioperative blood management. Practice guidelines for perioperative blood management. An updated report by the American Society of Anesthesiologists Task Force on perioperative blood management. Anesthesiology. 2015;122(2):241–75.
44. Stone ME, Soong W, Krol M, et al. The anesthetic considerations in patients with ventricular assist devices presenting for noncardiac surgery: a review of eight cases. Anesth Analg. 2002;95(1):42–9.
45. Mabvuure NT, Rodrigues JN. External cardiac compression during cardiopulmonary resuscitation of patients with left ventricular assist devices. Interact Cardiovasc Thorac Surg. 2014;19(2):286–9.
46. Rottenberg EM, Heard J, Hamlin R, et al. Abdominal only CPR during cardiac arrest for a patient with an LVAD during resternotomy: a case report. J Cardiothorac Surg. 2011;6:91.
47. Mancini D, Lietz K. Contemporary reviews in cardiovascular medicine. Selection of cardiac transplantation candidates in 2010. Circulation. 2010;122(2):173–83.

48. Esmailian F, Kobashigawa JA, Naka Y, et al. The PROCEED II International Heart Transplant Trial with the Organ Care System Technology (OCS). In process.
49. Latchana N, Peck JR, Whitson B, et al. Preservation solutions for cardiac and pulmonary donor grafts: a review of the current literature. J Thorac Dis. 2014;6(8):1143–9.
50. Apfelbaum JL, Connis RT, Nickinovich DG, et al. Practice advisory for preanesthesia evaluation: an updated report by the American Society of Anesthesiologists Task Force on preanesthesia evaluation. Anesthesiology. 2012;116(3):522–38.
51. Fleisher LA, Fleischmann KE, et al. ACC/AHA guideline on perioperative cardiovascular evaluation and management of patients undergoing noncardiac surgery. J Am Coll Cardiol. 2014. 2014;64(22):e77–e137.
52. Herre JM, Barnhart GR, Llano A. Cardiac pacemakers in the transplanted heart: short term with the biatrial anastomosis and unnecessary with the bicaval anastomosis. Curr Opin Cardiol. 2000;15(2):115–20.
53. Pavri BB, O'Nunain SS, Newell JB, et al. Prevalence and prognostic significance of atrial arrhythmias after orthotopic cardiac transplantation. JACC 1999. 1995;25(7):1673.
54. Valerio R Jr, Durra O, Gold ME. Anesthetic considerations for an adult heart transplant recipient undergoing noncardiac surgery: a case report. AANA J. 2014;82(4):293–9.
55. Lindenfeld JA, Miller GG, Shakar SF, Zolty R, Lowes BD, Wolfel EE, Mestroni L, Page RL, Kobashigawa J. Drug therapy in the heart transplant recipient. Circulation. 2004;110(25):3858–65.
56. Wilson W, Taubert KA, Gewitz M, American Heart Association, et al. Prevention of infective endocarditis: guidelines from the American Heart Association: a guideline from the American Heart Association Rheumatic Fever, Endocarditis and Kawasaki Disease Committee, Council on Cardiovascular Disease in the Young, and the Council on Clinical Cardiology, Council on Cardiovascular Surgery and Anesthesia, and the Quality of Care and Outcomes Research Interdisciplinary Working Group. J Am Dent Assoc. 2008;139(Suppl):3S–24S.
57. Kostopanagiotou G, Smyrniotis V, Arkadopoulos N, et al. Anesthetic and perioperative management of adult transplant recipients in nontransplant surgery. Anesth Analg. 1999;89(3):613–22.
58. Bengel FM, Ueberfuhr P, Ziegler SI, et al. Serial assessment of sympathetic reinnervation after orthotopic heart transplantation. A longitudinal study using PET and C-11 hydroxyephedrine. Circulation 13. 1999;99(14):1866–71.
59. Blasco LM, Parameshwar J, Vuylsteke A. Anaesthesia for noncardiac surgery in the heart transplant recipient. Curr Opin Anesthesiol. 2009;22(1):109–13.
60. Costanzo MR, Dipchand A, Starling R, et al. The International Society of Heart and Lung Transplantation, guidelines for the care of heart transplant recipients. J Heart Lung Transplant. 2010;29(8):914–56.
61. Bjerke RJ, Mangione MP. Asystole after intravenous neostigmine in a heart transplant recipient. Can J Anaesth. 2001;48(3):305–7.
62. Orthotopic heart transplant. by Jer5150 – Roediger JE. Licensed under CC BY-SA 3.0 via Commons. https://commons.wikimedia.org/wiki/File:Orthotopic_Heart_Transplant.png#/media/File:Orthotopic_Heart_Transplant.png.

Chapter 20
A Minor Hiccup: Singultus, Regurgitation, and Aspiration Under Anesthesia

Sonya M. Seshadri and Jonathan L. Benumof

Case Presentation

A 46-year-old male (weight 97 kg, height 6′1″, BMI 29) was scheduled for an outpatient right inguinal hernia repair. The patient had no significant past medical history or allergies. His surgical history consisted of a previous right inguinal hernia repair at 6 months of age. Induction of anesthesia proceeded with 150 mcg IV fentanyl, 100 mg IV lidocaine, and 200 mg IV propofol in anticipation of placement of a laryngeal mask airway (LMA). Once the patient was apneic, he began to have hiccups which made laryngeal mask airway placement and ventilation via mask difficult **(Lesson I)**.

The patient then regurgitated clear secretions into his oropharynx **(Lesson II)**. The anesthesiologist turned the head to the right side to suction the oropharynx, deepened anesthesia with 100 mg IV propofol, and paralyzed the patient with 150 mg IV succinylcholine to prepare for endotracheal intubation. The patient regurgitated clear secretions a second time, and the airway was suctioned for a second time. Ventilation via mask was possible at this point. The anesthesiologist performed direct laryngoscopy with cricoid pressure and intubated the patient uneventfully with an 8.0 mm endotracheal tube. A suction catheter was placed through the endotracheal tube, and an orogastric tube was placed in the stomach with no significant return of material through either conduit **(Lesson III)**. The lungs were clear to auscultation bilaterally, and breath sounds were equal throughout the lung fields. During the 70 min case, the patient's oxygen saturation ranged from

S. M. Seshadri (✉)
Department of Anesthesiology, Southern California Permanente Medical Group, San Diego, CA, USA
e-mail: sonya.m.seshadri@kp.org

J. L. Benumof
Department of Anesthesiology, University of California, UCSD Medical Center, UCSD School of Medicine, San Diego, CA, USA

J. L. Benumof, G. R. Manecke (eds.), *Clinical Anesthesiology II*,
https://doi.org/10.1007/978-3-030-12365-9_20

97% to 100% on 50% FiO2. At the end of the case, the anesthesiologist extubated the patient fully awake. During the patient's 3 h postoperative care unit (PACU) stay, his oxygen saturation was 94–97% on 2 L/min nasal cannula which was eventually weaned to room air. The patient had no apparent respiratory distress and was discharged home in stable condition.

On postoperative day 1, the patient came to the emergency department with wheezing, a productive cough with thick brownish-colored sputum, and a fever to 103 °F. Physical exam revealed wheezing and crackles on the right side which correlated with a right middle lobe consolidation on chest radiograph **(Lesson IV)**. The patient was admitted to the hospital for a course of intravenous antibiotics to treat aspiration pneumonia. He was discharged home with oral antibiotics on hospital day 3 after he had been afebrile for 48 h with improvement of his wheezing and cough.

Lesson I: Hiccups Under Anesthesia

Lesson IA: What Is the Definition of a Hiccup?

A hiccup (singultus) is an episodic spasm of the diaphragm and intercostal muscles followed by closure of the vocal cords. During a hiccup, the diaphragm contracts and flattens, and the external intercostal muscles contract, simulating a forceful inspiration [1]. Thirty-five milliseconds after spasm of the respiratory muscles, the vocal cords close suddenly preventing the movement of air into the lungs [2]. The closure of the vocal cords is what creates the characteristic sound of a hiccup [3].

Lesson IB: What Causes Hiccups Under Anesthesia?

Hiccups can occur for many reasons related to anesthesia and surgery. Causes related to anesthesia include gastric distention (i.e., from ventilation via mask) and side effects from induction agents such as propofol [2, 4]. A few case reports have suggested that epidural anesthesia with long-acting local anesthetics such as bupivacaine and ropivacaine can cause hiccups in a dose-dependent manner. This effect could be due to alterations in gastrointestinal, diaphragmatic, or abdominal wall innervation and reflexes [5, 6]. Hiccups appear to occur more frequently in certain types of surgical procedures such as those with direct manipulation of the diaphragm, gastrointestinal surgery, and respiratory procedures such as bronchoscopy and tracheostomy [1]. Another rare but important cause of hiccups is phrenic nerve irritation along its course. Atrial pacing, ablation procedures for atrial fibrillation, and placement of central venous catheters have been reported to cause hiccups due to the anatomical proximity of the right atrium to the right branch of the phrenic nerve [7–9].

Lesson IC: What Is the Reflex Pathway That Causes Hiccups?

Regardless of the triggering event, the common pathway for hiccups is a reflex that is incompletely understood. This reflex consists of afferent input from the vagus nerve, phrenic nerve, and sympathetic fibers from T6 to T12. These afferents synapse in the cervical spinal cord at C3-C5 and in the brainstem (likely at the medulla). The efferent output of the reflex is from the phrenic nerve to the diaphragm and respiratory muscles (Fig. 20.1) [1, 2, 10–12]. Neurotransmitters involved in this process include gamma-aminobutyric acid (GABA) and dopamine [3, 13].

Lesson ID: What Are the Treatments for Hiccups Under Anesthesia?

Hiccups are generally self-limited, but treatment may be needed if vocal cord closure or patient movement is preventing a procedure from proceeding. Support for most treatments is largely empirical rather than evidence-based. Therapies are primarily aimed at blocking the reflex discussed above at the level of the gastrointestinal (GI) triggers, respiratory muscles, autonomic nervous system, or neurotransmitters.

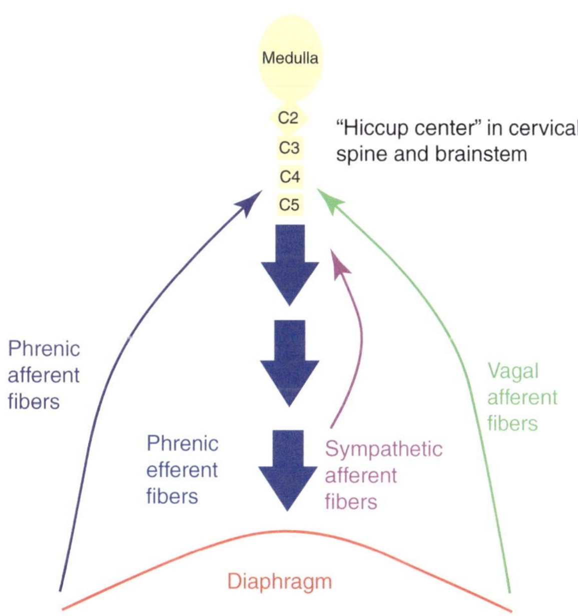

Fig. 20.1 A schematic of the contributions to the reflex arc of a hiccup

Many diverse pharmacological interventions can be used to treat hiccups. To attenuate GI triggers for hiccups such as gastric distention and GI reflux, prokinetic agents such as metoclopramide (Reglan) and proton pump inhibitors (omeprazole) can be used [2, 13]. Neuromuscular blockade is one way to attenuate respiratory muscle and vocal cord movement from hiccups in an anesthetized patient [10]. Baclofen may have an antispasmodic effect on respiratory muscles. Furthermore, baclofen and gabapentin are GABA agonists that may inhibit vagal impulses in the hiccup reflex [14, 15]. Dopaminergic antagonists such as chlorpromazine (Thorazine), the only FDA-approved treatment for hiccups, may also act on brainstem modulation of the hiccup reflex. The suggested dose of Thorazine for this purpose is 25–50 mg IV or IM. Other antidopaminergic agents such as prochlorperazine (Compazine) and droperidol (Inapsine) have been used to treat hiccups in the dosages used for postoperative nausea and vomiting [2]. Medications that inhibit and overcome afferent vagal impulses of the hiccup reflex include sympathomimetic agents such as ketamine and ephedrine and local anesthetics such as lidocaine that may anesthetize vagal afferents [10].

There are also nonpharmacological treatments for hiccups. Airway irritants such as smelling salts or nasopharyngeal stimulation may interrupt vagal afferents in the hiccup reflex [10, 16]. Increased arterial $PaCO_2$ has been shown to decrease the frequency of hiccups which may explain why breath holding may stop hiccups [1, 12]. Breath holding can be simulated under anesthesia with mild hypoventilation, sigh breaths, and continuous positive airway pressure (CPAP). These actions may also stop hiccups by breaking diaphragmatic spasm and restoring phrenic nervous rhythms [1, 2]. The efficacy of blocking vagal afferents may also explain the utility of acupuncture and phrenic nerve blockade for persistent hiccups [1, 10] (Table 20.1).

Table 20.1 Summary of treatment options for hiccups

Acute pharmacologic	*Acute nonpharmacologic*
Muscle relaxants	Nasopharyngeal stimulation
Prokinetic agents: metoclopramide (Reglan)	Mild hypoventilation
Proton pump inhibitors (omeprazole)	Sigh breaths
Antidopaminergic agents: chlorpromazine, prochlorperazine, droperidol	Continuous positive airway pressure (CPAP)
	Chronic therapy for refractory hiccups
	Acupuncture
Sympathomimetic agents: ketamine, ephedrine	Phrenic nerve block
IV or nebulized lidocaine	GABA agonists: baclofen, gabapentin
Smelling salts (ammonium chloride)	

Lesson II: Regurgitation

Lesson IIA: What Determines Whether Regurgitation Will Occur?

Regurgitation is the backward, passive expulsion of ingested material or secretions into the oropharynx from the stomach or esophagus [17]. Because regurgitation is a passive process, the movement of material relies primarily on pressure gradients. The three barriers to regurgitation are the following: (1) the lower esophageal sphincter (LES), (2) the upper esophageal sphincter (UES), and (3) the protective laryngeal reflexes [18].

Lesson IIB: Why Are Patients Prone to Regurgitation Under General Anesthesia?

The LES spans the diaphragm and separates the stomach from the esophagus. The tendency to regurgitate from the stomach to the esophagus depends primarily on the barrier pressure, the pressure gradient between the intragastric pressure (normally 5 mm Hg) and the LES pressure (normally 10–25 mm Hg) (Fig. 20.2) [10, 17]. A lower barrier pressure predisposes to regurgitation by creating a gradient favorable for movement of material from the stomach to the esophagus [10]. A typical anesthetic with opioids, muscle relaxants, and inhaled anesthetics decreases lower esophageal sphincter pressure and therefore decreases the barrier pressure [19]. Furthermore, cricoid pressure and laryngeal mask airways (LMAs) seem to reflexively decrease LES and barrier pressure. LMAs, but not cricoid pressure, also appear to increase reflux of materials from the stomach though this is not significant at the level of the upper esophagus unless the patient is placed in lithotomy position [20–22].

The tendency to regurgitate from the esophagus to the hypopharynx is related to the UES. The UES is a band of the cricopharyngeus muscle at the level of the cricoid cartilage that is continuous with the upper esophagus [18]. Most inhaled and intravenous anesthetic techniques, with the notable exception of ketamine, decrease the UES tone from approximately 40 mm Hg to less than 10 mm Hg [23, 24].

Airway reflexesare the final barrier to protect the lungs from aspiration of regurgitated substances. The four protective airway reflexes are (1) apnea with laryngospasm or closure of both the true and false vocal cords, (2) coughing during which a prolonged and forceful expiration follows a brief rapid flow inspiration, (3) sudden isolated expiration with opening of the false vocal cords, and (4) spasmodic panting or shallow breathing with rapid glottic opening and closing [18]. Patients

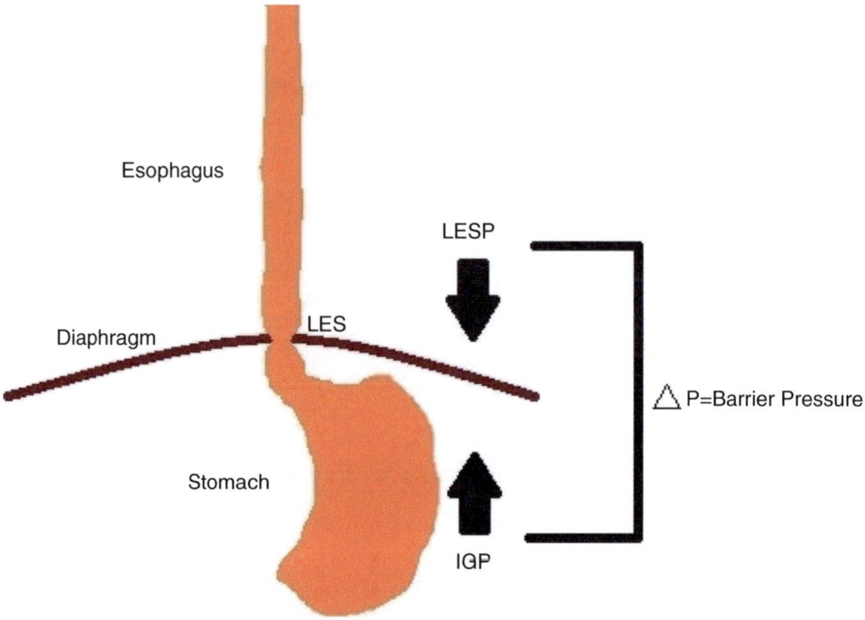

Fig. 20.2 An illustration of barrier pressure, the difference between the lower esophageal sphincter pressure and the intragastric pressure. LES lower esophageal sphincter, LESP lower esophageal sphincter pressure, IGP intragastric pressure

can have depressed airway reflexes preoperatively due to depressed levels of consciousness, advanced age, and premedication. Inhaled and intravenous general anesthetics also significantly diminish these reflexes both intraoperatively and postoperatively even after other measures of recovery are met [25–27].

Lesson III: Aspiration

Lesson IIIA: What Are Preoperative Risk Factors for Regurgitation and Aspiration?

The main risk factors for regurgitation are increased gastric volume, altered LES tone or anatomy, and loss of protective laryngeal reflexes. Increased gastric volume can arise from delayed gastric emptying which occurs during pregnancy (especially labor), autonomic dysfunction from diabetes mellitus, and conditions that cause peristaltic abnormalities of the gastrointestinal tract (i.e., obstruction, infection, or increased sympathetic tone). Clinical conditions with reduced LES tone include pregnancy and gastroesophageal reflux (GERD). The functionality of the LES may also be altered by anatomical displacement above the diaphragm in pregnancy, obesity, and the presence of a hiatal hernia [10]. Loss of protective laryngeal reflexes occurs from trauma, depressed consciousness, and premedication [18].

Lesson IIIB: How Can One Decrease the Possibility of Regurgitation and Subsequent Aspiration in Patients Who Are at Risk?

An anesthesiologist can decrease the possibility of regurgitation in a patient who is at risk by attempting to reduce the patient's gastric volume and maintain LES tone. The severity of pulmonary damage caused by aspirated gastric contents can also be reduced by increasing the pH of gastric contents (making them less acidic). The ways to accomplish these goals include nil per os (NPO) guidelines, mechanically decompressing the stomach, and specific pharmacologic agents [10, 18, 28].

The two nonpharmacological ways to decrease gastric volume are NPO guidelines and tube decompression of the stomach. NPO guidelines give recommendations regarding the duration of patient fasting for various liquids and solids prior to surgery (Table 20.2) [28]. If NPO guidelines must be by passed and the patient has clear evidence of severely overfilled gastrum (i.e., bowel obstruction, recent oral contrast ingestion), it is advisable to place an 18 French nasogastric (NG) tube and thoroughly suction gastric contents through the tube prior to induction of anesthesia to reduce the risk of aspiration (see Table 20.3). Placement of an NG tube may be complicated by patient discomfort and bleeding from the nasal mucosa. Patient discomfort can be overcome with 4% lidocaine spray to the oropharynx, lidocaine-soaked pledgets into the nare, and serial dilation of the nasal passageway with nasopharyngeal airways of increasing size coated in 5% lidocaine ointment. Bleeding can be avoided by spraying oxymetazoline (Afrin) into the nare. The NG tube should be removed prior to induction of anesthesia to prevent difficulty with preoxygenation and mask ventilation due to the NG tube breaking the seal between the mask and the patient's face. Furthermore, material can travel backward along the sides of the NG tube from the stomach to the oropharynx once the patient is under general anesthesia ("wick effect"). Finally, the NG tube may decrease the efficacy of cricoid pressure. After removal of the NG tube prior to the induction of general anesthesia (for all of the above reasons), a rapid sequence induction (RSI) should still be performed in this setting [29].

Pharmacologic aspiration prophylaxis is not routinely recommended unless a patient has one or more of the regurgitation and aspiration risk factors described

Table 20.2 Summary of NPO guidelines from the American Society of Anesthesiologists [28]

Ingested material	Interval of fasting prior to elective procedure	Additional comments
Clear liquids	2 h	Excludes alcohol
Human breast milk	4 h	
Nonhuman infant formula	6 h	Low-fat or low-protein foods
Light meal		
Heavy meal	8 h	Fatty or fried foods

Table 20.3 Placement of nasogastric tube in an awake patient prior to the induction of general anesthesia in a patient at high risk for aspiration due to full stomach

<table>
<tr><th>Positive consideration</th><th colspan="2">Negative considerations</th></tr>
<tr><td rowspan="10">Greatly reduce the risk of aspiration of high volume of gastric contents during the induction of general anesthesia</td><td>Specific negative consideration</td><td>Solution to negative consideration</td></tr>
<tr><td rowspan="3">Noxious stimulus</td><td>1. Spray nare with lidocaine</td></tr>
<tr><td>2. Place series of soft nasopharyngeal airways lubricated with lidocaine ointment</td></tr>
<tr><td>3. Spray posterior oropharynx with lidocaine</td></tr>
<tr><td>May cause nose bleed</td><td>Spray oxymetazoline (Afrin) into nare</td></tr>
<tr><td>May decrease effective preoxygenation by mask</td><td rowspan="4">After thoroughly suctioning gastric contents through NGT, remove the NGT prior to the induction of general anesthesia</td></tr>
<tr><td>May decrease effective ventilation by mask if needed</td></tr>
<tr><td>May decrease effectiveness of cricoid pressure</td></tr>
<tr><td>“Wick effect”</td></tr>
<tr><td>Still need to perform RSI</td><td>Risk of aspiration prior to securing airway has been reduced</td></tr>
</table>

above [28]. Pharmacologic options include prokinetic agents (metoclopramide or Reglan), histamine antagonists (H2Bs, ranitidine or Pepcid), proton pump inhibitors (PPIs, omeprazole or Prilosec), and nonparticulate antacids (sodium citrate or Bicitra). Metoclopramide (Reglan) reduces gastric volume via a prokinetic effect mediated by muscarinic agonism, dopaminergic antagonism, and serotonergic antagonism. H2Bs and PPIs decrease gastric volume and increase gastric pH at the level of the parietal cells in the stomach, via histamine receptors and H+/K+ ATPases, respectively. H2Bs work within a few hours of administration, while PPIs should be given in two successive doses starting the night before surgery. Nonparticulate antacids such as sodium citrate (Bicitra) neutralize stomach acid immediately but may slightly increase gastric volume. Antacids and Reglan have also been shown to increase LES tone [18]. There is limited evidence that combining multiple agents increases their efficacy [18, 28]. A summary of aspiration risk reduction can be seen in Fig. 20.3.

The interventions in Fig. 20.3 are listed in the American Society for Anesthesiologists (ASA) “Practice Guidelines for Preoperative Fasting and the Use of Pharmacologic Agents to Reduce the Risk of Pulmonary Aspiration.” It is important to note that these guidelines are based largely on expert opinion rather than randomized controlled trials. Furthermore, while the available scientific evidence

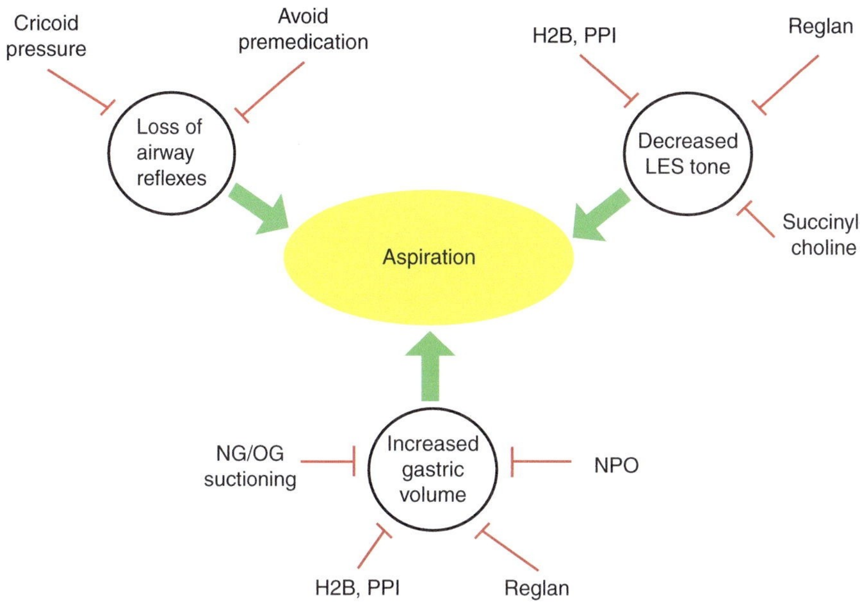

Fig. 20.3 Risk factors for regurgitation and aspiration are indicated by green arrows, and prophylactic measures for each risk factor are indicated with red flathead arrows. H2B H2 blocker, PPI proton pump inhibitor, NPO nil per os, NG/OG nasogastric/orogastric

shows decreased gastric volumes and increased gastric pH when NPO guidelines and appropriate pharmacologic prophylaxis are used, there is inadequate evidence to address the relationship between these measures and the risk of perioperative aspiration into the lungs [28].

Lesson IIIC: What Is an Appropriate Action Plan to Manage a Witnessed Aspiration Event?

The immediate treatment of witnessed or suspected aspiration in an anesthe tized patient includes turning the patient's head to the right side, suctioning the oropharynx, and tracheal intubation with a cuffed endotracheal tube. As soon as tube placement is confirmed with end- tidal carbon dioxide (EtCO2), the trachea should be suctioned through the endotracheal tube with a 14 French soft suction catheter. It is highly desirable to examine the tracheobronchial tree with a fiber-optic bronchoscope following a known or suspected aspiration and perform localized, small volume saline lavage and suctioning of the inhaled gastric contents under the control of an appropriately sized fiber-optic bronchoscope. Blind saline lavage of the airway is never recommended. Alkali lavage of the tracheobronchial tree is also not recommended because the toxic effect of gastric aspirate on the airways is immediate [30].

Disposition of a patient who aspirates gastric contents before or during anesthesia depends on the patient's level of clinical stability. A patient with compromised oxygenation or cardiovascular instability after aspiration should remain intubated and be admitted to the intensive care unit (ICU) for observation, pulmonary toilet, and repeated fiber-optic examinations. Occasionally, aspiration can lead to pneumonia, acute respiration distress syndrome (ARDS), multi-organ failure, sepsis, and death [31]. A stable patient can be extubated after anesthesia provided the patient is observed for 4–6 h after extubation for the development of cough, wheezing, and hypoxemia. Outpatient follow-up may be appropriate if none of these symptoms develop and the patient is given explicit instructions to return to a medical facility if symptoms of pneumonia arise. Inpatient monitoring may be needed after extubation if the likelihood of severe aspiration is high or the patient has significant comorbidities such as preexisting lung disease. Treatment of aspiration with corticosteroids is not helpful and may increase the risk of bacterial infection. Prophylactic treatment with antibiotics is not indicated because not all aspiration results in pneumonia and unnecessary antibiotics may facilitate the colonization of resistant organisms [30].

Lesson IV: Aspiration Pneumonia

Lesson IVA: How Do You Diagnose and Treat Aspiration Pneumonia?

Bacterial pneumonia can develop after aspiration due to the transference of nasopharyngeal, oropharyngeal, and gastrointestinal bacteria into the airways. Aspiration pneumonia usually has a rather indolent course because the causative agents are oral anaerobes and streptococci which are less virulent than the bacteria that cause other types of pneumonia. The onset of symptoms of pneumonia such as fever and productive cough after aspiration is typically days to weeks. The presence of purulent or malodorous sputum is regarded as diagnostic of anaerobic infection [32]. The treatment for aspiration pneumonia is a 7–10 day course of antibiotics. Regimens include clindamycin, amoxicillin-clavulanate, or a penicillin plus metronidazole (Flagyl) for 7–10 days [33–35]. While this clinical course is common in mild to moderate aspiration in a healthy patient, occasionally, aspiration pneumonia can be severe and lead to ARDS, sepsis, and death as mentioned above.

The differential diagnosis for postoperative aspiration pneumonia includes chemical pneumonitis and atelectasis. Chemical pneumonitis occurs when bile and stomach acid cause an acute (within 2 h) inflammatory process in lungs that leads to hypoxemia and respiratory distress. Clinical recovery from pneumonitis occurs in 24–36 h of aspiration [31, 36]. Atelectasis, or collapse of the lung parenchyma, occurs during almost all inhaled and intravenous anesthetics due to compression of lung tissue by altered chest wall and diaphragm mechanics, slower rate of gas entry into the alveolus than absorption of gas into the blood, and altered surfactant function. While atelectasis from surgery improves within 24 h, it can be a significant cause of hypoxemia and even mild fever [37]. The treatment for both pneumonitis and atelectasis is supportive care of pulmonary function (deep breathing, coughing, noninvasive positive pressure ventilation) unless there is progression of symptoms or development of superimposed pneumonia.

While all of the above diagnoses cause hypoxemia and respiratory distress, aspiration pneumonia can be differentiated from pneumonitis and atelectasis by its clinical progression with high fevers, elevated white blood cell count, and purulent sputum. However, these symptoms may take days to develop after aspiration. A chest radiograph may be diagnostically useful to differentiate early pneumonia from atelectasis due to differences in their pathophysiology (Fig. 20.4). Generally, chest radiograph from aspiration shows bilateral air space opacification without volume loss. Opacification from atelectasis is often accompanied by signs of volume loss including diaphragm elevation and displacement of ribs, fissures, or mediastinal structures toward the area of collapse [38].

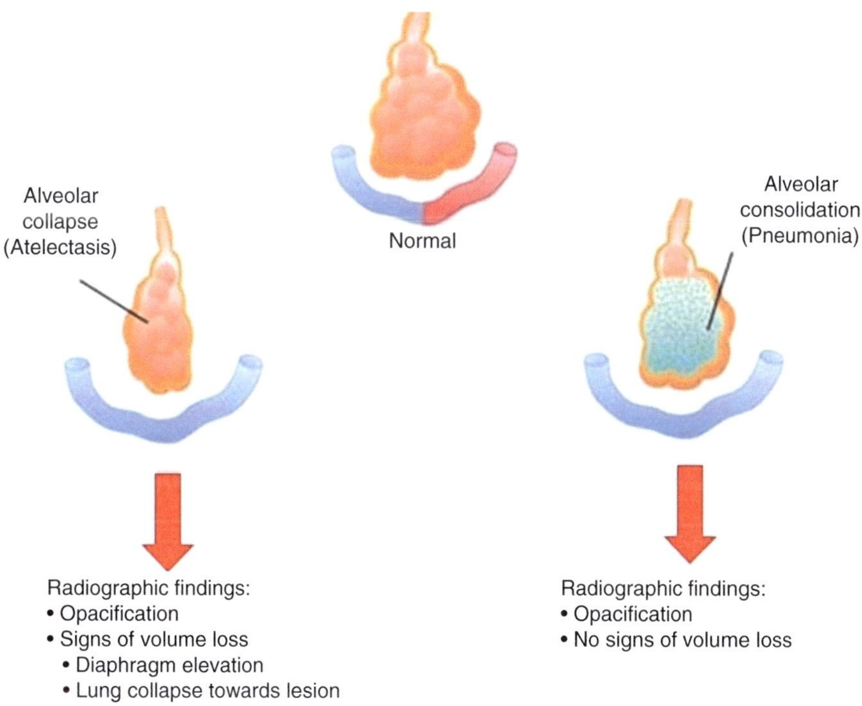

Fig. 20.4 Illustration of how atelectasis and pneumonia differ at the level of the alveoli which creates the differences apparent on chest radiography

Summary of Key Teaching Points

- A hiccup is an episodic spasm of the diaphragm followed by vocal cord closure that is caused by activation of a reflex involving phrenic and vagal afferents, integration in the spinal cord and brainstem, and phrenic efferents.
- Hiccups can be caused by a number of anesthetic and surgical factors, and the treatment of hiccups under anesthesia includes dopamine antagonists, muscle paralysis, prokinetic agents, breath holding, and maneuvers to inhibit vagal impulses.
- Regurgitation under anesthesia occurs when the development of a favorable pressure gradient allows gastric contents to move backward by overcoming the lower esophageal sphincter, the upper esophageal sphincter, and the protective airway reflexes.
- Risk factors for regurgitation and aspiration include increased gastric volume, decreased LES tone, and loss of protective airway reflexes. NPO guidelines, awake NG tube gastric emptying, and appropriate pharmacologic prophylaxis are measures for risk reduction.
- Witnessed or suspected aspiration under anesthesia should be treated with right lateral head positioning, oral suctioning, and endotracheal intubation. Tracheal lavage, corticosteroids, and prophylactic antibiotics are not indicated.
- The differential diagnosis for hypoxemia and respiratory distress after aspiration is chemical pneumonitis, atelectasis, and aspiration pneumonia. These can be distinguished by clinical course and radiological findings.
- On chest radiography, aspiration pneumonia will show infiltrates but no volume loss, while atelectasis will show infiltrates with evidence of volume loss.

References

1. Chang FY, Lu CL. Hiccup: mystery, nature and treatment. J Neurogastroenterol Motil. 2012;18:123–30.
2. Howes D. Hiccups: a new explanation for the mysterious reflex. BioEssays. 2012;34:451–3.
3. Becker DE. Nausea, vomiting, and hiccups: a review of mechanisms and treatment. Anesth Prog. 2010;57:150–6.
4. Landers C, Turner D, Makin C, Zaglul H, Brown R. Propofol associated hiccups and treatment with lidocaine. Anesth Analg. 2008;107:1757–8.
5. Bagdure DN, Reiter PD, Bhoite GR, Dobyns EL, Laoprasert P. Persistent hiccups associated with epidural ropivacaine in a newborn. Ann Pharmacother. 2011;45:e35.
6. Mcallister RK, Mcdavid AJ, Meyer TA, Bittenbinder TM. Recurrent persistent hiccups after epidural steroid injection and analgesia with bupivacaine. Anesth Analg. 2005;100:1834–6.
7. Doshi H, Vaidyalingam R, Buchan K. Atrial pacing wires: an uncommon cause of postoperative hiccups. Br J Hosp Med. 2008;69:534.

8. Sacher F, Monahan KH, Thoas SP, et al. Phrenic nerve injury after atrial fibrillation catheter ablation: characterization and outcome in a multicenter study. J Am Coll Cardiol. 2006;47:2498–503.
9. Sav T. Hiccups, a rare complication arising from use of a central venous catheter. Hemodial Int. 2010;14:337–8.
10. Kirby RR. Clinical anesthesia practice. 2nd ed. Philadelphia: Saunders; 2002. p. 86.
11. Kim M. Has science solved the mystery of the hiccup? Don't hold your breath. https://www.theguardian.com/science/2014/jun/06/scientific-research-hiccups-cure-cause. The Washington Post, 6 June 2014. Web. 8 Sept 2015.
12. Davis JN. An experimental study of hiccup. Brain. 1970;93:851–72.
13. Steger M, Schneemann M, Fox M. Systemic review: the pathogenesis and pharmacological treatment of hiccups. Aliment Pharmacol Ther. 2015;42:1037–50.
14. Ramirez FC, Graham DY. Treatment of intractable hiccup with baclofen: results of a double-blind randomized, controlled, cross-over study. Am J Gastroenterol. 1992;87:1789–91.
15. Thompson DF, Brooks KG. Gabapentin therapy of hiccups. Ann Pharmacother. 2013;47:897–903.
16. Salem MR. Treatment of hiccups by pharyngeal stimulation in anesthetized and conscious subjects. JAMA J Am Med Assoc. 1967;202:126–30.
17. Chaudry MA, Thrumurthy SG, Mughal M. Gastric and oesophageal surgery. Oxford: Oxford University Press; 2014.
18. Ng A, Smith G. Gastroesophageal reflux and aspiration of gastric contents in anesthetic practice. Anesth Analg. 2001;93:494–513.
19. Cotton BR, Smith G. The lower oesophageal sphincter and anesthesia. Br J Anaesth. 1984;56:37–57.
20. Tournadre JP, Chassard D, Berrada KR, Bouletreau P. Cricoid cartilage pressure decreases lower esophageal sphincter tone. Anesthesiology. 1997;86:7–9.
21. Rabey PG, Murphy PJ, Lancgton JA, et al. Effect of the laryngeal mask airway on lower oesophageal sphincter pressure in patients during general anaesthesia. Br J Anaesth. 1992;69:346–8.
22. McCrory CR, McShane AJ. Gastroesophageal reflux during spontaneous respiration with the laryngeal mask airway. Can J Anaesth. 1999;46:268–70.
23. Vanner RG, Pryle BJ, O'Dwyer JP, Reynolds F. Upper oesophageal sphincter pressure and the intravenous induction of anesthesia. Anesthesia. 1992;47:371–5.
24. Vanner RG, Pryle BJ, O'Dwyer JP, Reynolds F. Upper oesophageal sphincter pressure during inhalational anesthesia. Anesthesia. 1992;47:950–4.
25. Murphy JP, Langton JA, Simth G. Effect of oral diazepam on the sensitivity of upper airway reflexes. Br J Anaesth. 1993;70:131.
26. Erskne RJ, Murphy PJ, Langton JA, Smith G. Effect of age on the sensitivity of upper airway reflexes. Br J Anaesth. 1993;70:574–5.
27. Caranza R, Nandwani N, Tring JP, et al. Upper airway reflex sensitivity following general anesthesia for day case surgery. Anaesthesia. 2000;55:367–70.
28. Practice guidelines for preoperative fasting and the use of pharmacologic agents to reduce the risk of pulmonary aspiration, application to healthy patients undergoing elective procedures: an updated report by the American Society of Anesthesiologists Committee on Standards and Practice Parameters. Anesthesiology. 2011;114:495–511.
29. Sinclair RC, Luxton MC. Rapid sequence induction. Contin Educ Anaesth Crit Care Pain. 2005;5:45–8.
30. Barash P, Cullen B, Stoelting R. Postoperative pulmonary dysfunction. In: Clinical anesthesia. Philadelphia: Lippincott Williams & Wilkins; 2006. p. 1569.
31. Menelson CL. The aspiration of stomach contents into the lungs during obstetric anesthesia. Am J Obstet Gynecol. 1946;52:191.
32. Bartlett J. Aspiration pneumonia in adults. www.uptodate.com. 06 July 2015. Web. 01 Oct 2015.

33. Kadowaki M, Demura Y, Mizuno S, et al. Reappraisal of clindamycin IV monotherapy for treatment of mild-to-moderate aspiration pneumonia in elderly patients. Chest. 2005;127:1276.
34. Eykyn SJ. The therapeutic use of metronidazole in anaerobic infection: six years' experience in a London hospital. Surgery. 1983;93:209.
35. Germaud P, Poirier J, Jacqueme P, et al. Monotherapy using amoxicillin/clavulanic acid as treatment of first choice in community-acquired lung abscess. Apropos of 57 cases. Rev Pneumol Clin. 1993;49:137.
36. Bynum LJ, Pierce AK. Pulmonary aspiration of gastric contents. Am Rev Respir Dis. 1976;114:1129.
37. Magnusson L. New concepts of atelectasis during general anaesthesia. Br J Anaesth. 2003;91:61–72.
38. Collins J, Stern EJ. Chest radiology, the essentials. Philadelphia: Lippincott Williams & Wilkins; 2007.

Chapter 21
Myasthenia Gravis

Daniel J. Sisti

Case Narrative

A 74-year-old man, weighing 54 kg, height 159 cm, BMI 21, was admitted to the hospital for dysphagia and weight loss. His past medical history was significant for coronary artery disease (with coronary artery bypass graft surgery done 7 years previously), hypertension, and nephrolithiasis. He had been in his usual state of health until 3 weeks prior to admission, when he began having progressive difficulty with swallowing. He presented to the hospital after having choking episodes while eating that day.

Workup by his primary team led to a diagnosis of myasthenia gravis suggested by electromyography and confirmed by seropositivity of acetylcholine receptor antibodies on laboratory testing (**L-1,2,3**). During this admission, he was started on pyridostigmine, prednisone, and mycophenolate mofetil. He was also given a course of intravenous immunoglobulin (IVIG) (**L-4**). He improved and was asymptomatic at discharge, though video laryngoscopy still demonstrated moderate oropharyngeal dysphagia.

Approximately 6 weeks after discharge, the patient presented to the emergency department with sudden onset of severe abdominal pain radiating to his back. The emergency medicine department evaluated him, and a plain film abdominal x-ray revealed free air under the diaphragm (Fig. 21.1). General surgery was consulted, and the decision was made to bring him to the operating room for an emergent exploratory laparotomy.

Preoperative examination by the anesthesiologist (**L-5**) showed a heart rate of 84 beats per minute, blood pressure 147/84 mmHg, respiratory rate 16 breaths per minute, and oxygen saturation 97% on room air. Examination demonstrated a favorable Mallampati class I airway, ability to prognath, normal extension of the neck, and thyromental distance of 5 cm. Lungs were clear and cardiovascular exam was

D. J. Sisti (✉)
Department of Anesthesiology, University of California, San Diego, CA, USA

J. L. Benumof, G. R. Manecke (eds.), *Clinical Anesthesiology II*,
https://doi.org/10.1007/978-3-030-12365-9_21

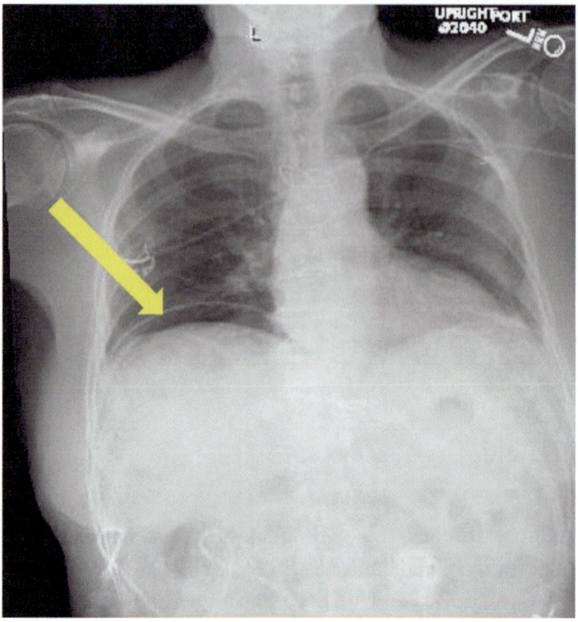

Fig. 21.1 The patient's chest x-ray demonstrating subdiaphragmatic free air (yellow arrow)

normal. Laboratory values (Table 21.1) were significant for creatinine of 1.92 mg/dl, which was near his baseline at the time.

The patient was brought into the operating room, preoxygenated, and standard ASA monitors were placed. Induction was accomplished with etomidate, fentanyl, and 20 mg of rocuronium (**L-6**). Intubation was successful, and the operation proceeded smoothly. The surgical team discovered a perforated prepyloric ulcer which was oversewn. At the conclusion of the operation, train-of-four monitoring again showed four twitches. Neuromuscular blockade reversal was administered, consisting of 2.5 mg of neostigmine and 0.5 mg of glycopyrrolate. Four twitches were again seen, and the patient had sustained tetany for 5 s without fade. While still intubated, the patient had tidal volumes of approximately 400 cc with a respiratory rate of 12 (**L-7**). He was subsequently extubated and brought to PACU for recovery. His PACU course was uneventful. He had stable vital signs, adequate analgesia, no residual weakness, and was transferred to a monitored bed (**L-8**).

Lesson 1: Pathophysiology of Myasthenia Gravis

Myasthenia gravis is an autoimmune disorder that affects the neuromuscular junction [1] (NMJ; see Fig. 21.2). In the normal state of the NMJ, a nerve impulse results in acetylcholine released from the nerve terminal. Binding of acetylcholine to nicotinic acetylcholine receptors (NAChRs) on the motor end plate causes influx of sodium into the muscle cell, triggering a cascade of molecular events that transiently increase intracellular calcium, leading to muscle contraction. Acetylcholinesterase within the cleft of the NMJ quickly degrades the acetylcholine, allowing muscle relaxation [2].

Table 21.1 Laboratory data

Variable	On admission	Reference range
Sodium (mmol/l)	134	136–145
Potassium (mmol/l)	4.8	3.5–5.1
Chloride (mmol/l)	102	98–107
Carbon dioxide (mmol/l)	18	22–29
Urea nitrogen (mg/dl)	47	6–20
Creatinine (mg/dl)	1.92	0.67–1.17
Glucose (mg/dl)	177	70–115
Calcium (mg/dl)	8.8	8.5–10.6
Aspartate aminotransferase (U/l)	32	0–40
Alanine aminotransferase (U/l)	30	0–41
Alkaline phosphatase (U/l)	89	40–129
Total bilirubin (mg/dl)	0.3	<1.20
White-cell count (per mm^3)	11,900	4000–10,000
Differential count (%)		
Neutrophils	89	34–71
Lymphocytes	9	19–53
Monocytes	1	5–12
Eosinophils	2	2
Basophils	1	0–2
Hemoglobin (g/dl)	12.1	13.7–17.5
Hematocrit (%)	36.0	40–50
Platelet count (per mm^3)	133	140,000–370,000
International normalized ratio	1.1	
Partial thromboplastin time (s)	30.8	25.0–34.0

The most common form of myasthenia gravis involves autoantibodies directed against acetylcholine receptors, leading to their destruction by the patient's immune system (Fig. 21.3). Acetylcholine is released and is quickly cleaved by acetylcholine esterase normally, but there is less muscle contraction because of the decreased acetylcholine receptor density. Clinically this presents as weakness. Most commonly weakness appears first with ocular symptoms such as ptosis and diplopia. This can progress to generalized weakness and/or bulbar weakness with difficulty swallowing or weight loss. The hallmark of myasthenia gravis is fatigability, with weakness getting worse with more activity [3].

Lesson 2: Diagnosis of Myasthenia Gravis

The first step in diagnosis of myasthenia gravis requires a sufficient degree of clinical suspicion. There is a small battery of tests that can be used to make the diagnosis. The first is repetitive nerve stimulation, which involves electrically stimulating muscles and recording compound muscle action potentials (CMAPs) that are generated in response to the stimulus [4]. To ensure that the entire muscle group is

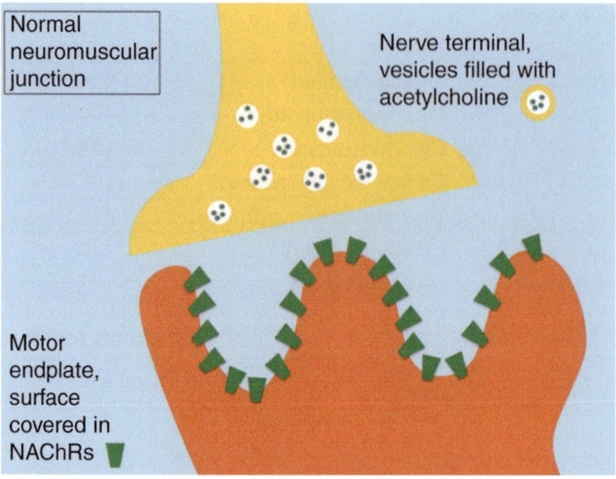

Fig. 21.2 Normal neuromuscular junction. Acetylcholine is released into the NMJ cleft via exocytosis. These molecules bind to their respective receptors, causing muscular contraction. NAChR nicotinic acetylcholine receptor

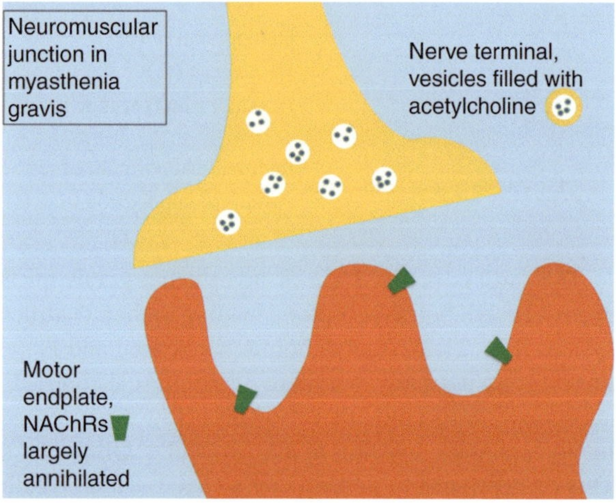

Fig. 21.3 Neuromuscular junction in myasthenia gravis. The motor end plate is nearly denuded of NAChRs. When acetylcholine is released from the nerve terminal, it is quickly cleaved by acetylcholinesterase, and muscular contraction is ineffectual. NAChR nicotinic acetylcholine receptor

recruited, the nerve is supramaximally stimulated in a train of 6–10 stimuli, with a rate of 2–3 Hz. Note that different amounts of stimulating current are needed depending on what muscle is being tested. In the normal state, the CMAP amplitude will be the same throughout the test. In myasthenia gravis, the recorded CMAPs will demonstrate a decremental response to the train of stimuli (Fig. 21.4).

A second test is the edrophonium test. A patient with clinical signs of weakness (e.g., unilateral ptosis) is given an intravenous bolus of edrophonium, a short-acting acetylcholinesterase inhibitor. Edrophonium increases the availability of acetylcholine in the NMJ, thereby allowing activation of NAChRs leading to effective muscular contraction. Thus, a positive edrophonium test will result in temporary resolution of the weakness.

Another test that is sometimes used is single-fiber electromyography (SFEMG). When a motor neuron triggers a muscle contraction, there is a normal, predictable delay from the release of acetylcholine into the NMJ to the compound muscle action potential that is generated in response to that molecular signal. In SFEMG, a specialized recording needle is inserted between two individual muscle fibers, and the patient is asked to hold a steady contraction, while the SFEMG machine records 100 consecutive CMAPs. Displayed graphically and superimposed on one another, there is minimal variation, or "jitter," between the action potentials in normal physiology [4–6] (Fig. 21.5).

With the loss of NAChRs in myasthenia gravis, the time to recruit muscle fiber after release of acetylcholine into the NMJ becomes unreliable. Many nerve impulses fail to trigger muscle contraction, and the time to contract one muscle fiber after another becomes markedly variable. The resulting SFEMG graph will show a spread of action potentials (increased jitter, Fig. 21.6).

SFEMG is a very sensitive test for myasthenia gravis, but it is not specific. You can see a similar jitter in other neuromuscular disorders such as amyotrophic lateral sclerosis, polymyositis, or Lambert-Eaton syndrome [2].

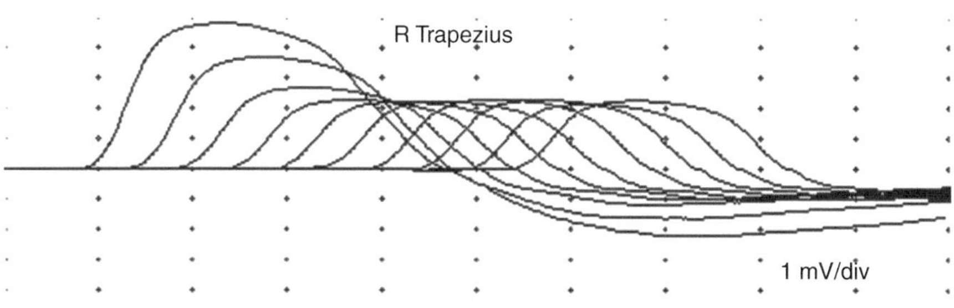

Fig. 21.4 Repetitive nerve stimulation test in myasthenia gravis. There is a quick decline in compound muscle action potential in response to nerve stimulation. (Copyright © 2010, VC Juel)

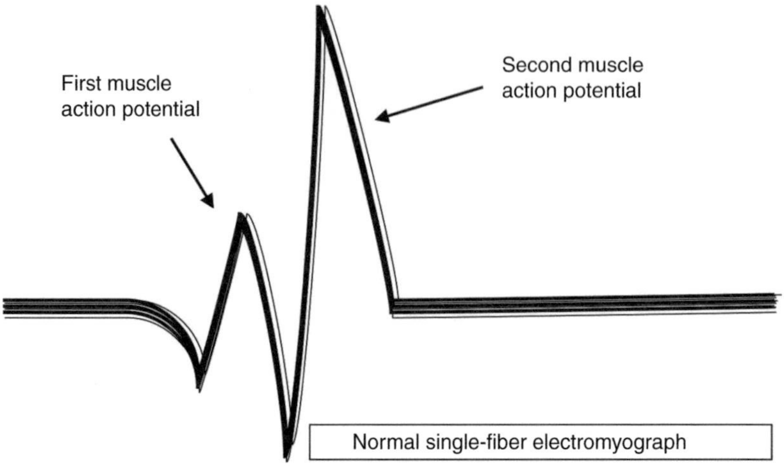

Fig. 21.5 Normal single-fiber electromyography. Recording of multiple stimuli shows consistent latencies in the tested muscle fiber. (Courtesy of Daniel J. Sisti, MD)

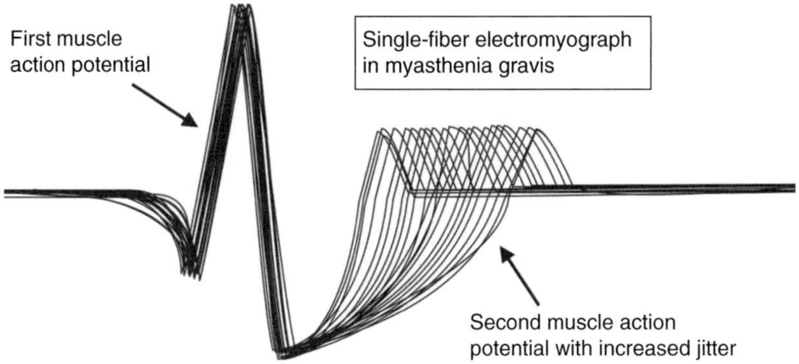

Fig. 21.6 Single-fiber electromyography in myasthenia gravis. Increased jitter characteristic of myasthenia gravis. (Courtesy of Daniel J. Sisti, MD)

A test that is very specific for myasthenia gravis is the detection of autoimmune antibodies (Table 21.2). Myasthenia gravis is a prototypical autoimmune disease, where the patient's immune system attacks self-antigens. Most commonly, myasthenia gravis patients have antibodies directed against the NAChR. A recently recognized form of myasthenia gravis has antibodies directed against muscle-specific tyrosine kinases, which are involved in the normal organization of acetylcholine receptors in the NMJ [7]. A smaller subset of patients present with clinical myasthenia gravis but without recognized autoantibodies.

Table 21.2 Forms of myasthenia gravis

Antibody type	Incidence
Nicotinic acetylcholine receptor	80%
Muscle-specific tyrosine kinase	15%
Unknown ("seronegative")	5%

Table 21.3 Osserman classification of myasthenia gravis

Class	Clinical presentation
I	Ocular symptoms
IIa	Generalized weakness
IIb	Generalized moderate weakness and/or bulbar symptoms
III	Fulminating presentation with respiratory distress/failure
IV	Late, severe symptoms

Lesson 3: Classification of Myasthenia Gravis

Clinicians may use one of many extant variations of the Osserman classification (Table 21.3) to designate the severity of myasthenia gravis. These classes range from type I with ocular symptoms alone to type IV, with severe disease and profound weakness [1]. This classification scheme does not carry any connotation of the prognosis of a patient's disease. Criticisms of the classification have argued that the scheme overly relies on subjective clinical impressions and lacks quantification [3].

Lesson 4: Treatment of Myasthenia Gravis

First-line treatment for myasthenia (Table 21.4) is the use of long-acting acetylcholinesterase inhibitors, typically pyridostigmine. Acetylcholinesterase inhibitors treat symptoms by increasing the amount of acetylcholine in the NMJ, thereby activating the remaining receptors. Side effects are primarily cholinergic, such as bradycardia, nausea, and diarrhea.

Steroids are used to treat the underlying pathophysiology by suppressing the immune system. Side effects of long-term steroid use include myopathy, glucose intolerance, osteoporosis, and many others. Other immune modulators such as azathioprine or cyclosporine are commonly used, as well.

Exacerbations of myasthenic symptoms can be treated with intravenous immunoglobulin infusions. This is thought to interfere with antibody-mediated destruction of acetylcholine receptors. In case a patient has a history of allergy or intolerance to IVIG, plasmapheresis is an alternative [3].

Table 21.4 Treatment of myasthenia gravis

Therapy	Mechanism of action	Complications
Acetylcholinesterase inhibitors	Increase acetylcholine in NMJ	Cholinergic effects: bradycardia, increased gut motility, secretions
Steroids	Immune suppression, slows disease progression	Myopathy, glucose intolerance, osteoporosis, infection, etc.
Immune modulators (e.g., azathioprine, cyclosporine, mycophenolate)	Immune suppression, slows disease progression	Variable depending on agent
Intravenous immunoglobulin	Short-term immune modulation	Headaches, allergy, thromboembolism
Plasmapheresis	Autoantibody clearance	Vascular access placement complications (e.g., pneumothorax, hematoma), infection, thrombosis, central vein stenosis
Thymectomy: videoscopic, transcervical, or transsternal	Removal of antigenic stimulus	Postoperative ventilation, incomplete resection

Thymectomy has been recognized for decades as a means to achieve long-term remission in a significant subset of patients. Good candidates for this are typically younger patients or patients with thymomas. While it is not fully understood why thymectomy leads to remission of myasthenia gravis, it likely involves removal of an antigenic stimulus that triggers the production of autoantibodies. When patients undergo thymectomy, a significant consideration is they will typically not have immediate disease remission and may have postoperative myasthenic exacerbations and require postoperative mechanical ventilation.

Lesson 5: Preoperative Management of Myasthenia Gravis

There are a number of important considerations prior to beginning any anesthetic in a patient with myasthenia gravis (Fig. 21.7). First, is the disease optimized? If the patient has significant symptoms and the case is elective, the patient may benefit from a course of preoperative IVIG and appropriate adjustment of medication. Close follow-up with their primary neurologist should be routine before surgery.

A careful review of medical history is critical as approximately 12% of myasthenic patients have coexisting autoimmune disease [3]. These may include autoimmune thyroiditis, rheumatoid arthritis, and others that may substantially affect your anesthetic plan (Table 21.5).

Some practitioners would consider pulmonary function testing, which may serve as a baseline for ICU management in case postoperative mechanical ventilation should be required. Optimally, the anesthesiologist should have a frank discussion

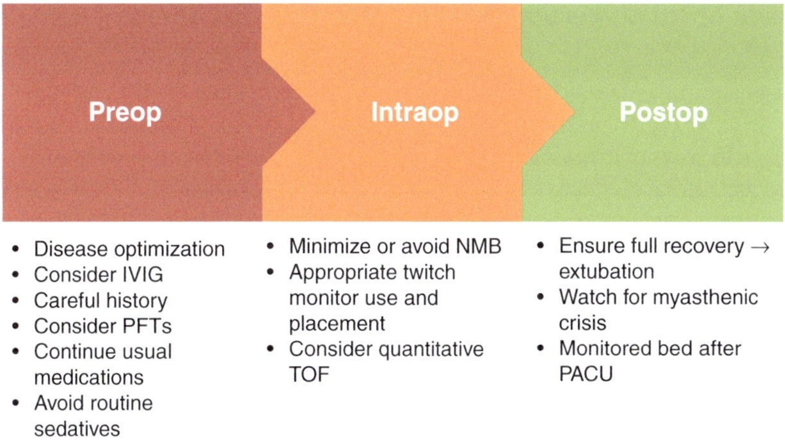

Fig. 21.7 Summary of anesthetic management of myasthenia gravis. IVIG intravenous immunoglobulin, PFT pulmonary function test

Table 21.5 Autoimmune diseases coexisting with myasthenia gravis

Disease	Sequelae with anesthetic implications
Rheumatoid arthritis	Atlantoaxial instability, TMJ dysfunction, pericarditis, coronary arteritis, aortic insufficiency, pulmonary fibrosis, pleural effusions
Systemic lupus erythematosus	Renal dysfunction, esophageal dysmotility, cardiac conduction abnormalities, coronary arteritis, pulmonary hypertension, antiphospholipid antibodies
Scleroderma	Myofibrosis, heart failure, pulmonary hypertension, renal dysfunction, esophageal dysmotility, limited mouth opening, limited neck mobility
Inflammatory myopathies	Sensitivity to non-depolarizing muscle blockade, hyperkalemia from succinylcholine, cardiac dysfunction
Grave's disease	Dysrhythmias, heart failure, hypertension, thyroid storm
Autoimmune thyroiditis	Bradycardia, decreased cardiac contractility, hypotension, hypothermia
Addison's disease	Refractory hypotension, hyperkalemia

TMJ temporomandibular joint

with the patient about what to expect at the end of surgery, so that the patient is mentally prepared to remain intubated, while strength and responsiveness is assessed in the operating room.

In terms of medication regimen, most authors recommend continuing their usual regimen without any changes the day of surgery. Routine acetylcholinesterase taken by the patient should not affect the dose of reversal given for any intraoperative neuromuscular blockade. Finally, it is probably wisest to avoid any sedatives preoperatively in case the patient has subtle, subclinical oropharyngeal or respiratory compromise.

Lesson 6: Intraoperative Management of Myasthenia Gravis

Myasthenic patients are relatively resistant to succinylcholine [8] and extremely sensitive to nondepolarizing neuromuscular blockers [9–11]. Careful thought should be given to ways of avoiding neuromuscular blockade. Neuraxial and regional anesthesia are safe and effective alternatives to general anesthesia [1, 12]. If general is required, neuromuscular blockade may be possible to avoid altogether. Good intubating conditions can be obtained with an inhalational induction or high-potency opioids. Volatile anesthetics have inherent muscle-relaxing properties, while boluses of alfentanil or remifentanil are induction agents that provide moderately good intubating conditions when avoidance of neuromuscular blockade is needed [13–17].

Despite these alternatives, neuromuscular blockade may be necessary to improve surgical conditions. The need for effective monitoring of blockade depth and recovery cannot be overemphasized.

Typical sites of monitoring neuromuscular blockade depth are the facial and ulnar nerves. The former is convenient, and loss of facial twitching is a reliable indicator of adequate intubating conditions for induction. The adductor pollicis muscle regains function after the diaphragm, so the ulnar nerve is a good site to monitor for emergence. A commonly unrecognized factor in train-of-four monitoring is the correct polarity of the lead placement (Fig. 21.8). Correct placement ensures maximum response to the applied stimulus.

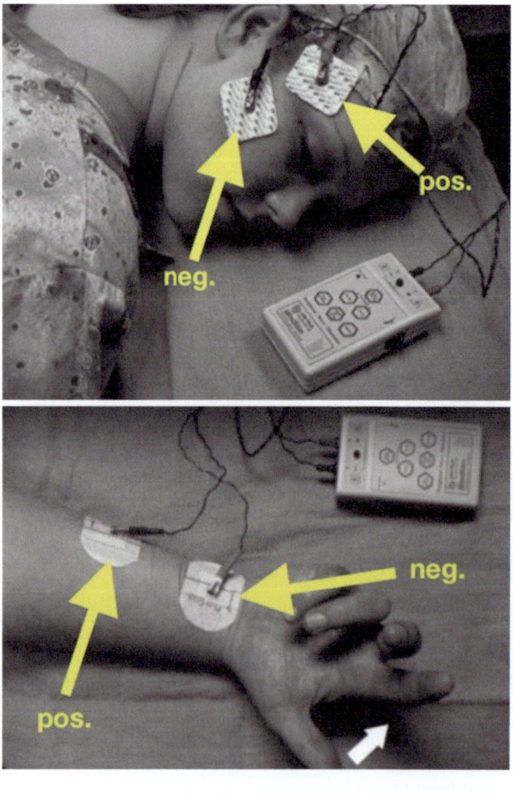

Fig. 21.8 Twitch monitor placement. Monitoring facial nerve (top panel) and ulnar nerve (bottom panel). Depicted polarity ensures maximal response. (Adapted from Dillon [3]. With permission from Thieme)

Monitoring neuromuscular blockade recovery is essential, especially in patients who are already at risk of having postoperative weakness. There are several tests used today for monitoring recovery: crude strength testing such as sustained head or leg lift, qualitative train-of-four, sustained tetany, and quantitative train-of-four. The literature is rife with studies demonstrating that subjective tests of recovery (i.e., qualitative train-of-four, sustained tetany, head lift) can be unreliable indicators of full recovery [18–20]. Conversely, multiple recent studies have shown that quantitative train-of-four monitoring significantly reduces the risk of residual paralysis in surgical patients [21–23].

Lesson 7: Myasthenia Gravis and Risk of Postoperative Ventilation

Leventhal and colleagues published a landmark paper in 1980 that identified risk factors for postoperative ventilation in patients undergoing transsternal thymectomy (Table 21.5). In order of significance, these risk factors were disease duration greater than or equal to 6 years, history of chronic respiratory disease, daily pyridostigmine dose greater than 750 mg, and vital capacity less than 2.9 l [24]. These risk factors formed the basis of risk assessment for anesthesiologists from that point forward.

These exact criteria may not be broadly applicable to myasthenic patients undergoing other surgical procedures or the more commonly performed transcervical or videoscopic thymectomy, which are associated with less respiratory dysfunction [25, 26]. Nevertheless, the Leventhal criteria serve as a good foundation of risk assessment for the anesthesiologist.

Lesson 8: Myasthenic Crisis and Cholinergic Crisis

Myasthenic crisis is a sudden and life-threatening exacerbation of myasthenia gravis with respiratory distress or failure. It can be precipitated by physiologic stress such as surgery, infection, or emotional stress. During myasthenic crisis cholinesterase inhibitors often have decreased effectiveness.

Cholinergic crisis is characterized by excess acetylcholine at the NMJ due to excessive cholinesterase inhibitor dose. This can cause generalized weakness and even respiratory failure in severe cases.

The two crises can be difficult to differentiate. The first step in differentiation is a careful history. Patients with recent up-titration of pyridostigmine are at higher risk of cholinergic crisis. Postoperatively, myasthenic crisis is more common as the patient has undergone a major recent stressor. When in doubt, the two crises can at times be differentiated by giving a small dose of edrophonium. In myasthenic crisis, edrophonium may temporarily improve symptoms, while it will worsen a cholinergic crisis [12].

Both myasthenic and cholinergic crises may require mechanical ventilation for respiratory failure. In myasthenic crisis, treatment may involve IVIG, steroids, and supportive therapy. In cholinergic crisis, the treatment is simply withdrawing anti-cholinesterase drugs.

Since patients with myasthenia gravis are at risk from developing myasthenic crisis or postoperative respiratory difficulty, it is best that they are transferred to a monitored bed after recovery in the PACU.

References

1. Baraka A. Anaesthesia and myasthenia gravis. Can J Anaesth. 1992;39:476–86.
2. Hirsch NP. Neuromuscular junction in health and disease. Br J Anaesth. 2007;99:132–8.
3. Dillon FX. Anesthesia issues in the perioperative management of myasthenia gravis. Semin Neurol. 2004;24:83–94.
4. Juel VC. Evaluation of neuromuscular junction disorders in the electromyography laboratory. Neurol Clin NA. 2012;30:621–39.
5. Sanders DB, Stålberg EV. AAEM minimonograph #25: single-fiber electromyography. Muscle Nerve. 1996;19:1069–83.
6. Selvan VA. Single-fiber EMG: a review. Ann Indian Acad Neurol. 2011;14:64–7.
7. Hoch W, et al. Auto-antibodies to the receptor tyrosine kinase MuSK in patients with myasthenia gravis without acetylcholine receptor antibodies. Nat Med. 2001;7:365–8.
8. Eisenkraft JB, Book WJ, Mann SM, Papatestas AE. Resistance to succinylcholine in myasthenia gravis: a dose-response study. Anesthesiology. 1988;69:760–2.
9. Abel M, Eisenkraft JB. Anesthetic implications of myasthenia gravis. Mt Sinai J Med. 2002;69:31–7.
10. Smith CE, Donati F, Bevan DR. Cumulative dose-response curves for atracurium in patients with myasthenia gravis. Can J Anaesth. 1989;36:402–6.
11. Eisenkraft JB, Book WJ, Papatestas AE. Sensitivity to vecuronium in myasthenia gravis: a dose-response study. Can J Anaesth. 1990;37:301–6.
12. Blichfeldt-Lauridsen L, Hansen BD. Anesthesia and myasthenia gravis. Acta Anaesthesiol Scand. 2012;56:17–22.
13. Morgan JM, Barker I, Peacock JE, Eissa A. A comparison of intubating conditions in children following induction of anaesthesia with propofol and suxamethonium or propofol and remifentanil. Anaesthesia. 2007;62:135–9.
14. McNeil IA, Culbert B, Russell I. Comparison of intubating conditions following propofol and succinylcholine with propofol and remifentanil 2 μg kg–1 or 4 μg kg–1. Br J Anaesth. 2000;85:623–5.
15. Imani F, Alebouyeh M-R, Taghipour-Anvari Z, Faiz SH-R. Use of remifentanil and alfentanil in endotracheal intubation: a comparative study. Anesth Pain. 2011;1:1–5.
16. Fotopoulou G, Theocharis S, Vasileiou I, Kouskouni E, Xanthos T. Management of the airway without the use of neuromuscular blocking agents: the use of remifentanil. Fundam Clin Pharmacol. 2011;26:72–85.
17. Aouad MT, Karam VY, Mallat CE, et al. The effect of adjuvant drugs on the quality of tracheal intubation without muscle relaxants in children: a systematic review of randomized trials. Pediatr Anesth. 2012;22:616–26.
18. Mikatti El N, Wilson A, Pollard BJ, Healy TE. Pulmonary function and head lift during spontaneous recovery from pipecuronium neuromuscular block. Br J Anaesth. 1995;74:16–9.
19. Capron F, Fortier L-P, Racine SB, Donati FO. Tactile fade detection with hand or wrist stimulation using train-of-four, double-burst stimulation, 50-hertz tetanus, 100-hertz tetanus, and acceleromyography. Anesth Analg. 2006;102:1578–84.

20. Murphy GS, Brull SJ. Residual neuromuscular block: lessons unlearned part I: definitions, incidence, and adverse physiologic effects of residual neuromuscular block. Anesth Analg. 2010;111:1–9.
21. Brull SJ, Murphy GS. Residual neuromuscular block: lessons unlearned. Part II. Methods to reduce the risk of residual weakness. Anesth Analg. 2010;111:1–12.
22. Murphy GS, et al. Intraoperative acceleromyography monitoring reduces symptoms of muscle weakness and improves quality of recovery in the early postoperative period. Anesthesiology. 2011;115:946–54.
23. Todd MM, Hindman BJ, King BJ. The implementation of quantitative electromyographic neuromuscular monitoring in an academic anesthesia department. Anesth Analg. 2014;119:323–31.
24. Leventhal SR, Orkin FK, Hirsh RA. Prediction of the need for postoperative mechanical ventilation in myasthenia gravis. Anesthesiology. 1980;53:26–30.
25. de Perrot M, Bril V, McRae K, Keshavjee S. Impact of minimally invasive trans-cervical thymectomy on outcome in patients with myasthenia gravis. Eur J Cardiothorac Surg. 2003;24:677–83.
26. Eisenkraft JB, et al. Predicting the need for postoperative mechanical ventilation in myasthenia gravis. Anesthesiology. 1986;65:79–82.

Chapter 22
Massive Hemorrhage After Dilatation and Curettage

Jessica G. Hollingsworth and Luis M. Rivera

In anesthetic practice sometimes even minor procedures can result in life-threatening situations. In this chapter the diagnosis and management of massive uterine bleeding after dilation and curettage is discussed.

Case Description

The patient is a 38-year-old woman, with a history significant for a self-reported severe bleeding episode during a prior breast augmentation. This was thought to be secondary to an underlying, undiagnosed bleeding disorder, although testing for this was not done (**L-1**). Her family history was negative for any bleeding disorders. The patient denied taking any current medications or having any drug allergies. She had a dilation and evacuation with curettage at 16 weeks of gestation under ultrasound guidance at an outside clinic and had brisk vaginal bleeding immediately following the procedure. The patient was given 0.2 mg methylergonovine (methergine) intramuscularly, misoprostol 800 mcg per-rectum, and oxytocin intravenously, and a uterine balloon was placed with 80 ml of normal saline to help tamponade the bleed. The patient was then sent to our facility for definitive treatment of postsurgical vaginal bleeding.

The patient was admitted to the floor unit. Initial laboratory results including hemoglobin (Hgb), hematocrit (Hct), platelets (PLT), fibrinogen (FGN), international normalized ratio (INR), prothrombin time (PT), partial thromboplastin time (PTT), and hemodynamic values all remained stable and within acceptable limits

J. G. Hollingsworth · L. M. Rivera (✉)
Department of Anesthesiology, University of California, San Diego, CA, USA
e-mail: LMRivera@ucsd.edu

J. L. Benumof, G. R. Manecke (eds.), *Clinical Anesthesiology II*,
https://doi.org/10.1007/978-3-030-12365-9_22

for the first hospital day. Since the bleeding had seemed to cease, the obstetrics team slowly deflated the uterine balloon on hospital day 2. Shortly after the balloon was deflated, the patient had sudden vaginal hemorrhage, with approximately 2 l of blood in the bed. She was taken emergently to the operating room for a dilation and curettage (D&C).

General endotracheal anesthesia was induced uneventfully. The patient had two large-bore peripheral IVs attached to fluid warmers, placed prior to induction, and an arterial line placed after induction. Two units of packed red blood cells (PRBCs) and one unit of fresh frozen plasma (FFP) were administered shortly after induction. As the patient was being prepared for surgery, the surgical team notified the anesthesiologist that there was continued "oozy, watery" bleeding. Additional methergine and carboprost tromethamine (hemabate) were administered intramuscularly, and a massive transfusion protocol was initiated (**L-2**).

Approximately 20 min into the case, the patient had an acute drop in blood pressure with mean arterial pressures dropping from 80 to 40 mmHg. In addition, there appeared to be a slight upslant in the capnogram waveform that had previously been flat. During this event, the patient's heart rate remained in the range of 80 90 beats per minute and remained in normal sinus rhythm, and pulse oximetry readings remained at 100% saturation. At this time, the patient was immediately placed on 100% fractional inspired oxygen concentration (FiO2), and phenylephrine and vasopressin boluses were given with recovery of mean arterial pressure to a value of 80 mmHg. While transfusions continued to be given, an additional 14-gauge peripheral IV was placed in the external jugular vein. Blood specimens were sent to the laboratory, extra anesthesia help was called for, and a transesophageal echocardiogram (TEE) was brought into the room.

As continued resuscitation was underway, a second anesthesia provider assisted with TEE, which showed adequate wall motion function, an adequate volume status, and no valvular or structural abnormalities. Lab results were significant for a fibrinogen decreased from 248 to 152 mg/dL, platelets decreased from 128 to 68×10^9/L, a hemoglobin stable at 8 g/dL, and a hematocrit stable at 24%. A thromboelastogram (TEG®) was interrupted before the fibrinolysis phase had concluded and, therefore, was inconclusive. However, it showed an initial shortened R interval with a normal alpha angle and maximum amplitude (MA) (**L-3, L-4**).

Meanwhile, the surgical team continued to experience surgical bleeding, and the decision was made to convert from a D&C to an open hysterectomy (**L-5, L-6**). The surgeons then saw evidence of a partial perforation of the right posterior uterine wall near the broad ligament. At the completion of the hysterectomy, the bleeding had ceased. The patient's trachea was extubated at the end of the procedure, and the patient was taken to the postanesthesia recovery area.

During the surgical course, the patient received a total of eight units of packed red blood cells, four units of platelets, seven units of fresh frozen plasma, two units of cryoprecipitate, and 1.5 L of lactated ringers, with an estimated blood loss of 4.6 l. Subsequent hospital course was uneventful with no further bleeding. The patient was discharged home on postoperative day 3.

Lessons Learned

L-1: General Causes of Intraoperative Bleeding and a Review of von Willebrand Disease (vWD)

There are many possible reasons for intraoperative bleeding. These include surgical trauma, other trauma, inherited coagulopathies, and acquired coagulopathies. Acquired coagulopathies can result from ingestion of medications (e.g., aspirin), herbal supplements (e.g., excessive garlic), pathologic processes (e.g., disseminated intravascular coagulation, primary fibrinolysis, and iatrogenic dilutional from fluid resuscitation).

Although our patient did not have any significant family history or laboratory testing to verify a preexisting bleeding disorder, her personal history of excessive bleeding with prior surgical procedures could be an indicator of an underlying disorder of hemostasis. von Willebrand disease (vWD) is one of the most common causes of inherited bleeding disorders with about 1% of the population being affected [1]. von Willebrand factor (vWF) is a protein which is synthesized in endothelial cells and secreted into the vessel lumen. vWF serves as a carrier for factor VIII. In addition, it plays a role in platelet adhesion and binding to endothelial components, serving an essential role in hemostasis [2]. vWD results from a qualitative or quantitative deficiency of vWF, leading to impaired hemostasis and subsequently to an increased propensity for bleeding.

vWD can be inherited or acquired. There are three types of inherited vWD (see Table 22.1).

Type 1 vWD

Type 1 vWD has an autosomal dominant inheritance and is the most common form of vWD. It is characterized by a partial quantitative deficit of vWF. Treatment

Table 22.1 Classification of inherited von Willebrand disease subtypes

<table>
<tr><th>Type</th><th>Inheritance</th><th>Pathophysiology</th><th>Effect of DDAVP</th></tr>
<tr><td>Type 1</td><td>Autosomal dominant</td><td>Partial quantitative deficiency of vWF</td><td>DDAVP helpful</td></tr>
<tr><td rowspan="5">Type 2 (2A, 2B, 2M, 2N)</td><td rowspan="5">Autosomal dominant</td><td>Qualitative defects</td><td>2A: DDAVP helpful</td></tr>
<tr><td>2A: dysfunction in platelet adhesion</td><td>2B: DDAVP contraindicated will cause thrombocytopenia</td></tr>
<tr><td>2B: increased platelet binding, leading to thrombocytopenia</td><td>2M: DDAVP may help</td></tr>
<tr><td>2M: dysfunction in platelet adhesion</td><td rowspan="2">2N: DDAVP may help</td></tr>
<tr><td>2N: decreased affinity and levels of factor VIII</td></tr>
<tr><td>Type 3</td><td>Autosomal recessive</td><td>Complete quantitative deficiency of vWF</td><td>DDAVP unlikely to help</td></tr>
</table>

involves administration of desmopressin (DDAVP) prior to elective surgical procedures. DDAVP causes increased vWF release from endothelial cells and increased levels of factor VIII for up to 12 h [2].

Type 2 vWD

Type 2 vWD has an autosomal dominant inheritance pattern as well; however it results in a qualitative defect in vWF. There are four type 2 subtypes depending on the functional deficit (2A, 2B, 2M, 2N). 2A and 2M are both variants in which defective vWF activity results in problems with platelet adhesion. Types 2A and 2M show variable responses to DDAVP treatment [2]. However, DDAVP treatment is still recommended.

Type 2B is characterized by a defective vWF that has enhanced affinity for receptors on the surface of platelets [1]. The increased binding of this defective vWF to platelets results in increased cleavage and clearance of the complexes, leading to thrombocytopenia [1]. **Treatment of type 2B vWD with DDAVP is** *contraindicated* as it will release more dysfunctional vWF, promoting thrombocytopenia.

Type 2N involves a defective vWF with decreased ability to bind factor VIII. This results in a marked decrease in serum factor VIII levels and associated issues with hemostasis [1]. Because of the associated decrease in factor VIII, type 2N subtype is often confused with hemophilia A. DDAVP may show some benefit for type 2N vWD.

Type 3 vWD

Type 3 vWD has an autosomal recessive inheritance pattern and is the most rare form of vWD. It is characterized by a complete to severely depressed quantitative deficit of vWF and a significant reduction in factor VIII [3]. Patients with type 3 may present with history of spontaneous bleeding and/or severe bleeding in response to trauma. Because the quantitative deficit of vWF is so severe in type 3, DDAVP is unlikely to show any benefit. These patients will need treatment with plasma-derived vWF, and factor VIII concentrates in response to bleeding.

Acquired vWD

Impaired function of vWF can be acquired secondary to various disease processes such as certain malignancies, leukemias, or autoimmune disorders. It has also been seen in association with some drug side effects and in high vascular flow states such as with ventricular assist devices or extracorporeal membrane oxygenation [2]. Treatment involves discontinuing the offending drug and/or treating the underlying precipitating disease process. DDAVP or antifibrinolytic administration may also be helpful in limiting perioperative bleeding [1].

Depending on the subtype and severity, many patients with vWD may not have clinically significant bleeding issues, allowing their disease to go undiagnosed. Most cases of vWD are not diagnosed until after a work up is done in the setting of recurrent bruising or prolonged bleeding from minor surgeries or menstruation [2]. There are three primary criteria for the diagnosis of vWD (1) a history of mucosal bleeding, prolonged bleeding after surgical procedures or postpartum hemorrhage, (2) a family history of bleeding disorders, and (3) a reduced activity of vWF demonstrated by laboratory assays [1].

In the case being discussed, the patient had only one of the criteria used to diagnose vWD. It is best to have a definitive diagnose of vWD and the subtype prior to treatment with DDAVP. Depending on the subtype, DDAVP may not help at all or, at worst, as is the case with subtype 2B, will exacerbate bleeding and thrombocytopenia. Therefore, blind administration of DDAVP for an unknown coagulopathy should not be done.

In our case, there is uncertainty as to whether the patient's coagulopathy has a component of an inherited vWD, another acquired coagulopathy, or a coagulopathic process due to massive blood loss and transfusion (**L-2, L-4, L-5**). Surgical treatment of the bleeding source or of the underlying hemostasis disorder, if known, should be done. In our case, surgical hysterectomy, after the discovery of the uterine perforation, facilitated hemostasis. Blood product and factor replacement was dictated by blood loss in our case, and this may be the best plan for a patient until a definitive diagnosis for the coagulopathy can be obtained.

L-2: Coagulopathies Associated with Massive Transfusion

There are variable definitions of massive transfusion.

The most practical definition from the perspective of an anesthesiologist in an intraoperative setting is the requirement of greater than four units of packed red blood cells (PRBCs) infused over a 1-h period with an ongoing need for transfusion [4].

Although massive hemorrhage in itself can induce coagulopathies (see **L-5**), the process of massive transfusion can also impair hemostasis. The phases of resuscitation with potential for aggravation of coagulopathies can be broken down into two main categories: (1) Initial fluid resuscitation and the steps taken during sudden massive bleeding. (2) Problems associated with the transfusion of large amounts of blood products.

Initial Fluid Resuscitation

Intravenous fluids (IVF) are often the first approach to compensate for blood loss prior to the arrival of blood products. Both crystalloids and colloids in large amounts will dilute coagulation factors, hemoglobin, and platelets [5]. In addition, rapid administration of unwarmed fluids can cause hypothermia, which will slow down enzymatic functions essential to the coagulation cascade. It is estimated that there is a 10% reduction in coagulation function for every 1 °C decrease in temperature [6].

Beyond hemodilution and hypothermia, the administration of crystalloids and colloids can impair coagulation in other ways. With excessive administration of isotonic crystalloids such as sodium chloride (NaCl), a hyperchloremic, non-anion-gap metabolic acidosis can develop. This is due to dilution of the preexisting bicarbonate, high chloride levels, and a decrease in renal bicarbonate reabsorption as a result of volume expansion. This acidosis will affect enzyme kinetics essential for the proper function of the coagulation cascade.

Colloids, in general, have the same risks of hemodilution and hypothermia as crystalloids. Colloids, including hydroxyethyl starch solution, gelatins, and dextrans (although no longer widely used), have some disadvantages relating to hemostasis. The mentioned colloids can impair platelet function by reducing glycoprotein IIb/IIIa availability, inhibit fibrin polymerization, and induce an acquired vWD (see **L-1**) by causing a reduction in factor VIII and vWF [5]. The more widely used colloid, human albumin, demonstrates decreased clot growth and strength on TEG® analysis, however not to the same degree as the previously mentioned colloids [7]. Despite the decreased clot strength demonstrated in the setting of human albumin, this has not shown to affect the degree of blood loss when compared to crystalloid solutions [8].

Withholding fluids is not a recommended option as this leads to low tissue perfusion. Low perfusion states result in interstitial edema, lactic acidosis, and impairment of microcirculation [6]. In addition, hypoperfusion leads to increased thrombomodulin expression which then complexes with thrombin, decreasing production of fibrin and increasing production of the anticoagulant protein C, all of which worsen coagulopathy (see **L-5**) [4].

In the case being discussed, prior to the arrival of replacement blood products, temporizing measures utilized to treat hypotension included both resuscitation with crystalloid fluids and treatment with vasopressor medications. The early use of vasopressors during hemorrhage has a useful role in quickly restoring hemodynamics and vital organ perfusion. In addition, small doses of vasopressors reduce the overall fluid requirement and the complications associated with initial fluid replacement as discussed above [9]. Although vasopressors may serve a beneficial temporizing role during hemorrhage, balanced fluid and blood product administration remains the mainstay of treatment [9].

Resuscitation with Blood Products

As is the case with the rapid administration of unwarmed crystalloids and colloids, the rapid administration of unwarmed blood products can lead to a hypothermia that can impair coagulation. Relative dilution of coagulation factors and platelets is also a concern in the case of unbalanced product administration. In the setting of massive transfusion, early use of FFP, PRBCs, and platelets is supported. However the American Association of Blood Banks does not endorse a preset FFP:PRBC ratio [5].

Transfusions of large volumes of stored blood can lead to various metabolic consequences, which can impair coagulation. Citrate is added to stored blood products as an anticoagulant. Normally, the liver is able to metabolize the citrate in blood products. However, with excess citrate during a massive transfusion, the liver cannot keep up, and citrate toxicity can develop. Unmetabolized citrate binds serum calcium and magnesium leading to hypocalcemia and hypomagnesemia [4]. Because adequate magnesium levels are needed for release of serum calcium, hypomagnesemia exacerbates hypocalcemia. Low serum calcium not only depresses cardiac function, but calcium is also essential for the formation of coagulation factors. Therefore, deficits in calcium can promote increased bleeding. The longer blood is stored, the higher the acid content of the product becomes. This is secondary to glycolysis by red blood cells over time. Acidosis impairs enzyme activity and depresses the activity of both the extrinsic and intrinsic coagulation pathways, contributing to impaired hemostasis [4].

In the case being discussed, massive hemorrhage was encountered leading to hemodynamic instability. Both the act of fluid and blood product resuscitation and the physiology of massive hemorrhage in itself (see **L-3**) can impair coagulation and worsen bleeding. Despite this, there are steps that can be taken to lessen these effects.

1. Avoiding hypothermia

   Fluid warmers should be utilized for large-volume fluid and product replacements or when blood loss is anticipated. In addition, forced air surface warmers or a warmed operating room can help to reduce radiative and convective heat losses.
2. Avoiding hemodilution

   Balanced fluid and early use of blood products is recommended. Initiation of a massive transfusion protocol, as seen in our case, helps to expedite delivery of blood products. Calling for an extra anesthesia provider to help place IVs, drawing blood specimens for laboratory analysis, and verifying correct compatibility of blood products can also facilitate the resuscitation process.
3. Avoiding hypoperfusion

   Low perfusion states worsen coagulopathy and may cause end-organ dysfunction. Balanced fluid and blood product administration are ideal treatment for volume loss due to bleeding. However, as seen in our case, temporizing measures with vasopressor administration may help in avoiding low perfusion states that could potentially cause end-organ ischemia and aggravate coagulopathy. Arterial line placement when anticipating large blood loss is helpful in closely monitoring hemodynamics and serial blood sampling. In the case being discussed, large-bore IV access established prior to induction, and the additional large-bore 14-gauge peripheral IV access placed in the external jugular vein, facilitated rapid volume resuscitation and avoidance of prolonged hypoperfusion.
4. Avoiding metabolic disturbances

   Acidosis impairs enzyme function and worsens coagulopathy. Being cognizant of the risk of a potential metabolic acidosis with large-volume NaCl or with aging blood products is important. Severe acidosis may have to be corrected with bicarbonate. Early administration of magnesium and calcium with the anticipation of hypomagnesemia and hypocalcemia, respectively, when multiple blood products are given, is also necessary. Having an arterial line placed early facilitates frequent blood chemistry monitoring and early correction of any developing metabolic disturbances.

L-3: What Is a Thromboelastogram (TEG®) and What Is Its Utility During Massive Hemorrhage?

As opposed to other methods of measuring the degree of blood coagulation, which look at static components of the coagulation cascade in isolation, TEG® evaluates the dynamic process of hemostasis by recording clot development, stabilization, and dissolution in whole blood. The test is done by obtaining a sample of whole blood, which is then placed in a heated cup containing a sensor pin. In a TEG®, a cup containing the blood sample moves around a pin, whereas in a rotational thromboelastogram (ROTEM®), the cup remains static, while the pins move around, while the blood clots. The resistance to oscillation with clot formation is transmitted in the sensor pin and converted into an electrical signal. A computer uses this signal to create a graphical and numerical depiction of clot formation [1]. Although the two systems operate differently and use different terminology, they provide clinically equivalent information.

A graphical representation of a TEG® (see Fig. 22.1) can be used to evaluate different stages of coagulation. Parameters of measurement on the TEG® include R-time, K-time, alpha (α) angle, maximum amplitude (MA), and clot lysis at 30 min (LY30).

- R-time: The R interval measures the time of initial fibrin clot formation. The crosslinking of fibrin depends on the function of coagulation factors and thus the r-time is a reflection of this.
- K-time: The K-time represents the time required to achieve a clot strength of 20 mm. Amplification and buildup of the clot is also a reflection of the function of coagulation factors.
- α-Angle: Measures the slope between the R and K values representing the rate of clot formation. This speed is a reflection of fibrin buildup, crosslinking, fibrinogen function, and coagulation factors.
- Maximum amplitude: MA, which is the widest portion of the tracing, represents the overall strength of the fibrin clot. It is the result of fibrin and platelet binding and correlates clinically to platelet function.
- LY30: LY30 is the percentage of amplitude decrease 30 min after the peak of the MA. LY30 therefore represents clot stability and the dynamic process of fibrinolysis.

TEG® analysis has been shown to be useful for guiding transfusion therapy and reducing the use of blood products in both liver transplantation and cardiac surgery

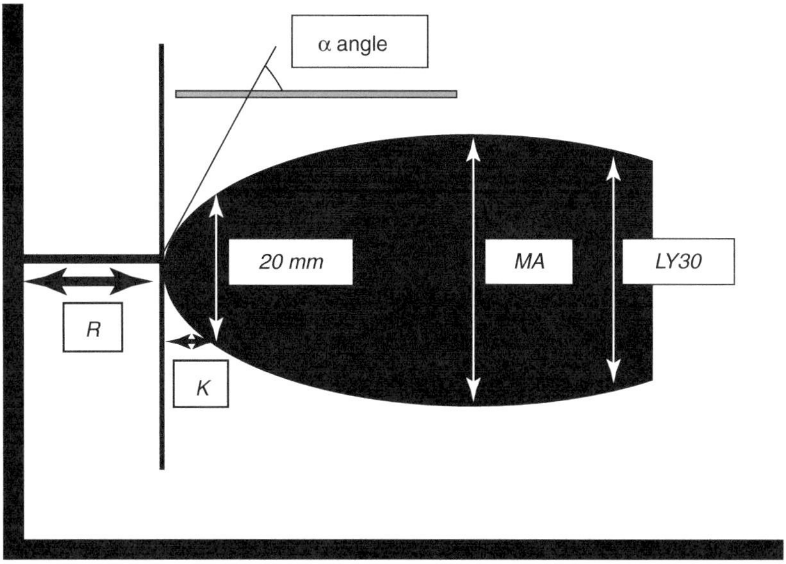

Fig. 22.1 A graphical representation of a normal TEG®. (Adapted from da Luz et al. [10]. With permission from Creative Commons License 2.0: https://creativecommons.org/licenses/by/2.0/)

[10]. In addition, TEG can help in dictating appropriate transfusion therapy in other situations involving complex bleeding such as massive hemorrhage with consumptive or dilutional coagulopathy [1]. However, threshold TEG® values justifying transfusion in trauma bleeding have not been conclusively identified [10]. TEG® is not a substitute for conventional lab tests of hemostasis. It is, however, an additional tool that may be useful in guiding appropriate transfusion therapy for trauma and massive hemorrhage.

In the case being discussed, TEG® was an additional test used to aid in resuscitation. The shortened R interval, indicating rapid clot onset, could be a reflection of the hypercoagulable state of pregnancy or of the recent transfusions that had been given. The normal MA, despite the lab values showing a quantitative decrease in platelets, indicates adequate strength of the fibrin clot and a qualitative reflection of platelet function. Because the TEG® analysis from the blood sample sent intraoperatively was interrupted, there is not a value given for LY30, and the degree of fibrinolysis is unable to be interpreted.

L-4: Disseminated Intravascular Coagulation (DIC)

DIC is a process resulting in systemic activation of pathways regulating coagulation [11]. This non-focal response of the coagulation cascade provokes a dynamic state, which can result in both uncontrolled bleeding from multiple sites and thrombosis

Table 22.2 ISTH scoring criteria for diagnosing DIC

Clinical condition predisposing to DIC?	Essential
Platelet count (×10^9/L)	>100=0, <100=1, <50=2
Fibrin degradation-related markers	Mod increase=2, strong increase=3
Fibrinogen (g/L)	>1=0, <1= 1
PT (s)	<3=0, 3–6= 1, >6=2
DIC diagnosis	≥5

leading to microvascular ischemia or end-organ damage [12]. Identifying DIC clinically is not always straightforward since other coagulopathic disorders can present similarly with either hypocoagulation or hypercoagulation. For this reason, the International Society of Thrombosis and Hemostasis (ISTH) has developed a widely validated scoring criteria for identifying overt DIC which takes into consideration both clinical and laboratory data (Table 22.2).

DIC does not occur in isolation. An underlying clinical disorder is an essential requirement for the diagnosis of DIC. Conditions predisposing to DIC include, but are not limited to, sepsis, amniotic fluid embolism, preeclampsia, malignancy, and placental abruption. Tissue damage from trauma and hypoperfusion from blood loss are also factors that can worsen DIC and are relevant in the surgical setting [12]. In addition, the International Society on Thrombosis and Haemostasis (ISTH) scoring criteria (vide infra) takes into consideration particular coagulation tests: platelet count, fibrin degradation products, fibrinogen levels, and prothrombin time (PT).

Laboratory studies in isolation for the diagnosis of DIC are not adequate. However, as established by the ISTH algorithm, there are common laboratory abnormalities associated with DIC. A downward trend in platelet count is the most common laboratory finding associated with DIC, with thrombocytopenia occurring in 98% of cases [11].

Fibrin degradation products (D-Dimers) may be increased in DIC. However, many conditions can cause an increase in fibrin degradation markers, including pregnancy and recent surgery. Therefore this test is less specific in the diagnosis of DIC.

Fibrinogen levels are also commonly assessed in the evaluation of DIC. Decreased fibrinogen levels are expected in the presence of DIC, which causes ongoing consumption of coagulation factors. However, fibrinogen is also an acute-phase reactant-increased production of fibrinogen can be observed during physiological stress. Therefore, decrease in fibrinogen level has low (28%) sensitivity in the diagnosis of DIC [11].

Consumption of coagulation factors and low perfusion damage to the liver resulting in impaired coagulation factor synthesis are both events that can contribute to a prolonged PT. However, increased production of clotting factors in the setting of a bleeding diathesis can result in a normal or shortened PT. Low PT is seen in around 50–60% of DIC cases [11].

TEG® analysis, with its dynamic evaluation of hemostasis, could be helpful in guiding transfusion therapy. However, cutoff points in establishing a diagnosis for DIC have not yet been identified (see **L-3**).

In the case being discussed, the diagnosis of DIC could not be clearly established. Known coagulation changes are seen in normal pregnancy, including elevations in numerous coagulation factors. Specifically, a woman in the second trimester would be expected to have a fibrinogen level elevated to about 291–538 mg/dL, as opposed to 233–496 mg/dL in a nonpregnant individual [13].

In order to adjust for the coagulation changes seen during pregnancy, a revision to the ISTH DIC scoring system was proposed by Clark et al. [14]. Their scoring criteria eliminate the need for fibrin markers, which are universally elevated in pregnancy and the postpartum period. In addition, they increase the cutoff for fibrinogen levels to compensate for the increased levels seen in pregnancy [14].

With these revised criteria, the diagnosis for DIC in our case becomes a possibility. A definitive diagnosis, however, is unable to be made in the setting of likely coagulation profile changes seen in the setting of massive hemorrhage and massive transfusion (see **L-2, L-5**).

L-5: Coagulopathy Associated with Massive Hemorrhage

Problems with hemostasis during massive hemorrhage are more than just the consequences of resuscitation with fluids, colloids, and blood products as mentioned above (see **L-2**). Although clotting factors can become depleted in massive hemorrhage, the coagulopathy associated with major blood loss is sometimes seen without major depletion of factors and in the absence of significant fluid administration or hypothermia [14].

The coagulopathy secondary to massive hemorrhage is multifactorial. Although the exact mechanism causing the coagulation derangements is unknown, it is thought that tissue trauma and systemic hypoperfusion cause a global anticoagulated and hyperfibrinolytic state [15].

Tissue hypoperfusion diverts thrombin from fibrin formation to the production of activated protein C generation [15]. Activated protein C exerts an anticoagulant effect by inactivating factor Va and factor VIIIa [6]. In addition, increased activated protein C will deactivate plasminogen activator inhibitor (PAI-1), causing increased fibrinolysis. Plasma tissue plasminogen activator (tPA), an anticoagulant, has an increased effect due to decreased breakdown by PAI-1.

Increased tPA production is also seen secondary to the stress response, as it is released directly from the endothelium and from the production of epinephrine, vasopressin, bradykinin, and other substances [5]. Overall, the coagulopathy seen secondary to massive hemorrhage results in a systemic pathologically anticoagulated state and excessive fibrinolysis.

L-6: Strategy for When Encountering Intraoperative Coagulopathy with an Unknown Cause

The contributors to a coagulopathic state during massive hemorrhage can be multifactorial. Oftentimes, it is impossible to pinpoint an exact cause of a worsening coagulopathy. Prevention of a coagulopathy and treatment of identifiable contributors is the goal. Perioperative treatment with specific blood coagulation factors in a patient with a known coagulopathy, such as DDAVP, for specific subtypes of vWD would be ideal (see **L-1**). Balanced fluid and blood product administration, while staying aware of coagulopathic issues inherent with massive transfusion and massive hemorrhage, can prepare the anesthesiologist and ensure proper planning and treatment (see **L-2, L-5**). Adequate temperature and acid-base balance control are mandatory.

Ultimately, surgical control of the bleeding source, which in our case was done with a hysterectomy after the discovery of a uterine wall laceration, is essential for bleeding control and preventing the spiral of a worsening coagulopathy.

References

1. Barash PG, Cullen BF, Stoelting RK, Cahalan MK, Stock MC, Ortega R. Clinical anesthesia. 7th ed. Philadelphia: Lippincott Williams & Wilkins; 2013.
2. Sabih A, Babiker HM. Von Willebrand disease. [Updated 2017 Oct 22]. StatPearls [Internet]. Treasure Island: StatPearls Publishing; 2018. Available from: https://www.ncbi.nlm.nih.gov/books/NBK459222/.
3. Bryckaert M, Rosa J, Denis CV, Lenting PJ. Of von willebrand factor and platelets. Cell Mol Life Sci. 2015;72:307–26. https://doi.org/10.1007/s00018-014-1743-8.
4. Patil V, Shetmahajan M. Massive transfusion and massive transfusion protocol. Indian J Anesth. 2014;58(5):590–5. https://doi.org/10.4103/0019-5049.144662.
5. Bollinger D, Gorlinger K, Tanaka D. Pathophysiology and treatment of coagulopathy in massive hemorrhage and hemodilution. Anesthesiology. 2010;113:1205–19.
6. Meibner A, Schlenke P. Massive bleeding and massive transfusion. Transfus Med Hemother. 2012;39(2):73–84. https://doi.org/10.1159/000337250.
7. Winstedt DW, Hanna JH, Schott US. Albumin-induced coagulopathy is less severe and more effectively reversed with fibrinogen concentrate than is synthetic colloid induced coagulopathy. Crit Care. 2013;17(Suppl 2):P734. https://doi.org/10.1196/cc12312.
8. Rasmussen KC, Hojskov M, Secher NH. Impact of albumin on coagulation competence and hemorrhage during major surgery. Medicine. 2016;95(9):e2720.
9. Gupta B, Garg N, Ramachandran R. Vasopressors: do they have any role in hemorrhagic shock? J Anesthesiol Clin Pharmacol. 2017;33(1):3–8. https://doi.org/10.4103/0970-9185.202185.
10. da Luz LT, Nascimento B, Rizoli S. Thromboelastography (TEG): practical considerations on its clinical use in trauma resuscitation. Scand J Trauma Resusc Emerg Med. 2013;21:29. https://doi.org/10.1186/1757-7241-21-29.
11. Levi M, Toh CH, Thachil J, Watson HG. Guidelines for the diagnosis and management of disseminated intravascular coagulation. Br J Haematol. 2009;145:24–33. https://doi.org/10.1111/j.1365-2141.2009.07600.x.
12. Thachil J. Disseminated intravascular coagulation: a practical approach. Anesthesiology. 2016;125(1):230–6. https://doi.org/10.1097/ALN.0000000000001123.

13. Abbassi-Ghanavati M, Greer L, Cunningham FG. Pregnancy and laboratory studies: a reference table for clinicians. Obstet Gynecol. 2010;115(2 Pt 1):387.
14. Clark SL, Romero R, Dildy GA, et al. Proposed diagnostic criteria for the case definition of amniotic fluid embolism in research studies. Am J Obstet Gynecol. 2016;215(4):408–12. https://doi.org/10.1016/j.ajog.2016.06.037.
15. Davenport R. Pathogenesis of acute traumatic coagulopathy. Transfusion. 2013;53:23S–7S.

Chapter 23
Intraoperative Bradycardia and Asystole

Jessica G. Hollingsworth and Luis M. Rivera

Patient factors, surgical manipulation, and medications can all lead to sudden bradycardia and asystole in surgical patients. Preparedness, both cognitive and physical, is essential in the successful diagnosis and treatment of these potentially life-threatening dysrhythmias.

Case Description

The patient is a 71-year-old man, weighing 121 kg, with a body mass index (BMI) of 33 kg/m^2. His history was significant only for Barrett's esophagus and esophageal cancer. He was scheduled for laparoscopic robotic-assisted transhiatal esophagectomy with endoscopic pyloric botox injection. He had no previous history of allergies or anesthetic complications.

An epidural catheter for postoperative pain was not offered as the procedure was intended to be performed laparoscopically. General anesthesia was induced intravenously, and an endotracheal tube (ETT) was placed without incidence. His vital signs remained stable during induction. A radial arterial line was then placed and surgery began. General anesthesia was maintained with sevoflurane in air and oxygen. The patient remained hemodynamically stable throughout the beginning of surgery. However, the surgeons commented that surgical dissection was proving to be very difficult with the laparoscopic technique due to the patient's obesity.

The decision was then made by the surgeons to convert to an open technique in an attempt to mobilize the esophagus through incisions in the mediastinum and the neck. As the surgeons started to tunnel through the mediastinum, there was an acute, 1–2 s, episode of severe bradycardia during which the patient's heart rate dropped

J. G. Hollingsworth · L. M. Rivera (✉)
Department of Anesthesiology, University of California, San Diego, CA, USA
e-mail: LMRivera@ucsd.edu

J. L. Benumof, G. R. Manecke (eds.), *Clinical Anesthesiology II*,
https://doi.org/10.1007/978-3-030-12365-9_23

from approximately 60 beats per minute (BPM) to 30 BPM (**L-1, L-2**). The anesthesiologist alerted the surgeons of the incident, the surgeons ceased their manipulation, and the patient's heart rate returned to 60 BPM. The surgeons acknowledged that they were near the vagus nerve at the time. As a precaution in case of subsequent events, the anesthesiologist then obtained atropine from the anesthesia cart and placed it nearby (**L-7**).

Surgery continued for another 4 h, while the surgeons continued their dissection of the esophagus. Once the surgeons believed the esophagus was adequately mobilized, an 8 cm subxiphoid incision was made. With one surgeon at the patient's chest and one at the neck, they attempted to free the distal esophagus by pushing up through the mediastinum and pulling the esophagus up proximally through the neck. As the surgeon pushed up through the mediastinum, there were occasional episodes of hypotension, with stable heart rate. During these hypotensive episodes, the patient's blood pressure was supported adequately using intravenous (IV) phenylephrine, ephedrine, and IV fluid boluses (**L-3**).

The surgeons then communicated that the esophagus was "stuck," and at this point they then began to use more force to push and pull on the esophagus from above and below. At this time, the anesthesiologist prepared dilute epinephrine and placed it nearby. Suddenly, the esophagus was violently freed from the neck. During the forceful liberation of the esophagus, the heart rate dropped from 80 BPM, to the 40 BPM range, to 0 BPM over about six to ten heart beats, and the arterial line tracing became flat, indicative of hemodynamic collapse (**L-4**). The surgeons were initially unaware of the acute hemodynamic change during their manipulation. However, the anesthesia provider immediately alerted them that the patient was asystolic and stated they need to begin chest compressions (**L-5, L-6, L-7**). As chest compressions were begun, 100 mcg of epinephrine was administered IV, yielding a return to normal sinus rhythm and blood pressure waveform within 20 s. The patient's blood pressure and heart rate peaked post epinephrine to a maximum of about 220/100 mmHg and 140 BPM, respectively. A bolus of propofol was then given to counter these effects, and the patient's blood pressure and heart rate returned to baseline after about 2 min. The rest of the case was uneventful. The patient's trachea was left intubated at the end of the lengthy surgery, and the patient was transported to the intensive care unit. Postoperatively, he remained in stable condition, and his trachea was extubated the next day.

Lessons Learned

L-1: Managing Intraoperative Bradycardia

There are many mechanisms that can lead to intraoperative bradycardia (see **L-2**). One of the anesthesiologist's most important roles is to quickly recognize hemodynamic aberrations and treat them appropriately (Table 23.1).

Table 23.1 Simultaneous interventions to be performed when managing intraoperative bradycardia

Determine hemodynamic significance
Scan surgical field and notify surgeon of hemodynamic changes
Ensure adequate ventilation and oxygenation
Provide pharmacological treatment or transcutaneous pacing as required

Sinus bradycardia is defined as a heart rate less than 60 BPM originating at the sinoatrial (SA) node. The first step when identifying intraoperative bradycardia is to assess its hemodynamic significance. Since an anesthetized patient is unable to communicate symptoms, the anesthesiologist must look for signs of poor perfusion caused by the bradycardia such as hypotension, reduction in the expired end-tidal carbon dioxide (ETCO2) concentration, decreases in oxygen saturation (O2sat), and other cardiac dysrhythmias. Concurrent conditions such as hypotension may also guide medication choices when treating bradycardia. Dysrhythmias such as third-degree heart block or ST segmental changes in the electrocardiogram (EKG) may prompt transcutaneous pacing or treatment for myocardial ischemia, respectively.

The surgical field should be scanned for contributing causes and the surgical team notified of the bradycardic event, especially if it is severe or associated with signs of inadequate perfusion. There may be surgical stimuli such as insufflation of the abdominal cavity during laparoscopy, viscus manipulation, pressure to the eye, or vena cava compression contributing to the hemodynamic change. The surgeon should be asked to cease the inciting stimulus until symptoms are treated. Timely discussion with the surgical team may prompt alterations in surgical approach when appropriate.

Treatment of symptomatic or hemodynamically significant bradycardia should not be delayed. Many of the steps discussed below must be performed simultaneously as treatment is underway (Table 23.1). Adequate ventilation must be confirmed and maintained, and the fraction of inspired oxygen (FIO2) should be increased to 100% oxygen if not contraindicated. A call for help may be required to prepare medications or bring necessary equipment such as transcutaneous pacemaker or transthoracic echocardiogram (TTE) to the operating room (OR). Pharmacological treatment for symptomatic bradycardia should be initiated per ACLS guidelines [1], tailored to the intraoperative environment (Fig. 23.1). The initial treatment depends upon the severity of the hemodynamic compromise. In most cases, particularly those resulting from vagal activity, an atropine dose of 0.5 mg IV bolus along with asking the surgeons to discontinue the vagal stimulus is sufficient. Atropine may be repeated every 3–5 min up to a total of 3 mg. If atropine is unsuccessful, chronotropic agents such as dopamine IV infusion of 2–10 mcg/kg/min or epinephrine IV infusion of 2–10 mcg/min can be started. Alternatively, transcutaneous pacing may be initiated. If neither transcutaneous pacing nor chronotropic agents resolve the symptoms, steps should be taken to prepare for transvenous pacing.

In the case being discussed, the initial bradycardic event was relatively mild and was managed by simply having the surgeons discontinue traction on the esophagus.

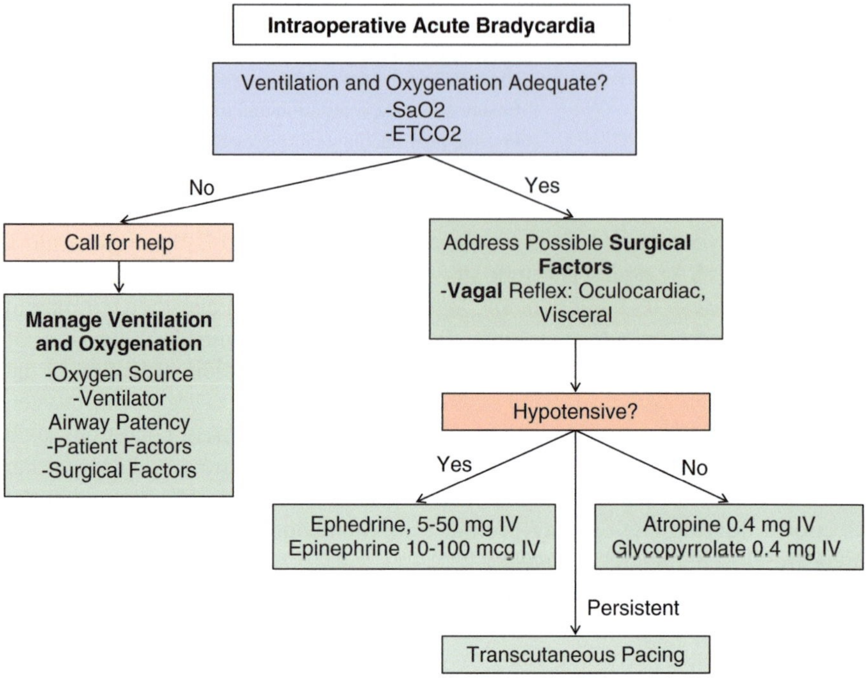

Fig. 23.1 General algorithm for management of acute intraoperative bradycardia. Medication doses vary according to the severity of the situation, with the dose of epinephrine being as high as 1 mg IV for severe, persistent cases. Severe, persistent bradycardia, asystole, or severe hypotension should prompt full ACLS resuscitation. Pharmacologic support may be needed, while airway/ventilation/oxygenation issues are addressed

Bringing the situation to the attention of the surgeons allowed them to identify the probable cause of the bradycardic event.

The later event was severe (asystole) with hemodynamic collapse, so it was immediately treated with an IV bolus of epinephrine.

L-2: Discussion of Vagal Reflexes Causing Bradycardia

There are multiple possible etiologies for intraoperative bradycardia (see **L-4**). One important cause, which was relevant to this case, is vagal reflex. Traction applied to organs directly innervated by the vagus nerve or stimulation that activates a vagal efferent response as part of a reflex arc can result in sudden bradycardia. Specifically, the vagal-mediated responses discussed below include direct vagal nerve traction, oculocardiac reflex, the Bezold-Jarisch reflex, and the baroreceptor reflex.

1. Vagus Nerve Traction

   Applying traction to the peritoneum and viscera innervated by the vagus nerve (esophagus, intestines, testicles, ovaries, uterus), during surgical manipulation, can result in a profound parasympathetic response resulting in bradycardia or even asystole. This reflex bradycardia has been described during tissue deformation of viscera with various abdominal surgeries and during dilation and curettage (D&C) procedures involving peritoneal stretch and cervical dilation [2]. Rapid peritoneal insufflation may be a factor in triggering this response. However, in some instances direct surgical manipulation of abdominal viscera without pneumoperitoneum can result in a severe vagal reaction [3]. Frequently, ceasing the surgical stimulus that incited the event is enough to allow hemodynamics to return to baseline, as was seen with the initial esophageal stimulation in our case. However, it is of utmost importance for the anesthesiologist to communicate significant hemodynamic changes with the surgeons and to prepare for further intervention if needed.

2. Oculocardiac Reflex

   The oculocardiac reflex describes a reflex arc involving the trigeminal nerve at the afferent limb and the vagus nerve at the efferent limb. The reflex is triggered by pressure to the globe via external pressure or trauma, pressure from local anesthetic accumulation during a retrobulbar block, or by traction of extraocular muscles or orbital structures. Sensory nerve endings at the trigeminal nerve send neuronal signals via the gasserian ganglion. These afferent fibers continue to the reticular formation where they connect with the efferent pathway in the motor nucleus of the vagus nerve. The cardioinhibitory efferent fibers from the vagus nerve then terminate on SA and AV nodes and the myocardium, provoking a negative chronotropic and inotropic response, resulting in bradycardia [4].

   Although the oculocardiac reflex wasn't involved in the case described, it is an important etiology to consider when encountering sudden bradycardia during ophthalmologic or sinus surgeries. The incidence of occurrence during provoking surgeries is 16–82% depending on the study, with a higher incidence seen in the pediatric population [5]. Control of this dysrhythmia should first be managed as any intraoperative bradycardic event (see **L-1**). Frequently however, asking the surgeon to stop the inciting stimulus while ventilatory and anesthetic depth are optimized will be sufficient to return heart rate and rhythm to baseline [5].

3. Bezold-Jarisch Reflex

   The Bezold-Jarisch reflex (BJR) involves chemoreceptors and mechanoreceptors in the left ventricular (LV) wall. These receptors, when stimulated, communicate via unmyelinated vagal fibers that increase parasympathetic tone and inhibit sympathetic outflow resulting in the triad of hypotension, bradycardia, and peripheral vasodilation [6]. Mechanical mediators include an underfilled LV, such as the paradoxical bradycardia following profound hypovolemia seen during severe acute hemorrhage. Another common mechanical mediator is cardiac wall deformations, which can be characteristic of an MI or during coronary reperfusion, in which case the BJR is thought to be cardioprotective [6]. Chemoreceptor activation of the reflex is less common intraoperatively and has been described in the setting of veratrum alkaloids and insect venoms. Treatment includes rapid restoration of volume deficits provoking the reflex. Pharmacologic management may often begin with an anticholinergic medication such as atropine, however because concomitant hypotension and vasodilation often occur with BJR, drugs that are both chronotropic and inotropic, such as ephedrine or epinephrine, may be indicated.

4. Baroreceptor Reflex

   Arterial baroreceptor reflexes serve as a negative feedback loop for short-term blood pressure buffering in response to abrupt changes in blood volume, cardiac output, or peripheral resistance. Afferent receptors are found in the carotid sinus innervated by the glossopharyngeal nerve and in the aortic arch by the vagus nerve. Afferent receptors react to increases in stretch caused by elevations in blood pressure. Impulses carried by afferent fibers synapse at the medullary vasomotor center activating the efferent limb, which travels via the vagus nerve. Efferent vagal fibers then send signals inhibiting sympathetic outflow and increasing the parasympathetic response [4]. The end result of the increased stretch to the baroreceptors is vasodilation, lowered heart rate, and lowered blood pressure. Hemodynamic changes due to baroreceptor reflex are usually transient, however should be approached as any intraoperative bradycardia event (see **L-1**). After assuring adequate ventilation, oxygenation, and anesthesia, identifiable causative factors such as sustained intrathoracic pressures should be corrected and pharmacologic treatment with chronotropic agents initiated as appropriate.

L-3: What Are Possible Mechanisms for Rhythm Changes During the Esophageal Manipulation Phase of Surgery?

During a transhiatal approach for esophagectomy, the esophagus is mobilized through a subxiphoid incision and neck incisions. This is done through blind manipulation through the posterior mediastinum using blunt dissection. Thus, the patient is susceptible to dysrhythmias, while the surgeon manipulates the structures close to the heart (see Fig. 23.2). Dysrhythmias occur in 50–78% of patients during the manipulation phase of surgery [7, 8]. The contributors to rhythm changes seen during transhiatal esophagectomy can be attributed to three main categories: stimulation of the pericardium, vagal nerve stimulation, and atrial pressure or heart rotation.

1. Touching the pericardium can induce dysrhythmias. The most commonly induced dysrhythmias seen are premature atrial contractions (PACs) and premature ventricular contractions (PVCs) [8].

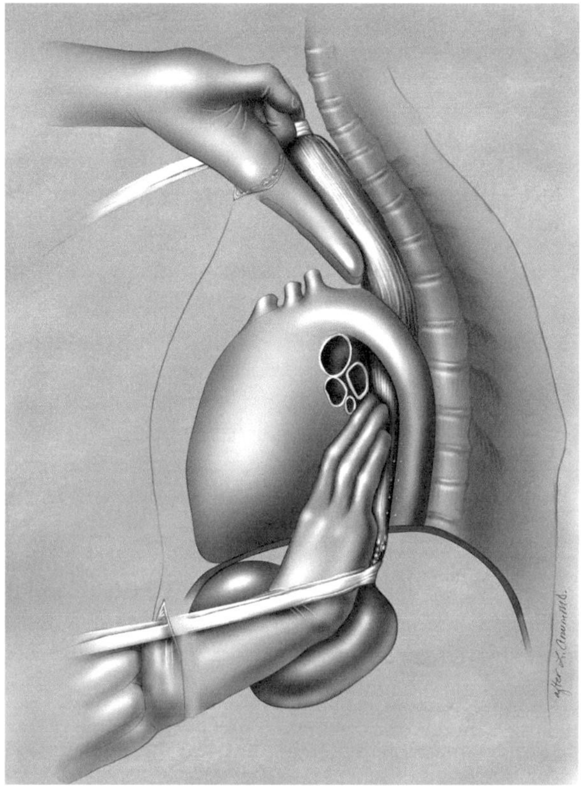

Fig. 23.2 Blunt dissection of esophagus through the posterior mediastinum during transhiatal esophagectomy is a blind procedure [9]. (Reprinted from Orringer [9]. With permission from Elsevier)

2. Vagal nerve stimulation can induce dysrhythmias. The posterior surface of the pericardium is supplied by vagal input from the esophageal plexus. Stimulation during blunt dissection can cause bradycardia or rarely cardiac arrest [7, 8]. This was likely the predominant mechanism in the case being discussed.
3. Blind surgical manipulation can cause atrial pressure and heart rotation leading to dysrhythmias. Atrial pressure interferes with cardiac filling and cardiac output leading to arterial hypotension. Prolonged or severe hypotension can result in impaired heart function or impaired coronary blood flow resulting in various associated cardiac rhythm changes [7].

Although surgical manipulation is unavoidable, it is the responsibility of the anesthesiologist to support hemodynamic changes and maintain effective communication with the surgeon. Some of the perturbations seen in our case during the manipulative phase include bradycardia and occasional hypotension. The anesthesiologist supported these changes effectively with occasional fluid boluses, phenylephrine boluses, and ephedrine boluses. If necessary, the surgeon should be notified of when manipulation should be paused, as hemodynamic changes are usually rapidly corrected with ceasing manipulation [7].

L-4: What Are Some Common Causes of Intraoperative Bradycardia Leading to Hemodynamic Collapse?

Acute bradycardia can rapidly progress to asystole if left unmanaged. It is important to consider common causes of bradycardia leading to hemodynamic collapse (see Table 23.2) as it may direct subsequent management. Causes can be broken down into five main categories:

1. Hypoxia: Problems with oxygenation and ventilation leading to hypoxia can result in severe bradycardia and cardiac arrest. An example is unrecognized esophageal intubation. Treatment with medications will not be successful until ventilation and oxygenation are restored.
2. Medications: Many of the medications administered during anesthesia can result in bradycardia. They include beta blockers, digoxin, amiodarone, procainamide, calcium channel blockers, opioids, alpha 2 agonists, phenylephrine, succinylcholine, anticholinesterases, and overdose of local anesthetic (see Table 23.2).

   Knowing a specific drug to be a causative agent can help guide secondary treatment, for example, beta blocker overdose can be treated with beta agonists or glucagon and local anesthetic toxicity with intralipid. In addition, an anaphylactic reaction can be precipitated by many medications and can lead to rapid hemodynamic collapse.
3. Acute vagal stimulation: Vagal reflex arcs leading to bradycardia are discussed previously (see **L-2**) and include oculocardiac reflex, Bezold-Jarisch reflex, and baroreceptor reflex. However, other mechanisms of vagal stimulation can occur such as with direct cardiac manipulation (see **L-3**), peritoneal distension secondary to insufflation, bowel or gonadal manipulation, laryngoscopy, and bladder catheterization.
4. Neuraxial anesthesia: A high spinal or epidural anesthetic can result in blockade of the cardiac accelerator fibers at levels T1-T4, resulting in uninhibited vagal response and resultant bradycardia. Apnea and loss of consciousness is attributed to decreased blood flow to the brain and the medullary ventilatory centers [10].

Table 23.2 Medication causes of bradycardia

Beta blockers (propranolol, metoprolol, esmolol, etc.)	Calcium channel blockers (diltiazem, verapamil, etc.)
Digoxin	Amiodarone
Procainamide	Flecainide
Adenosine	Lithium
Alpha 2 agonists (clonidine, dexmedetomidine, methyldopa)	Opioids (fentanyl, alfentanil, etc.)
Phenylephrine	Succinylcholine
Anticholinesterases (neostigmine, physostigmine, etc.)	Overdose of local anesthetics (lidocaine, bupivacaine, etc.)

5. Acute cardiac event: An acute myocardial infarction (MI) that affects blood supply to the SA node, the primary pacemaker of the heart, or a high degree AV node block may cause a bradycardia. Also consider acute pacemaker failure in patients who have implanted devices.

L-5: How Should Sudden Cardiovascular Collapse Be Managed in the OR?

Sudden intraoperative cardiovascular collapse is an emergency that requires quick identification and action on the part of the anesthesiologist. The complexity of the situation requires a team approach, as multiple goals may need to be fulfilled at the same time. When faced with a situation with a plurality of goals, it is important to be able to prioritize [11]. There may be multiple variables involved leading to an asystolic event in the OR, and ongoing problem-solving will ensue. However, the amount of time available for decision-making is scarce, and any delay can result in poor patient outcomes. Therefore, the anesthesiologist must strictly adhere to basic guidelines, allowing cognitive resources to focus on knowledge-based problem-solving behavior [11]. Outlined below are some immediate simultaneous actions that should be performed during cardiovascular collapse, while cognitive resources focus on higher-level problem-solving.

1. Verify that there is no pulse.

   A spurious failure of a single monitor can easily be identified by looking at the other monitors. For instance, the arterial line tracing may disappear and indicate 0/0 mmHg, while the ETCO2 and O2sat tracings remain unchanged, indicative of an arterial line failure, not asystole. It is essential to quickly survey all monitors including the pulse oximeter, ETCO2 wave form, arterial line, noninvasive BP cuff, EKG monitor, and leads, as well as to palpate for a pulse or ask the surgeon to do so if they have better access.
2. Notify the surgeons and the OR staff of cardiac arrest.

   Call for extra help to the OR to assist with additional vascular access if necessary, prepare medications, and gather equipment. Call for a defibrillator ("crash cart") and have the defibrillator pads applied. Call for someone to bring the echocardiogram machine and probes to the OR. While the esophagus was not accessible for transesophageal echocardiogram (TEE) in the case being discussed, TTE may still be performed if necessary.
3. Ensure adequate ventilation and oxygenation.

   Increase FIO2 to 100% oxygen. Arterial blood gases (ABG) can be sent in order to assess ventilation and oxygenation. Correct endotracheal tube placement should be verified by auscultation, examining the ETCO2 waveform, and looking for changes in peak ventilator pressure changes that may result from decreased lung compliance. Suctioning of the endotracheal tube or readjustment of the tube may be necessary.

4. Drugs or agents capable of producing hypotension such as all volatile and intravenous anesthetics and any other IV infusions of drugs that may cause hypotension should be stopped.
5. Start Advanced Cardiovascular Life Support (ACLS) interventions.
   Assign and delegate tasks. Initiate high-quality chest compressions. Ensure emergency drugs are readily available. Do not delay defibrillation in the presence of a shockable rhythm.
6. Search for treatable causes of pulseless electrical activity (PEA)/asystole (see **L-6**).

L-6: What Are Some Treatable Causes of Pulseless Electrical Activity (PEA) or Asystole?

Initiation of high-quality cardiopulmonary resuscitation (CPR) and restoration of a perfusing rhythm are paramount when encountering sudden PEA or asystole in the operating room. Identifying a treatable cause is fundamental in successful resuscitation. During the management of PEA/asystole, the anesthesiologist should consider what has long been referred to as the Hs and Ts of PEA/asystole (see Table 23.3) that may be hindering resuscitative efforts [1].

1. Hypovolemia
   Hypovolemia is one of the most common causes of hypotension, whether due to excessive fluid losses or inadequate fluid administration. Fluid losses can be in the form of free water or blood and can be hemodynamically significant when the losses result in impaired venous return and cardiac output. By communicating with the surgeons and surveying the surgical field, the anesthesiologist can quickly assess for acute hemorrhage. The presence of occult hemorrhage with blood pooling in places such as the retroperitoneum, in the patient's drapes, under the OR table, or in other inconspicuous locations should also be considered.
   An account of the surgical approach and anesthetic management may also reveal factors that can contribute to a decreased preload such as surgical pressure on the vena cava, insufflation of the peritoneum, neuraxial anesthesia, or anesthetics. Contributing factors should be treated as appropriate with fluid boluses, blood products, left uterine displacement, releasing peritoneal insufflation, releasing visceral retraction, and turning down or off the anesthetics.

Table 23.3 Treatable causes of PEA/asystole

Hypovolemia	Tamponade
Hydrogen ions (acidosis)	Thrombosis
Hypothermia	Toxins and tablets
Hypoxia	Tension pneumothorax
Hyper/hypokalemia	

2. Hydrogen ions
   Either metabolic or respiratory acidosis can lead to cardiac arrest. An ABG sample and a blood chemistry panel should be evaluated, adequate ventilation ensured, and pH disturbances treated as appropriate.
3. Hypothermia
   Hypothermia can cause cardiac depression, myocardial ischemia, dysrhythmias, leftward shift of the oxyhemoglobin dissociation curve, coagulopathies, acidosis, and a blunted response to catecholamines [10]. Maintenance of normothermia is cardioprotective. Measures such as forced air warmer, warmed IV fluids, and warmed room should be taken in order to provide normothermia.
4. Hypoxia
   Adequate oxygenation is essential in order to maintain hemodynamic stability and attempt to maximize oxygen delivery during hemodynamic collapse. The patient should be ventilated with 100% FiO2 and all volatile anesthetics turned off. One must also ensure proper placement of endotracheal tube by auscultation and possibly direct laryngoscopy. Keep in mind that there will not be confirmation of ETCO2 if there is no cardiac output. Other actions include suctioning or repositioning of the endotracheal tube and treating bronchospasm with a beta-agonist.
5. Hyperkalemia or hypokalemia
   Maintaining a normal potassium gradient across cell membranes is essential in ensuring normal transmission of action potentials and resting membrane potentials in myocardial cells. Significant changes in potassium levels can result in cardiac instability. Other electrolyte disturbances can also disrupt gradients across cell membranes. Therefore a complete metabolic panel including sodium, potassium, chloride, bicarbonate, magnesium, calcium, and glucose should be drawn and disturbances corrected as warranted.
6. Cardiac tamponade
   Increased pressure in the pericardium, as seen with cardiac tamponade, can result in decrease filling of the right heart. Without adequate cardiac filling, the result is decreased cardiac output leading to rapid cardiovascular collapse. Relief of cardiac tamponade can be achieved with either pericardiocentesis or surgery (pericardial "window" or median sternotomy). TEE (or TTE if the esophagus is inaccessible) should be called to the OR to assist with diagnosis. Anesthetic goals include maintaining venous return with adequate volume, avoiding drugs that may cause vasodilation or myocardial depression, preserving systemic blood pressure, and maintaining a relative tachycardia [5].
7. Thrombosis
   Coronary artery thrombus or pulmonary emboli (PE) (secondary to clot, fat, or amniotic fluid) can lead to severe hemodynamic decompensation and cardiac arrest. TTE or TEE may be used to identify regional wall motion abnormalities and can assist in the diagnosis of coronary thrombus. PE can be difficult to diagnose under general anesthesia. American Heart Association (AHA) recommendations suggest empirical fibrinolytic therapy when a PE is suspected [1]. Prior

to initiation, however, fibrinolytic therapy should be discussed with the surgical team in order to weigh the risks of anticoagulation during surgery. Other advanced treatment options include extracorporeal membrane oxygenation (ECMO).

8. Toxins and tablets

   Poisonings or overdose of prescription medications should be considered in the nonsurgical patient. However, during general anesthesia, the anesthesiologist should consider all medications administered as potential contributors to hemodynamic collapse. Iatrogenic causes leading to bradycardia (see **L-4**) can also lead to cardiac collapse if left uncorrected. Anaphylactic reactions to anesthetic drugs can also precipitate PEA/asystole. Offending medications should be discontinued and reversal agents or antidotes administered as appropriate.

9. Tension pneumothorax

   Tension pneumothorax can cause pressure on the heart and great vessels leading to decreased filling, decreased cardiac output, and ultimately cardiac collapse. Diagnosis of pneumothorax can be difficult under general anesthesia. The presence of unilateral breath sounds, tracheal deviation, and information obtained with a TEE or TTE examination can assist in the intraoperative diagnosis. Surface pulmonary ultrasound can also be useful, showing absent pulmonary tissue and loss of the "sliding sign" on the side affected. If a tension pneumothorax is suspected, nitrous oxide (N2O) should be discontinued, insufflation should be terminated, and immediate needle decompression should be performed on the affected side. Decompression in adults is done with a large-bore needle or angiocatheter at the second intercostal space, midclavicular line.

L-7: Importance of Vigilance, Teamwork, and Communication in the OR

Constant vigilance on the part of the anesthesiologist is paramount to patient safety. The concept of vigilance is reinforced repeatedly in the profession, and the word "vigilance" is even found on the American Society of Anesthesiologists seal. The anesthesiologist must be able to continually assess the situation and environment for changes yet simultaneously focus on specific tasks during a crisis situation. This level of mental attention can at times be taxing due to stress, fatigue, monotony of task, or other factors [11]. In an attempt to optimize performance, St Pierre et al. suggest taking the effects of fatigue seriously. Frequent breaks or relief should be requested if needed, as performance deficits often precede the feelings of fatigue. In addition, developing a degree of situational awareness allows one to assess a situation and anticipate future clinical developments [11].

Beyond vigilance however, the anesthesiologist has a responsibility to communicate with the surgical team about acute physiologic events during the operative procedure and in this sense has a role in guiding surgical management. At times during a crisis, it is necessary for the anesthesiologist to take the lead in communicating roles and functions to other physicians and staff to successfully manage the situation. This type of communication and fortitude helps team members to function effectively together during an otherwise chaotic situation. Although there are many barriers to effective communication, there are strategies to help promote good communication. Practicing active listening, clearly conveying concerns, establishing relationships with members of the team, and using congruent body language are just a few methods that can be employed in everyday situations to ensure effective communication during a crisis [11].

Oftentimes, in the intraoperative setting, there are multiple demands and responsibilities that may lead to a setting that verges on chaos. It is critical, therefore, to have an interdisciplinary approach to cope with the demands of this environment. The operating room team, including the surgeon, anesthesiologist, nurses, support staff, and patient, should be knowledgeable about their environment and comfortable with open communication among team members in order to facilitate success. A breakdown in teamwork and communication in the healthcare team has repeatedly been shown to be a key factor in poor care and the occurrence of medical errors [11]. In a high-stakes environment such as the OR, performance as a team will exceed the sum of individual abilities. Congruence among OR team members is essential, because ultimately all players involved have the same goal, to guide the patient safely and successfully through the surgery. All operating rooms should have a pre-approved plan for handling emergencies, with policies and procedures to cover such events.

Multiple times, throughout the case being discussed, the anesthesiologist demonstrated vigilance to the changing surgical and physiologic environment. Early in the case, when the patient was experiencing episodes of bradycardia, she notified the surgery team. The surgery team then showed cognizance of the manipulations they were performing, including vagal nerve stimulation, that were contributing to the event. Later, when the surgeons communicated difficulty with removal of the esophagus, the anesthesiologist was cued to prepare epinephrine, realizing that this may be a critical time for adverse hemodynamic events. Immediate communication by the anesthesiologist with the surgical team, by prompt announcement of the asystolic event, resulted in rapid initiation of chest compressions, which was critical in the successful resuscitation of the patient. These scenarios demonstrate the importance of vigilance on the part of the anesthesiologist, the role of effective interdisciplinary communication, and the indispensable function of teamwork in the OR.

References

1. American Heart Association. Web-based integrated guidelines for cardiopulmonary resuscitation and emergency cardiovascular care – part 7: adult advanced cardiovascular life support. ECCguidelines.heart.org. American Heart Association, Inc. 2015.
2. Doyle DJ, Mark PW. Reflex bradycardia during surgery. Can J Anaesth. 1990;37(2):219–22.
3. Valentin M, Tulsyan N, Dolgin C. Recurrent asystolic cardiac arrest and laparoscopic cholecystectomy: a case report and review of the literature. JSLS. 2004;8(1):65–8.

4. Schaller B, Cornelius JF, Prabhaker H, et al. The trigemino-cardiac reflex: an update of the current knowledge. J Neurosurg Anesthesiol. 2009;21(3):187–95.
5. Barash PG, Cullen BF, Stoelting RK, Cahalan MK, Stock MC, Ortega R. Clinical anesthesia. 7th ed. Philadelphia: Lippincott Williams & Wilkins; 2013.
6. Campagna J, Carter C. Clinical relevance of the bezold-jarisch reflex. Anesthesiology. 2003;98(5):1250–8.
7. Nikbakhsh N, Parviz M, Asdollah S, et al. Changes in blood pressure and heart rhythm during transhiatal esophagectomy. Caspian J Intern Med. 2012;3(4):541–5.
8. Ahmadinejad M, Hashemi M, Tabatabai A, et al. Incidence and risk factors of an intraoperative arrhythmia in transhiatal esophagectomy. Iran Red Crescent Med J. 2015;17(12):e22053.
9. Orringer M. Transhiatal esophagectomy without thoracotomy. Oper Tech Thorac Cardiovasc Surg. 2005;10(1):63–83.
10. Miller RD, Pardo MC. Basics of anesthesia. 6th ed. Philadelphia: Elsevier Saunders; 2011.
11. St. Pierre M, Hofinger G, Beurschaper C. Crisis management in acute care settings: human factors and team psychology in a high stakes environment. Berlin: Springer; 2008.

Chapter 24
Anesthesia for the Obese Parturient

Ryan W. Hill and Leon Chang

Case Description

The patient was a 27-year-old woman Gravida 2 Para 1, 5′10″, 158 kg (BMI 44), with a past medical history significant for asthma, hypertension, poorly controlled diabetes mellitus type 2, morbid obesity, slipped capital femoral epiphysis repair as a teenager, anemia, and homelessness. The patient was pregnant at 36 weeks gestation with diamniotic, dichorionic twins. The pregnancy was complicated by group B streptococcus vaginal colonization and severe preeclampsia. The patient was initially admitted for glycemic control that was achieved by an insulin sliding scale. Subsequently she developed severely elevated blood pressure, which improved with labetalol and a magnesium sulfate infusion, to the 140s/80s range. The patient was later scheduled for cesarean section (C-section) because of malpresentation of twin A.

The patient's airway exam revealed macroglossia; an inter-incisor distance of greater than 4 cm; Mallampati score of 2; thyromental distance of 5–6 cm; a short, thick neck; and the ability to prognath. Laboratory studies were significant for hemoglobin of 9.9 g/dl, platelets of 240,000/microL, and magnesium of 3.6 mg/dl (reference range 1.6–2.6). She was type and cross-matched for two units of packed red blood cells and had a negative antibody screen.

A combined spinal and epidural anesthetic was planned as the patient did not yet have an epidural catheter in situ, and the obstetricians felt that the surgery would likely take longer than 2 h given the patient's body habitus.

R. W. Hill
Department of Anesthesiology, University of California, San Diego, CA, USA

L. Chang (✉)
Department of Anesthesiology, University of California, San Diego Medical Center, San Diego, CA, USA
e-mail: lchang@ucsd.edu

J. L. Benumof, G. R. Manecke (eds.), *Clinical Anesthesiology II*,
https://doi.org/10.1007/978-3-030-12365-9_24

The patient was brought to the operating room (OR) and positioned seated upright on the OR table. She was prepped and draped in sterile fashion, and the skin was anesthetized using 3 ml of 1% lidocaine via a 25 g needle. The epidural space was located with difficulty, requiring two attempts using a 17 g Touhy needle. On the second attempt, a loss of resistance was achieved; however, a 25 g spinal needle was passed through the Tuohy, and no "pop" or return of CSF was obtained. At this point the patient became increasingly agitated, felt "sick," and requested to lie down. The Tuohy needle was removed and the patient asked to bear one more attempt. The same loss of resistance occurred, but again CSF return or "pop" of the spinal needle breaching the dura was lacking. As the patient was becoming increasingly agitated, the spinal portion was abandoned, the epidural catheter was quickly and easily threaded, and the patient was allowed to lie down and positioned for surgery.

The epidural catheter was dosed with 10 ml of 2% lidocaine with bicarbonate and 1:200,000 epinephrine. The onset of anesthesia was slow and another 10 ml of the same medication was given. After a few minutes, the patient's degree of anesthesia was again tested, with the patient endorsing loss of cold sensation up to the T6 dermatome level. After another few minutes, the level was tested a final time, but this time she reported that she could feel cold at all levels. Given a very unclear and contradictory sensory exam, the obstetricians were allowed to prepare and drape; the plan was to perform a more definitive and patient-blind test with a surgical clamp. There was a high suspicion that the block would be inadequate for surgery and a general anesthetic would be required. The patient's pannus was taped up over her shoulders for surgical exposure. The clamp test was then performed and the patient did not have an adequate surgical block.

The need to convert to general anesthesia was then discussed with the patient who agreed to proceed. Preoxygenation was performed for approximately 3 min, with end-tidal oxygen >85% and SpO_2 at 100%. General anesthesia was induced with propofol and succinylcholine and intubation attempted, and a grade 4 view was obtained (neither epiglottis nor glottis could be visualized). There was considerable difficulty placing the laryngoscope into the mouth due to macroglossia and proximity of the chest wall to the handle of the laryngoscope. Direct laryngoscopy was again attempted by a more senior practitioner, also yielding a grade 4 view. The patient's oxygen saturation began to fall, and mask ventilation was begun successfully; however, ventilation was difficult and would likely not be able to be continued indefinitely. Help was called for and the taped pannus was released. A Cookgas air-Q® LMA was placed with improvement in ventilation. However, the patient's oxygenation was very slow to improve, remaining at or below 90% for approximately 5 min despite sufficient ventilation and tidal volumes ~350 ml through the LMA. Help arrived with a fiber-optic bronchoscope (FOB). An intermediate (4.0 mm OD) FOB with an Aintree® catheter loaded to the most proximal part of the FOB was passed through the LMA into the trachea down to the carina. The FOB was then removed, leaving the

Aintree® well within the trachea and the LMA still in place. The LMA was removed by securing the proximal portion of the Aintree® catheter while backing up the LMA and then fixing the catheter as soon as possible at the teeth, while the LMA was completely removed. At this point, the Aintree® catheter remained in the trachea, 25 cm at the teeth. A 7.0 ETT was advanced over the catheter. Once near the teeth, the catheter was backed up minimally until the proximal portion could again be controlled. The tube was then advanced over the catheter using counterclockwise rotation into the trachea, and the catheter was removed. Tracheal placement was confirmed via sustained end-tidal CO_2.

The endotracheal tube allowed larger tidal volumes and recruitment maneuvers to be performed, which in turn resulted in return of SpO_2 to 100%. No gastric contents were noted in either the oropharynx or tracheobronchial tree, and an orogastric tube was placed in the stomach and suctioned. The remainder of the case and emergence were uneventful, with no apparent anesthetic complications.

L-1: Anesthetic Options: Advantages and Disadvantages

It is important to first describe the anesthetic options and the benefits and disadvantages of each technique. Five possible techniques will be discussed, including single-shot spinal, epidural, combined spinal epidural, continuous spinal, and general anesthesia.

L-1a: Single-Shot Spinal

A single-shot spinal involves a one-time injection of local anesthetic +/− adjuncts such as opiates or clonidine into the intrathecal space. The advantages of this technique include relative ease of placement, fast onset, and a dense and reliable bilateral block. There is also low risk of local anesthetic toxicity due to small total amounts of local anesthetic administered (e.g., 10–15 mg of bupivacaine).

Disadvantages include limited duration (generally 2–3 h in parturients), which may be inadequate for longer surgical procedures. Hypotension is also relatively common – this may occur from a rapid sympathectomy resulting in arterial and venous dilation. In the extreme, this could progress to cardiovascular collapse in the case of a "high spinal." Finally, like all neuraxial procedures, there is a risk of bleeding (with potentially devastating complications such as spinal or epidural hematoma), infection (e.g., epidural abscess, CNS infection), and damage to surrounding structures. Finally, there is approximately 1% chance of a post-dural puncture headache (PDPH) in this patient population.

L-1b: Epidural

Epidural anesthesia typically involves threading a small catheter into the epidural space through which local anesthetic and adjuncts can be injected. Advantages of this technique include a virtually unlimited duration of anesthesia, the ability to titrate medications in controlled fashion (which in turn can yield less hemodynamic effects), and versatility – anesthesia can be provided for a myriad of needs, including analgesia for labor and delivery, surgical anesthesia for C-sections, and postoperative pain control.

Disadvantages of this technique include relatively slower onset than a spinal, combined spinal epidural, or general anesthetic. Therefore, epidural anesthesia may not be the best choice in an emergency. In addition, there is a higher risk of systemic local anesthetic toxicity than a single shot spinal, given the larger volumes of local anesthetic necessary to produce analgesia and the vascular nature of the epidural space. This vascularity may be especially pronounced in parturients. Epidurals are also characteristically less reliable than a spinal or general anesthetic for surgical anesthesia, with "patchy," incomplete, or one-sided blocks being fairly common. This procedure carries the usual risks of bleeding, infection, and damage to surrounding nerves. Because a large needle is used, epidural attempts carry a higher risk of PDPH than spinal, should an inadvertent dural breach occur.

L-1c: Combined Spinal and Epidural (CSE)

The combined spinal and epidural (CSE) technique involves first finding the epidural space and then passing a spinal needle through the larger bore epidural needle, achieving CSF flow, and then administering medication into the intrathecal space. The spinal needle is then removed, and the epidural catheter is threaded into the epidural space. This technique captures the benefits of both spinal and epidural in a single procedure. These include the fast onset of action of a spinal, with a virtually unlimited duration of action, as the epidural can be dosed prior to and after the spinal wearing off. Performing a CSE can also improve the likelihood that the epidural catheter will be properly placed, as it confirms that the needle is midline. Indeed, some practitioners will utilize the CSE technique as a diagnostic tool to aid epidural placement only, without administering medication through the spinal needle. The combined spinal epidural can also be used for both blood pressure stability and fast onset by giving a small spinal dose and then early titrated medication via the epidural catheter.

Disadvantages of this procedure include the inability to test the epidural immediately if a spinal dose is given. One could then be faced with a situation in which the spinal wears off, only to find out that there is a nonfunctioning or inadequate epidural. There is also a higher risk of local anesthetic toxicity than spinal alone given the larger volumes of local anesthetic administered and the vascular nature of the epidural space. Finally, there are the same risks as other neuraxial procedures, as discussed above.

L-1d: Continuous Spinal

This technique involves finding the intrathecal space with an epidural needle and placing a catheter into this space. The advantages of this method are essentially all those of a single-shot spinal, with the added ability to titrate medication slowly and to re-dose if necessary.

Disadvantages include a high risk of PDPH (50%) as compared to spinal or epidural because of the large bore needle breaching the dura and leaving a passage for CSF leakage once the catheter is removed. There is also a higher risk of serious CNS infection such as meningitis given the continuous tract from the skin to the intrathecal space. In addition, most practitioners have less experience with this technique because it is not as commonly performed as either spinal, epidural, or CSE. Finally, all the previously discussed generic risks of neuraxial procedures apply.

L-1e: General Anesthesia

It is important to remember that general anesthesia is an option for cesarean section, although it is usually not preferred. The advantages of general anesthesia include potentially the fastest onset of any technique, the ability to tailor the duration of anesthesia to surgical requirement, minimal to no risk of local anesthetic toxicity, and reliable surgical anesthesia. General anesthesia also does not carry the risks associated with a neuraxial procedure such as PDPH.

The drawbacks to general anesthesia are potentially severe, and the mortality rate associated with general anesthesia in parturients is higher than that of regional anesthesia. The airway must be instrumented, and this patient population is at particular risk for both aspiration and a difficult airway. Additionally, there may be delivery of anesthetics to the baby, and there is the potential for increased uterine relaxation from volatile anesthetics. This relaxation can be resistant to maneuvers to increase uterine tone. There may be hemodynamic instability on induction, and finally, the mother, not being awake, is unable to participate in the birth of her baby.

L-2: Causes of Failed Spinal

There are a number of reasons for a failed spinal. Most of the reasons fall into two categories: the inability to identify (procure CSF) and inject medication into the subarachnoid space and an inadequate dose of spinal medication.

L-2a: Failure to Identify (Procure CSF) the Subarachnoid Space

This problem is often operator dependent and is more common in the trainee than the experienced anesthesiologist. However, no matter the experience level of the practitioner, this type of failure is more common in the obese, anxious, or moving patient. In the obese patient, it may be difficult to palpate landmarks and locate the midline. Patient positioning is crucial in the obese patient, as poor positioning can make a difficult spinal placement even more challenging. Incorrect needle trajectory with poor positioning is likely the most common cause of inability to locate the intrathecal space. A helpful tip is that if the bone is encountered relatively superficially, this is likely spinous process, and the needle should be redirected cranially or caudally; on the other hand, if the bone is encountered more deeply, this is likely lamina, and the needle should be adjusted left or right. In the case of the moving or anxious patient, speaking with them ahead of time and answering questions may help calm them; small doses of anxiolytics and making sure the skin is thoroughly anesthetized may also be useful. Advancing the spinal needle without the stylet in place can be problematic as a tissue plug or clot can occlude the lumen of the needle, and CSF will not be obtained even if the needle enters the intrathecal space. Abnormalities of the spine may also make successful placement difficult. These include prior back surgery with instrumentation, scoliosis, kyphosis, and calcified ligaments. It is also possible to get return of clear fluid that is not CSF. In some cases, this could be previously placed local anesthetic or saline (e.g., recently dosed or attempted epidural, too much local anesthetic when numbing up the skin and soft tissue). Finally, there are very rare causes such as a congenital arachnoid cyst.

L-2b: Inadequate Spinal Dose

Inadequate dose as a cause of spinal failure is most often due to a misplaced injection of local anesthetic [1]. The misplacement of local anesthetic may be as simple as having fluid leakage between the needle hub and syringe if the syringe is not adequately secured. It is also possible for the spinal needle position to migrate superficially or deep when attaching the syringe. More nuanced occurrences are the possibility of the pencil-point needle lumen straddling the dura so that some local anesthetic is injected epidurally and some subarachnoid as pictured below (Fig. 24.1).

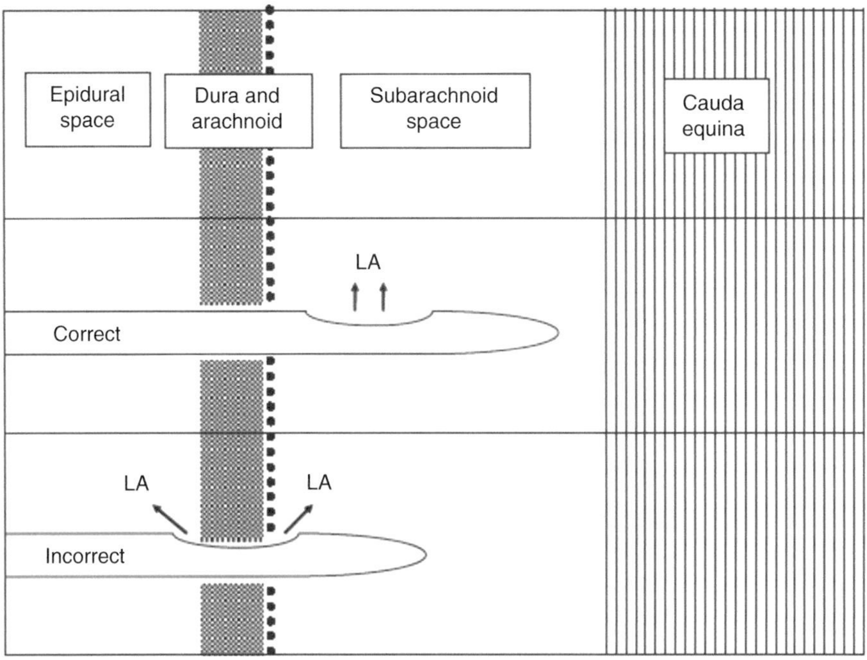

Fig. 24.1 Possible positions of the tip of a pencil-point needle. In the upper image, all the local anesthetic solution will reach the subarachnoid space, but if the opening straddles the dura (lower image), some solution will be deposited in the epidural space. (Reprinted from Fettes et al. [1]. With permission from Elsevier)

Another possibility is the dura acting as a flap so that during aspiration, the dura and arachnoid layers are pulled back and CSF enters the needle, but upon injection, the flap is pushed forward, and the dose is not delivered to the intrathecal space. A variant of this situation is the dura and arachnoid layers separating so that the injected dose of local anesthetic goes subdural as illustrated below.

L-3: Causes of Failed Epidural

Causes of failed epidurals can be divided into three main categories: initial misplacement of the epidural needle, suboptimal catheter position upon threading or migration during labor, and patient anatomic variations.

In considering epidural needle or catheter position, there are four areas where the needle tip could be. The first is subcutaneous and is likely the most common cause of complete epidural failures. In obese patients with a large amount of soft tissue present, it may be easier to obtain a false “loss of resistance” while still in the subcutaneous space. This may result from engaging interspinous ligament at some point and thus encountering resistance, followed by the needle crossing midline into subcutaneous tissue with a subsequent tactile loss of resistance. Obesity is a risk factor for threading an epidural catheter into this space. Arendt$_2$ describes the locations where an epidural catheter or needle may wind up and explains why a failed epidural might initially be missed in a laboring patient. A laboring patient may initially endorse analgesia, possibly from a transient decrease in contractions from pausing an oxytocin infusion or pre-epidural fluid loading. If opioids are added to the epidural mixture, there can be some systemic opioid absorption leading to slight analgesia. Finally, there is a possible placebo effect from placing an epidural, which may lead the patient to report improvement in their pain score even in the case of a misplaced epidural.

Secondly, the epidural needle can inadvertently enter the intrathecal space, known as a "wet tap"; typically, the practitioner observes free-flowing CSF out the hub of the needle, but this is not always the case. If a dose meant for the epidural space is delivered via either catheter or needle into the intrathecal space, a profound block and a high spinal can result.

Another possible mal-location is the subdural space (Fig. 24.2). If dosed, this may lead to patchy, incomplete block with variable sensory, motor, and autonomic effects. Presentation not unlike a high spinal is possible as the subdural space cannot

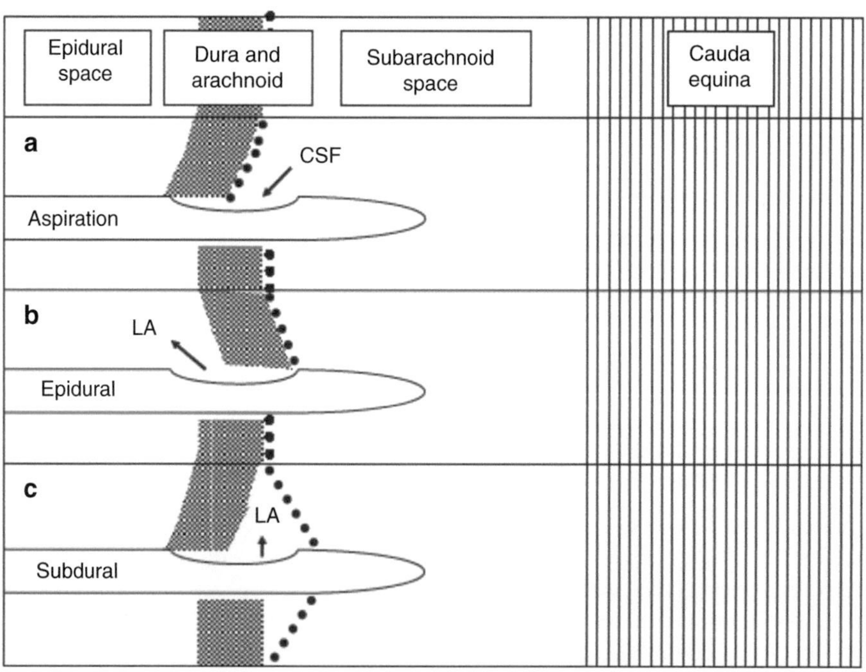

Fig. 24.2 The dura or arachnoid mater may act as a flap valve across the opening of a pencil-point needle. During aspiration (**a**) the dura/arachnoid is pulled back allowing CSF to enter the needle. During injection the dura (**b**) or arachnoid (**c**) is pushed forward and the local anesthetic enters the epidural or subdural space. (Reprinted from Fettes et al. [1]. With permission from Elsevier)

accommodate the same volume of fluid as the epidural space and marked spread in the cranial direction is possible.

The final possibility is intravascular needle or catheter placement. This is more likely in the pregnant population because the gravid uterus compresses the IVC, causing dilation of collateral veins in the epidural space. Intravascular placement may but not always be detected by the return of blood into the catheter or needle. It is thus important to aspirate gently before injecting local anesthetic and to provide small doses incrementally. If an unrecognized large dose is given, local anesthetic toxicity may result. During labor the parturient is likely to readjust position frequently, and this may lead to migration of an initially well-placed epidural into any one of the abovementioned, non-epidural spaces.

As with spinal anesthetics, variations in patient anatomy may interfere with successful epidural placement. The epidural space is notoriously heterogeneous, with epidural fat and engorged blood vessels that can affect the spread of local anesthetic. This heterogeneity can be one of the causes of patchy anesthetic coverage. A dorsal median connective tissue band has been described in some patients that can act as a partition down the midline of the epidural space. If the catheter is on one side of that tissue band, there may not be spread to the other side resulting in unilateral block. More likely causes of unilateral block are patient positioning (settling of local anesthetic on one side due to gravity) or an epidural that is threaded too far and migrates to one side. Repositioning the patient or pulling the epidural catheter back slightly and re-securing it can often remedy these situations.

L-4: Risks of Re-attempting Neuraxial Anesthesia

When faced with a failed epidural or spinal, most practitioners would recommend re-attempting the procedure at a different level. Even though in most cases this is a reasonable approach, re-attempting a spinal or epidural is not without increased risk. To begin, subsequent attempts may be more technically difficult than the initial attempt for a number of reasons. The patient may have been sitting up for some time and may tire of remaining still in this position. In the case of a failed epidural that had been recently dosed, there may be pockets of local anesthetic in the patient's back that could contribute to a false loss of resistance on the second attempt. Should a spinal be attempted, this may contribute to obtaining local anesthetic that appears to be CSF (false positive CSF). Furthermore, if a "wet tap" were to occur, there is a chance that pre-existing local anesthetic in or near the epidural space could enter the intrathecal space resulting in a high spinal. Local anesthetic toxicity is also a risk when re-attempting an epidural after dosing of a previous epidural because an even larger amount of local anesthetic that may approach or exceed toxic ranges is being introduced into a highly vascular region. Finally, the dose to administer if attempting a spinal after a patient has had an epidural may be very unclear. Pregnant women already have a lower requirement for intrathecal local anesthetic because the engorged epidural vessels push the CSF more cranially by putting pressure on the intrathecal sac. By adding local anesthetic volume to the epidural space, this compression is increased and can lead to a high spinal at doses that would not normally cause this problem. The chosen dose must be adjusted accordingly.

L-5: Physiology of the Obese Parturient

Relevant physiology of the obese pregnant patient will be discussed in this section. These include factors contributing to maternal hypoxemia and hastening time to oxyhemoglobin desaturation, namely, shunt and cardiovascular compromise from aortocaval compression. The parturient's difficult airway compared to baseline, full stomach considerations after 20 weeks gestation, and the effects of pregnancy on CSF volume will be discussed as well.

L-5a: Cardiopulmonary

Functional residual capacity (FRC) decreases by approximately 20% in pregnancy, and an obese patient's FRC will be further reduced compared to their non-obese counterparts. This magnifies the reduction in oxygen reserve, causing a "two-pronged insult" (pregnancy plus obesity) that greatly hastens oxyhemoglobin desaturation. Obesity itself also causes a decrease in chest wall compliance and increases the work of breathing. These factors all contribute to increased shunt (areas of the lung that are perfused, but not ventilated). Further, aortocaval compression by the gravid uterus (in our case study *twin* gravid uterus) and, in the case of the obesity, further weight of a large pannus cause compression of the great vessels at the level of the uterus, impeding venous return to the heart. This decreases cardiac output and thus increases tissue oxygen extraction ratio. When the increasingly deoxygenated venous blood mixes through normal physiologic shunts (and others secondary to decreased FRC) with the fully oxygenated blood coming from the lungs, the arterial oxygen content is lowered, leading to arterial oxygen desaturation. Finally, the pregnant patient has increased oxygen consumption due to fetal oxygen consumption and requirements. If a patient is also obese, they have overall more tissue that consumes oxygen (although the oxygen requirement for adipose tissue is generally lower than more metabolically active tissue). The following diagrams illustrate the downward spiral of oxygen saturation from shunt and decreased cardiac output from aortocaval compression. This physiology not only hastens the time to desaturation but can also increase the time it takes for the patient's SpO2 to recover after a desaturation. This was very apparent in the case presented in this chapter (Fig. 24.3)

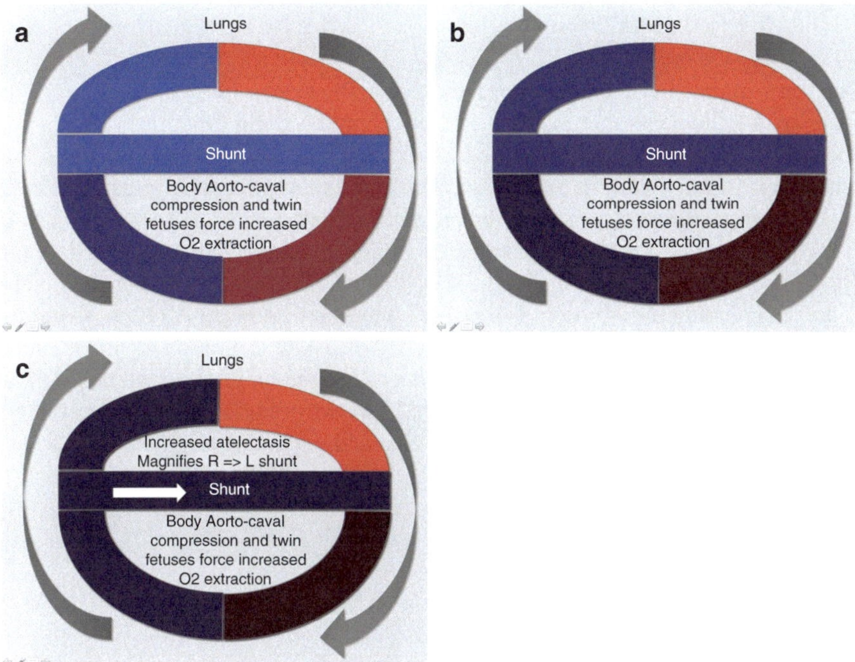

Fig. 24.3 (**a**) Aortocaval compression (**b**) increased intrapulmonary shunt and (**c**) increased peripheral oxygen utilization combine to cause rapid arterial oxyhemoglobin desaturation in the parturient

L-5b: Airway

Parturients are notorious for having an airway that is more difficult to manage than it would be in their nonpregnant state. One reason for the increased difficulty of ventilating and intubating parturients is that they often have airway edema from engorged capillary veins all along the airway. In addition, their oral and nasal mucosa is more friable than baseline, which can lead to a bloody airway with minimal instrumentation, making visualization of the vocal cords even more challenging. The obese parturient in this case presented further airway difficulty, with a thick neck and increased pharyngeal soft tissue available to collapse around the airway. In these patients, positioning is even more important as laryngoscopy must be optimized for the first attempt. In addition, it is common at the authors' institution for the obstetricians to tape the patient's pannus up for surgical exposure prior to induction of anesthesia. The tape is anchored over the patient's shoulders, pulling the belly upwards and applying pressure to the thorax. This increases atelectasis and further decreases FRC, hastening the time to oxyhemoglobin desaturation. Desaturation occurs very quickly in this circumstance despite 3–5 min of thorough preoxygenation.

L-5c: Gastrointestinal

Pregnant patients have a number of factors that affect their GI system, but we will focus on the elements that increase risk of aspiration during induction of general anesthesia. First, they have decreased lower esophageal sphincter tone due to the high levels of circulating progesterone. This makes them especially susceptible to gastrointestinal reflux (GERD) during pregnancy. Next, they have decreased gastric emptying such that at any given time their stomach is more full than those of their nonpregnant counterparts. Finally, the gravid uterus puts pressure on the abdominal contents including the stomach, increasing intragastric pressure. All of these physiologic changes cause the parturient to be at higher risk of aspiration on induction of anesthesia. These changes are more pronounced later in pregnancy, and therefore it is mandatory that all pregnant patients over 20 weeks gestation be treated as if they have full stomachs. A rapid sequence induction and intubation must be performed if general anesthesia is induced.

L-5d: Neurological

As previously mentioned, pregnant patients have lower local anesthetic requirements during spinal anesthesia. This is because pregnancy decreases CSF volume (vide supra). The decrease in CSF volume may be even more pronounced in the obese parturient. The gravid uterus and the patient's excess soft tissue cause compression of the inferior vena cava (IVC), which increases blood flow through the lumbar vertebral plexus causing engorgement of the epidural veins. This increases pressure on the intrathecal sac, displacing fluid cranially and lowering the overall space the CSF occupies. With less space, it is possible to obtain increased spread of local anesthetic and a higher than anticipated level of anesthesia. This must be taken into account, especially if a spinal is to be attempted after an epidural because additional fluid injected into the epidural space may further displace the intrathecal sac and reduce overall space (Fig. 24.4).

L-6: Considerations for Converting to General Anesthesia

Although general anesthesia is usually not the preferred method for C-section, there are many situations that necessitate conversion from a neuraxial technique to a general as was presented in the case description. There are a number of considerations to be aware of when it becomes necessary to perform a general anesthetic in an obese parturient, especially if this was not the originally intended method of anesthesia. The first factor to address is overcoming plan change inertia. This means getting organized for the new anesthetic as if it were the original plan and going

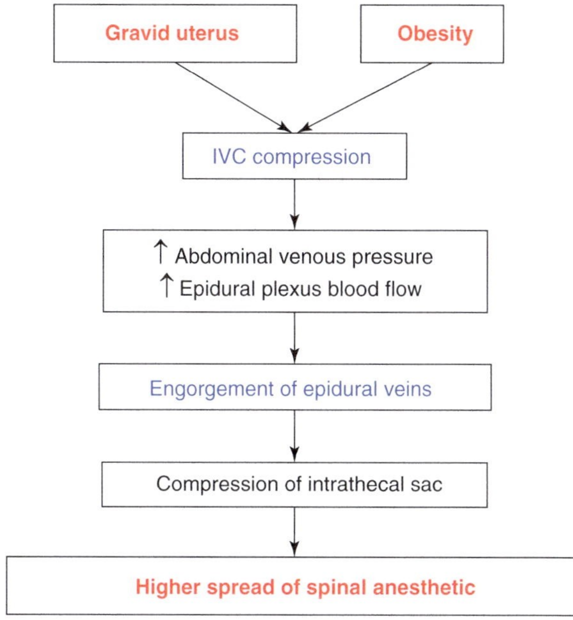

Fig. 24.4 Factors leading to enhanced spread of spinal anesthetic in the obese parturient

through the normal checklists to have the machine, medications, airway equipment, etc. ready before induction. Although this may seem obvious, there is a real phenomenon whereby practitioners tend to not be as well-prepared when changing quickly to an anesthetic that was not initially planned. The next consideration is optimizing patient positioning. If a neuraxial was intended, there may not have been as much care to place the patient in an ideal "sniffing" position in preparation for intubation. This is doubly important in an obese parturient who is at higher risk for having a difficult airway and has a shortened time to desaturation if the airway is not immediately established. The patient should be ramped until the sternal angle is parallel with the external auditory meatus; this has been shown to optimize the direct laryngoscopy view. In addition, if the patient's pannus has been taped up, strong consideration should be given to releasing it prior to induction. Adequate preoxygenation is also crucial. It may be worthwhile to preoxygenate these patients in the sitting position as this has been shown to provide approximately one extra minute before desaturation to 90% [2].

The laryngeal mask airway (LMA) is an established early rescue option on the ASA difficult airway algorithm for "cannot intubate, cannot ventilate" situations. A number of LMAs (e.g., Cookgas LMA®) are also designed to facilitate intubation via fiber-optic bronchoscopy, and several different intubation techniques exist. In this case, the LMA provided both the critical ability to ventilate and served as a useful conduit for intubation. All anesthesia practitioners should be proficient at placing an LMA to rescue ventilation and at using an LMA as a tool for intubation. Further discussion and videos can be found at https://www.cookmedical.com/products/cc_caeaic_webds/.

The next consideration when converting to a general anesthetic for C-section is the effect of volatile anesthetics in decreasing uterine tone, which can lead to hemorrhage and an unstable patient. This should be taken into account especially when the patient has other risk factors for uterine atony including multiparity, multiple gestations, prolonged labor, macrosomia, or other factors such as a magnesium infusion. In this case, both magnesium and a twin gestation were potential risk factors, although uterine atony did not occur. If in a situation where general anesthesia is necessary with risk factors for uterine atony, the practitioner should reevaluate IV access and monitors; consideration should be given to placing extra large bore IVs, an arterial line, and even central access if massive hemorrhage is anticipated.

Conclusion

When planning an anesthetic for obstetrical surgery in the obese parturient, there are many considerations, including urgency, length of surgery, whether an epidural is in situ, and the pros and cons of each possible anesthetic technique. It is important to be able to recognize a failed or inadequate neuraxial anesthetic in order to properly troubleshoot or avoid pitfalls. Importantly, provider tendency to accept suboptimal conditions for neuraxial or general anesthesia should be resisted with the utmost scrupulousness. Finally, it is crucial to be familiar with the altered physiology of the obese parturient and how it might affect the planned anesthetic.

References

1. Fettes PDW, et al. Failed spinal anaesthesia: mechanisms, management, and prevention. Br J Anaesth. 2009;102(6):739–48.
2. Altermatt FR, et al. Pre-oxygenation in the obese patient: effects of position on tolerance to apnoea. Br J Anaesth. 2005;95(5):706–9.

Suggested Reading

1. Arendt K, Segal S. Why epidurals do not always work. Rev Obstet Gynecol. 2008;1(2):49–55.
2. Greenland KB, et al. External auditory meatus-sternal notch relationship in adults in the sniffing position: a magnetic resonance imaging study. Br J Anaesth. 2010;104(2):268–9.
3. Hawkins JL, Chang J, Palmer SK, Gibbs CP, Callaghan WM. Anesthesia-related maternal mortality in the United States: 1979–2002. Obstet Gynecol. 2011;117(1):69–74.
4. Mcculloch WJD, Littlewood DG. Influence of obesity on spinal analgesia with isobaric 0.5% bupivacaine. BJA Br J Anaesth. 1986;58(6):610–4. Web.
5. OpenAnesthesia. Physiologic changes of pregnancy. 2018. Retrieved from: https://www.openanesthesia.org/physiologic_changes_of_pregnancy/.
6. Vimeo. OpenAnesthesia virtual grand rounds in OB anesthesia. April 2016. Retrieved from: https://vimeo.com/163447989.

Chapter 25
Management of Intracardiac Thrombus During Orthotopic Liver Transplant

Claire Soria, Richard Bellars, Ramon Sanchez, Anush Minokadeh, and Gerard R. Manecke

Case Presentation

History of Present Illness

A 46-year-old man with end-stage liver disease due to hepatocellular carcinoma (HCC), hepatitis C, and a history of alcohol abuse was scheduled for orthotopic liver transplant (**L1**). As a bridge to liver transplantation, he had undergone drug-eluting bead transarterial chemoembolization (DEB-TACE) therapy three times, and his last treatment was 2 months prior to admission. Secondary to his liver disease, he had esophageal varices, ascites, and portal hypertensive gastropathy. He had no cardiac or pulmonary disease (**L2**), and his exercise tolerance was >4 METs. Transthoracic echocardiogram (TTE) 1 year prior to admission demonstrated normal biventricular size and function, with a late positive agitated saline contrast study suggesting an intrapulmonary shunt (**L3**).

Two years prior to admission, he had been declined for transplant listing due to a low Model of End-Stage Liver Disease (MELD) score but since then was diagnosed with stage T2 hepatocellular carcinoma. The presence of his hepatocellular carcinoma was an exception to the standard MELD scoring and increased his score from a 10 to a 22 (**L4**). The donor was hepatitis C positive. The patient qualified to receive this liver because he also was hepatitis C positive (**L5**). Preoperative thromboelastogram (TEG) showed R-time 1.6 min, K-time 3.2 min, angle degree 53.3°, MA 47.0 mm, and LY30 0.0%. Labs were notable for platelet count 54,000/L, hemoglobin 15.1 g/dL, international normalized ratio (INR) 1.3, prothrombin time (PT) 14.1, partial thromboplastin time (PTT) 38.7 s, and fibrinogen 197 mg/dL.

C. Soria (✉) · R. Bellars · R. Sanchez · A. Minokadeh
Department of Anesthesiology, University of California, San Diego, CA, USA

G. R. Manecke
Department of Anesthesiology, University of California, UCSD Medical Center, UCSD School of Medicine, San Diego, CA, USA

J. L. Benumof, G. R. Manecke (eds.), *Clinical Anesthesiology II*,
https://doi.org/10.1007/978-3-030-12365-9_25

Narrative

Anesthetic Induction

Standard ASA monitors were placed, and the patient was preoxygenated for 5 min prior to induction. A total of 10 mg of midazolam IV and 1000 mcg of fentanyl IV were titrated to patient response followed by induction with propofol 50 mg IV and succinylcholine 120 mg IV (**L6**). Intubation was uneventful with a 7.0 ETT and MAC3, with a grade 2 view (**L7**).

Transesophageal echocardiography (TEE) and line placement: Initial TEE exam showed normal biventricular function, normal valvular function, and no evidence of intracardiac clot (**L8**). A right internal jugular introducer sheath was placed on the first attempt, with confirmation of placement using manometry and TEE. A pulmonary artery catheter (PAC) was inserted on the first attempt, with placement confirmed via pulmonary artery waveform and TEE visualization in the proximal right pulmonary artery. An additional venous sheath was placed in the left internal jugular vein using ultrasound guidance on the first attempt. A left radial and left femoral arterial lines were then placed uneventfully. Central line placement was confirmed again with intraoperative chest x-ray prior to the start of surgery. Initial cardiac output, pulmonary artery pressure, systemic vascular resistance, and pulmonary vascular resistance values were within normal limits.

Maintenance

Pre-anhepatic

The patient was hemodynamically stable post induction, (**L9**) maintained on 0.5 MAC sevoflurane. Epinephrine 0.1 mcg/kg/min and phenylephrine 20–60 mcg/min were started to augment cardiac output and maintain a mean arterial pressure (MAP) of 65–70 (**L10**) during the dissection phase. The hepatectomy portion was complicated due to inflammation and scar tissue (**L11**). During mobilization of the retrohepatic vena cava, the surgeons reported massive surgical bleeding, resulting in a dramatic drop in systolic blood pressure (SBP) 100 (MAP 70) to SBP 40 (MAP 35). This period of hypotension lasted for about 7 min, during which time the surgeons obtained hemostasis and the anesthesia team resuscitated the patient with rapid transfusion of packed red blood cells and fresh frozen plasma using a Belmont Rapid Infuser, as well as inotropic and pressure support. Hemodynamic stability was obtained and bleeding was eventually controlled. A total of 50 units of PRBCs, 31 units of FFP, 10 units of platelets, and 55 units (11 packs) of cryoprecipitate were administered.

Anhepatic

Prior to placement of vena cava clamp, hemodynamics were optimized, and venous clamping was tolerated. At our institution the preferred surgical technique is the "piggyback method," where the liver is dissected off of the retrohepatic vena cava and partial clamping is done to preserve venous return. Serial ABGs were checked during this phase to assist in optimizing transfusion and electrolyte management. TEG (Haemonetics, Niles, Il, USA) was used to guide coagulation management. Vasopressors and inotropes were titrated to maintain a MAP of 65–70. The TEE was monitored continuously in the four-chamber view, and echocardiographic changes such as decreased contractility or hypovolemia were treated appropriately with inotropic support and volume.

Reperfusion

Close communication was maintained between the surgeons and anesthesiologists regarding timing of the reperfusion. A repeat TEG and ABG were sent just prior to reperfusion and were notable for a hemoglobin of 5.0 g/dL. Roles were assigned to monitor for evidence of hemodynamic instability. Continuous monitoring of TEE, arterial line, and pulmonary artery catheter during unclamping was utilized.

Immediately post reperfusion, the patient was hemodynamically stable, with a heart rate in the 70s in normal sinus rhythm and SBP 100s (MAP 70s). The RV and LV appeared to be contracting well, with no evidence of intracardiac thrombi. Within 5 min, multiple events occurred simultaneously. First the SBP dropped to 50s (MAP 40s), then the patient's rhythm converted from normal sinus rhythm to a wide complex tachycardia at a rate of 100–130 beats per minute. At the same time, the perfusionist reported a high-pressure alarm on the Belmont suddenly, and the infusion rate automatically dropped to a safe, slower rate of 50 ml/min. Review of the TEE now showed a new, large, approximately 4×4 cm clot in the right atrium which was not present at the start of reperfusion (**L12, L13, L14, L15**). The right ventricle and left ventricle appeared to be contracting appropriately initially. There was no evidence of right heart failure, with no tricuspid regurgitation and no distension of right ventricle. The left ventricle appeared to be underfilled. The radial arterial line then quickly showed a flattened waveform, and the femoral arterial waveform was lost from aortic compression by the surgeon in an attempt to augment blood pressure. There continued to be ongoing bleeding at the same time as the RV thrombus and the surgeons continued to attempt to obtain surgical control of bleeding. The patient initially was in normal sinus rhythm and then quickly progressed to various arrhythmias, including ventricular tachycardia, ventricular fibrillation, and torsades de pointes (Fig. 25.1).

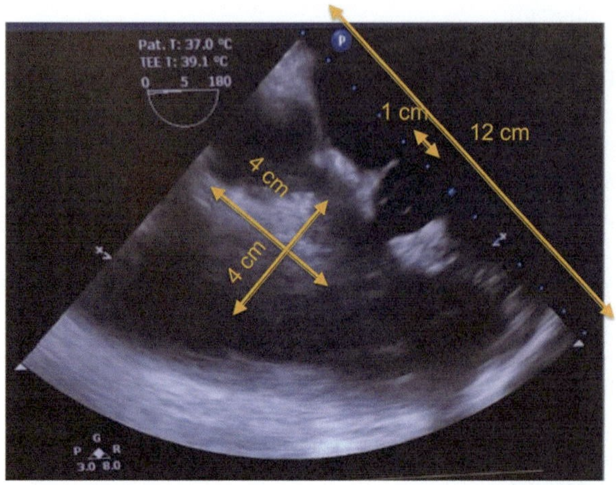

Fig. 25.1 TEE image of right atrial clot, measuring approximately 4 × 4 cm

Call for Help

Anesthesia STAT (our institutional code, calling for emergency anesthesiology and technical support to the room) was called immediately.

Hemodynamic Instability/Arrhythmia/Unclear Pulsatility

The working diagnosis at this point was cardiac arrest secondary to an acute, large right atrial thrombus. Chest compressions and aortic compression were done by our surgeons. Multiple rounds of epinephrine 1 mg were administered, as well as calcium chloride and sodium bicarbonate to support contractility and treat metabolic acidosis. The patient's rhythm fluctuated rapidly between ventricular tachycardia, ventricular fibrillation, and torsades de pointes, staying in each rhythm for approximately 10–20 s at a time. It was difficult to identify whether the patient had a pulse because the radial arterial line was flattened and the femoral arterial line was absent due to surgeon compression of the aorta. The patient was first given an unsynchronized cardioversion for ventricular tachycardia with a pulse. The patient then went into ventricular fibrillation and torsades de pointes, so defibrillation was performed. The patient then went back into ventricular tachycardia with a pulse, so another unsynchronized cardioversion was performed. The patient then had return of spontaneous circulation with normal sinus rhythm. In between cardioversions, amiodarone 150 mg was loaded, and an infusion was started at 1 mg/min. Lidocaine 100 mg and magnesium sulfate 2 g were also given.

Massive Transfusion/Belmont Troubleshooting

The Belmont infusion machine was inspected from the reservoir to the patient, and there was no evidence of obstruction or other cause for a high-pressure alarm (**L16**). Manual transfusion of blood products was continued using different ports on the right IJ and left IJ central lines. Since there was no evidence of obstruction within the Belmont system, and there was no resistance using different ports manually, the Belmont system was connected to a different port on another central line. The high-pressure alarm then resolved, and the Belmont continued to be used for massive transfusion at a rate of 200 ml/min. The suspected cause is that the large right atrial clot was obstructing the lumens of our right IJ central line, and the port we happened to be using for the Belmont was connected to the lumen being occluded by the right atrial clot. By switching the Belmont to a different port on the left IJ central line, whose lumen opened more proximal to the right atrial clot, there was no longer an obstruction of flow and a high-pressure alarm.

Return of Spontaneous Circulation

Within 7 min of the initial cardiac arrest, the patient had return of spontaneous circulation, with rebound hypertension and systolic blood pressure of 180 mm/Hg. A nicardipine infusion was titrated to lower SBP to 120s. Blood pressure eventually stabilized to SBP 100–130s using epinephrine 0.05 mcg/kg/min and phenylephrine gtt at 100 mcg/min to support biventricular function and low SVR post reperfusion. TEE showed appropriately full and well-contracting right and left ventricles. The anesthesiology team discussed possible etiologies of the intracardiac thrombus with the surgical team. Differential diagnoses included embolic material from the new liver, the inferior vena cava surgical anastomosis, and central lines or pulmonary artery catheters. Since the patient had stabilized and was now coagulopathic, the teams decided to watch the clot and not attempt to dissolve the clot with anticoagulant medications. The large right atrial clot gradually disappeared spontaneously within 30 min.

Coagulopathy

The surgeons reported persistent clinical coagulopathy post-resuscitation. This was not unexpected, given sequence of events of hemorrhage, intracardiac clot, and resuscitation. Repeat TEGs showed early fibrinolysis (degradation of the amplitude) and a low mean amplitude, consistent with thrombocytopenia. This resolved with administration of multiple rounds of PRBC, FFP, platelets, cryoprecipitate, K-Centra (prothrombin complex concentrate), tranexamic acid (TXA), and protamine (**L17, L18**). The patient's baseline TEG at the start of surgery was notable for a low mean amplitude that correlated with baseline thrombocytopenia. Most likely in this patient with a low MELD score and HCC, his coagulation status was initially fairly normal or possibly hypercoagulable. Massive hemorrhage intraoperatively then led to dilutional coagulopathy. Attempts at resuscitation with blood products may have contributed to thrombus formation. With reperfusion, then there was a combination of dilutional coagulopathy, fibrinolysis, and possible liver dysfunction.

Postoperative

The patient's trachea remained intubated, and he was transported to the surgical intensive care unit. The patient was neurologically intact, alert, and oriented × 3. On POD#3, he was extubated, and he was transferred to the floor on POD#10. On POD#20, the patient was discharged to home with family.

Lessons Learned

1. What is an orthotopic liver transplant? What are the indications and contraindications to liver transplantation?

Liver transplantation is the only definitive treatment for patients with irreversible acute or chronic liver failure. The donor liver organ is carefully selected, removed, preserved, and prepared for transport. It typically must be transplanted into the recipient within 12–18 h [1, 2]. The two approaches to transplant are live donor liver transplant and cadaveric. The advantage of live donor transplantation is greater availability of fresh donor organs. This allows patients who might not otherwise receive a transplant (e.g., with lower MELD score and better physiology) to undergo transplantation. The disadvantage of living donor transplant is potential risk to an altruistic donor. With cadaveric transplant, there is a longer wait time for an available organ and thus risk of death while on the transplant list.

Patients are considered for liver transplantation in the following situations: fulminant hepatic failure, life-threatening systemic complication of liver disease, liver-based metabolic defect, cirrhosis with complications like hepatic encephalopathy, hepatocellular carcinoma, ascites, hepatorenal syndrome, bleeding, or portal hypertension [1, 2]. Contraindications to liver transplantation include active extrahepatic malignancy or hepatic malignancy with diffuse invasion, active and uncontrolled infection, active substance or alcohol abuse, severe cardiopulmonary comorbidities, psychosocial barriers, and brain death.

2. What are the manifestations of end stage liver disease?

End-stage liver disease has multiple systemic complications that can impact anesthetic management. These are described in the following table by system [3].

3. What is the role of pre-operative echocardiogram in liver transplants? What is the significance of an intrapulmonary shunt?

Preoperative TTE (transthoracic echocardiography) is essential for screening for cardiac disease as well as estimating pulmonary artery pressure. Elevated RVSP (right ventricular systolic pressure) greater than 50 mmHg warrants a right heart catheterization to rule out portopulmonary hypertension (PVR >240 dyne.sec. cm^{-5}). This must be differentiated from pulmonary hypertension from high cardiac output and volume overload. Baseline evaluation should be done within 1 year prior to liver transplant [4]. Coronary artery disease is also an area of interest. Those with significant risk factors should undergo dobutamine stress echo or SPECT (single-photon emission computed tomography technetium-99 sestamibi scan). Cardiac catheterization is considered the gold standard for assessment of occlusive coronary artery disease and may be indicated.

Patients may have concomitant cardiovascular disease, end-stage liver disease secondary to cardiovascular disease, or secondary cardiovascular effects. This last phenomenon is known as "cirrhotic cardiomyopathy," which includes cardiac structural changes, diastolic dysfunction, and supernormal cardiac output with impaired contractile reserve in response to stress [4]. Overt heart failure is rarely seen preoperatively because the peripheral vasodilation from the ESLD masks any underlying left ventricular dysfunction – the left ventricle faces a low systemic vascular resistance preoperatively. Then, intraoperatively, under physiological and pharmacological stress, an impaired ventricular response finally manifests. Liver transplant surgery involves significant hemodynamic stress, and up to 70% of patients undergoing liver transplantation will have a cardiovascular event intraoperatively [5].

4. What is the MELD scoring system?

MELD is the Model for End-Stage Liver Disease. It is a measure of mortality risk in patients 12 years and older who have end-stage liver disease [6]. The MELD score is used as a disease severity index to stratify patients who are awaiting liver transplant. Donor organs are provided to listed patients with the highest estimated short-term mortality [2]. It predicts mortality in the following situations: (1) after transjugular intrahepatic portosystemic shunt (TIPS); (2) cirrhotic patients undergoing non-transplantation surgical procedures; (3) acute alcoholic hepatitis; and (4) acute variceal hemorrhage. Scores range from 6 to 40, with higher scores indicating more severe liver disease and higher mortality. It is based on serum creatinine, bilirubin, international normalized ratio (INR), serum sodium level, and whether the patient is undergoing dialysis. There are exceptions to the scoring system, including hepatocellular carcinoma, hepatopulmonary syndrome, and portopulmonary hypertension, among others. Policy and medical recommendation updates on using the MELD score can be found through the United Network for Organ Sharing [6].

5. How should a patient be evaluated pre-operatively for liver transplant, both immediately before surgery and while awaiting transplant availability?

During evaluation for liver transplantation, patients undergo extensive work-up. General assessment includes past medical and surgical history, physical examination, vaccinations, psychosocial assessment, and evaluation by a hepatologist and transplant surgeon. It is now recommended that liver transplant programs formally include an experienced liver transplant anesthesiologist in the selection and longer-term preoperative evaluation process. Early involvement of an anesthesiologist provides the unique perspectives the anesthesiologist brings, including management and optimization of cardiac and pulmonary issues. It also improves pre-planning of the anesthetic/perioperative care. Laboratory work-up includes type and screen, testing for antibodies, complete blood count, coagulation studies, basic metabolic panel, liver function tests, thyroid studies, tumor markers, urinalysis, and testing for hepatitis and communicable diseases like HIV and tuberculosis. Imaging often includes chest x-ray, CT scan of thorax and abdomen, and liver ultrasound. Cardiac evaluation includes an electrocardiogram and echocardiogram. Based on these results and associated comorbidities, the patient may be referred to a cardiologist and other specialists while still on the waiting list for a liver transplant [7, 8].

Due to the unscheduled nature of liver transplantation, the anesthesiologist who will care for the patient likely will not know of the case until 12 h prior to surgery. Patients are usually admitted for preoperative lab work-up and are kept NPO. The anesthesiologist should evaluate the patient in person as soon as possible. Table 25.1 lists specific anesthetic considerations unique to ESLD. The anesthesiologist should also inquire about potential contraindications to liver transplantation, including undiagnosed, unstable arrhythmias, such as atrial fibrillation with rapid ventricular response, and severe pulmonary hypertension. Since most patients will not have seen an anesthesiologist prior to admission, the provider should evaluate the airway and prepare for possible difficult intubation. Depending on the patient's NPO status, degree of ascites, gastroesophageal reflux disease, or other causes of delayed gastric mobility, the patient may need a rapid sequence induction or an awake fiber-optic intubation to protect against aspiration.

6. What monitors and access should be used for a liver transplant? Is transesophageal echocardiography (TEE) necessary? Can a TEE probe be safely used in the presence of esophageal varices?

Monitors: Routine American Society of Anesthesiology (ASA) monitors are used, including pulse oximetry, blood pressure, 5-lead electrocardiogram, ETCO2, and core temperature. Urine output is monitored as well [7, 8]. Additionally, invasive blood pressure monitoring in the form of both a radial arterial line and a femoral

Table 25.1 Manifestations of end-stage liver disease and their anesthetic impact

System	Characteristics	Anesthetic impact
Neurological	Hyperammonemia → hepatic encephalopathy, coma, asterixis, altered mental status, seizures	
	In fulminant liver failure → cerebral edema → increased intracranial pressure (ICP) → herniation; intracerebral hemorrhage	Caution with factors that increase ICP
	Most liver failure patients will die of intracerebral hemorrhage	
Cardiovascular	Low systemic vascular resistance	*Cardiac effects:*
	Portal hypertension	Decrease SVR + central hypovolemia = hyperdynamic circulatory state
	Splanchnic and peripheral vasodilation	
	Cirrhotic cardiomyopathy	Cardiac dysfunction can be masked by the ESLD (LV faces low SVR)
		Supernormal cardiac output, with impaired contractile reserve in response to stress
		Vascular Effects: Expansion and redistribution of blood volume → relative splanchnic hypervolemia and effective central hypovolemia
	Occasionally, ESLD is due to underlying cardiac disease	Preoperative EKG and echocardiogram within 1 year prior to surgery should be obtained to evaluate baseline cardiac function
	ESLD → left ventricular hypertrophy, myocardial fibrosis, and subendothelial edema → myocardial stiffness	Left ventricular diastolic dysfunction
	Undiagnosed coronary artery disease due to associated risk factors (age, male, HTN, T2DM, non-alcohol-related etiology of cirrhosis)	Unrecognized, asymptomatic CAD → intraoperative or postoperative MI
Pulmonary	Ascites → restrictive lung physiology, decreased functional residual capacity	Decreased respiratory reserve, faster oxygen desaturation
	Ascites → pleural effusions, right > left	
	Pulmonary edema	
Hepatopulmonary syndrome	Vascular endothelial growth factor (VEGF) not cleared by liver → arteriovenous malformations → increased shunting within the intrapulmonary vasculature → hypoxemia	Hypoxemia on ABG

(continued)

Table 25.1 (continued)

System	Characteristics	Anesthetic impact
Portopulmonary hypertension	Toxic mediators not cleared by the liver → increase in pulmonary vascular resistance → pulmonary hypertension	Right heart strain/failure
		Contraindication to transplantation if moderate-severe
Gastrointestinal	Ascites	Higher aspiration risk despite NPO status. Rapid sequence induction recommended
	Esophageal varices	Caution with TEE probe placement. Potential for bleeding risk
	Peptic ulcer disease	
	Massive splanchnic vasodilation	
Renal	Hepatorenal syndrome: massive splanchnic vasodilation → low renal perfusion pressure → renal system attempts to vasoconstrict by activating the renin-angiotensin-aldosterone system → salt and water retention	Potentially overall fluid-overloaded. Caution with fluid resuscitation, as distended IVC is suboptimal for surgeon
Hematologic	All clotting factors are disordered	
	Fragile equilibrium between being hypercoagulable and prothrombotic	Cannot interpret coagulation status by lab values alone. Must send frequent ABGs and TEGs intraoperatively
Endocrine/metabolic	Impaired glucose homeostasis, decreased gluconeogenesis → hypoglycemia	Frequent serum glucose measurements
	Electrolyte imbalances, malnourished, chronic hyponatremia (water > sodium), hypokalemia, hypomagnesemia	
	High volume of distribution	Theoretically need a higher dosage of induction agents, but also have impaired hepatic metabolism of drugs
Infectious disease	Prone to infection, bacterial translocation across cut well	Spontaneous bacterial peritonitis
	Most common infection is actually pneumonia	

arterial line should be used. The radial arterial line may be placed prior to or after anesthetic induction, depending on the patient's underlying cardiac and pulmonary function. For example, a patient with concomitant severe pulmonary hypertension or aortic stenosis would be predicted to have greater hemodynamic instability during induction than a patient with no cardiac disease. A femoral arterial line is beneficial because the radial arterial waveform may become dampened during the case due to vasoplegia or peripheral vasoconstriction. It is important to monitor core temperature, such as esophageal or bladder temperature. During reperfusion, the surgeons perform a staged unclamping of the inferior vena cava. The surgeons and anesthesiologist will carefully monitor the decrease in temperature associated with reperfusion of cold blood into the systemic circulation.

Intravenous access: Large-bore intravenous (IV) access should be established at the start of the case in anticipation of massive transfusion and fluid resuscitation. This usually includes one or two central lines in the right and/or left internal jugular veins or femoral veins if cannulation is difficult. One central line can be connected to a rapid infuser such as the Belmont. A second central line or a large-bore 14 G or 16 G peripheral IV can be used for cryoprecipitate and platelets. This decreases the risk of clotting off the largest central venous access line.

Pulmonary artery (PA) catheter: Overall, there is a trend away from utilizing PA catheters during liver transplantation. Risks associated with PA catheters include delaying the start of the case in the event of difficult placement, atrial or ventricular arrhythmias, clot formation, migration with position changes, and traumatic placement leading to myocardial wall damage. Benefits of the PA catheter include detection of pulmonary hypertension and right ventricular failure and improved assessment of volume status and hemodynamic changes. PA catheters are especially useful postoperatively when the patient goes to the intensive care unit (ICU). However, proper use of PA catheters does require expertise, and providers must know how to accurately interpret pulmonary artery pressures, cardiac output, and venous blood gases.

Transesophageal echocardiography (TEE): Whether or not a TEE probe is inserted at the start of the case largely depends on the provider's preference and the patient's underlying cardiac and pulmonary disease. Even if a TEE probe is not inserted prior to the start of surgery, most anesthesiologists will at least have a TEE probe and machine available in the room. If an intraoperative complication occurred, such as suspected cardiac arrest or suspected pulmonary embolism, the provider would then be able to place the TEE probe. The benefit of placing the TEE probe early on is that a provider can conduct an initial survey of the four chambers and assess contractility and valvular function. The provider could then monitor cardiac function in real time and make more informed treatment decisions. Echocardiographic changes such as new regional wall motion abnormalities indicating myocardial ischemia or acute tricuspid regurgitation suggesting pulmonary embolism or pulmonary hypertension provide invaluable information.

TEE probes can be difficult to place in some patients. In the patient who is already prepped, draped, and secured in position for surgery, it can be even more challenging to insert a TEE probe without disrupting the surgical field. Risks of placing the TEE probe are largely due to traumatic insertion causing dental damage, swelling or laceration of the oropharynx and larynx, and esophageal damage. In ESLD patients who may have esophageal varices, there is a significant concern for variceal rupture leading to undetected hemorrhage. In this situation, the provider could gently place the TEE probe and leave the probe in the mid-esophageal four-chamber view. The four-chamber view would provide a global assessment of cardiac function. Minimizing manipulation of the TEE probe would theoretically decrease the risk of esophageal trauma and variceal rupture.

7. What is a safe method of induction?

There are multiple ways to induce anesthesia in a liver transplant patient. The safest induction achieves the following: (1) secure the airway quickly and with minimal trauma; (2) avoid gastric aspiration; (3) avoid hemodynamic instability; and (4) ensure amnesia and analgesia. The choice of induction agents ultimately depends on the provider's preference. Common induction agents include propofol, etomidate, and ketamine, with some combination of benzodiazepines and opiates such as fentanyl. Each agent has its pros and cons, including amnesia, analgesia, muscle relaxation, and sympathetic blockade [2, 7, 8].

As with all anesthetics, the provider must consider the patient's underlying cardiac and respiratory function. Usually, patients with ESLD have hyperdynamic hearts with a low systemic vascular resistance and high cardiac output. They may also have hepatopulmonary syndrome and/or portopulmonary hypertension. This can result in rapid oxygen desaturation and acute right heart failure with exacerbators like hypoxemia and hypercarbia from apnea. Depending on whether the patient has acute or chronic liver failure, they may be in septic shock, be coagulopathic and bleeding already, have cerebral edema and elevated intracranial pressure, or be hemodynamically unstable.

Given the timing of transplants, a patient's NPO status may warrant a rapid sequence induction. Patients with ESLD also may have significant ascites, which decreases the functional residual capacity, decreases time to oxygen desaturation, and increases the risk of aspiration. The patient may not have been seen in anesthesia preoperative clinic for an airway evaluation and other discussions about the anesthetic plan. The provider caring for the patient on the day of surgery must evaluate the patient in person as soon as possible. If a difficult airway is anticipated, the provider must have backup airway equipment available and may need to consider an awake intubation. The largest-sized endotracheal tube (ETT) that can smoothly be placed past the vocal cords should be used, in case the provider needs to perform a fiber-optic bronchoscopy emergently. Possible difficult perioperative situations in which suctioning and fiber-optic examination of the airways may be useful include pulmonary edema, bleeding in the airway, and mucus plugging. A silver-coated ETT is often used to decrease bacterial growth during a prolonged ICU course.

8. Which TEE views are most helpful in a non-cardiac surgery?

TEE can be invaluable tool when used in the appropriate patient in the appropriate context. Liver transplantation, which is characterized by periods of rapid and variable hemodynamic instability, is a good situation to have TEE available. For the non-cardiac anesthesiologist who does not regularly use TEE for monitoring, TEE can be intimidating. The value lies not in the act of obtaining many images but in the acquisition and interpretation of a few basic ones. Inordinate amounts of time should not be spent attempting to optimize the images, but effort should be applied to interpreting them and applying the TEE results to the clinical situation [4].

For non-cardiac surgery, eight basic TEE views usually suffice:

1. Mid-esophageal aortic valve short axis
2. Mid-esophageal aortic valve long axis
3. Bicaval
4. Mid-esophageal RV inflow/outflow
5. Mid-esophageal four-chamber
6. Mid-esophageal two-chamber
7. Mid-esophageal long axis
8. Transgastric short axis

The purpose of TEE for non-cardiac surgery to look at two things: (1) structure and (2) function. A basic survey can be used to guide management and resuscitation (Table 25.2):

Signs of pulmonary hypertension include a thickened RV wall (chronic), dilated RV or RA, tricuspid regurgitation, interventricular septum shift toward the left ventricle, and dilated pulmonary artery. Normally, the RV is half the size of the LV and is wedge-shaped on the mid-esophageal four-chamber view.

9. What are the anesthetic challenges of the pre-anhepatic, anhepatic, and reperfusion phases of liver transplant?

There are three stages to a liver transplant: (1) pre-anhepatic, when the surgeons dissect and remove the native liver; (2) anhepatic, when the surgeons insert the donor liver into the patient and create surgical anastomoses to connect the new liver to the recipient's hepatobiliary system; and (3) reperfusion, when the surgeons gradually release vascular clamps and establish blood flow into the new liver [3, 8]. Each phase

Table 25.2 Basic survey approach to transesophageal echocardiography

Question	Answer	Utility
Is there volume?	Yes, it's full	Don't give fluid
	No, it's empty	Give fluid
Is the heart contracting well overall?	Yes, it looks normal/ hyperdynamic	Don't give inotrope
	No	Give inotrope
Is there a regional wall motion abnormality?	Yes	High suspicion for intraoperative myocardial ischemia/infarct
	Don't need to identify which coronary artery has the lesion	Consider consulting cardiologist and going to cath lab
	At least try to identify lateral wall, inferior wall, interventricular septum, etc.	
	No	Low suspicion for intraoperative MI
Is there regurgitation?	Yes (aortic, mitral, tricuspid, pulmonic)	Variable, most useful is TR indicating acute R heart failure or acute pulmonary HTN or pulmonary embolism

of the liver transplant is characterized by specific events, each with its own complications. Undoubtedly the most dangerous period is reperfusion. However, it is important to understand the unique events and anesthetic complications of all three phases. As with other routine anesthetics, the anesthesiologist's responsibility is to help optimize operating conditions for the surgeon, anticipate and prevent complications, and react to complications in a timely, organized fashion [2, 7, 8] (Table 25.3).

10. What drugs and blood products should be prepared for a liver transplant?

Routine medications, including narcotics, standard induction agents, muscle relaxants, and pressors, should be prepared. Liver transplants can be characterized by periods of rapid hemodynamic instability and major adverse events. These changes can occur quickly. It is recommended that additional inotropes and pressors such as epinephrine, norepinephrine, and vasopressin, as well as emergency drugs such as calcium chloride, sodium bicarbonate, atropine, and lidocaine be readily available. Many institutions have a designated "Anesthesia Liver Cart" that contains larger stocks of these medications. The following table lists the recommended drug preparations [2, 7, 8] (Table 25.4).

Regarding blood products, patients will frequently require dozens of units of packed red blood cells (PRBCs), fresh frozen plasma (FFP), and platelets, and potentially cryoprecipitate. Each institution has its own standardized protocol for

Table 25.3 Phases of liver transplant

Phase	Event	Impact
Pre-anhepatic	Abdomen opened	Release ascites
	Ascites released	Improvement in FRC and lung compliance
	Loss of tamponade effect on splanchnic vessels	Hemodynamic changes (hypotension, bradycardia)
		Hypovolemia from loss of ascites fluid
	Usually coagulopathic	Surgeon may request preemptive FFP and platelet transfusion to decrease bleeding during dissection
	Adhesions/scar tissue	Difficult dissection
	Portal hypertension	High risk of traumatic injury to liver or blood vessels with hemorrhage
	Engorged splanchnic vessels	May preemptively start pressors or give blood products
		Check ABG/TEG q20min minimum
		Keep volume low (low CVP) to decrease IVC distension and venous bleeding, and improve surgical view
	Lifting of the liver	Lose preload and therefore cardiac output
		Anticipate by watching surgeons carefully and giving pressors
	Acute vs. chronic liver failure	Acute liver failure: no time for collaterals; volume depleted
		Chronic liver failure: lots of collaterals

Table 25.3 (continued)

Phase	Event	Impact
Anhepatic	Clamp vessels	Thrombus formation in IVC
		Significant drop in preload
	Anhepatic: no liver to make clotting factors or clear toxins	Massive bleeding potential, very high EBL
		Acidosis: give bicarbonate, maintain adequate ventilation
		Coagulopathy: give blood products
		Frequent ABG/TEG q20min
		Glucose: hypoglycemia
		Hypocalcemia: massive transfusion; high citrate leading to calcium chelation
		Hyperkalemia: hyperventilation, bicarbonate
		Vasoplegia: lose arterial waveform, hypotension
		Cold: bair hugger on, warmed room; cold temperature worsens coagulopathy
	Waiting for surgeons to anastomose new liver	Organize anesthesia workstation
		Have a couple syringes of epinephrine, bicarbonate, and calcium setup
		Dilute epinephrine 10 mcg/ml in line ready to bolus
		Carefully watch TEE, EKG, and arterial lines
Reperfusion	Cold, acidotic, hyperkalemic, high lactate, and high citrate blood is reperfused and recirculated	This is when bad things happen (cardiac arrest, acute RV failure, MI, etc.)
		Hypocalcemia → hypotension
	Staged reperfusion: surgeons slowly unclamp	Hyperkalemia → arrhythmias
		Cold → arrhythmias, coagulopathy
		Massive blood loss → coagulopathy
		Acidosis → arrhythmias, myocardial ischemia/infarction, coagulopathy, hypotension
		Thrombi → arrhythmias, hypotension, pulmonary hypertension

liver transplants. It is routine to notify the hospital blood bank of the scheduled liver transplant. The blood bank will prepare batches of PRBcs, FFP, and platelets. Typically there is a designated fridge in the operating room specifically for blood storage. It is important to check frequently on the stock of blood products and call the blood bank to send more as needed.

11. How can major adverse events be detected in a timely fashion? What is the value of communication between surgeons, anesthesiologists, nurses, technicians, and perfusionists?

Liver transplantation is a particularly dynamic surgery. Hemodynamic changes due to surgical events can occur very quickly. It is critical that all providers in the

Table 25.4 Recommended medications to prepare for liver transplant

Narcotics	Midazolam 10 cc
	Fentanyl 20 cc
Induction agents	Etomidate 10 cc
	Propofol 20 cc
Paralytic	Succinylcholine 10 cc
	Rocuronium 10 cc
Steroids	Methylprednisolone 500 mg × 1 (at beginning and end of case)
Antibiotics	Ampicillin-sulbactam 3 g
Uppers (inotropes, pressors)	Ephedrine 10 cc syringe
	Phenylephrine 10 cc syringe
	Epinephrine gtt (preprogram to 0.02 mcg/kg/min)
	Phenylephrine gtt (preprogram to 20 mcg/min)
	Norepinephrine gtt (preprogram to 1 mg/min)
Downers (antihypertensives)	Nicardipine gtt (preprogram to 1 mg/h)
	Nitroglycerin gtt (preprogram to 20 mcg/min)
Emergency drugs	Vasopressin 1 unit/ml
Most institutions have a designated	Epinephrine 10 mcg/ml in 10 cc syringe
	Epinephrine 1 mg/10 ml in 10 cc syringe
"Anesthesia liver cart" containing these drugs	Atropine 1 mg/10 ml in 10 cc syringe
	Lidocaine 100 mg/10 ml in 10 cc syringe
	Calcium chloride 1000 mg/10 ml in 10 cc syringe
	Sodium bicarbonate 50 meq/50 ml in 50 ml syringe
	Multiple boxes stacked on top of the anesthesia cart/ machine very close by
Fluids	500 cc bottles of albumin
	100 cc and 250 cc bags of normal saline to dilute medications
	1 L bags of normal saline spiked and on fluid warmers

room communicate clearly, including surgeons, anesthesiologists, nurses, technicians, and perfusionists. Closed loop communication is essential. Major intraoperative events must be relayed to either side of the drapes in a timely fashion.

12. How does an intracardiac thrombus form? What is the incidence of intracardiac thrombi during orthotopic liver transplant?

Intracardiac thrombosis is a rare but dreaded complication of orthotopic liver transplantation. The reported incidence ranges from 1.2% to 6.2%. It is associated with an intraoperative mortality of 30% and an in-hospital mortality of 45%. The true incidence is limited by the use of TEE, as not all hospitals use TEE routinely for liver transplantation. Eighty-five percent of thrombi will occur during the reperfusion phase. The mechanism for intracardiac thrombus formation is thought to be an imbalance of prothrombotic and coagulopathic states, as well as resulting from low-flow circumstances. Traditionally, liver patients are primarily thought of as being prone to bleeding. End-stage liver disease is now known to have a fragile coagulopathy that is prone to both bleeding and thrombosis. Theoretically, clots can form anywhere in the body and embolize to the heart, resulting in hemodynamic consequences. In the particular case described above, the clot was thought to have formed in a large vessel such as the inferior vena cava, given the size of the clot. Clots can also form on central lines and pulmonary artery catheters, but tend to be associated with prolonged catheter duration. Close monitoring of the coagulation status is thus essential, to avoid excessive bleeding (inadequate blood product administration) as well as hypercoagulability (too much blood product and coagulation factor administration) [9–15].

13. What are the potential complications of an intracardiac thrombus?

An intracardiac thrombus can occlude the tricuspid valve (ball and valve locking mechanism), obstruct cardiac flow through the right atrium. The thrombus can break off into smaller clots, which can then embolize into the pulmonary circulation, leading to pulmonary hypertension, acute right ventricular failure, and pulmonary edema. If the patient has an atrial septal defect or patent foramen ovale, which 20% of patients do, the clot may embolize from the right to left heart, to the systemic circulation including the cerebral arteries, and cause ischemic strokes [10–12, 14–17].

14. What are the options to treat an intracardiac thrombus?

Treatment is primarily aimed at hemodynamic support with vasopressors and inotropic agents and possibly extracorporeal membrane oxygenation. Providers may also consider systemic thrombolytic therapy, such as heparin or recombinant tissue plasminogen activator, or surgical thrombectomy. The challenge with administering thrombolytic therapy is that most commonly, after transplantation of the donor liver, the primary problem encountered is maintaining hemostasis and managing coagulopathy. Administration of a large dose of thrombolytic medication may dissolve the intracardiac thrombus, but lead to systemic bleeding particularly at the site of the new liver graft [11–12, 14–17].

15. How is acute massive blood loss managed intraoperatively?

The following table summarizes guidelines for management of acute massive blood loss intraoperatively. Primary goals include calling for help, notifying the surgeons and blood bank, establishing large-bore IV access, administering blood products, supporting hemodynamics to maintain end-organ perfusion, and continually reassessing coagulopathic state with labs. Providers should know their hospital's massive transfusion protocol and how to initiate it in a timely fashion (Table 25.5).

16. What is the Belmont rapid infuser? What checks and balances are in place to prevent clot formation and embolization?

The Belmont Infuser is a rapid infusion system used for high blood loss surgical procedures, trauma resuscitations, and any situation where rapid replacement and warming of blood or fluids may be needed. It is a useful tool that enables rapid infusion of products while freeing the provider's hands for other tasks [18].

Table 25.5 Guidelines for acute massive blood loss

Goal	Intervention	Comments
Call for help	Blood bank	Blood bank mobilizes 45 U PRBC, 45 U FFP, 4–6 U platelets ASAP[a]
	OR RN	Blood bank supplies batches of 10 U PRBC, 10 U FFP, 1–2 U Plt to OR ASAP[a]
	OR runner	
	Massive transfusion protocol	
Restore volume	Large-bore IV access, central line	
	Crystalloid, colloid	Caution with dilutional anemia
		Caution with coagulopathy
		Monitor CVP
	Blood products	Blood loss is often underestimated
		Caution with coagulopathy
		Caution with hypothermia
		Caution with hypocalcemia
	Maintain normal BP and UOP	Pressors, inotropes
Arrest bleeding	Early surgical intervention	
Monitor labs	CBC, coagulation studies (PT, PTT, INR), fibrinogen, TEG, ABG, BMP	

[a]Based on Blood Bank Manual at University of California, San Diego

The Belmont machine is quick and easy to prepare. It consists of a reservoir chamber to collect blood and a machine to warm blood and detect air and clots. Simple instructions appear on the machine's screen when it is first powered on. The provider can program infusion rates based on the catheter size connected to the Belmont tubing. For example, a 12 G catheter can tolerate an infusion rate of 1000 ml/min, whereas a 20 G catheter can accept a rate of 100 ml/min. To minimize clot formation, lactated ringers, platelets, and cryoprecipitate cannot be infused through the Belmont machine.

There are multiple system checks to stop air and blood clots. Within the machine itself, there are two air detectors that automatically detect, remove, and release air into the environment. A pressure sensor continuously detects and displays pressure within the system. If there is an acute increase in pressure or a pressure greater than 300 mmHg, a high-pressure alarm will sound until the obstruction is resolved. The machine automatically slows the flow rate to a safe line pressure. Additionally, there is a high-speed peristaltic pump that breaks up clots and a warmer to prevent cooling and clot formation. The machine automatically recirculates blood while actively infusing or in standby mode. The provider can also manually recirculate blood at a higher rate of 200 ml/min by pressing a recirculation button.

17. What is in a blood product?

The following diagram illustrates one method of the separation of blood products:

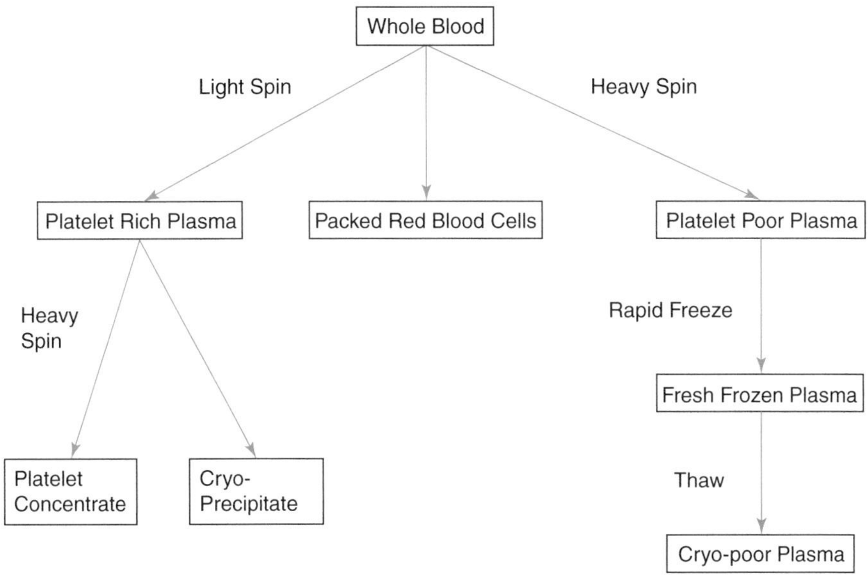

Fig. 25.2 Simplified diagram showing components of blood products and their origins

Cryoprecipitate consists of factor VIII, factor XIII, von Willebrand factor, and fibrinogen. One unit of FFP contains twice the amount of fibrinogen and twice the amount of factor VIII as one unit of cryoprecipitate. Typical ratios for transfusion are 2:2:1 of PRBC/FFP/platelet or 3:3:1 of PRBC/FFP/platelet [19] (Fig. 25.2).

18. How is coagulation status assessed intraoperatively?

Depending on the institution, CBC, coagulation studies, fibrinogen, and BMP can take up to an hour to result. Thus, they are of limited utility in the more acute intraoperative setting. Also, coagulation studies may indicate a coagulopathic or prothrombotic state that does not actually correlate with the clinical picture. This is because in end-stage liver disease, multiple clotting factors are abnormal. The more useful tool will be the thromboelastogram (TEG), which is a viscoelastic hemostatic assay that measures whole blood clot formation [19–20] (Table 25.6).

Liver transplantation is one of the most complex surgeries performed, requiring extensive preparation and seamless communication in the operating room. Managing the coagulation status of patients undergoing liver transplantation is complex, with continuous risks of hypo- and hypercoagulability. Diagnosing an intracardiac thrombus requires vigilant hemodynamic monitoring and skilled use of transesophageal echocardiography. When a cardiac or great vessel thrombus occurs, aggressive resuscitation is often required, as well as continued monitoring and management of coagulation status.

Table 25.6 Thromboelastogram interpretation

Component	Definition	Normal range	Problem	Treatment
R-time	Time to start forming clot	5–10 min	Coagulation factors	FFP
K-time	Time until clot reaches a fixed strength	1–3 min	Fibrinogen	Cryoprecipitate
Alpha angle	Speed of fibrin accumulation	53–72°	Fibrinogen	Cryoprecipitate
Maximum amplitude (MA)	Highest vertical amplitude of the TEG	50–70 mm	Platelets	Platelets and/or DDAVP
Lysis at 30 min (LY30)	Percentage of amplitude reduction 30 min after maximum amplitude	0–8%	Excess fibrinolysis	Tranexamic acid and/or aminocaproic acid

References

1. Farkas S, Hackl C, Schlitt HJ. Overview of the indications and contraindications for liver transplantation. Cold Spring Harb Perspect Med. 2014;4(5).
2. O'Leary JG, Lepe R, Davis GL. Indications for liver transplantation. Gastroenterology. 2008;134(6):1764–76.
3. Stoelting RK, Hines RL, Marshall KE. Chapter 13: Diseases of the liver and biliary tract, Stoelting's Anesthesia and Co-Existing Disease. 6th ed. Philadelphia: Saunders/Elsevier; 2012.
4. Garg A, Armstrong WF. Echocardiography in liver transplant candidates. JACC Cardiovasc Imaging. 2013;6(1):105–19.
5. Steadman RH. Anesthesia for liver transplant surgery. Anesthesiol Clin N Am. 2004;22:687–711.
6. United Network for Organ Sharing. Questions & answers for transplant candidates about MELD and PELD. 2008. https://www.unos.org/wp-content/uploads/unos/MELD_PELD.pdf.
7. Johns Hopkins Comprehensive Transplant Center. Liver transplant program. 2018. http://www.hopkinsmedicine.org/transplant/programs/liver/index.html.
8. Jaffe RA, Schmiesing C, Golianu B. Chapter 7.12: Liver/kidney/pancreas transplantation, Anesthesiologist's Manual of Surgical Procedures. 4th ed. Philadelphia: Lippincott Williams & Wilkins; 2009.
9. Goldflam K, et al. Focus on: inferior vena cava ultrasound. American College of Emergency Physicians News. 2011. https://www.acep.org/Content.aspx?id=80791.
10. Edwards Lifesciences Corporation. Central venous access. 2018. http://www.edwards.com/eu/products/central-venous-access.
11. Lisman T, Porte RJ. Rebalanced hemostasis in patients with liver disease: evidence and clinical consequences. Blood. 2010;12:878–86.
12. Peiris P, et al. Intracardiac thrombosis during liver transplant: a 17-year single-institution study. Liver Transpl. 2015;21:1280–5.
13. Prince MR, et al. The diameter of the inferior vena cava and its implications for the use of vena caval filters. Radiology. 1983;149:687–9.
14. Sakai T, et al. Pulmonary thromboembolism during adult liver transplantation: incidence, clinical presentation, risk factors, and diagnostic predictors. Br J Anesth. 2011;108(3):469–77.
15. Sanchez R, Kim BA, Aryafar H, Schmidt U, Berumen J. Transesophageal echo guided thrombus extraction and catheter-directed thrombolytic therapy during orthotopic liver transplantation: a case report. J Cardiothorac Vasc Anesth. 2017; https://doi.org/10.1053/j.jvca.2017.04.042.

16. Protin C, et al. Emergent management of intracardiac thrombosis during liver transplantation. Case Rep Transplant. 2016:2016;6268370.
17. Warnaar N. Intraoperative pulmonary embolism and intracardiac thrombosis complicating liver transplantation: a systematic review. J Thromb Hemost. 2007;6:297–302.
18. Belmont Instrument Corporation. Belmont rapid infuser. 2018. http://www.belmontinstrument.com/.
19. Holcom JB, et al. Transfusion of plasma, platelets, and red blood cells in a 1:1:1 vs a 1:1:2 ratio and mortality in patients with severe trauma; the PROPPR randomized clinical trial. JAMA. 2015;313(5):471–82.
20. Stainsby D, MacLennan S, Hamilton PJ. Management of massive blood loss: a template guideline. Br J Anesth. 2000;85(3):487–91.

Chapter 26
Preventing Perioperative Complications of Epidermolysis Bullosa

Claire Soria and Mark Greenberg

Case Presentation

An 11-year-old girl, 3′10″, 17 kg, with severe epidermolysis bullosa dystrophica (**L1**) with chronic sloughing, bilateral hand contractures, and syndactyly (**L2**), presented for outpatient surgery. She was scheduled for left-hand skin excision; de-cocooning, with first web space deepening; syndactyly releases (**L3**); and full-thickness skin grafting. Significant preoperative findings included generalized scars, blisters, and joint contractures. Chronic pain control was a challenge, as she developed gastrointestinal upset with NSAIDs and did not tolerate opioids well. She had developed itching, mood irritability, and severe constipation with all opioids. The pruritus was especially concerning as this led to scratching and severe skin ulcers in the past. She was being followed by the UCSD Pain Service as an outpatient. At home, her pain management regimen included taking modest amounts of oral morphine and ibuprofen and spreading cannabidiol oils over her skin. The cannabinoid was most effective and was her mainstay of therapy. Airway assessment revealed Mallampati II, thyromental distance 3 cm, full range of motion of neck, and 3 cm interincisor distance. Mouth opening was limited but intubation had not been a problem in the past.

Additional past medical history included previous admission at 6 years of age for daily wound care and allograft placement over her anterior and posterior torso due to mechanical trauma suffered from uncontrolled itching/scratching of her skin. She underwent esophageal dilation for esophageal stricture during that time. Eventually she required gastric tube placement due to failure to thrive, which was later removed due to skin breakdown at the insertion site. At the time of presentation for her current surgery, she was able to eat soft foods by mouth. She could ambulate independently for short periods of time and used a powered wheelchair

C. Soria (✉) · M. Greenberg
Department of Anesthesiology, University of California, San Diego, CA, USA
e-mail: mgreenberg@ucsd.edu; csoria@ucsd.edu

J. L. Benumof, G. R. Manecke (eds.), *Clinical Anesthesiology II*,
https://doi.org/10.1007/978-3-030-12365-9_26

for longer distances. She was cognitively intact, was homeschooled by her mother, and enjoyed playing with her electronic digital tablet.

In preparation for surgery, significant operating room coordination was necessary. The anesthesia, surgery, nursing staff, and wound care team all met in the OR to discuss the important points of skin protection which were as follows: preventing lateral skin shearing forces, minimizing direct physical contact with the patient, thoroughly padding all pressure points, avoiding stickers or tight wraps around the skin, thoroughly lubricating equipment that would touch skin with petroleum jelly, providing a layer of gauze or other cloth protection between equipment and skin if possible, lifting or repositioning the patient very gently, and double-checking padding. A supply cart full of Xeroform®, cushions, Aquaphor® ointment, and Vaseline® gauze was kept in the room throughout the case.

Preoperative Evaluation (L4)

On examination, the patient had no evidence of oral sores or bleeding in the mouth. No evidence of new blistering was noted. The anesthesia team discussed pain management with the patient and her mother. For pain management, the plan was to avoid opioids as much as possible. The patient was cooperative and no premedication was necessary. Although she came in to the hospital in a motorized wheelchair, she was able to walk herself from the preoperative area to the OR and, with a stool, crawled up onto the OR table and positioned herself appropriately with verbal guidance (**L5**).

Monitors

The monitors used were coated with Aquaphor®, including the clip-on pulse oximeter probe (**L6**). A sticker pulse oximetry monitor was not used. EKG leads were avoided in order to prevent new skin lesions. EKG needle electrodes were available in the OR for emergency use. To monitor blood pressure, a noninvasive cuff was wrapped around her calf, which was coated with Aquaphor® ointment and gauze, and the cuff was cycled every 10 min. For protection of her scalp, a gel pad was used instead of a foam pad, which was also covered in Aquaphor® ointment. Foam padding and gauze covered with Aquaphor® and/or Xeroform® were applied around all pressure points such as the elbows, heels, and knees. Neuromuscular blockade was not monitored.

Induction

Due to the patient's skin disease, intravenous access would have been difficult to obtain, thus the decision was made to perform an inhalational induction. The circuit facemask was prepared to be a soft cushion, which was liberally coated with Aquaphor®. Anesthesia was induced with 8% sevoflurane and 70% nitrous oxide (**L7**). A light chin lift was applied to assist with ventilation during induction. Care was taken to minimize pressure on the chin by lifting the finger and applying pressure lightly as needed. During this time, a 22 G peripheral IV was placed in the hand (**L8**). The catheter was secured with Xeroform® and Aquaphor® wrapping the catheter circumferentially and covered lightly with self-adherent wrap (Coban®). The anesthesia was then deepened with propofol, and the patient's muscles were relaxed with vecuronium. Her trachea was intubated using a Miller 2 laryngoscope and a cuffed 4.5 ETT, both of which had been coated in Aquaphor® (**L9**). The cuff was inflated with the minimal volume of air needed for an adequate seal. The tube was secured with twill, which was covered with Xeroform and Aquaphor applied to the face and then tied in place. The eyes were protected with eye lubricant and not taped.

Maintenance

Anesthesia was maintained with a combination of a propofol infusion 200 mcg/kg/min, low-dose sevoflurane, vecuronium, and dexmedetomidine. Muscle relaxant dosing with vecuronium was based on the appearance of spontaneous breaths over the pressure-controlled ventilation settings. Cefazolin was given as antibiotic prophylaxis. Additionally, she was given weight-based dosing of ketorolac and acetaminophen at the end of the case (**L10**). For prophylaxis of postoperative nausea and vomiting, she received weight-based dosing of metoclopramide and ondansetron.

Emergence

The propofol infusion was discontinued 45 min prior to extubation, and sevoflurane was discontinued 30 min prior. The patient was given appropriate weight-based dosing of neostigmine and glycopyrrolate for reversal. A lubricated ten French suction catheter was used to gently suction the mouth. The decision was made to extubate her while deep anesthetized to decrease the risk of trauma from the endotracheal tube from coughing (**L11**). Emergence was unremarkable, with no pain issues or no recall of events. The issues related to epidermolysis bullosa management were reviewed with the nursing staff and the anesthesia team remained with the patient until the patient was awake and stable.

Lessons Learned

1. What is epidermolysis bullosa?

Epidermolysis bullosa (EB) is a rare genetic mechanobullous disorder characterized by excessive fragility of skin and mucous membranes [1]. Mutations in genes coding for collagen, responsible for epidermal adherence, cause the disease. The type of epidermolysis bullosa is defined by where in these layers the blisters form. This can be diagnosed by skin biopsy for immunofluorescent mapping to identify the layer of skin and proteins involved [2]. Genetic testing can confirm the diagnosis but is expensive. Families with histories of EB may consider prenatal testing and genetic counseling. Most forms of EB are inherited and appear in infancy or early childhood, although some patients do not develop signs and symptoms until adolescence or early adulthood. Siblings with epidermolysis bullosa can present clinically with different severities of the disease.

Shearing forces and friction lead to intradermal fluid accumulation and resultant bullae formation [3]. Compressive forces are better tolerated than shearing forces, but can still lead to bullae formation. Blisters can form in response to even minor injury, including heat, friction from rubbing, scratching, or adhesives. The blisters form not only on external skin but also inside the body, such as the lining of the mouth or the intestines. There is no correlation between the degree of skin involvement and the severity of the disease internally in the pharynx and esophagus.

Most patients die during childhood due to malnutrition. Malnutrition leads to hypoproteinemia, anemia, and electrolyte imbalance, which can affect pharmacodynamics of anesthetic agents. Infection is common because patients have poor immunity and are often on long-term corticosteroid treatment [1]. There is no cure for EB at this time. Treatment addresses symptoms such as infection and itching, pain control, and wound care (Table 26.1).

2. What are the complications of epidermolysis bullosa? [2–4, 6]

Patients with EB present for multiple surgeries to treat complications of EB, especially skin infection and esophageal and tracheal stenosis from scarring (Table 26.2).

3. What types of surgeries will EB patients require?

EB patients will present for multiple surgeries throughout their lifetimes, most commonly for wound care and extensive dressing changes. These include plastic surgeries to correct pseudosyndactyly of hands and feet, release of joint contrac-

Table 26.1 Most common types of epidermolysis bullosa

	Junctional epidermolysis bullosa	Epidermolysis bullosa dystrophica
Incidence	1–2 in 1,000,000	1–2 in 1,000,000
Life expectancy	1–5 years old	Early 20s
When clinical signs appear	Severe, apparent at birth	Starts in birth or early childhood
Characteristic clinical features	Blisters, scars on vocal cords	Progressive scarring and deformity
	Notable for laryngotracheal and genitourinary tract involvement	Oropharyngeal and esophageal involvement
Genetic cause	Autosomal recessive mutation in fibrils	Autosomal dominant or recessive mutation in collagen
Cause of death	Sepsis	Metastatic squamous cell carcinoma
	Failure to thrive	Sepsis
	Respiratory failure	Pneumonia
	Renal failure	Cardiomyopathy
		Renal failure

Based on data from Refs. [1, 2, 4, 5]

Table 26.2 Clinical signs, symptoms, and complications of epidermolysis bullosa

Signs and symptoms	Complications
Fluid-filled blisters on skin due to friction	Bacterial infection
	Atrophic scarring
	Squamous cell carcinoma
Deformity or loss of fingernails, toenails	Pseudosyndactyly
	Joint contractures
Internal blistering: vocal cords, upper airway	Oral and pharyngeal scarring
	Limited mouth opening
	Laryngotracheal scarring
Internal blistering: esophagus	Esophageal strictures
	Dysphagia
	Malnutrition
	Anemia
	Failure to thrive
	Growth retardation
	Impaired wound healing
	Dehydration
	Constipation
Scalp blistering	Scarring alopecia
Eye inflammation	Corneal erosion
	Blindness
Poorly formed dental enamel	Tooth decay

tures, and release procedures to increase mouth opening [6]. Due to scarring of the esophagus, patients may require upper endoscopy or esophageal dilation in order to eat. If patients are unable to tolerate oral intake, they will need gastrostomy tube placement to prevent malnutrition and failure to thrive [2].

4. What are the goals of safe anesthetic management?

    1. Prevent the formation of new lesions.
    2. Optimize pain control.
    3. Avoid airway trauma, especially with induction and emergence.

To achieve these goals, it is essential to have an anesthetic plan carefully prepared before the starting the case. Holding a preoperative meeting with all OR personnel is critically important to success. During this time, it is key that staff members review how to move the patient and what supplies will be needed for the case. Retaining a cart that has large stocks of the necessary skin care products will help the case progress smoothly.

The importance of avoiding creating new lesions in the skin, airway, or esophagus cannot be overemphasized. The formation of a new lesion can have debilitating consequences. For example, if, intraoperatively, the patient developed a new esophageal bulla from a temperature probe, or a new oropharyngeal lesion from a traumatic intubation, then the child would not be able to eat for days to weeks until that lesion healed. This would exacerbate the child's already poor nutritional status and make pain control even more challenging. EB patients are malnourished and require a high number of calories and proteins to continually heal their lesions. Respiratory tract lesions incurred during airway management can also lead to edema and stricture. This may result in delayed extubation, respiratory difficulty, prolonged hospitalization, and increased risk of infection.

5. How should an epidermolysis bullosa patient be positioned on the OR table? How should the patient be repositioned during surgery? (Fig. 26.1)

Extreme caution must be used when positioning a patient to avoid creating new lesions. If the patient is able to walk and follow verbal instructions, the patient can walk into the OR and position himself on the OR table. This avoids staff members inadvertently placing pressure and tension on the patient's skin. The patient can also then identify which position is most comfortable. Once the patient is anesthetized, all patient repositioning must be coordinated with the members of the OR team. All movements should be slow, gentle, and well coordinated to avoid placing any tension on the skin.

There should be no direct contact between the patient's skin and the OR table. This can be achieved by applying a layer of lubricated gauze or other cloth protection between the skin and table or equipment where possible. Lubricated cushions can be applied at each pressure point, such as the heels, elbows, and occiput. No stickers or tight wraps should be used on the skin. Each piece of equipment that may touch the skin must be thoroughly lubricated.

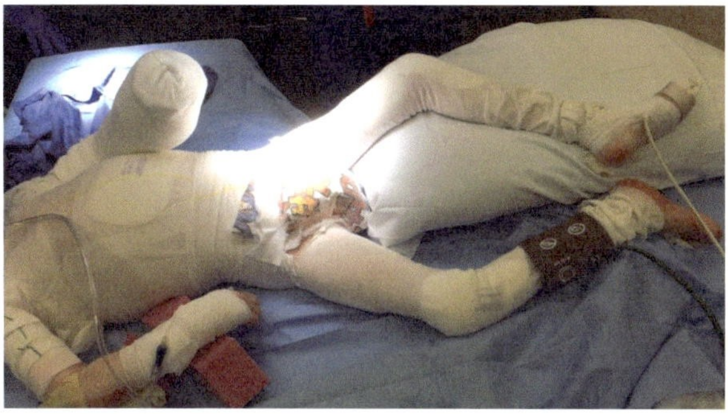

Fig. 26.1 Padding pressure points. The sterile blue drape underneath the patient was used as a hammock to move the patient intraoperatively. Lubricated foam pads, pillows, and Xeroform® gauze were placed at all pressure points including the heels and elbows. Monitoring interfaces and IV access were secured with lubricated gauze, not tape on the skin. Wherever possible, there was no direct contact between monitors and skin

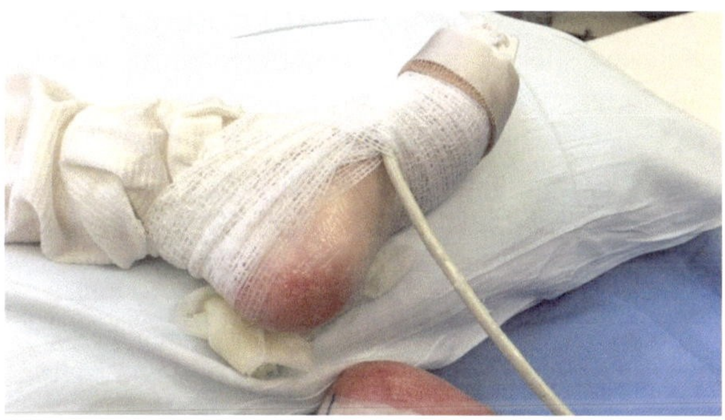

Fig. 26.2 Pulse oximeter. A layer of lubricant was placed between the patient's skin and the clip-on pulse oximeter probe. To reduce tension of the clip-on probe on the skin, the pulse oximeter cable was wrapped with lubricated gauze around the patient's foot and ankle. Note that the tape and Coban® dressing are not in contact with skin

6. Which monitors should be used during surgery? How can monitors and lines be secured? (Figs. 26.2 and 26.3)

    1. Monitoring pulse oximetry is necessary to assess oxygenation status. Pulse oximeters with adhesive stickers should not be used. Using a clip-on pulse oximeter is acceptable and if well lubricated will not cause blisters. Lubricant should be applied all around the monitor including the inside of the clip where it touches the patient's skin. With all monitors, extra slack must be applied on the cables in the event that someone accidentally pulls on the cable. This adverse event can cause shearing of the skin.
    2. EKG leads may be optional depending on the patient's comorbidities and the type of surgery being performed. For example, if the patient has cardiac

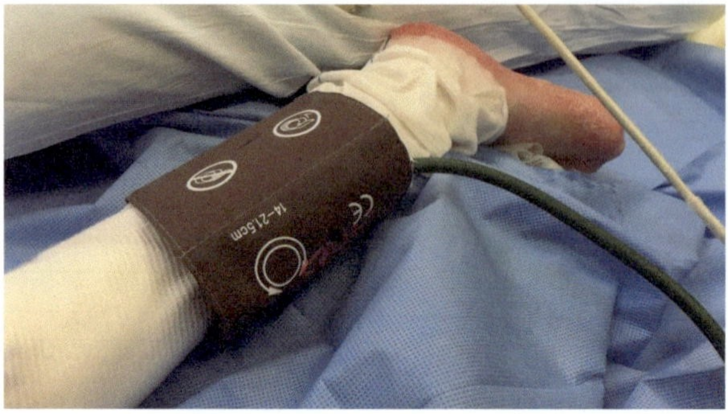

Fig. 26.3 Blood pressure cuff. The blood pressure cuff was placed on the patient's calf because the surgeons were operating on the patient's upper extremities. The cuff was wrapped over the patient's dressing and more loosely than usual to minimize compressive forces. Inflation of the cuff alone should not cause lesions, but excess inflation should be avoided

disease or there is concern for the development of arrhythmias intraoperatively, EKG leads may be necessary. The most commonly available EKG leads are adhesive stickers, which are not recommended in EB patients. If it is necessary to use EKG leads, needle electrodes are safer than adhesives. Needle electrodes can also damage the skin and may not be readily available at every institution. An alternative method to safely apply standard silver EKG electrodes is to remove all of the adhesive and then place them on the skin. The electrodes can then be secured to the extremities with Vaseline® gauze and Kling® wrap gauze.

3. A blood pressure cuff is necessary for measuring hemodynamic stability. It is important to not wrap the cuff directly around the skin. As the cuff tightens, it can pinch the skin. The compressive force can also cause skin trauma. A safer method is to wrap the cuff loosely around the extremity with a protective layer of lubricated gauze in between the cuff and skin. Depending on the degree of hemodynamic changes expected, the cuff can be cycled less frequently than usual, for example, every 5–10 min rather than every 2.5 min. Since the cuff is wrapped more loosely, the blood pressure reading will be falsely low. Therefore, it is necessary to follow the trends, not just the absolute readings, when assessing hypertension or hypotension.
4. To monitor neuromuscular blockade with a nerve stimulator, as with EKG leads, stickers should not be used. If neuromuscular monitoring is deemed absolutely essential, metallic electrodes can be placed lightly on lubricated skin.
5. A temperature probe is not absolutely necessary. There is a significant risk of shear forces leading to esophageal lesions when a temperature probe is blindly inserted, even if it is well lubricated. Discuss with OR staff about keeping the room warm and minimizing loss of heat through exposure. EB patients can become hypothermic quickly during surgery due to heat loss from their extensive skin lesions.

7. How can a patient with epidermolysis bullosa be mask ventilated safely?

It is important to use extreme caution with finger placement and pressure while mask ventilating a patient with EB. Patients can easily develop blisters even from compressive forces. There should be a layer of lubricant between the anesthesiologist's fingers and the patient's skin. Only minimal compressive force should be applied for a chin lift and jaw thrust. The anesthesiologist must lift his fingers intermittently, avoid creating shearing force or tension while masking, and frequently check for signs of blister formation while mask ventilating. Nasopharyngeal and oropharyngeal airways should not be routinely placed unless absolutely needed for difficult mask ventilation. If airway adjuncts are needed, lubricant should be applied and the airway adjunct gently inserted. There is a significant risk of shearing forces creating bullae in the nasopharynx and oropharynx during insertion and removal.

8. How is intravenous access established in a patient with EB? (Fig. 26.4)

The majority of EB patients are children and young adults. If the patient does not come to the operating room with intravenous access, mask induction before gaining IV access is preferred, especially in young children. Due to the patient's parchment-thin skin, peripheral veins are usually well visualized even without a tourniquet. That being said, it is best to have the most experienced anesthesiologist place the IV to minimize repeated trauma to the skin from less experienced providers. If a tourniquet is needed for IV placement, lubricated gauze should be wrapped around the extremity and the tourniquet placed over the gauze, using as minimal pressure needed. Tegaderm® and other bio-occlusive dressings should not be used.

9. How does the anesthesiologist choose the safest airway management technique? How is an epidermolysis bullosa patient safely intubated? (Fig. 26.5)

There is no contraindication to endotracheal intubation in EB patients. As with all anesthetic plans, the decision to intubate will depend on the patient and the type

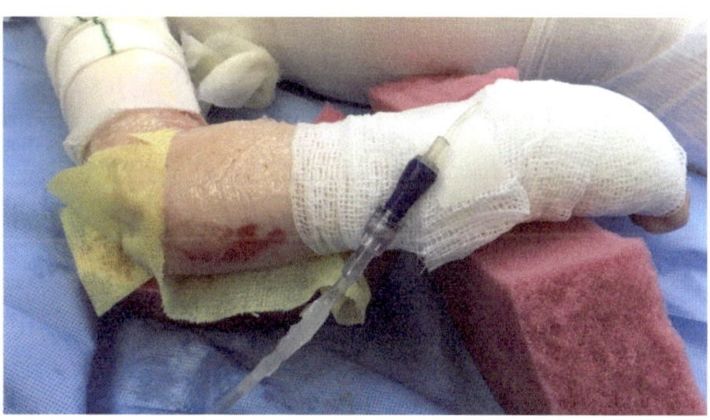

Fig. 26.4 Peripheral IV. The peripheral IV was secured with lubricated gauze gently wrapped several times around the hand. Adhesive tape was only applied to the gauze externally to secure the wrapping. The IV tubing was lubricated as well in case it came into contact with the skin under the drapes

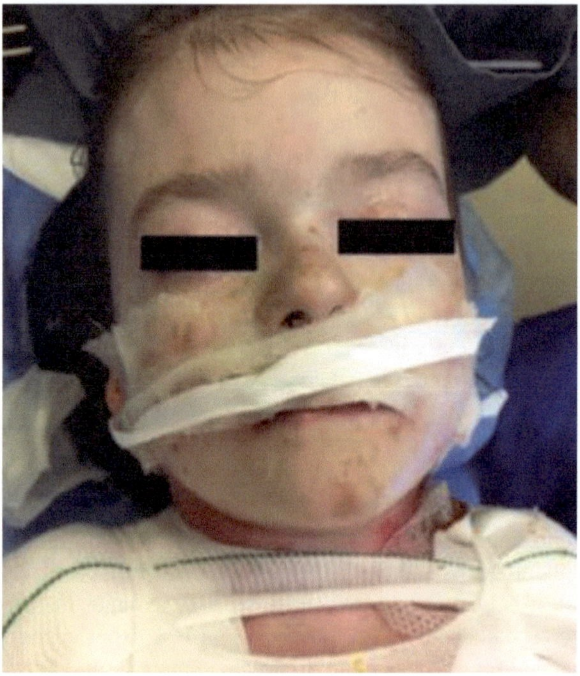

Fig. 26.5 Endotracheal tube securement. Prior to induction, a lubricated silicone head cushion was placed underneath the patient's head. Lubricated gauze was wrapped circumferentially around the patient's head, and the twill tape was used over this layer to secure the ETT without directly touching the skin. Adhesive tape, traditionally used for securing endotracheal tubes, cannot be used in EB patients. Eye lubricant was placed over the eyelids to prevent abrasions. No adhesive tape was used to tape the eyelids closed. Extra slack was provided on the circuit tubing. The tubing was loosely connected to the ETT so that in the event of tension, it would disconnect from the ETT rather than pull on the ETT and create shearing forces within the patient's airway

of surgery. The anesthesiologist should conduct a proper airway exam and anticipate a difficult airway in advance. It is pivotal that all airway equipment be prepared ahead of time and readily available in the event of a difficult mask ventilation or intubation. Carefully outlined backup plans are essential to avoid an uncontrolled situation that may result in trauma.

Any instrument that goes into the nasopharynx or oropharynx, including laryngoscopes and endotracheal tubes, must be generously lubricated. Irritation of the columnar mucosa of the nares, larynx, and trachea can cause laryngeal and subglottic stenosis. Intubations should be done cautiously. Using minimal force on direct laryngoscopy and avoiding shearing forces as much as possible will minimize airway trauma. If a difficult airway is anticipated, a fiber-optic intubation may be the first choice rather than direct laryngoscopy. Limiting the number of intubation attempts will reduce trauma. Although laryngeal mask airways have been used in EB patients in other case reports, LMAs are not recommended. As a large silicone structure sitting in the larynx, the LMA has a high risk of causing mucosal damage with blind insertion. Mouth opening also is reduced in EB patients, so insertion of an LMA into the oropharynx alone can cause trauma to the lips and tongue.

10. What are the options for providing postoperative analgesia?

It is important to ensure adequate postoperative analgesia to enable faster recovery from surgery, patient comfort, and earlier discharge to home. Consequences of poorly controlled pain in the immediate postoperative period include emotional and physical distress, sleep disturbance, impaired respiratory function due to pain from coughing, increased metabolic requirements, and impaired gastrointestinal motility. In particular, if children with EB emerge from anesthesia in significant pain, they may thrash around and scratch their skin, exacerbating or creating new skin lesions. Long-term effects of uncontrolled pain include chronic pain, behavioral changes such as difficulty sleeping or mood changes, and poor wound healing. The impact of uncontrolled pain is especially great for EB patients, as they already suffer from chronic pain and malnutrition due to extensive skin lesions [7, 8].

Multimodal analgesia employs a strategy of opioid and non-opioid analgesics, including neuraxial techniques and regional blockade, to improve pain control and minimize side effects of narcotics. Better pain control results from targeting multiple different receptors involved in nociception. Parents of children with EB are helpful resources for the anesthesiologist in deciding on pain management. In caring for their children at home with wound dressing changes, parents know which medications work well and which cause significant side effects (Table 26.3).

Table 26.3 Opioid and non-opioid intravenous analgesics

Class of drugs	Examples and dosing	Side effects
Opioids	Fentanyl (0.5–1 mcg/kg)	Drowsiness and sedation
	Hydromorphone (0.015 mg/kg)	Postoperative nausea and vomiting
	Morphine (0.1 mg/kg)	Pruritus
		Urinary retention
		Constipation
		Respiratory depression
NSAIDs	Ketorolac (0.5 mg/kg)	Platelet dysfunction
		Gastrointestinal bleeding
Alpha-2 adrenergic agonists	Clonidine (0.5–2 mcg/kg)	Hypotension
	Dexmedetomidine (0.25–1 mcg/kg)	Bradycardia
		Sedation
N-methyl-D-aspartate antagonists	Ketamine (0.1–0.5 mg/kg)	Hallucinations
		Excessive sedation
		Nightmares
Glucocorticoids	Dexamethasone (0.1 mg/kg)	Osteoporosis
		Inhibition of bone growth
Acetaminophen	Acetaminophen (15 mg/kg)	Hepatotoxicity

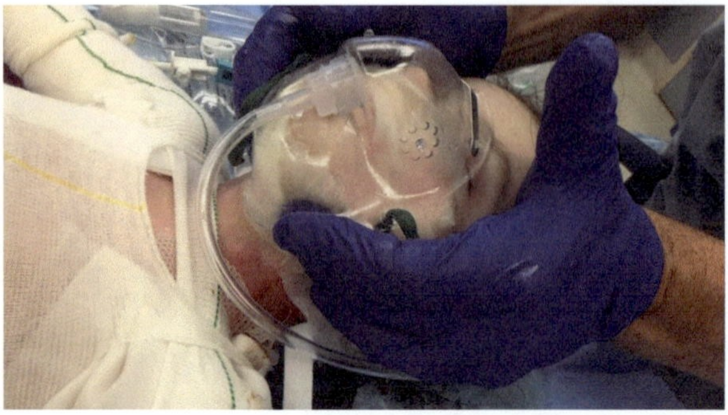

Fig. 26.6 Emergence. Strips of lubricated gauze were placed on the face at any possible point of contact between the patient's skin and the simple face mask. A deep extubation was performed, and a gentle chin lift, with intermittent lifting of the fingers to alleviate pressure points, was provided to assist with ventilation

11. What methods can be used to ensure safe emergence from general anesthesia? (Fig. 26.6)

The goal is to have a smooth emergence with minimal trauma. Pain and agitation should be controlled with appropriate agents such as benzodiazepines and alpha-2 agonists so that the patient does not wake up writhing in pain and causing new skin lesions. Using propofol instead of sevoflurane can help decrease emergence delirium. Avoiding traumatic extubations and re-intubations will decrease the incidence of blister formation. When suctioning oropharyngeal secretions prior to extubation, a soft flexible suction catheter is gentler than a rigid Yankauer tube. When placing a simple face mask over the patient's face, direct contact with the skin should be avoided. This can be achieved by placing several strips of well-lubricated gauze to place over the patient's face as a barrier between the skin and face mask. As with mask ventilation on induction, minimal pressure should be applied for chin lift as the patient emerges from anesthesia.

References

1. Culpepper TL. Anesthetic implications in epidermolysis bullosa dystrophica. J Am Assoc Nurse Anesth. 2001;69(2):114–8.
2. Denyer JPE. Best practice guidelines for skin and wound care in epidermolysis bullosa. Int Consens DEBRA 2012.
3. Nandi R, Howard R. Anesthesia and epidermolysis bullosa. Dermatol Clin. 2010;28(2):319–24. https://doi.org/10.1016/j.det.2010.01.011.
4. Fine J-D. Inherited epidermolysis bullosa. Orphanet J Rare Dis. 2010;5(1):12. https://doi.org/10.1186/1750-1172-5-12.
5. Iohom G, Lyons B. Anaesthesia for children with epidermolysis bullosa: a review of 20 years' experience. Eur J Anaesthesiol. 2001;18(11):745–54. https://doi.org/10.1046/j.1365-2346.2001.00916.x.

6. Saraf SV, Mandawade NJ, Gore SK, Padhye UD, Pereira CS. Epidermolysis bullosa: careful monitoring and no touch principle for anesthesia management. J Anaesthesiol Clin Pharmacol. 2013;29(3):390–3. https://doi.org/10.4103/0970-9185.117112.
7. Buvanendran A. Multimodal analgesia for perioperative pain management. ASA Refresh Courses Anesthesiol. 2012;40(1):1–6. https://doi.org/10.1097/ASA.0b013e318261324e.
8. Sivrikaya GU. Multimodal analgesia for postoperative pain management, pain management - current issues and opinions. Racz G, editors. InTech; 2012. ISBN: 978-953-307-813-7, Available from: http://www.intechopen.com/books/pain-management-current-issues-and-opinions/multimodalanalgesia-forpostoperative-pain-management.

Index

J. L. Benumof, G. R. Manecke (eds.), *Clinical Anesthesiology II*,
https://doi.org/10.1007/978-3-030-12365-9

MIX
Papier aus verantwortungsvollen Quellen
Paper from responsible sources
FSC® C105338

If you have any concerns about our products,
you can contact us on
ProductSafety@springernature.com

In case Publisher is established outside the EU,
the EU authorized representative is:
Springer Nature Customer Service Center GmbH
Europaplatz 3, 69115 Heidelberg, Germany

Printed by Libri Plureos GmbH
in Hamburg, Germany